COVID-19 Coagulopathy: Advances on Pathophysiology and Therapies

COVID-19 Coagulopathy: Advances on Pathophysiology and Therapies

Editors

Alexandru Schiopu
Emil Marian Arbănași
Eliza Russu

MDPI

Basel • Beijing • Wuhan • Barcelona • Belgrade • Novi Sad • Cluj • Manchester

Editors
Alexandru Schiopu
Department of Translational Medicine
Lund University
Lund
Sweden

Emil Marian Arbănași
Departament of Vascular Surgery
George Emil Palade University of Medicine, Pharmacy, Science and Technology of Targu Mures
Targu Mures
Romania

Eliza Russu
Departament of Vascular Surgery
George Emil Palade University of Medicine, Pharmacy, Science and Technology of Targu Mures,
Targu Mures
Romania

Editorial Office
MDPI
St. Alban-Anlage 66
4052 Basel, Switzerland

This is a reprint of articles from the Special Issue published online in the open access journal *International Journal of Molecular Sciences* (ISSN 1422-0067) (available at: www.mdpi.com/journal/ijms/special_issues/S571AL81D8).

For citation purposes, cite each article independently as indicated on the article page online and as indicated below:

Lastname, A.A.; Lastname, B.B. Article Title. *Journal Name* **Year**, *Volume Number*, Page Range.

ISBN 978-3-7258-0964-6 (Hbk)
ISBN 978-3-7258-0963-9 (PDF)
doi.org/10.3390/books978-3-7258-0963-9

Contents

About the Editors . . . . **vii**

Preface . . . . **ix**

Eliza Russu, Emil-Marian Arbănaşi and Alexandru Șchiopu
Special Issue "COVID-19 Coagulopathy: Advances on Pathophysiology and Therapies"
Reprinted from: *Int. J. Mol. Sci.* **2024**, *25*, 3548, doi:10.3390/ijms25063548 1

Eszter-Anna Dho-Nagy, Attila Brassai, Patrick Lechsner, Corina Ureche and Erika-Gyöngyi Bán
COVID-19 and Antipsychotic Therapy: Unraveling the Thrombosis Risk
Reprinted from: *Int. J. Mol. Sci.* **2024**, *25*, 818, doi:10.3390/ijms25020818 7

David E. Scheim, Paola Vottero, Alessandro D. Santin and Allen G. Hirsh
Sialylated Glycan Bindings from SARS-CoV-2 Spike Protein to Blood and Endothelial Cells Govern the Severe Morbidities of COVID-19
Reprinted from: *Int. J. Mol. Sci.* **2023**, *24*, 17039, doi:10.3390/ijms242317039 23

Iulia Făgărășan, Adriana Rusu, Horațiu Comșa, Tudor-Dan Simu, Damiana-Maria Vulturar and Doina-Adina Todea
IL-6 and Neutrophil/Lymphocyte Ratio as Markers of ICU Admittance in SARS-CoV-2 Patients with Diabetes
Reprinted from: *Int. J. Mol. Sci.* **2023**, *24*, 14908, doi:10.3390/ijms241914908 58

Mónika Szilveszter, Sándor Pál, Zsuzsánna Simon-Szabó, Orsolya-Zsuzsa Akácsos-Szász, Mihály Moldován, Barbara Réger, et al.
The Management of COVID-19-Related Coagulopathy: A Focus on the Challenges of Metabolic and Vascular Diseases
Reprinted from: *Int. J. Mol. Sci.* **2023**, *24*, 12782, doi:10.3390/ijms241612782 71

Biju Bhargavan and Georgette D. Kanmogne
SARS-CoV-2 Spike Proteins and Cell–Cell Communication Induce P-Selectin and Markers of Endothelial Injury, NETosis, and Inflammation in Human Lung Microvascular Endothelial Cells and Neutrophils: Implications for the Pathogenesis of COVID-19 Coagulopathy
Reprinted from: *Int. J. Mol. Sci.* **2023**, *24*, 12585, doi:10.3390/ijms241612585 89

Elisabeth Zechendorf, Christian Beckers, Nadine Frank, Sandra Kraemer, Carolina Neu, Thomas Breuer, et al.
A Potential Association between Ribonuclease 1 Dynamics in the Blood and the Outcome in COVID-19 Patients
Reprinted from: *Int. J. Mol. Sci.* **2023**, *24*, 12428, doi:10.3390/ijms241512428 111

Beatrice Ragnoli, Beatrice Da Re, Alessandra Galantino, Stefano Kette, Andrea Salotti and Mario Malerba
Interrelationship between COVID-19 and Coagulopathy: Pathophysiological and Clinical Evidence
Reprinted from: *Int. J. Mol. Sci.* **2023**, *24*, 8945, doi:10.3390/ijms24108945 124

Antonio G. Solimando, Max Bittrich, Endrit Shahini, Federica Albanese, Georg Fritz and Markus Krebs
Determinants of COVID-19 Disease Severity–Lessons from Primary and Secondary Immune Disorders including Cancer
Reprinted from: *Int. J. Mol. Sci.* **2023**, *24*, 8746, doi:10.3390/ijms24108746 145

About the Editors

Alexandru Schiopu

Șchiopu Alexandru , MD, PhD, is a Consultant at the Internal Medicine Clinic SUS Lund. He is also the Principal Investigator and research team manager of the Cardiac Inflammation Research Group at the Department of Translational Medicine, Lund University. Dr. Șchiopu completed a full-time Ph.D. at the Malmö Department of Clinical Sciences at Lund University, Sweden in 2006. His research was focused on developing a passive immunization strategy against atherosclerosis. He has also held postdoctoral positions at reputable institutions, such as the Atherosclerosis Research Center at Cedars Sinai Medical Center in Los Angeles, USA, and the Transplantation Research Immunology Group at the University of Oxford, UK. His academic achievements include securing numerous research grants from prestigious organizations such as the Swedish Heart and Lung Foundation, Novo Nordisk Foundation, Vetenskapsr, etc. He has been recognized for his outstanding contributions to the field through awards such as the "Erik K. Fernström" prize for successful young promising researchers at Lund University and the "Rising Star" award from Skane University Hospital Research Committee. Furthermore, he has actively contributed to academia through the supervision of PhD students and postdoctoral fellows, teaching activities, and editorial roles in scientific journals. He has served as a reviewer and editor for various journals, and has been involved in grant review assignments and faculty oppositions. Through his dedication to cardiovascular research and commitment to advancing medical science, Dr. Alexandru Șchiopu has made significant contributions to the field and continues to drive innovation in cardiovascular medicine.

Emil Marian Arbănași

Emil Marian Arbănași is a Resident Doctor of Vascular Surgery at the Emergency County Hospital in Targu Mures, Romania, and also a University Research Assistant at the George Emil Palade University of Medicine, Pharmacy, Science, and Technology of Targu Mures, Department of Vascular Surgery. He is currently pursuing his Ph.D. study at the Doctoral School of Medicine and Pharmacy in Târgu Mureș, his research interests are primarily focused on the development of new strategies based on UVA ultraviolet radiation in the biomechanical stabilization and strengthening of the abdominal aortic aneurysmal wall, venous graft and arteriovenous fistula. Dr. Arbănași Emil Marian was actively involved in several research projects, which materialized with numerous publications and international recognition, and is a review board member of numerous journals. As a result of his hard work and achievements, he was awarded a research scholarship at the Cardiac Inflammation Research Group at the Department of Translational Medicine at Lund University, under the guidance of Dr. Alexandru Șchiopu. Dr. Arbănași Emil Marian has actively participated in national and international conferences and seminars. With a strong background in medicine and a dedication to advancing vascular surgery research, Arbănași continues to make valuable contributions to the field.

Eliza Russu

Eliza Russo, MD, Ph.D., is a Senior surgeon at the Vascular Surgery Clinic of the Targu Mures Emergency County Hospital and Lecturer in the Vascular Surgery Department of the Targu Mures University of Medicine, Pharmacy, Science and Technology George Emil Palade. Working in the field of vascular surgery since 2003, Dr. Russu's general interests have been extraanatomical revascularizations (the subject of her PhD thesis), graft infections (studied during her post-PhD project) and several technical innovative solutions in the world of grafting. Amongst Dr. Russu's scientific interests worth mentioning are vascular access, biomechanical properties of the aortic wall and venous grafts, coagulopathies and the predictive values of systemic inflammatory biomarkers in various situations, as well as the role of computed tomography angiography markers as predictors of abdominal aortic aneurysm rupture. Serving as a mentor for last-year students of the Alma Mater, she has supervised several graduation theses and many scientifical research papers, some of them awarded by national student congresses. Participation and papers from her research has led to national awards granted during Surgery Congresses. Some of her current developing projects are the experimental study of the role of UV-A radiation in the prophylaxis of aortic aneurysmal rupture, and ultrasonography markers, nutritional status and inflammatory status in vascular access dysfunction.

Preface

This Special Issue is Guest-Edited by Dr. Alexandru Schiopu (Department of Clinical Sciences Malmo, Lund University) who is specialized in cardiovascular research and cardiology, and vascular surgeons Dr. Eliza Russu and Dr. Emil Marian Arbanasi (Department of Vascular Surgery, George Emil Palade University of Medicine, Pharmacy, Science and Technology of Targu Mures). The distinguished authors of the 14 published papers come from 10 different countries and research groups.

Despite intensive worldwide efforts, the underlying mechanisms of COVID-19-induced coagulopathy remain largely unknown. This collection provides insights into the modifications of normal coagulation patterns during the acute and late scenarios of COVID-19. The authors aimed to shed light on the pathophysiology of the virus-induced coagulopathy and discuss, from this perspective, the role of the addressed therapies. The purpose was to publish relevant papers presenting some of the most important current advances in understanding the molecular pathways and clinical manifestations of thrombo-embolic events in COVID-19 patients. As we published the results of our own work, presenting our Vascular Surgery Clinic data during the pandemic, and as Dr. Schiopu is a prominent researcher with significant contributions to the field of molecular pathways, we united our efforts in research focused on the coagulation malfunction which arises in this viral infection as one of its major complications.

We wish for this research to be available to all medical personnel, students or researchers wanting to stay up-to-date on these topics.

Alexandru Schiopu, Emil Marian Arbănași, and Eliza Russu
Editors

International Journal of
Molecular Sciences

MDPI

Editorial

Special Issue "COVID-19 Coagulopathy: Advances on Pathophysiology and Therapies"

Eliza Russu [1,2], Emil-Marian Arbănaşi [1,2,3,4,*] and Alexandru Şchiopu [5,6,7]

1 Clinic of Vascular Surgery, Mures County Emergency Hospital, 540136 Targu Mures, Romania; eliza.russu@umfst.ro
2 Department of Vascular Surgery, George Emil Palade University of Medicine, Pharmacy, Science and Technology of Targu Mures, 540139 Targu Mures, Romania
3 Doctoral School of Medicine and Pharmacy, George Emil Palade University of Medicine, Pharmacy, Science and Technology of Targu Mures, 540142 Targu Mures, Romania
4 Centre for Advanced Medical and Pharmaceutical Research (CCAMF), George Emil Palade University of Medicine, Pharmacy, Science, and Technology of Targu Mures, 540139 Targu Mures, Romania
5 Department of Translational Medicine, Lund University, 22100 Lund, Sweden; alexandru.schiopu@med.lu.se
6 Department of Internal Medicine, Skåne University Hospital Lund, 22185 Lund, Sweden
7 Nicolae Simionescu Institute of Cellular Biology and Pathology, 050568 Bucharest, Romania
* Correspondence: emil.arbanasi@umfst.ro

Citation: Russu, E.; Arbănaşi, E.-M.; Şchiopu, A. Special Issue "COVID-19 Coagulopathy: Advances on Pathophysiology and Therapies". *Int. J. Mol. Sci.* **2024**, *25*, 3548. https://doi.org/10.3390/ijms25063548

Received: 12 March 2024
Accepted: 14 March 2024
Published: 21 March 2024

The Special Issue on COVID-19 coagulopathy initiated one year ago aimed to shed light on the mechanisms underlying the changes in the coagulation status making SARS-CoV-2 infection such a tough adversary for every one of the medical specialties encountering it, along with overseeing the therapeutic applications derived from the current understanding of these mechanisms.

Every emergency and ICU compartment admitting critical patients during the SARS-CoV-2 pandemic fought against the clinical manifestations of arterial and venous thrombosis, along with a variety of severe disorders affecting almost all organs and systems [1–5].

Bacterial infections are associated with disseminated intravascular coagulation (DIC), but COVID-19 coagulopathy differs from DIC occurring during severe bacterial infections and sepsis. In sepsis-associated DIC, disease severity and mortality were associated with a low platelet count and platelet time (PT) prolongation, whereas severe COVID-19 coagulopathy was best reflected by increased levels of D-dimers. Laboratory, clinical, and histopathologic findings suggested that COVID-19 coagulopathy is characterized by dysregulated hemostasis, leading to the formation and degradation of micro- and macrovascular thrombi [6]. There appears to be a close link between severe systemic inflammation and dysregulated hemostasis in the pathophysiology of the disease [7]. COVID-19-related coagulopathy is also associated with thrombocytopenia. In a meta-analysis of 7613 COVID-19 patients, Julien Maquet et al. [8] have shown that thrombocytopenia was worse in the critically ill group compared to patients with mild forms of the disease.

The "two-path unifying theory" of hemostasis and endotheliopathy aimed to explain the imbalance between coagulation and inflammation. Viral protein S adhesion to endothelial membrane angiotensin-converting enzyme (mACE2) is a widely recognized pathway for viral penetration into the cells [9]. ACE-2 polymorphisms, alongside gender, race and age differences, are the major factors contributing to the wide variability in COVID-19 deaths, as Wooster et al. [10], Santosh et al. [11], and Srivastava et al. [12] have shown in their reports.

The main role of ACE-2 is the degradation of angiotensin II at the endothelial surface, counteracting its potent vasoconstrictor and pro-inflammatory effects [13]. Experimental studies have shown how the injection of the recombinant SARS spike protein led to elevated levels of angiotensin II in mice, possibly via the downregulation of ACE-2 expression on the endothelium. In turn, treatment of the mice with angiotensin II receptor type

1 (AT1R) blockers reduced disease severity [14]. Thus, understanding the role of the interplay between ACE-2, ACE, and their receptors in the pathogenesis of COVID-19 is very important. The downregulation of endothelial ACE2 as a consequence of SARS-CoV-2 infection inhibits the vasodilator, anti-inflammatory, and anti-coagulant effects of the enzyme, leading to endothelial dysfunction, vasoconstriction and a prothrombotic status. Recombinant human ACE-2 has been tested as a potential therapy for acute lung injury, as it may act as a decoy receptor for SARS-CoV-2 in the circulation and prevent the binding of the virus to the endothelium [15,16].

The virus invades type II pulmonary alveolar and endothelial cells, releasing danger-associated molecular patterns (DAMPs), proinflammatory cytokines, and chemokines. The subsequent activation of leukocytes and platelets leads to a cytokine storm, characterized by a potent release of interleukin-1, -6, -8, -10, and -12 (IL-1, IL-6, IL-8, IL-10, Il-12), tumor necrosis factor-alpha (TNF-α), interferon-γ, C–X–C motif chemokine 10, and monocyte chemoattractant protein-1 [7]. These inflammatory mediators trigger the further recruitment and activation of leukocytes and platelets, activation of the coagulation cascade, and generation of intravascular thrombin in a continuous loop [7].

COVID-19-associated microthrombosis is initiated via the endothelial exocytosis of ultra-large von Willebrand factor multimeric glycoproteins and antihemophilic globulins A from the Weibel–Palade bodies. If the ADAMTS-13 levels are insufficient to cleave the large vWF multimers, the latter will activate intravascular thrombosis by anchoring to the damaged endothelial cells and recruiting platelets, triggering the formation of "microthrombi strings" [17]. The generation of antibodies against ADAMTS13 appears to be a frequent and unique finding in COVID-19, supporting "COVID-19 immunothrombosis", a term coined recently to embed both micro- and macrovascular thrombotic events associated with the disease [18].

COVID-19-associated pulmonary thrombosis is an in situ immunothrombosis not related to venous thromboembolism, in which similar mechanisms involving endothelial injury and a loss of anticoagulant properties can be incriminated [19].

It has also been proposed that the virus may trigger complement activation by acting as a cofactor to enhance lectin pathway activation [20]. The terminal complement complex C5b-C9 (MAC—membrane attack complex) causes the formation of pores on the membranes of the endothelial cells leading to endothelial damage when the MAC-inhibitor CD59 is under-expressed and cannot properly exhibit its regulatory function [21]. C5a can stimulate the release of TF and plasminogen activator inhibitor-1 (PAI-1) and activate neutrophils, which release cytokines and neutrophil extracellular traps (NETs). NETs are structures of DNA, histones, and antimicrobial proteins that bind and kill pathogens. The excessive production of NETs can facilitate microthrombosis by creating a scaffold for platelet aggregation, thus contributing to the vicious pro-thrombotic circle [22].

The link between coagulopathy in viral infections and COVID-19 is discussed in a recent review published in a Special Issue by Ragnoli et al. [23]. Two possible mechanisms implicated in the pathogenesis of coagulation dysfunction during SARS-CoV2 infection are reviewed here: the cytokine storm and virus-specific mechanisms related to the virus interaction with the renin–angiotensin system and the fibrinolytic pathway. The role of IL-1 and IL-6, as well as IL-18 is emphasized. Moreover, a reduction in endothelial nitric oxide synthase activity and nitric oxide levels is cited as a possible pathogenic culprit of endothelial dysfunction. They also discuss the very interesting topic of thrombocytopenia induced by COVID-19 vaccination. In rare cases, the immune thrombotic thrombocytopenia (VITT) syndrome was induced by the vaccine, particularly by the ChAdOx1 nCoV-19 vaccine (COVID-19 Vaccine AstraZeneca) [23]. The hypothesis is the possible recruiting of antibodies against platelet factor 4 (PF4), inducing massive platelet activation and immune thrombotic thrombocytopenia [24].

SARS-CoV-2 penetration into the cells is dependent on glycans with sialic acid (SA) terminal moieties found on the viral spike protein (SP), which serve as the initial attachment anchors to red blood cells (RBCs), platelets, leukocytes, and endothelial cells. Hemagglutination is a defense mechanism used by RBCs and platelets against pathogens expressing SA terminal moieties, involving pathogen attachment, followed by delivery to leukocytes for phagocytosis, in a process termed "immune adherence". The capacity of this initial defense mechanism is surpassed in severe COVID-19 infections, leading to high levels and sizes of RBC rouleaux (stacked clumps) exceeding the leukocyte capacity to sequester them, as discussed in the review by Sheim et al. [25]. The risk factors of increased age, diabetes, and obesity associated with COVID-19 were found to also be associated with significantly increased RBC aggregation, another valuable conclusion by Sheim et al. [25]. SARS-CoV-2 SP attachments to RBCs were demonstrated directly by Lam et al. [26] through immunofluorescence imaging. In this Special Issue, Boschi et al. [27] show that SARS-CoV-2 SP from various strains induced hemagglutination when mixed with human RBCs. These results are in line with other studies documenting associations between RBC aggregation and microvascular occlusion in severe COVID-19 [28,29].

Microthrombi in the heart, kidneys, and liver were also frequently observed in autopsy examinations of COVID-19 patients, suggesting that these may have contributed to multi-organ damage and failure. A report from Koutsiaris et al. [30] demonstrated the persistence of microthrombosis even after recovery, as demonstrated by video capillaroscopy of the ocular microvessels of severe COVID-19 patients within 28 days post-discharge.

Wada et al. [31] reviewed some of the most studied mechanisms of thrombosis as important factors leading to a negative COVID-19 patient evolution: old age, long-time bed rest and comorbidities, inflammation, cytokine storms, vascular endothelial injuries, PTE, hypoventilation, a hypercoagulable state (including activation of the TF pathway), NETs, hypofibrinolysis, and platelet activation. The authors illustratively compare the mechanism underlying thrombosis in COVID-19 and bacterial infections.

The molecular mechanisms of direct and indirect effects of the spike protein on the expression of adhesion molecules, markers of endothelial injury, and elevated inflammation are presented in the work of Bhargavan and Kanmogne [32]. According to Wada et al. [31], among the most valuable routine biomarkers for the evaluation of thrombosis in COVID-19 are CWA-APTT (clot waveform analysis of activated partial thromboplastin time) and TF-induced factor IX activation assay (sTF/FIXa) Although D dimer is useful for the exclusion of VTE in COVID-19 patients, it is too unspecific for VTE diagnosis, as its cut-off level is low in these patients.

Soluble platelet membrane glycoprotein VI (sGPVI) and soluble C-type lectin-like receptor 2 (sCLEC-2) were also proposed as platelet activation biomarkers [33]. The presence of activated platelets causing severe microangiopathy in patients with COVID-19 may be detected by the release of large amounts of sCLEC-2 into the blood [33]. Studies have also detected a mild decrease in ADAMTS-13 in plasma, but the clinical significance of this finding remains unclear [34].

Increased fibrinogen and PAI-I levels have been found to be the biomarkers of hypo-fibrinolysis, reducing the capacity to dissociate thrombi. In advanced COVID-19 patients, vascular endothelial cell injury markers such as soluble thrombomodulin (sTM), VWF, and PAI-I are high, while AT (antithrombin) levels are low [35]. It is thought that the ensuing hypo-fibrinolysis may contribute to organ failure in these patients [35].

The early recognition of a hyperinflammatory and hypercoagulation state would allow for the timely application of preventive measures against a fulminant disease evolution. In their study, Făgărașan et al. [36] demonstrated that IL-6 and the neutrophil–lymphocyte ratio (NLR) predicted disease severity in COVID-19 patients with diabetes mellitus (DM). Significant associations between IL-6 levels and disease evolution have also been described in non-diabetics [37]. Further studies are needed to elucidate the role of IL-6 in this context to determine the cut-off values associated with worse outcomes and explore the potential of IL-6 as a treatment target in COVID-19 [37].

A number of studies emphasized the procoagulant profile of COVID-19 patients during the acute phase of the illness, but less is known about the short- and long-term effects. The long-term persistence of COVID-19-related coagulopathy, along with long-lasting lung dysfunction, have been noted since the beginning of the pandemic [38–40].

Of particular interest for this Special Issue is the anti-coagulant therapy in COVID-19. As the pathogenesis of SARS-CoV-2-induced coagulopathy is incompletely understood and multifactorial, the use of antithrombotic therapy is difficult to standardize. Three pivotal phase III randomized clinical trials regarding antithrombotic agents were conducted, starting from 2020: INSPIRATION, Remap/cap/ACTIV-4a/ATTACC, and RECOVERY INSPIRATION Investigators [41–43]. The studies showed a lack of improvement in the outcome of critically ill patients receiving intermediate-dose prophylactic anticoagulants. This outlined the superiority of the therapeutic anticoagulant dose compared to the prophylactic dose for the survival of non-critically ill patients, but not in the critically ill ones, and the failure of Aspirin to reduce the 28-day mortality or progression to mechanical ventilation/death in hospitalized patients [42]. Similarly, the ACTIVE-4a trial showed that the use of P2Y12 receptor inhibitors did not improve the number of organ support-free days in patients with mild forms of COVID-19 [44]. Importantly, the use of antithrombotic therapies requires the careful balancing of thrombotic and bleeding risks. The measurement of serum AT-III activity is recommended in the algorithm of evaluating SARS-CoV-2-infected patients, as emphasized by the review of Szilveszter et al. [45].

According to guidelines, a prophylactic or therapeutic dose of low-molecular-weight heparin (LMWH) should be administered to all patients as prophylaxis against venous thromboembolism (VTE) and PTE, particularly in those with a high thrombosis risk (that is, patients with elevated D-dimer levels) and a low bleeding risk [46]. For patients who are transferred to an intensive care unit, increasing from a prophylactic to a therapeutic LMWH dose is recommended. Patients with heparin resistance caused by AT-III deficiency may be treated with direct thrombin inhibitors, such as Argatroban. The use of oral anticoagulants is not recommended in COVID-19 [46]. Considering the substantial contribution of inflammation to COVID-19-associated coagulopathy, the development of anti-inflammatory therapies to treat COVID-19 might interfere with anticoagulation, raising the risk of bleeding. The combined use of anti-inflammatory and anticoagulant drugs must be evaluated in further clinical trials [47].

As underlined by the studies discussed above, we are happy to conclude that the Special Issue "COVID-19 Coagulopathy: Advances in Pathophysiology and Therapies" has brought important contributions to understand the underlying mechanisms of SARS-CoV-2-induced coagulopathy to define diagnostic and prognostic biomarkers for COVID-19 patients, and discuss the potential anti-coagulant and anti-thrombotic therapies in this complex disease.

Author Contributions: Conceptualization, A.Ș. and E.R.; writing—original draft, E.R.; writing—review and editing, A.Ș., E.R. and E.-M.A.; supervision, A.Ș. and E.R.; Project Administration, A.Ș., E.R. and E.-M.A. All authors have read and agreed to the published version of the manuscript.

Acknowledgments: The Guest Editors of the current Special Issue want to express their gratitude to all contributors for their unique and outstanding articles. Additionally, special credit should be given to all reviewers for their comprehensive analysis and their overall effort in improving the quality of the published articles.

Conflicts of Interest: The authors declare no conflicts of interest.

References

1. Cheruiyot, I.; Kipkorir, V.; Ngure, B.; Misiani, M.; Munguti, J.; Ogeng'o, J. Arterial Thrombosis in Coronavirus Disease 2019 Patients: A Rapid Systematic Review. *Ann. Vasc. Surg.* **2021**, *70*, 273–281. [CrossRef]
2. Piazza, G.; Morrow, D.A. Diagnosis, Management, and Pathophysiology of Arterial and Venous Thrombosis in COVID-19. *JAMA* **2020**, *324*, 2548–2549. [CrossRef]
3. Arbănași, E.-M.; Kaller, R.; Mureșan, A.V.; Voidăzan, S.; Arbanasi, E.-M.; Russu, E. Impact of COVID-19 Pandemic on Vascular Surgery Unit Activity in Central Romania. *Front. Surg.* **2022**, *9*, 883935. [CrossRef]
4. Mureșan, A.V.; Russu, E.; Arbănași, E.M.; Kaller, R.; Hosu, I.; Arbănași, E.M.; Voidăzan, S.T. Negative Impact of the COVID-19 Pandemic on Kidney Disease Management—A Single-Center Experience in Romania. *J. Clin. Med.* **2022**, *11*, 2452. [CrossRef]

5. Stoian, A.; Bajko, Z.; Stoian, M.; Cioflinc, R.A.; Niculescu, R.; Arbănași, E.M.; Russu, E.; Botoncea, M.; Bălașa, R. The Occurrence of Acute Disseminated Encephalomyelitis in SARS-CoV-2 Infection/Vaccination: Our Experience and a Systematic Review of the Literature. *Vaccines* **2023**, *11*, 1225. [CrossRef]
6. Colling, M.E.; Kanthi, Y. COVID–19-Associated Coagulopathy: An Exploration of Mechanisms. *Vasc. Med.* **2020**, *25*, 471–478. [CrossRef]
7. Conway, E.M.; Pryzdial, E.L.G. Is the COVID-19 Thrombotic Catastrophe Complement-connected? *J. Thromb. Haemost.* **2020**, *18*, 2812–2822. [CrossRef]
8. Maquet, J.; Lafaurie, M.; Sommet, A.; Moulis, G. Thrombocytopenia Is Independently Associated with Poor Outcome in Patients Hospitalized for COVID-19. *Br. J. Haematol.* **2020**, *190*, e276–e279. [CrossRef]
9. Ni, W.; Yang, X.; Yang, D.; Bao, J.; Li, R.; Xiao, Y.; Hou, C.; Wang, H.; Liu, J.; Yang, D.; et al. Role of Angiotensin-Converting Enzyme 2 (ACE2) in COVID-19. *Crit. Care* **2020**, *24*, 422. [CrossRef]
10. Wooster, L.; Nicholson, C.J.; Sigurslid, H.H.; Cardenas, C.L.L.; Malhotra, R. Polymorphisms in the ACE2 Locus Associate with Severity of COVID-19 Infection. *MedRxiv* **2020**. [CrossRef]
11. Sidhwani, S.K.; Mirza, T.; Khatoon, A.; Shaikh, F.; Khan, R.; Shaikh, O.A.; Nashwan, A.J. Angiotensin-Converting Enzyme 2 (ACE2) Polymorphisms and Susceptibility of Severe SARS-CoV-2 in a Subset of Pakistani Population. *Virol. J.* **2023**, *20*, 120. [CrossRef]
12. Srivastava, A.; Bandopadhyay, A.; Das, D.; Khanam, N.; Srivastava, N.; Singh, P.P.; Sultana, G.N.N.; Chaubey, G. Genetic Association of ACE2 Rs2285666 Polymorphism With COVID-19 Spatial Distribution in India. *Front. Genet.* **2020**, *11*, 564741. [CrossRef]
13. Liu, M.-Y.; Zheng, B.; Zhang, Y.; Li, J.-P. Role and Mechanism of Angiotensin-Converting Enzyme 2 in Acute Lung Injury in Coronavirus Disease 2019. *Chronic Dis. Transl. Med.* **2020**, *6*, 98–105. [CrossRef]
14. Kuba, K.; Imai, Y.; Rao, S.; Gao, H.; Guo, F.; Guan, B.; Huan, Y.; Yang, P.; Zhang, Y.; Deng, W.; et al. A Crucial Role of Angiotensin Converting Enzyme 2 (ACE2) in SARS Coronavirus–Induced Lung Injury. *Nat. Med.* **2005**, *11*, 875–879. [CrossRef]
15. Shirbhate, E.; Pandey, J.; Patel, V.K.; Kamal, M.; Jawaid, T.; Gorain, B.; Kesharwani, P.; Rajak, H. Understanding the Role of ACE-2 Receptor in Pathogenesis of COVID-19 Disease: A Potential Approach for Therapeutic Intervention. *Pharmacol. Rep.* **2021**, *73*, 1539–1550. [CrossRef]
16. Khan, A.; Benthin, C.; Zeno, B.; Albertson, T.E.; Boyd, J.; Christie, J.D.; Hall, R.; Poirier, G.; Ronco, J.J.; Tidswell, M.; et al. A Pilot Clinical Trial of Recombinant Human Angiotensin-Converting Enzyme 2 in Acute Respiratory Distress Syndrome. *Crit. Care* **2017**, *21*, 234. [CrossRef]
17. Fujimura, Y.; Holland, L.Z. COVID-19 Microthrombosis: Unusually Large VWF Multimers Are a Platform for Activation of the Alternative Complement Pathway under Cytokine Storm. *Int. J. Hematol.* **2022**, *115*, 457–469. [CrossRef]
18. Shaw, R.J.; Bradbury, C.; Abrams, S.T.; Wang, G.; Toh, C.-H. COVID-19 and Immunothrombosis: Emerging Understanding and Clinical Management. *Br. J. Haematol.* **2021**, *194*, 518–529. [CrossRef]
19. Niculae, C.-M.; Hristea, A.; Moroti, R. Mechanisms of COVID-19 Associated Pulmonary Thrombosis: A Narrative Review. *Biomedicines* **2023**, *11*, 929. [CrossRef]
20. Malaquias, M.A.S.; Gadotti, A.C.; da Silva Motta-Junior, J.; Martins, A.P.C.; Azevedo, M.L.V.; Benevides, A.P.K.; Cézar-Neto, P.; do Carmo, L.A.P.; Zeni, R.C.; Raboni, S.M.; et al. The Role of the Lectin Pathway of the Complement System in SARS-CoV-2 Lung Injury. *Transl. Res.* **2021**, *231*, 55–63. [CrossRef]
21. Couves, E.C.; Gardner, S.; Voisin, T.B.; Bickel, J.K.; Stansfeld, P.J.; Tate, E.W.; Bubeck, D. Structural Basis for Membrane Attack Complex Inhibition by CD59. *Nat. Commun.* **2023**, *14*, 890. [CrossRef]
22. Chen, Z.; Zhang, H.; Qu, M.; Nan, K.; Cao, H.; Cata, J.P.; Chen, W.; Miao, C. Review: The Emerging Role of Neutrophil Extracellular Traps in Sepsis and Sepsis-Associated Thrombosis. *Front. Cell. Infect. Microbiol.* **2021**, *11*, 653228. [CrossRef]
23. Ragnoli, B.; Da Re, B.; Galantino, A.; Kette, S.; Salotti, A.; Malerba, M. Interrelationship between COVID-19 and Coagulopathy: Pathophysiological and Clinical Evidence. *Int. J. Mol. Sci.* **2023**, *24*, 8945. [CrossRef]
24. Aleem, A.; Nadeem, A.J. Coronavirus (COVID-19) Vaccine-Induced Immune Thrombotic Thrombocytopenia (VITT). In *StatPearls*; StatPearls Publishing: Treasure Island, FL, USA, 2023.
25. Scheim, D.E.; Vottero, P.; Santin, A.D.; Hirsh, A.G. Sialylated Glycan Bindings from SARS-CoV-2 Spike Protein to Blood and Endothelial Cells Govern the Severe Morbidities of COVID-19. *Int. J. Mol. Sci.* **2023**, *24*, 17039. [CrossRef]
26. Lam, L.K.M.; Reilly, J.P.; Rux, A.H.; Murphy, S.J.; Kuri-Cervantes, L.; Weisman, A.R.; Ittner, C.A.G.; Pampena, M.B.; Betts, M.R.; Wherry, E.J.; et al. Erythrocytes Identify Complement Activation in Patients with COVID-19. *Am. J. Physiol.-Lung Cell. Mol. Physiol.* **2021**, *321*, L485–L489. [CrossRef]
27. Boschi, C.; Scheim, D.E.; Bancod, A.; Militello, M.; Bideau, M.L.; Colson, P.; Fantini, J.; Scola, B.L. SARS-CoV-2 Spike Protein Induces Hemagglutination: Implications for COVID-19 Morbidities and Therapeutics and for Vaccine Adverse Effects. *Int. J. Mol. Sci.* **2022**, *23*, 15480. [CrossRef]
28. Li, H.; Deng, Y.; Li, Z.; Gallastegi, A.D.; Mantzoros, C.S.; Frydman, G.H.; Karniadakis, G.E. Multiphysics and Multiscale Modeling of Microthrombosis in COVID-19. *PLOS Comput. Biol.* **2022**, *18*, e1009892. [CrossRef]
29. Ackermann, M.; Verleden, S.E.; Kuehnel, M.; Haverich, A.; Welte, T.; Laenger, F.; Vanstapel, A.; Werlein, C.; Stark, H.; Tzankov, A.; et al. Pulmonary Vascular Endothelialitis, Thrombosis, and Angiogenesis in COVID-19. *N. Engl. J. Med.* **2020**, *383*, 120–128. [CrossRef]

30. Koutsiaris, A.G.; Riri, K.; Boutlas, S.; Panagiotou, T.N.; Kotoula, M.; Daniil, Z.; Tsironi, E.E. COVID-19 Hemodynamic and Thrombotic Effect on the Eye Microcirculation after Hospitalization: A Quantitative Case-Control Study. *Clin. Hemorheol. Microcirc.* **2022**, *82*, 379–390. [CrossRef]
31. Wada, H.; Shiraki, K.; Shimpo, H.; Shimaoka, M.; Iba, T.; Suzuki-Inoue, K. Thrombotic Mechanism Involving Platelet Activation, Hypercoagulability and Hypofibrinolysis in Coronavirus Disease 2019. *Int. J. Mol. Sci.* **2023**, *24*, 7975. [CrossRef]
32. Bhargavan, B.; Kanmogne, G.D. SARS-CoV-2 Spike Proteins and Cell-Cell Communication Induce P-Selectin and Markers of Endothelial Injury, NETosis, and Inflammation in Human Lung Microvascular Endothelial Cells and Neutrophils: Implications for the Pathogenesis of COVID-19 Coagulopathy. *Int. J. Mol. Sci.* **2023**, *24*, 12585. [CrossRef]
33. de Oliveira Sales, L.; de Oliveira, L.L.B.; da Silva, J.B.S.; de Moraes Filho, M.O.; de Moraes, M.E.A.; Montenegro, R.C.; Moreira-Nunes, C.A. The Role of Platelet Molecules in Risk Stratification of Patients with COVID-19. *Hemato* **2023**, *4*, 364–383. [CrossRef]
34. Martín-Rojas, R.M.; Chasco-Ganuza, M.; Casanova-Prieto, S.; Delgado-Pinos, V.E.; Pérez-Rus, G.; Duque-González, P.; Sancho, M.; Díez-Martín, J.L.; Pascual-Izquierdo, C. A Mild Deficiency of ADAMTS13 Is Associated with Severity in COVID-19: Comparison of the Coagulation Profile in Critically and Noncritically Ill Patients. *Blood Coagul. Fibrinolysis* **2021**, *32*, 458. [CrossRef]
35. Andrianto; Al-Farabi, M.J.; Nugraha, R.A.; Marsudi, B.A.; Azmi, Y. Biomarkers of Endothelial Dysfunction and Outcomes in Coronavirus Disease 2019 (COVID-19) Patients: A Systematic Review and Meta-Analysis. *Microvasc. Res.* **2021**, *138*, 104224. [CrossRef]
36. Făgărășan, I.; Rusu, A.; Comșa, H.; Simu, T.-D.; Vulturar, D.-M.; Todea, D.-A. IL-6 and Neutrophil/Lymphocyte Ratio as Markers of ICU Admittance in SARS-CoV-2 Patients with Diabetes. *Int. J. Mol. Sci.* **2023**, *24*, 14908. [CrossRef]
37. McElvaney, O.J.; Curley, G.F.; Rose-John, S.; McElvaney, N.G. Interleukin-6: Obstacles to Targeting a Complex Cytokine in Critical Illness. *Lancet Respir. Med.* **2021**, *9*, 643–654. [CrossRef]
38. Townsend, L.; Fogarty, H.; Dyer, A.; Martin-Loeches, I.; Bannan, C.; Nadarajan, P.; Bergin, C.; O'Farrelly, C.; Conlon, N.; Bourke, N.M.; et al. Prolonged Elevation of D-dimer Levels in Convalescent COVID-19 Patients Is Independent of the Acute Phase Response. *J. Thromb. Haemost.* **2021**, *19*, 1064–1070. [CrossRef]
39. Kalaivani, M.; Dinakar, S. Association between D-Dimer Levels and Post-Acute Sequelae of SARS-CoV-2 in Patients from a Tertiary Care Center. *Biomark. Med.* **2022**, *16*, 833–838. [CrossRef]
40. Fan, B.E.; Wong, S.W.; Sum, C.L.L.; Lim, G.H.; Leung, B.P.; Tan, C.W.; Ramanathan, K.; Dalan, R.; Cheung, C.; Lim, X.R.; et al. Hypercoagulability, Endotheliopathy, and Inflammation Approximating 1 Year after Recovery: Assessing the Long-Term Outcomes in COVID-19 Patients. *Am. J. Hematol.* **2022**, *97*, 915–923. [CrossRef]
41. INSPIRATION Investigators. Effect of Intermediate-Dose vs Standard-Dose Prophylactic Anticoagulation on Thrombotic Events, Extracorporeal Membrane Oxygenation Treatment, or Mortality among Patients with COVID-19 Admitted to the Intensive Care Unit: The INSPIRATION Randomized Clinical Trial. *JAMA* **2021**, *325*, 1620–1630. [CrossRef]
42. Duncan, A.; Halim, D.; Kholy, K.E. The RECOVERY Trial: An Analysis and Reflection Two Years On. *Eur. J. Intern. Med.* **2022**, *105*, 111–112. [CrossRef]
43. Therapeutic Anticoagulation with Heparin in Noncritically Ill Patients with COVID-19. *N. Engl. J. Med.* **2021**, *385*, 790–802. [CrossRef]
44. Berger, J.S.; Kornblith, L.Z.; Gong, M.N.; Reynolds, H.R.; Cushman, M.; Cheng, Y.; McVerry, B.J.; Kim, K.S.; Lopes, R.D.; Atassi, B.; et al. Effect of P2Y12 Inhibitors on Survival Free of Organ Support among Non–Critically Ill Hospitalized Patients with COVID-19: A Randomized Clinical Trial. *JAMA* **2022**, *327*, 227–236. [CrossRef]
45. Szilveszter, M.; Pál, S.; Simon-Szabó, Z.; Akácsos-Szász, O.-Z.; Moldován, M.; Réger, B.; Dénes, L.; Faust, Z.; Tilinca, M.C.; Nemes-Nagy, E. The Management of COVID-19-Related Coagulopathy: A Focus on the Challenges of Metabolic and Vascular Diseases. *Int. J. Mol. Sci.* **2023**, *24*, 12782. [CrossRef]
46. Cuker, A.; Tseng, E.K.; Nieuwlaat, R.; Angchaisuksiri, P.; Blair, C.; Dane, K.; Davila, J.; DeSancho, M.T.; Diuguid, D.; Griffin, D.O.; et al. American Society of Hematology Living Guidelines on the Use of Anticoagulation for Thromboprophylaxis in Patients with COVID-19: May 2021 Update on the Use of Intermediate-Intensity Anticoagulation in Critically Ill Patients. *Blood Adv.* **2021**, *5*, 3951–3959. [CrossRef]
47. Murakami, N.; Hayden, R.; Hills, T.; Al-Samkari, H.; Casey, J.; Del Sorbo, L.; Lawler, P.R.; Sise, M.E.; Leaf, D.E. Therapeutic Advances in COVID-19. *Nat. Rev. Nephrol.* **2023**, *19*, 38–52. [CrossRef]

International Journal of
Molecular Sciences

MDPI

Review

COVID-19 and Antipsychotic Therapy: Unraveling the Thrombosis Risk

Eszter-Anna Dho-Nagy [1,*], Attila Brassai [1], Patrick Lechsner [1], Corina Ureche [2] and Erika-Gyöngyi Bán [1,*]

1 Department of Pharmacology and Clinical Pharmacology, Faculty of Medicine in English, Preclinical Research Laboratory, George Emil Palade University of Medicine, Pharmacy, Science, and Technology of Targu Mures, 540142 Targu Mures, Romania
2 Department of Internal Medicine, Faculty of Medicine, George Emil Palade University of Medicine, Pharmacy, Science, and Technology of Targu Mures, 540142 Targu Mures, Romania
* Correspondence: eszter-anna.dho-nagy@umfst.ro (E.-A.D.-N.); erika.ban@umfst.ro (E.-G.B.)

Abstract: In the context of the COVID-19 pandemic, this study investigates the potential correlation between the increased use of antipsychotic medications and the rising incidence of venous thromboembolism (VTE). As psychiatric disorders surged, the consequential escalation in antipsychotic drug use raised concerns about thrombotic risks. We conducted a comprehensive literature review using PubMed, focusing on articles that intersected COVID-19, antipsychotic medication, and thrombosis. This approach allowed for a nuanced examination of the historical and recent data on antipsychotic drugs and their association with thrombotic events. Our findings reveal a notable link between the use of antipsychotic medications, particularly second-generation antipsychotics, and an increased risk of VTE, including pulmonary embolism and deep vein thrombosis. This association was evident, despite variations in study designs and populations. The study underscores the need for cautious medication management in psychiatric care, especially during pandemic conditions like COVID-19, to mitigate thrombotic risks. It advocates a personalized approach to prescribing antipsychotics, considering individual patient factors and comorbidities, to balance the benefits against potential thrombotic complications.

Keywords: antipsychotic medications; thrombosis; COVID-19

Citation: Dho-Nagy, E.-A.; Brassai, A.; Lechsner, P.; Ureche, C.; Bán, E.-G. COVID-19 and Antipsychotic Therapy: Unraveling the Thrombosis Risk. *Int. J. Mol. Sci.* **2024**, *25*, 818. https://doi.org/10.3390/ijms25020818

Academic Editors: Eliza Russu, Alexandru Schiopu and Emil Marian Arbănaşi

Received: 16 December 2023
Revised: 4 January 2024
Accepted: 4 January 2024
Published: 9 January 2024

1. Introduction

In the shadow of the COVID-19 pandemic, a secondary crisis has emerged, marked by a significant rise in psychiatric disorders [1,2]. This increase has necessitated the escalated use of antipsychotic medications, a response that brings its own set of complexities and concerns. Concurrently, there has been a noticeable uptick in the incidence of venous thromboembolism (VTE), a condition characterized by the formation of blood clots in the venous system [1].

The parallel surge in both psychiatric disorders and VTE cases during this period has prompted a compelling question: is there a link between the increased use of antipsychotic medications and the heightened risk of venous thromboembolism?

Our research embarks on this quest, aiming to unravel the potential connections between the management of psychiatric illnesses with antipsychotic drugs and the occurrence of VTE. This exploration is not merely academic; it holds significant implications for public health, offering insights into managing the dual challenge of psychiatric care and thrombotic risks in the context of a global pandemic.

2. Materials and Methods

2.1. Literature Search Strategy

Our research commenced with an extensive literature review utilizing PubMed as our primary database. The initial search strategy was designed to explore the intersection between COVID-19, antipsychotic medication, and thrombosis. We employed a combination of the three keywords "COVID", "antipsychotic", and "thrombosis" to ensure a comprehensive capture of relevant studies. This initial query resulted in the identification of only four articles, indicating a scarcity of research directly addressing all three aspects simultaneously.

To broaden our research scope while maintaining relevance, we adjusted our search strategy to examine the links between keywords. A search combining "antipsychotics" and "thrombosis" was conducted, yielding a more substantial pool of 312 articles. This indicated a well-explored link between antipsychotic medication and thrombotic events in the existing literature.

In our review, we excluded studies reporting thromboembolic events in patients using antipsychotics who also suffered from end-stage diseases; these were omitted due to the inherently higher thrombotic risk in these populations, which could have confounded our assessment [3–5]. Additionally, we excluded studies focusing on postoperative patients, as the increased baseline risk for thromboembolism associated with surgery could potentially skew our analysis of antipsychotic-related risks [6–8].

2.2. Article Selection and Analysis

The selection process involved a preliminary screening of titles and abstracts to identify studies that directly addressed the research question. Full-text articles were then evaluated in depth. The inclusion criteria were centered on studies that provided empirical data or comprehensive reviews related to our key themes: the impact of COVID-19 on thrombotic risks and the role of antipsychotic medications in this context.

Our exclusion criteria encompassed studies involving antipsychotic use in patients with end-stage diseases, as well as those on postoperative patients, where thromboembolism risk could have biased our analysis.

Our analysis involved synthesizing findings from the selected publications, with a particular focus on identifying commonalities and discrepancies in the reported results. This process allowed us to construct a nuanced understanding of the current state of knowledge regarding the links between COVID-19, antipsychotic medication use, and thrombosis.

2.3. Inclusion of a Research Methodology Flow Chart

To enhance the clarity and transparency of our research methodology, we included a detailed flow chart that outlines our literature search and article selection process. This flow chart visually represents the step-by-step approach we employed, from the initial broad search to the final selection of relevant articles (Figure 1).

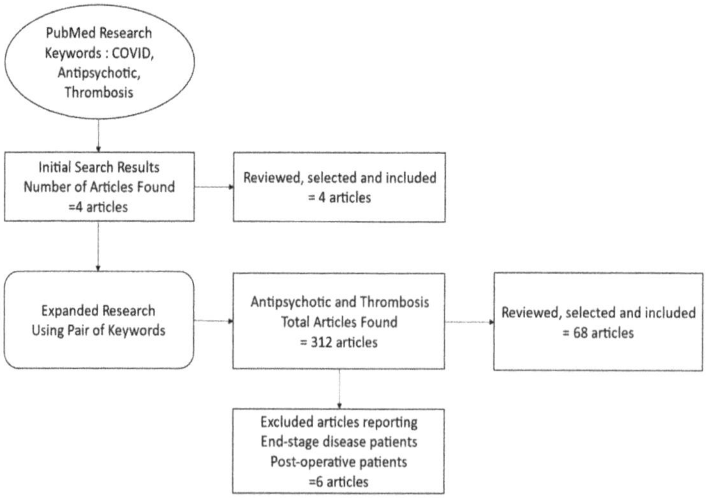

Figure 1. Flow chart outlining the literature search and article selection process.

3. Results

3.1. Historical Approach: Antipsychotic Medications and Venous Thromboembolic Risk

The historical literature on antipsychotic drugs reveals a longstanding awareness of their potential link to venous thromboembolism, particularly pulmonary embolism (PE). The discovery of chlorpromazine's antipsychotic properties in 1953 was quickly followed by German case reports citing fatal pulmonary embolism linked to its use, as noted by Brehmer & Ruckdeschel (1953) and Labhardt (1954) [9]. An early case series covering 1954–1957 reported venous thrombosis and pulmonary embolism in 3.3% of phenothiazine users, a notable contrast to a non-phenothiazine control group (Grahmann & Suchenwirth, 1959) [9,10].

Further studies continued to highlight this risk. In 1963, Mahmodian observed a threefold increase in thrombosis risk from 1958 to 1961 in psychiatric and neurological patients compared to earlier decades. Lal et al. (1966) reported a 10% prevalence of PE in autopsies of psychiatric patients, primarily diagnosed with schizophrenia and chronic brain syndrome, matching the general hospital population's prevalence, suggesting a high incidence of PE in these patients [11].

Kendel and Fodor (1969) found a 29% incidence of PE in psychiatric patients, with a notable association with acute psychiatric symptoms [10]. Scholz (1967) studied psychiatric patients with PE as the clinical cause of death, finding that many had used antipsychotic drugs without any explanatory comorbidity [10]. Ziegler (1977) noted that 4% of autopsy reports with PE as the sole cause of death had an underlying psychiatric disorder [10].

In a large observational study, Meier-Ewert et al. (1967) compared patients with schizophrenia or depression taking chlorpromazine, amitriptyline, or imipramine to similar patients not using these medications [12]. They observed a higher frequency of thromboembolic complications in the medication group (2.9% versus 0.59%) [12]. A study in 1984 reported deep venous thrombosis leading to fatal pulmonary embolism in women with schizophrenia after an acute psychotic phase, highlighting the risk in psychiatric patients [13].

Although there was a gap in the literature post-1984, the topic regained attention with studies by Walker et al. (1997) and Hagg et al. (2000), reflecting continued interest in and concern about the association between antipsychotic medication and venous thrombosis in psychiatric patients [14].

Various antipsychotic drugs, particularly phenothiazines, are known to increase platelet aggregation. However, clinical reports detailing deep vein thrombosis and other thromboembolic phenomena associated with antipsychotics are scarce. Dally noted that chlorpromazine might induce thrombosis in leg veins, especially in bedridden patients. Bernhardt and colleagues discussed four cases of pulmonary embolism linked to major tranquilizers and tricyclics, highlighting these drugs' roles in producing hyperaggregability. Singer and team reported three cases of pulmonary embolism in elderly women on major tranquilizers. This paper also presented three cases of thromboembolic events in ambulatory patients in good physical health, receiving similar medications [15].

3.2. Defining Antipsychotic Medications

Antipsychotic medications are broadly classified into two categories: traditional (first-generation) and novel (second-generation) antipsychotics. Traditional antipsychotics, encompassing classes such as butyrophenones (e.g., haloperidol), phenothiazines (e.g., chlorpromazine and thioridazine), and others, including indoles and thioxanthenes, were initially authorized in the 1950s, predominantly for schizophrenia management, with widespread application in a variety of psychiatric conditions [16].

In contrast, novel antipsychotics, introduced in the 1990s, comprise agents such as clozapine, risperidone, olanzapine, quetiapine, ziprasidone, aripiprazole, paliperidone, asenapine, and amisulpride. These medications exhibit considerable variability in their receptor-binding characteristics, indicating that they do not represent a uniform class of therapeutic agents. Initially sanctioned by the Food and Drug Administration exclusively for schizophrenia, these novel antipsychotics have also received approval for the treatment of bipolar mania, dementia, and large off-label practice [16].

Novel antipsychotics have increasingly been adopted as the preferred treatment option. This trend is attributed to their relative advantages over traditional antipsychotics, particularly in reducing the occurrence of extrapyramidal symptoms and tardive dyskinesia [16].

3.3. Defining Venous Thromboembolism

Antipsychotic medications are frequently used for managing behavioral and psychological symptoms, but they come with a range of adverse effects, impacting both the hematological and neurological systems [17]. Some of these drugs have been associated with an increased risk of venous thromboembolism, a condition that manifests primarily in two forms: pulmonary embolism and deep vein thrombosis (DVT) [18].

Pulmonary thromboembolism, often resulting from deep vein thrombosis and colloquially referred to as "economy-class syndrome", is a noted cause of sudden death in psychiatric patients, particularly those under physical restraint. The primary risk factors for DVT, known as the Virchow triad, include decreased venous blood flow, damage to vessel walls, and enhanced blood clotting [17]. Physical restraint is thought to impede venous blood flow, while antipsychotic drugs might promote blood clotting. Venous thromboembolism represents a complex condition with multiple contributing factors [10,19]. It ranks among the top three causes of mortality related to cardiovascular disease [20,21].

Therefore, preventive measures and early diagnosis are essential to avert sudden deaths due to DVT in these scenarios [22].

The exact causes of the heightened prescription of antipsychotic medications among patients remain uncertain. However, it is suggested that this trend could be linked to an escalation in behavioral and psychological symptoms in these individuals due to the constraints enforced during the pandemic, such as limited visitor access and the suspension of group activities. Global entities such as Alzheimer's Disease International have emphasized the augmented necessity for psychological support for those living with dementia amid the COVID-19 crisis [1].

Dispensation of antipsychotic drugs increased in the COVID-19 period compared to the pre-COVID era [1,23].

Our analysis indicated a significant association between COVID-19 and increased odds of thromboembolic events and all-cause mortality in dementia patients receiving antipsychotic medications [1].

Furthermore, it i's theorized that individuals affected by COVID-19 might experience a disruption in coagulation balance and an intensified inflammatory response, potentially leading to a "hypercoagulable state" and elevated thrombosis risk. A study published in July 2020 indicated that antipsychotic medication treatment could aggravate respiratory issues and heighten thromboembolism risks in COVID-19 patients [24].

3.4. Antipsychotics and Venous Thromboembolism

The examination of data from the Food and Drug Administration Adverse Event Reporting System (FAERS) reveals a notable correlation between the use of antipsychotic medications and an escalation in thromboembolic events [25]. This link is supported by substantial statistical evidence, manifesting in significant reporting odds ratios and information components [26]. These findings bring to light a pivotal concern in medical management: the heightened risk of venous thromboembolism connected to antipsychotic drug usage [25,27].

The investigation delving into the amplified risks found links with antipsychotic medication in dementia patients, particularly under the strains of the COVID-19 pandemic. Notably, increased mortality rates in patients treated with haloperidol and risperidone, especially those infected with COVID-19, call for meticulous medication management in this sensitive group. The varying impacts of distinct antipsychotics point to the importance of strategic medication selection to minimize risks [1,28,29].

Further research, including a meta-analysis, established a clear association between the usage of antipsychotics and an augmented risk of venous thromboembolism and pulmonary embolism, with no evidence of publication bias [28,30]. Our comprehensive review of antipsychotic drug usage indicates a trend, as of 2006, toward a predominance of second-generation antipsychotics, constituting over 78% of all antipsychotic prescriptions and overshadowing the usage of first-generation antipsychotics [18].

The study uncovers a significant link between the usage of neuroleptics and increased VTE risk, with odds ratios indicating a 3.5-fold elevation in VTE risk associated with antipsychotic drugs. In contrast, antidepressant use did not show a significant correlation with VTE risk. This hospital-based case-control study reinforces the view that antipsychotic drug exposure is a potential risk factor for VTE [28,30].

In dementia patients, who often consume other medications impacting serotonin receptors and platelet function, research on the peripheral vascular effects of antipsychotics is limited. A recent nested case-control analysis within a cohort of 72,591 dementia patients indicated that current antipsychotic users in this group had a significantly higher risk of VTE compared to controls [16].

3.5. Contributing Factors Increasing Thromboembolic Risk

In the realm of psychiatric care, particularly in the context of antipsychotic medication use, understanding the risk of thrombosis is crucial for effective patient management. The literature provides valuable insights into various risk factors, or contributory elements, that are thought to increase the likelihood of thrombotic events in individuals prescribed these medications [18,30,31]. These factors span physiological, pharmacological, and lifestyle domains, each contributing uniquely to the overall risk profile [30]. As we delve into these factors, it is important to recognize the multifaceted nature of thrombosis risk in the context of antipsychotic therapy. The following section will explore these key risk factors, as reported in the literature, shedding light on the complex interplay of elements that may predispose patients to thrombotic complications.

3.6. Mostly Involved Antipsychotic Medications

Multiple research studies have pinpointed a range of acquired risk factors for venous thromboembolism [26,31]. The most commonly reported antipsychotics were quetiapine, haloperidol, olanzapine, and risperidone. Other antipsychotics were less frequently used [1,32].

Our study highlights a significant risk of pulmonary embolism in patients undergoing antipsychotic drug treatment, showing an odds ratio (OR) of 1.2, which indicates a considerable statistical significance [18]. Particularly alarming are the 30-day all-cause mortality rates in patients treated with haloperidol, and the pronounced difference in mortality rates between COVID-19 positive and negative patients receiving risperidone, suggesting a heightened risk associated with these drugs [1].

In the context of olanzapine, a case of hyperprolactinemia linked to increased pulmonary thromboembolism has been reported [33]. Interestingly, our research indicates that the elevated risk of VTE in patients treated with antipsychotics is not necessarily tied to the known risks of these medications, such as metabolic abnormalities, sedation, or hyperprolactinemia [34].

Deep vein thrombosis has been recognized as a potential complication of antipsychotic therapy, particularly with atypical antipsychotics like risperidone [35]. Additionally, numerous case reports and studies have shown an increased risk of VTE with antipsychotic use. For example, a 51-year-old female patient with bipolar disorder developed a pulmonary embolism following chlorpromazine treatment, while instances of central retinal vein occlusion have been observed in patients administered olanzapine and risperidone [36,37]. Furthermore, a case of a 39-year-old woman with chronic schizophrenia who developed acute right hemiparesis and visual field loss during a switch to clozapine therapy has been reported, leading to a provisional diagnosis of ischemic stroke [38,39].

Acute bilateral coronary artery thrombosis and myocardial infarction have also been documented in a 25-year-old man after long-term oral clozapine treatment [40]. Notably, the risk of PE varies with the type of antipsychotic used, with clozapine showing the highest associated risk (OR = 1.54). Second-generation antipsychotics, such as risperidone and ziprasidone, also present a significant risk. While previous studies have already implicated second-generation antipsychotics, such as clozapine, risperidone, and olanzapine, in PE risk, our findings additionally identify ziprasidone as carrying a significant risk for PE, a revelation that stands in contrast to other studies [18,41].

3.6.1. Based on Duration of the Treatment

The duration of antipsychotic medication use is a critical factor in assessing the risk of thrombotic events, such as venous thromboembolism. This temporal correlation has been consistently observed in numerous studies, emphasizing the importance of monitoring the length of treatment when prescribing antipsychotics [35,42].

Commonly used antipsychotics, such as quetiapine, haloperidol, olanzapine, and risperidone, have been linked to an increased risk of thrombotic events, particularly with prolonged use. Our research indicates a heightened risk of pulmonary embolism in patients treated with these drugs over extended periods. This relationship points to a direct connection between the duration of antipsychotic therapy and the increased likelihood of developing thrombotic complications [18,30,42,43].

The study revealed that individuals using antipsychotic medications face a 32% higher risk of developing VTE compared to non-users. This risk escalates among current users (those with a prescription within the last three months) who experience a 56% increased risk. However, past users of antipsychotics did not show a significantly increased risk. Notably, new users of antipsychotic medications demonstrated a higher increase in VTE risk compared to those continuing with their existing medication [42].

Contrastingly, some studies found no correlation between the duration of antipsychotic drug use and the occurrence of VTE, suggesting a complex array of factors contributing to the risk [44,45]. Specifically, risperidone, a second-generation atypical antipsychotic, has been linked to cases of deep vein thrombosis, usually emerging within a period ranging from two weeks to a few months after treatment initiation [35].

Thromboembolic events have been documented within the first week of treatment with antipsychotics such as chlorpromazine and clozapine. While there are reports of risperidone-induced venous thrombosis occurring after two weeks of therapy, an extensive literature review did not reveal any cases of deep vein thrombosis specifically linked to the first week of risperidone treatment [35].

Among current users of antipsychotics, new users showed a higher risk of VTE compared to both prevalent and past users [16]. The median time frame for the diagnosis of VTE in one cohort was approximately 42 days, ranging from 16 to 94 days [46]. Our findings align with previous studies indicating that current users of antipsychotics face a greater risk of VTE than past users, suggesting that the underlying disease and the antipsychotic drugs themselves might be primary contributors to these thromboembolic events [34]. Interestingly, our study did not establish a significant dose–response relationship between the use of antipsychotic drugs and the occurrence of thromboembolic events [34].

In conclusion, the average onset time for thromboembolic conditions related to antipsychotic use was found to be about 7.49 months, with reported occurrences ranging from the third day to as late as 84 months following the initiation of treatment [20]. This underscores the need for careful monitoring of patients on antipsychotic medication, considering the varying risks associated with different durations of treatment.

3.6.2. First or Second Generation

The relationship between antipsychotic medication use and the risk of venous thromboembolism and pulmonary embolism presents a nuanced picture. A key finding from one study showed no significant differences in VTE risk between first-generation antipsychotics and second-generation antipsychotics when analyzed separately, suggesting that the risk of thromboembolic events might be a general concern across different generations of antipsychotic drugs [47]. Furthermore, the study did not delve into the risks associated with individual antipsychotic drugs [16].

Contrastingly, another study highlighted a significant association between the risk of VTE and PE and exposure to second-generation antipsychotics. The risk was found to be about twice as high in individuals exposed to second-generation antipsychotics as in those not exposed. Interestingly, second-generation antipsychotics seem to have a higher likelihood of causing PE compared to VTE [30,42]. This finding underscores the need for careful consideration when prescribing second-generation antipsychotics, particularly in patients with other risk factors for thromboembolic events.

Given these findings, it is crucial for medical professionals to conduct a thorough assessment of the risk factors for each patient before initiating antipsychotic treatment. This process should involve adherence to guidelines provided by regulatory bodies and a careful evaluation of the efficacy and safety of both typical and atypical antipsychotics. Such an assessment is particularly important in the context of the patient's specific clinical scenario, taking into account their overall health, pre-existing conditions, and potential risk factors for thromboembolic events [48].

This approach highlights the importance of individualized patient care in psychiatric treatment, emphasizing the need to weigh the benefits of antipsychotic therapy against the potential risks, especially concerning thrombotic complications.

3.6.3. Antipsychotic Medication Potency

The risk of venous thromboembolism associated with antipsychotic medications appears to be influenced by the potency of the drugs, affecting both first-generation antipsychotics and second-generation antipsychotics. Notably, low-potency first-generation antipsychotics have been linked to a higher risk of VTE compared to high-potency agents [30].

A study focusing on the use of traditional antipsychotic medications found a significant association with an increased risk of idiopathic VTE compared to non-use, demonstrating an adjusted odds ratio of 7.1. This heightened risk was particularly notable with lower potency drugs such as chlorpromazine and thioridazine, which showed a stronger association with VTE (OR 24.1) compared to higher potency drugs such as haloperidol (OR 3.3). The risk was most pronounced during the initial months of treatment with conventional antipsychotic medications [49].

Additionally, our research indicates that haloperidol, classified as a high-potency first-generation antipsychotic, is associated with an increased risk of pulmonary embolism. This finding underscores the significance of a specific antipsychotic drug in determining the risk of PE [18].

Moreover, patients prescribed low-potency antipsychotic drugs were found to face a higher risk of VTE compared to those on high-potency drugs, with the odds ratio being 1.99 for low-potency drugs and 1.28 for high-potency drugs [42].

This differentiation in risk based on the potency of the antipsychotic underscores the need for careful consideration when choosing the appropriate medication, especially in patients who may be at increased risk for thromboembolic events.

3.7. Antiphospholipid Antibodies

Furthermore, the use of some psychotropic drugs, including chlorpromazine and clozapine, correlates with increased levels of anti-phospholipid antibodies (aPLs), which are thrombogenic. Interestingly, increased aPL levels can also be a primary condition in schizophrenic patients. Research by Canoso et al. found a significantly higher prevalence of autoantibodies, such as antinuclear antibodies, aPLs, rheumatoid factor, and immunoglobulin M, in chronic psychiatric patients on long-term neuroleptic therapy compared to normal controls [44].

In contrast to observations in systemic lupus erythematosus and similar autoimmune conditions, chlorpromazine does not seem to correlate with a heightened incidence of thrombosis [50].

3.8. Endothelial Involvement

Endothelial dysfunction has emerged as a significant concern linked to the use of antipsychotic agents [45]. Atypical antipsychotics, in particular, have been implicated in elevating the risk of vascular dysfunctions, which, in turn, are associated with an increased susceptibility to cardiovascular diseases [21]. The intricate relationship between antipsychotic medications and endothelial health warrants an in-depth exploration of the multiple facets contributing to this connection [51,52].

Emerging research suggests that various drugs, including antipsychotic agents, have the capacity to impede the vasoprotective mechanisms maintained by the endothelium. By tampering with these mechanisms, these medications can potentially pave the way for the development of cardiovascular diseases. The specific pathways and molecular interactions through which antipsychotic agents influence endothelial function remain subjects of ongoing investigation [53,54].

Curiously, a study conducted on schizophrenia patients undergoing antipsychotic drug therapy explored the interplay between genetic variants and metabolic syndrome concerning endothelial function. The investigation unveiled noteworthy associations between genetic variants of endothelial nitric oxide synthetase and endothelial dysfunction [55]. This connection provides a critical link between the genetic makeup of patients and their response to antipsychotic treatment, shedding light on individualized approaches to care [56].

In the quest to understand the dynamics of endothelial function among somatically healthy schizophrenia patients treated with atypical antipsychotic agents, researchers made a significant discovery, revealing elevated levels of asymmetric dimethylarginine (ADMA), an endogenous inhibitor of nitric oxide synthase. Elevated ADMA levels serve as pertinent markers of endothelial dysfunction, emphasizing the elaborate cellular-level interactions influenced by antipsychotic medications [57].

An additional dimension of this multifaceted relationship is the observation that plasma levels of vascular endothelial growth factor (VEGF) exhibit variation in patients with schizophrenia, particularly prior to antipsychotic treatment. Research findings indicate that VEGF levels are lower in these patients before the commencement of treatment. However, a compelling shift occurs after the administration of antipsychotic agents, with VEGF levels showing a subsequent increase. This dynamic points to a complex interplay between antipsychotic treatment and the intricate mechanisms involved in endothelial health [58,59].

3.9. Platelet Aggregation

Recent investigations have uncovered an intriguing association between the use of clozapine and the occurrence of thrombosis. While clozapine's direct interaction with fibrinogen does not compromise its structural integrity, the drug markedly influences fibrin formation. Specifically, clozapine slows down the coagulation process and results in thinner fibrin fibers. This phenomenon suggests that clozapine may confer thrombogenic properties to fibrinogen, potentially in a dose-dependent manner. Consequently, the dosage of clozapine could be a pivotal factor in determining its influence on fibrinogen and the overall coagulation process within the body [45,60].

Contrary to the hypothesis that increased platelet aggregation due to activation of serotonin receptor 2A (5-HT2A) leads to venous thromboembolism, some findings do not support this theory. Aripiprazole and quetiapine, both of which act on 5-HT2A receptors, have not shown a significant increase in the risk of pulmonary embolism. Furthermore, in vitro studies have failed to demonstrate an increase in platelet aggregation with the use of antipsychotics, such as haloperidol, olanzapine, or risperidone. This indicates that the link between antipsychotic drug use and PE risk is multifaceted and cannot be solely attributed to the sedative effects or serotonin receptor activation [18].

Prolactin and leptin, hormones known for their involvement in various physiological processes, have been identified as significant coactivators in adenosine diphosphate (ADP)-dependent platelet aggregation and P-selectin expression. These findings suggest their potential role as risk factors in both arterial and venous thrombosis. Clinical conditions that typically elevate prolactin or leptin levels, such as pregnancy, obesity, or treatment with antipsychotic drugs, have also been associated with an increased risk of thromboembolic events [61]. This correlation underscores the importance of considering hormonal influences, particularly prolactin and leptin, in the context of thrombosis risk when using antipsychotic medications [61].

In summary, the role of platelets in thrombosis associated with antipsychotic drug use is complex and involves multiple pathways and factors. The impact of clozapine on fibrin formation, the lack of a direct link between 5-HT2A receptor activation and increased PE risk, and the potential involvement of hormones like prolactin and leptin in platelet aggregation all contribute to our understanding of thrombosis in the context of antipsychotic medication use [60,61]. These insights are crucial for guiding clinical decisions and risk assessments in patients undergoing antipsychotic therapy.

3.10. Immobilization

The hypothesis that sedation induced by antipsychotic drugs contributes to an increased risk of pulmonary embolism is a subject of ongoing research and debate. While all antipsychotics potentially have sedative effects, the intensity of these effects varies depending on the specific drug [62]. For example, quetiapine is known for its sedative properties, yet it does not seem to be associated with an increased risk of PE [63]. Interestingly, the sedative effect of quetiapine may diminish over time. In contrast, ziprasidone, which is not typically linked to sedation, has been found to show a significant risk of PE [18].

Sedation induced by certain antipsychotic drugs, such as chlorpromazine, clozapine, olanzapine, and quetiapine, can reduce patient movement, potentially contributing to blood stasis [64]. Blood stasis is a well-recognized risk factor for venous thromboembolism [44]. This sedative effect, therefore, could be a contributing factor to the increased risk of thrombotic events in patients treated with these medications [27].

In studies of venous thromboembolism, risk factors present in at least 15% of both studied cohorts included acute infection or rheumatologic disorder, obesity, and the use of antipsychotic medication. Notably, in one of the cohorts, the two most prevalent risk factors were the use of an antipsychotic agent (observed in 100% of cases) and reduced mobility [46]. This suggests a strong association between antipsychotic use, reduced mobility, and the risk of VTE [62,65].

Furthermore, the study highlights a significant link between prolonged physical immobilization and the risk of venous thromboembolism in psychiatric patients, especially those receiving antipsychotic therapy [63,66]. Autopsy findings in five patients where pulmonary thromboembolism was identified as the direct cause of death emphasize the critical need to monitor and manage periods of immobilization in these patients to mitigate the risk of VTE [67,68]. This underlines the importance of physical activity and mobility in patients undergoing antipsychotic treatment as preventive measures against thrombotic risks.

3.11. Obesity

The relationship between antipsychotic drug use and obesity is particularly noteworthy, as obesity itself is a known risk factor for deep vein thrombosis [46]. Antipsychotic agents, such as clozapine and olanzapine, are frequently associated with an increased risk of obesity. It was observed that obese individuals had higher levels of blood clotting factors VIII and IX compared to controls. This elevation in clotting factors among obese patients underscores the augmented risk of thrombosis in this population [44].

In a specific cohort, the presence of a body mass index (BMI) of 30 kg/m^2 or higher was noted in 30% of the participants. This prevalence of obesity within the cohort points to its significant role as a risk factor for venous thromboembolism [46]. The high incidence of obesity in this group further emphasizes the importance of considering body weight and related metabolic factors when assessing the risk of VTE [62].

Moreover, in individuals diagnosed with schizophrenia or bipolar disorder, the use of antipsychotic medications, such as olanzapine and clozapine, has been linked to various metabolic irregularities [69]. These include substantial weight gain, disruptions in lipid profiles, and alterations in glucose metabolism [16,21].

In this scenario, a case of branch retinal vein occlusion was reported in which a young patient, initially with normal lab results, experienced dyslipidemia after two years of quetiapine use. Given that such antipsychotics can lead to thrombotic episodes through metabolic imbalances, it is essential to monitor and address any signs of dyslipidemia and obesity promptly to prevent thrombotic complications [70].

3.12. Age

Age-related variations in the risk of venous thromboembolism in the context of antipsychotic and antidepressant drug use present a complex clinical picture. While some studies suggest a heightened risk, others indicate a more nuanced scenario [71]. For instance, research involving adults aged 65 and older found no significant increase in VTE risk associated with the use of these medications [72]. This finding challenges the commonly held perception of a universally elevated thromboembolic risk with antipsychotic drug use in older adults [73].

In a detailed study of the elderly population encompassing 111,818 patients, no substantial correlation was found between the current use of antipsychotics and the incidence of VTE. This indicates that the thromboembolic risk profile in the elderly may differ from that in other age groups, suggesting a distinct response to these medications in older patients. This study considered various factors, such as medication dosage and duration, yet still reported no increased risk [71].

Certain antipsychotic agents, particularly depot preparations of thioxanthenes such as zuclopenthixol and flupenthixol, have been linked to rare instances of hypocoagulability. This condition arises due to the development of autoantibodies against factor VIII, a critical component in the coagulation cascade. These antibodies, primarily of the immunoglobulin G4 subclass, inhibit factor VIII, leading to reduced clotting capability. This immune response, resulting in acquired hemophilia A, is a rare but significant hematological side effect of the prolonged use of these antipsychotics [74]. However, case reports indicate atypical occurrences where the expected clinical risk profiles for zuclopenthixol use are contradicted, suggesting a more intricate interplay of underlying mechanisms [75].

An estimation from a study suggested that there are an additional 4 cases of VTE per 10,000 patients treated annually across all ages, with the number rising to 10 per 10,000 in patients aged 65 and over. Interestingly, younger patients are found to have an approximately threefold higher risk of PE and VTE compared to older patients [72].

However, case reports provide evidence of exceptions where typical risk factors are absent, contradicting typical clinical expectations and risk profiles for the use of zuclopenthixol and indicating a more complex interplay of the underlying mechanisms [75].

In the context of COVID-19, mortality is influenced by several factors, including gender, and the presence of cardiovascular and metabolic comorbidities, such as diabetes, obesity, chronic renal failure, and chronic heart disease. Medications such as antipsychotics, antidepressants, and antiepileptics were found to be significantly associated with increased COVID-19 mortality in both the Aragon and Campania regions. This highlights the importance of considering chronic baseline treatments for conditions that predispose patients to systemic inflammation and thrombosis in managing COVID-19 patients [1,2].

Furthermore, a correlation was observed between the use of antipsychotic drugs and an increased occurrence of thrombotic events, especially in the very elderly [76]. Additionally, individuals over the age of 40 are recognized as having an elevated risk of VTE, with this risk doubling with each passing decade. This information underscores the necessity of a nuanced approach to assessing and managing thromboembolic risks associated with psychiatric medications, especially considering age-related factors [1,2].

It is commonly recognized as a primary determinant in the mortality associated with infections. Additional factors contributing to this include being male and the presence of cardiovascular and metabolic comorbidities, such as diabetes, obesity, chronic renal failure, and chronic heart disease. Central to both these conditions and the pathophysiology of COVID-19 is their impact on the body's inflammatory response and the functioning of both the immune and coagulation systems [2].

In Table 1, we summarized the main findings.

Table 1. Risk factor analysis table for VTE in patients on antipsychotic medication.

Risk Factor	Description	Associated Antipsychotics	Impact on VTE Risk
Prolonged Immobilization	Reduced mobility due to sedative effects of drugs	Various antipsychotics	Immobility increases the risk of blood stasis, leading to thrombosis
Hypercoagulability	Altered coagulation pathways	Various antipsychotics	Certain antipsychotics may promote blood clotting, enhancing thrombosis risk
Endothelial Dysfunction	Impairment of endothelial function	Atypical antipsychotics	Endothelial dysfunction can contribute to cardiovascular diseases
Genetic Predispositions	Interaction with genetic factors	Various antipsychotics	Genetic factors can interact with medications to heighten VTE risk
COVID-19 Infection	Exacerbation of VTE risk due to COVID-19	Various antipsychotics	COVID-19 may disrupt coagulation balance, increasing thrombosis risk
Age and Comorbidities	Higher risk in older patients and those with comorbidities	Various antipsychotics	Older age and comorbidities like obesity increase VTE risk
Specific Medication Types	Different risks associated with specific drugs	Clozapine, Risperidone	Some antipsychotics, like clozapine, have a higher associated risk of PE

4. Discussion

4.1. COVID-19 and Thrombosis

Thrombosis, a serious concern in COVID-19, affects approximately one-third of patients, most severely leading to pulmonary embolism [77,78]. The development of thrombosis is influenced by multiple interacting factors, commonly known as Virchow's triad, including vascular endothelial damage, venous stasis, and hypercoagulability [79]. There seems to be an underlying mechanism causing a response severe enough to still cause venous thromboemboli in prophylactically anticoagulated patients [80]. This, plus the thrombotic and microangiopathic thrombotic findings on COVID-19 patients' autopsies, confirms the importance of this topic [81].

Basically, all coagulation parameters have been shown to be potentially altered in COVID-19 infection, but not all of them show clear correlation with the extent of the disease process [82].

While immobilization in severe COVID-19 cases surely plays a role in venous stasis, other effects are not as straight forward and are yet to be explored in detail [82].

SARS-CoV2 can enter the body in a variety of ways but infects through the binding of its S-protein to the angiotensin converting enzyme 2 (ACE2) receptor. ACE2 can be found in a variety of organs, including the nose, bronchi, blood vessels, heart, kidney, and brain [83]. Physiologically, ACE2 converts angiotensin II to angiotensin 1-7. Since it is being used by the virus, it has been hypothesized that less ACE2 is available for normal bodily function, leading to an increase in angiotensin II and a decrease in angiotensin 1-7. Angiotensin II causes vasoconstriction, which can lead to capillary congestion, with microthrombi in the alveolar capillaries [79]. In addition, ATII is a potent pro-inflammatory peptide hormone that causes the accumulation of reactive oxygen species (ROS) through NAD(P)H oxidase. Reactive oxygen species, in turn, are known to play a role in vascular inflammation and contribute to endothelial dysfunction [84], while Angiotensin 1-7 actually has anti-inflammatory and anti-thrombotic effects [85]. This dysregulation of the Renin-Angiotensin-Aldosterone-System causes endothelial dysfunction not only by ROS, but also by overexpressing various factors and receptors, such as COX-2, VEGF, and LOX-1 [83]. Another potential culprit involved is von Willebrand factor. Physiologically, von Willebrand factor is found sub endothelially, where it is released through endothelial damage, aiding platelet aggregation and ultimately thrombosis. A single-center, cross-sectional study from Yale–New Haven Hospital found a greatly increased amount of von Willebrand factor in COVID-19 patients. This amount was correlated with disease severity (ICU vs. non-ICU patients) [86].

It was discovered fairly early that a major part of COVID-19′s pathological effects are caused by an excessive immune response, including but not limited to the complement system, neutrophil extracellular traps (NETs), and mitogen-activated protein kinases (MAPKs) pathways. Commonly implicated is the release of inflammatory cytokines, namely IL-1, IL-6, IL-8, and IL-17. Cytokine IL-6 plays a vital role in hypercoagulability by magnifying fibrinogen and platelet production and is positively correlated with COVID-19 severity [87]. The "cytokine storm" is not necessarily found system-wide, but can also be triggered locally in the lung, causing local thrombus formation. This will lead to the common picture of pulmonary emboli without DVTs, as we encounter it in COVID-19 [88]. While cytokines, von Willebrand factor, and fibrinogen are responsible for increased thrombotic factors, they also cause a state of hypercoagulability due to the increased number of plasma components [79].

In addition to the triggered immune response, hypoxia, which is commonly encountered in COVID-19 patients, also stimulates thrombosis. Hypoxia causes expression of hypoxia-inducible transcription factors, causing activation of thrombosis-related genes [82].

There are specific genetic factors that can elevate the risk of thrombosis. However, research exploring the connection between genetic mutations and COVID-19-related thrombosis produces conflicting results, necessitating further investigation [79,86,88].

4.2. Limitations and Future Research Directions

While our study provides important insights, it also has limitations. The observational nature of the study restricts our ability to establish causality. Some studies suggest that patients with schizophrenia experience a higher incidence of venous thromboembolism compared to the general population [31].

Future research should focus on longitudinal studies to better understand the long-term impacts of antipsychotic use in patients, especially in the context of pandemic-related stressors and restrictions. Additionally, more research is needed to explore the mechanisms behind the varying impacts of different antipsychotic medications in the context of COVID-19 [1,71,73].

4.3. Need for Cautious Medication Management

Given the heightened risk of adverse outcomes, particularly thromboembolic events and mortality, healthcare providers should exercise heightened caution when prescribing antipsychotics for patients during pandemic conditions like COVID-19. Alternatives to antipsychotics or strategies to minimize exposure may be beneficial, especially for patients with additional risk factors for severe COVID-19 outcomes [1,23].

Evidence indicates that complications arising from the use of antipsychotic drugs are not only common, but also incur substantial costs. This situation underscores the necessity for the introduction of an effective algorithm in clinical practice, particularly in psychiatry, to mitigate these complications. Implementing protocols is crucial to reducing both the frequency of these adverse events and the associated healthcare expenses [46].

New risk prediction algorithms are now incorporating the use of antipsychotics as specific predictor variables in assessing the risk of venous thromboembolism. These algorithms are designed to more accurately evaluate the potential of antipsychotics to induce VTE, reflecting the nuanced risks associated with the different types of these medications. This approach marks a significant advancement in personalized medical assessments, particularly for patients undergoing antipsychotic therapy [89,90].

4.4. Our Contribution

This study contributes to the growing body of evidence concerning the adverse health outcomes linked to some of the antipsychotic drugs. Recent research has already established the significantly heightened risks of severe events and mortality in patients treated with antipsychotics for behavioral issues [42]. However, our findings warrant further validation through replication in another database before any modifications in clinical practices are suggested. To accurately assess the risks associated with specific antipsychotics, larger datasets are necessary.

5. Conclusions

Subsequent studies should corroborate our results, thus advocating for a more cautious approach in prescribing antipsychotic drugs, particularly for conditions like nausea and agitation, and especially in patients with a high risk of thromboembolism. Patients should be well informed about the risk–benefit balance of these drugs prior to starting treatment.

Achieving this requires the development of new algorithms capable of estimating an individual's absolute risk of thromboembolism. These algorithms should incorporate individual-level factors, such as age, sex, socioeconomic status, smoking habits, comorbidities, and concurrent medication use. Such a tailored approach would enhance patient care by providing a more nuanced understanding of the risks associated with antipsychotic drug therapy and enabl us to select the best individualized treatment.

Author Contributions: Conceptualization, E.-A.D.-N. and E.-G.B.; methodology, E.-A.D.-N. and E.-G.B.; formal analysis, E.-A.D.-N. and E.-G.B.; resources, E.-A.D.-N. and C.U.; writing—original draft preparation, E.-A.D.-N. and P.L.; writing—review and editing, E.-A.D.-N. and E.-G.B.; supervision, A.B. All authors have read and agreed to the published version of the manuscript.

Funding: This research received no external funding.

Institutional Review Board Statement: Not applicable.

Informed Consent Statement: Not applicable.

Data Availability Statement: Data available upon request.

Conflicts of Interest: The authors declare no conflicts of interest.

References

1. Harrison, S.L.; Buckley, B.J.R.; Lane, D.A.; Underhill, P.; Lip, G.Y.H. Associations between COVID-19 and 30-day thromboembolic events and mortality in people with dementia receiving antipsychotic medications. *Pharmacol. Res.* **2021**, *167*, 105534. [CrossRef] [PubMed]
2. Bliek-Bueno, K.; Mucherino, S.; Poblador-Plou, B.; González-Rubio, F.; Aza-Pascual-Salcedo, M.; Orlando, V.; Clerencia-Sierra, M.; Ioakeim-Skoufa, I.; Coscioni, E.; Carmona-Pírez, J.; et al. Baseline Drug Treatments as Indicators of Increased Risk of COVID-19 Mortality in Spain and Italy. *Int. J. Environ. Res. Public Health* **2021**, *18*, 11786. [CrossRef] [PubMed]
3. Laporte, S.; Benhamou, Y.; Bertoletti, L.; Frère, C.; Hanon, O.; Couturaud, F.; Moustafa, F.; Mismetti, P.; Sanchez, O.; Mahé, I.; et al. Management of cancer-associated thromboembolism in vulnerable population. *Arch. Cardiovasc. Dis.* **2024**, *117*, 45–59. [CrossRef] [PubMed]
4. Sanchez, O.; Roy, P.-M.; Gaboreau, Y.; Schmidt, J.; Moustafa, F.; Benmaziane, A.; Elias, A.; Espitia, O.; Sevestre, M.-A.; Couturaud, F.; et al. Home treatment for patients with cancer-associated venous thromboembolism. *Arch. Cardiovasc. Dis.* **2024**, *117*, 16–28. [CrossRef]
5. Pavlovic, D.; Niciforovic, D.; Markovic, M.; Papic, D. Cancer-Associated Thrombosis: Epidemiology, Pathophysiological Mechanisms, Treatment, and Risk Assessment. *Clin. Med. Insights Oncol.* **2023**, *17*, 11795549231220297. [CrossRef]
6. Agnelli, G. Prevention of venous thromboembolism in surgical patients. *Circulation* **2004**, *110*, IV-4–IV-12. [CrossRef]
7. Turner, B.R.H.; Machin, M.; Salih, M.; Jasionowska, S.; Lawton, R.; Siracusa, F.; Gwozdz, A.M.; Shalhoub, J.; Davies, A.H. An Updated Systematic Review and Meta-analysis of the Impact of Graduated Compression Stockings in Addition to Pharmacological Thromboprophylaxis for Prevention of Venous Thromboembolism in Surgical Inpatients. *Ann. Surg.* **2024**, *279*, 29–36. [CrossRef]
8. Heit, J.A. Epidemiology of venous thromboembolism. *Nat. Rev. Cardiol.* **2015**, *12*, 464–474. [CrossRef]
9. Grahmann, H.; Suchenwirth, R. Thrombosis hazard in chlorpromazine and reserpine therapy of endogenous psychoses. *Nervenarzt* **1959**, *30*, 224–225.

10. Manoubi, S.A.; Boussaid, M.; Brahim, O.; Ouanes, S.; Mahjoub, Y.; Zarrouk, L.; Mesrati, M.A.; Aissaoui, A. Fatal pulmonary embolism in patients on antipsychotics: Case series, systematic review and meta-analysis. *Asian J. Psychiatr.* **2022**, *73*, 103105. [CrossRef]
11. Meyers, D. Treatment of calcinosis circumscripta and Raynaud's phenomenon. *Med. J. Aust.* **1976**, *2*, 457. [CrossRef] [PubMed]
12. Born, G.V.; Wehmeier, A. Possible approaches to the pharmacological prevention of myocardial ischaemia. *Acta Med. Scand. Suppl.* **1980**, *642*, 191–194. [CrossRef] [PubMed]
13. Tranzer, J.P.; Baumgartner, H.R. Filling gaps in the vascular endothelium with blood platelets. *Nature* **1967**, *216*, 1126–1128. [CrossRef]
14. Thomassen, R.; Vandenbroucke, J.P.; Rosendaal, F.R. Antipsychotic medication and venous thrombosis. *Br. J. Psychiatry* **2001**, *179*, 63–66. [CrossRef] [PubMed]
15. Varia, I.; Krishnan, R.R.; Davidson, J. Deep-vein thrombosis with antipsychotic drugs. *Psychosomatics* **1983**, *24*, 1097–1098. [CrossRef] [PubMed]
16. Trifiró, G.; Sultana, J.; Spina, E. Are the safety profiles of antipsychotic drugs used in dementia the same? An updated review of observational studies. *Drug Saf.* **2014**, *37*, 501–520. [CrossRef]
17. Chow, V.; Reddel, C.; Pennings, G.; Scott, E.; Pasqualon, T.; Ng, A.C.C.; Yeoh, T.; Curnow, J.; Kritharides, L. Global hypercoagulability in patients with schizophrenia receiving long-term antipsychotic therapy. *Schizophr. Res.* **2015**, *162*, 175–182. [CrossRef] [PubMed]
18. Allenet, B.; Schmidlin, S.; Genty, C.; Bosson, J.-L. Antipsychotic drugs and risk of pulmonary embolism. *Pharmacoepidemiol. Drug Saf.* **2012**, *21*, 42–48. [CrossRef]
19. Ferraris, A.; Szmulewicz, A.G.; Posadas-Martínez, M.L.; Serena, M.A.; Vazquez, F.J.; Angriman, F. The Effect of Antipsychotic Treatment on Recurrent Venous Thromboembolic Disease: A Cohort Study. *J. Clin. Psychiatry* **2019**, *80*, 12656. [CrossRef]
20. Pallares Vela, E.; Dave, P.; Cancarevic, I. Clozapine-Related Thromboembolic Events. *Cureus* **2021**, *13*, e16883. [CrossRef]
21. Reponen, E.J.; Ueland, T.; Rokicki, J.; Bettella, F.; Aas, M.; Werner, M.C.F.; Dieset, I.; Steen, N.E.; Andreassen, O.A.; Tesli, M. Polygenic risk for schizophrenia and bipolar disorder in relation to cardiovascular biomarkers. *Eur. Arch. Psychiatry Clin. Neurosci.* **2023**, *273*. *Online ahead of print*. [CrossRef] [PubMed]
22. Nishio, A.; Gotoh, T.M.; Ueki, H. Deep vein thrombosis in the psychiatric patients under physical restraint. *Seishin Shinkeigaku Zasshi* **2007**, *109*, 998–1007. [PubMed]
23. Nobili, A.; D'Avanzo, B.; Tettamanti, M.; Galbussera, A.A.; Remuzzi, G.; Fortino, I.; Leoni, O.; Harari, S.; Mannucci, P.M. Post-COVID condition: Dispensation of drugs and diagnostic tests as proxies of healthcare impact. *Intern. Emerg. Med.* **2023**, *18*, 801–809. [CrossRef] [PubMed]
24. Ostuzzi, G.; Papola, D.; Gastaldon, C.; Schoretsanitis, G.; Bertolini, F.; Amaddeo, F.; Cuomo, A.; Emsley, R.; Fagiolini, A.; Imperadore, G.; et al. Safety of psychotropic medications in people with COVID-19: Evidence review and practical recommendations. *BMC Med.* **2020**, *18*, 466–481. [CrossRef]
25. Yan, Y.; Wang, L.; Yuan, Y.; Xu, J.; Chen, Y.; Wu, B. A pharmacovigilance study of the association between antipsychotic drugs and venous thromboembolism based on Food and Drug Administration Adverse Event Reporting System data. *Expert Opin. Drug Saf.* **2023**, *22*, 1–6. [CrossRef] [PubMed]
26. Farah, R.E.; Makhoul, N.M.; Farah, R.E.; Shai, M.D. Fatal venous thromboembolism associated with antipsychotic therapy. *Ann. Pharmacother.* **2004**, *38*, 1435–1438. [CrossRef]
27. Wilkowska, A.; Kujawska-Danecka, H.; Hajduk, A. Risk and prophylaxis of venous thromboembolism in hospitalized psychiatric patients. A review. *Gen. Hosp. Psychiatry* **2018**, *52*, 421–435. [CrossRef]
28. Lacut, K.; Le Gal, G.; Couturaud, F.; Cornily, G.; Leroyer, C.; Mottier, D.; Oger, E. Association between antipsychotic drugs, antidepressant drugs and venous thromboembolism: Results from the EDITH case-control study. *Fundam. Clin. Pharmacol.* **2007**, *21*, 643–650. [CrossRef]
29. Li, K.J.; Greenstein, A.P.; Delisi, L.E. Sudden death in schizophrenia. *Curr. Opin. Psychiatry* **2018**, *31*, 169–175. [CrossRef]
30. Di, X.; Chen, M.; Shen, S.; Cui, X. Antipsychotic use and Risk of Venous Thromboembolism: A Meta-Analysis. *Psychiatry Res.-Neuroimaging* **2021**, *296*, 113691. [CrossRef]
31. Hsu, W.-Y.; Lane, H.-Y.; Lin, C.-L.; Kao, C.-H. A population-based cohort study on deep vein thrombosis and pulmonary embolism among schizophrenia patients. *Schizophr. Res.* **2015**, *162*, 248–252. [CrossRef] [PubMed]
32. Hägg, S.; Tätting, P.; Spigset, O. Olanzapine and venous thromboembolism. *Int. Clin. Psychopharmacol.* **2003**, *18*, 299–300. [CrossRef] [PubMed]
33. Toki, S.; Morinobu, S.; Yoshino, A.; Yamawaki, S. A case of venous thromboembolism probably associated with hyperprolactinemia after the addition of olanzapine to typical antipsychotics. *J. Clin. Psychiatry* **2004**, *65*, 1576–1577. [CrossRef] [PubMed]
34. Ferraris, A.; Angriman, F.; Szmulewicz, A.G. Antipsychotic use and psychiatric disorders in COVID-19. *Lancet Healthy Longev.* **2021**, *2*, e64. [CrossRef]
35. Konnakkaparambil Ramakrishnan, K.; George, M. Deep vein thrombosis on the fourth day of risperidone therapy. *BMJ Case Rep.* **2021**, *14*, e239569. [CrossRef]
36. Reed, M.J.; Comeau, S.; Wojtanowicz, T.R.; Sampathi, B.R.; Penev, S.; Bota, R. Case report: Chlorpromazine and deep venous thrombosis. *Ment. Illn.* **2019**, *11*, 16–19. [CrossRef]

37. Nowrouzi, A.; Kafiabasabadi, S.; Rodriguez-Calzadilla, M.; Benitez-Del-Castillo, J.; Soto-Guerrero, A.; Diaz-Ramos, A.; Marques-Cavalcante, K.V. Central retinal vein occlusion in a patient using the antipsychotic drug olanzapine: A case report. *J. Med. Case Rep.* **2021**, *15*, 307. [CrossRef]
38. Arthur, J.; Duran-Gehring, P.; Kumetz, C.; Chadwick, S.; McIntosh, M. Cerebral Venous Thrombosis: An Uncommon Cause of Papilledema on Bedside Ocular Ultrasound. *J. Emerg. Med.* **2019**, *56*, 288–293. [CrossRef]
39. Srinivasaraju, R.; Reddy, Y.C.J.; Pal, P.K.; Math, S.B. Clozapine-associated cerebral venous thrombosis. *J. Clin. Psychopharmacol.* **2010**, *30*, 335–336. [CrossRef]
40. Wang, Y.; Gong, Y.; Liu, Z.; Fu, Z.; Xue, Y.; Huang, G. Acute Bilateral Coronary Artery Thrombosis and Myocardial Infarction in a 25-Year-Old Man After Long-Term Oral Clozapine Treatment. *J. Clin. Psychopharmacol.* **2020**, *40*, 84–86. [CrossRef]
41. Mameli, A.; Natale, L.; Musu, M.; Finco, G.; Pisanu, A.; Marongiu, F.; Barcellona, D. Olanzapine-Associated Portal and Superior Mesenteric Vein Thrombosis. *Am. J. Ther.* **2020**, *27*, e419–e420. [CrossRef] [PubMed]
42. Parker, C.; Coupland, C.; Hippisley-Cox, J. Antipsychotic drugs and risk of venous thromboembolism: Nested case-control study. *BMJ* **2010**, *341*, c4245. [CrossRef] [PubMed]
43. Barnhorst, A.; Xiong, G.L. Pulmonary embolism in a psychiatric patient. *Am. J. Psychiatry* **2014**, *171*, 1155–1157. [CrossRef] [PubMed]
44. Masopust, J.; Bazantova, V.; Kuca, K.; Klimova, B.; Valis, M. Venous Thromboembolism as an Adverse Effect During Treatment With Olanzapine: A Case Series. *Front. Psychiatry* **2019**, *10*, 330. [CrossRef] [PubMed]
45. Zheng, C.; Liu, H.; Tu, W.; Lin, L.; Xu, H. Hypercoagulable state in patients with schizophrenia: Different effects of acute and chronic antipsychotic medications. *Ther. Adv. Psychopharmacol.* **2023**, *13*, 20451253231200257. [CrossRef] [PubMed]
46. Ruhe, A.M.; Hebbard, A.; Hayes, G. Assessment of venous thromboembolism risk and initiation of appropriate prophylaxis in psychiatric patients. *Ment. Health Clin.* **2018**, *8*, 68–72. [CrossRef] [PubMed]
47. Liperoti, R.; Pedone, C.; Lapane, K.L.; Mor, V.; Bernabei, R.; Gambassi, G. Venous thromboembolism among elderly patients treated with atypical and conventional antipsychotic agents. *Arch. Intern. Med.* **2005**, *165*, 2677–2682. [CrossRef]
48. Sacchetti, E.; Turrina, C.; Valsecchi, P. Cerebrovascular accidents in elderly people treated with antipsychotic drugs: A systematic review. *Drug Saf.* **2010**, *33*, 273–288. [CrossRef]
49. Zornberg, G.L.; Jick, H. Antipsychotic drug use and risk of first-time idiopathic venous thromboembolism: A case-control study. *Lancet* **2000**, *356*, 1219–1223. [CrossRef]
50. Canoso, R.T.; de Oliveira, R.M. Chlorpromazine-induced anticardiolipin antibodies and lupus anticoagulant: Absence of thrombosis. *Am. J. Hematol.* **1988**, *27*, 272–275. [CrossRef]
51. Pons, S.; Fodil, S.; Azoulay, E.; Zafrani, L. The vascular endothelium: The cornerstone of organ dysfunction in severe SARS-CoV-2 infection. *Crit. Care* **2020**, *24*, 353. [CrossRef] [PubMed]
52. Zhang, J.; Tecson, K.M.; McCullough, P.A. Endothelial dysfunction contributes to COVID-19-associated vascular inflammation and coagulopathy. *Rev. Cardiovasc. Med.* **2020**, *21*, 315–319. [CrossRef] [PubMed]
53. Rampino, A.; Annese, T.; Torretta, S.; Tamma, R.; Falcone, R.M.; Ribatti, D. Involvement of vascular endothelial growth factor in schizophrenia. *Neurosci. Lett.* **2021**, *760*, 136093. [CrossRef] [PubMed]
54. Jorgensen, A.; Knorr, U.; Soendergaard, M.G.; Lykkesfeldt, J.; Fink-Jensen, A.; Poulsen, H.E.; Jorgensen, M.B.; Olsen, N.V.; Staalsø, J.M. Asymmetric dimethylarginine in somatically healthy schizophrenia patients treated with atypical antipsychotics: A case–control study. *BMC Psychiatry* **2015**, *15*, 67. [CrossRef] [PubMed]
55. Nair, G.M.; Skaria, D.S.; James, T.; Kanthlal, S.K. Clozapine Disrupts Endothelial Nitric Oxide Signaling and Antioxidant System for its Cardiovascular Complications. *Drug Res.* **2019**, *69*, 695–698. [CrossRef]
56. Murphy, B.P.; Pang, T.Y.; Hannan, A.J.; Proffitt, T.-M.; McConchie, M.; Kerr, M.; Markulev, C.; O'Donnell, C.; McGorry, P.D.; Berger, G.E. Vascular Endothelial Growth Factor and Brain-Derived Neurotrophic Factor in Quetiapine Treated First-Episode Psychosis. *Schizophr. Res. Treat.* **2014**, *2014*, e719395. [CrossRef]
57. Nguyen, T.T.; Dev, S.I.; Chen, G.; Liou, S.C.; Martin, A.S.; Irwin, M.R.; Carroll, J.E.; Tu, X.; Jeste, D.V.; Eyler, L.T. Abnormal levels of vascular endothelial biomarkers in schizophrenia. *Eur. Arch. Psychiatry Clin. Neurosci.* **2018**, *268*, 849–860. [CrossRef]
58. Lee, B.-H.; Hong, J.-P.; Hwang, J.-A.; Ham, B.-J.; Na, K.-S.; Kim, W.-J.; Trigo, J.; Kim, Y.-K. Alterations in plasma vascular endothelial growth factor levels in patients with schizophrenia before and after treatment. *Psychiatry Res.* **2015**, *228*, 95–99. [CrossRef]
59. Misiak, B.; Stramecki, F.; Stańczykiewicz, B.; Frydecka, D.; Lubeiro, A. Vascular endothelial growth factor in patients with schizophrenia: A systematic review and meta-analysis. *Prog. Neuro-Psychopharmacol. Biol. Psychiatry* **2018**, *86*, 24–29. [CrossRef]
60. Gligorijević, N.; Vasović, T.; Lević, S.; Miljević, Č.; Nedić, O.; Nikolić, M. Atypical antipsychotic clozapine binds fibrinogen and affects fibrin formation. *Int. J. Biol. Macromol.* **2020**, *154*, 142–149. [CrossRef]
61. Wallaschofski, H.; Kobsar, A.; Sokolova, O.; Eigenthaler, M.; Lohmann, T. Co-activation of platelets by prolactin or leptin—pathophysiological findings and clinical implications. *Horm. Metab. Res.* **2004**, *36*, 1–6. [CrossRef] [PubMed]
62. Dijkstra, M.E.; van der Weiden, C.F.S.; Schol-Gelok, S.; Muller-Hansma, A.H.G.; Cohen, G.; van den Bemt, P.M.L.A.; Kruip, M.J.H.A. Venous thrombosis during olanzapine treatment: A complex association. *Neth. J. Med.* **2018**, *76*, 263–268. [PubMed]
63. Therasse, A.; Persano, H.L.; Ventura, A.D.; Tecco, J.M. Incidence and prevention of deep vein thrombosis in restrained psychiatric patients. *Psychiatr. Danub.* **2018**, *30*, 412–414. [PubMed]
64. Tripp, A.C. Nonfatal pulmonary embolus associated with clozapine treatment: A case series. *Gen. Hosp. Psychiatry* **2011**, *33*, 85.e5–85.e6. [CrossRef] [PubMed]

65. Purcell, A.; Clarke, M.; Maidment, I. Venous thromboembolism prophylaxis in mental health in-patient services: A qualitative study. *Int. J. Clin. Pharm.* **2018**, *40*, 543–549. [CrossRef]
66. Takeshima, M.; Ishikawa, H.; Umeta, Y.; Kudoh, M.; Umakoshi, A.; Yoshizawa, K.; Ito, Y.; Hosoya, T.; Tsutsui, K.; Ohta, H.; et al. Prevalence of Asymptomatic Venous Thromboembolism in Depressive Inpatients. *Neuropsychiatr. Dis. Treat.* **2020**, *16*, 579–587. [CrossRef]
67. Cecchi, R.; Lazzaro, A.; Catanese, M.; Mandarelli, G.; Ferracuti, S. Fatal thromboembolism following physical restraint in a patient with schizophrenia. *Int. J. Legal Med.* **2012**, *126*, 477–482. [CrossRef]
68. Nielsen, A.S. [Deep venous thrombosis and fatal pulmonary embolism in a physically restrained patient]. *Ugeskr. Laeger* **2005**, *167*, 2294.
69. Maempel, J.F.; Darmanin, G.; Naeem, K.; Patel, M. Olanzapine and pulmonary embolism, a rare association: A case report. *Cases J.* **2010**, *3*, 36. [CrossRef]
70. Yong, K.C.; Kah, T.A.; Ghee, Y.T.; Siang, L.C.; Bastion, M.-L.C. Branch retinal vein occlusion associated with quetiapine fumarate. *BMC Ophthalmol.* **2011**, *11*, 24. [CrossRef]
71. Kleijer, B.C.; Heerdink, E.R.; Egberts, T.C.G.; Jansen, P.A.F.; van Marum, R.J. Antipsychotic drug use and the risk of venous thromboembolism in elderly patients. *J. Clin. Psychopharmacol.* **2010**, *30*, 526–530. [CrossRef] [PubMed]
72. Ray, J.G.; Mamdani, M.M.; Yeo, E.L. Antipsychotic and antidepressant drug use in the elderly and the risk of venous thromboembolism. *Thromb. Haemost.* **2002**, *88*, 205–209. [PubMed]
73. Letmaier, M.; Grohmann, R.; Kren, C.; Toto, S.; Bleich, S.; Engel, R.; Gary, T.; Papageorgiou, K.; Konstantinidis, A.; Holl, A.K.; et al. Venous thromboembolism during treatment with antipsychotics: Results of a drug surveillance programme. *World J. Biol. Psychiatry* **2018**, *19*, 175–186. [CrossRef] [PubMed]
74. Stewart, A.J.; Manson, L.M.; Dasani, H.; Beddall, A.; Collins, P.; Shima, M.; Ludlam, C.A. Acquired haemophilia in recipients of depot thioxanthenes. *Haemophilia* **2000**, *6*, 709–712. [CrossRef] [PubMed]
75. Andole, S.N. An unusual presentation of cortical venous thrombosis and its association with typical antipsychotics. *BMJ Case Rep.* **2011**, *2011*, bcr0720114542. [CrossRef] [PubMed]
76. Catalani, F.; Campello, E.; Occhipinti, G.; Zorzi, A.; Sartori, M.; Zanforlini, B.M.; Franchin, A.; Simioni, P.; Sergi, G. Efficacy and safety of direct oral anticoagulants in older adults with atrial fibrillation: A prospective single-centre cohort study. *Intern. Emerg. Med.* **2023**, *18*, 1941–1949. [CrossRef] [PubMed]
77. Iba, T.; Wada, H.; Levy, J.H. Platelet Activation and Thrombosis in COVID-19. *Semin. Thromb. Hemost.* **2023**, *49*, 55–61. [CrossRef]
78. Zanini, G.; Selleri, V.; Roncati, L.; Coppi, F.; Nasi, M.; Farinetti, A.; Manenti, A.; Pinti, M.; Mattioli, A.V. Vascular "Long COVID": A New Vessel Disease? *Angiology* **2024**, *75*, 8–14. [CrossRef]
79. Sastry, S.; Cuomo, F.; Muthusamy, J. COVID-19 and thrombosis: The role of hemodynamics. *Thromb. Res.* **2022**, *212*, 51–57. [CrossRef]
80. Tiwari, N.R.; Phatak, S.; Sharma, V.R.; Agarwal, S.K. COVID-19 and thrombotic microangiopathies. *Thromb. Res.* **2021**, *202*, 191–198. [CrossRef]
81. Babkina, A.S.; Yadgarov, M.Y.; Volkov, A.V.; Kuzovlev, A.N.; Grechko, A.V.; Golubev, A.M. Spectrum of Thrombotic Complications in Fatal Cases of COVID-19: Focus on Pulmonary Artery Thrombosis In Situ. *Viruses* **2023**, *15*, 1681. [CrossRef] [PubMed]
82. Hadid, T.; Kafri, Z.; Al-Katib, A. Coagulation and anticoagulation in COVID-19. *Blood Rev.* **2021**, *47*, 100761. [CrossRef] [PubMed]
83. Ali, M.A.M.; Spinler, S.A. COVID-19 and thrombosis: From bench to bedside. *Trends Cardiovasc. Med.* **2021**, *31*, 143–160. [CrossRef] [PubMed]
84. Mehta, P.K.; Griendling, K.K. Angiotensin II cell signaling: Physiological and pathological effects in the cardiovascular system. *Am. J. Physiol.-Cell Physiol.* **2007**, *292*, C82–C97. [CrossRef] [PubMed]
85. Santos, R.A.S.; Sampaio, W.O.; Alzamora, A.C.; Motta-Santos, D.; Alenina, N.; Bader, M.; Campagnole-Santos, M.J. The ACE2/Angiotensin-(1–7)/MAS Axis of the Renin-Angiotensin System: Focus on Angiotensin-(1–7). *Physiol. Rev.* **2018**, *98*, 505–553. [CrossRef] [PubMed]
86. Goshua, G.; Pine, A.B.; Meizlish, M.L.; Chang, C.-H.; Zhang, H.; Bahel, P.; Baluha, A.; Bar, N.; Bona, R.D.; Burns, A.J.; et al. Endotheliopathy in COVID-19-associated coagulopathy: Evidence from a single-centre, cross-sectional study. *Lancet Haematol.* **2020**, *7*, e575–e582. [CrossRef] [PubMed]
87. Chen, X.; Zhao, B.; Qu, Y.; Chen, Y.; Xiong, J.; Feng, Y.; Men, D.; Huang, Q.; Liu, Y.; Yang, B.; et al. Detectable Serum Severe Acute Respiratory Syndrome Coronavirus 2 Viral Load (RNAemia) Is Closely Correlated With Drastically Elevated Interleukin 6 Level in Critically Ill Patients With Coronavirus Disease 2019. *Clin. Infect. Dis.* **2020**, *71*, 1937–1942. [CrossRef] [PubMed]
88. Cheng, N.M.; Chan, Y.C.; Cheng, S.W. COVID-19 related thrombosis: A mini-review. *Phlebology* **2022**, *37*, 326–337. [CrossRef]
89. Hippisley-Cox, J.; Coupland, C. Development and validation of risk prediction algorithm (QThrombosis) to estimate future risk of venous thromboembolism: Prospective cohort study. *BMJ* **2011**, *343*, d4656. [CrossRef]
90. Falconer, N.; Barras, M.; Abdel-Hafez, A.; Radburn, S.; Cottrell, N. Development and validation of the Adverse Inpatient Medication Event model (AIME). *Br. J. Clin. Pharmacol.* **2021**, *87*, 1512–1524. [CrossRef]

International Journal of
Molecular Sciences

MDPI

Review

Sialylated Glycan Bindings from SARS-CoV-2 Spike Protein to Blood and Endothelial Cells Govern the Severe Morbidities of COVID-19

David E. Scheim [1,*], Paola Vottero [2], Alessandro D. Santin [3] and Allen G. Hirsh [4]

1 US Public Health Service, Commissioned Corps, Inactive Reserve, Blacksburg, VA 24060, USA
2 Department of Biomedical Engineering, University of Alberta, Edmonton, AB T6G 1Z2, Canada; vottero@ualberta.ca
3 Department of Obstetrics, Gynecology & Reproductive Sciences, Yale School of Medicine, P.O. Box 208063, New Haven, CT 06520, USA; alessandro.santin@yale.edu
4 CryoBioPhysica Inc., Chevy Chase, MD 20815, USA; allenhir@earthlink.net
* Correspondence: dscheim@alum.mit.edu

Abstract: Consistent with well-established biochemical properties of coronaviruses, sialylated glycan attachments between SARS-CoV-2 spike protein (SP) and host cells are key to the virus's pathology. SARS-CoV-2 SP attaches to and aggregates red blood cells (RBCs), as shown in many pre-clinical and clinical studies, causing pulmonary and extrapulmonary microthrombi and hypoxia in severe COVID-19 patients. SARS-CoV-2 SP attachments to the heavily sialylated surfaces of platelets (which, like RBCs, have no ACE2) and endothelial cells (having minimal ACE2) compound this vascular damage. Notably, experimentally induced RBC aggregation in vivo causes the same key morbidities as for severe COVID-19, including microvascular occlusion, blood clots, hypoxia and myocarditis. Key risk factors for COVID-19 morbidity, including older age, diabetes and obesity, are all characterized by markedly increased propensity to RBC clumping. For mammalian species, the degree of clinical susceptibility to COVID-19 correlates to RBC aggregability with $p = 0.033$. Notably, of the five human betacoronaviruses, the two common cold strains express an enzyme that releases glycan attachments, while the deadly SARS, SARS-CoV-2 and MERS do not, although viral loads for COVID-19 and the two common cold infections are similar. These biochemical insights also explain the previously puzzling clinical efficacy of certain generics against COVID-19 and may support the development of future therapeutic strategies for COVID-19 and long COVID patients.

Keywords: SARS-CoV-2; spike protein; COVID-19; sialic acid; glycophorin A; hemagglutination; hemagglutinin esterase

Citation: Scheim, D.E.; Vottero, P.; Santin, A.D.; Hirsh, A.G. Sialylated Glycan Bindings from SARS-CoV-2 Spike Protein to Blood and Endothelial Cells Govern the Severe Morbidities of COVID-19. *Int. J. Mol. Sci.* **2023**, *24*, 17039. https://doi.org/10.3390/ijms242317039

Academic Editors: Eliza Russu, Alexandru Schiopu and Emil Marian Arbănași

Received: 31 October 2023
Revised: 24 November 2023
Accepted: 27 November 2023
Published: 1 December 2023

1. Introduction

The virus that caused COVID-19 was first named "severe acute respiratory syndrome coronavirus 2" (SARS-CoV-2) in February 2020 in recognition of the disease's pulmonary symptoms and the lung's role as its initial target organ, as with its SARS predecessor. Yet as clinical experience and histological findings accrued, the hypoxia which emerged as a key morbidity of severe COVID-19 was found in a large percentage of such patients to accompany nearly normal breathing mechanics and lung gas volume [1–6]. Although COVID-19 typically gains infectious penetration in the respiratory epithelium, microvascular occlusion is frequently observed in pulmonary septal capillaries and in other organ systems of COVID-19 patients [7–20], accompanying morbidities such as intravascular clotting and peripheral ischemia [2,3,8,18,21–23]. Lung inflammation and other pulmonary symptoms are common with COVID-19, yet in several cases of severe disease, histological examinations have revealed microthrombi and extensively damaged endothelium in the septal capillary microvasculature adjoining relatively intact alveoli [14,24].

Soon after the determination of SARS-CoV-2 as the viral cause of COVID-19, ACE2 was identified as the host cell receptor supporting its replication [25–27], with neurophilin-1 its replication receptor for astrocytes and possibly certain other cell types [28,29]. Yet ACE2 is one of a variety of host cell receptors that different coronavirus strains use for replication; other receptors include DPP4 for MERS, APN for HCoV-229E, and CEACAM1 for MHV [30]. The morbidities of SARS-CoV-2, in particular, as shown below, are less dependent on its host cell replication receptor, ACE2, than on glycans having sialic acid (SA) terminal moieties found on viral spike protein (SP) and host cells. For coronaviruses, these sialylated glycans on their SP serve as the initial points of viral attachment to the host cell surface [30–42], after which the virus can migrate to fuse with a replication receptor [40,42–49]. One clue to the centrality of glycan bindings to the morbidities of the five human betacoronaviruses is the expression by the two common cold strains, HKU1 and OC43, of hemagglutinin esterase (HE), which releases glycan bindings between viral SP and host cells [50–54]. These common cold infections are generally benign, while the SARS, SARS-CoV-2 and MERS viruses do not express HE [50–54] and are deadly, even though the viral loads for COVID-19 and these common cold infections are about the same [55].

The Molecular Composition of Glycans on SARS-CoV-2 SP and the RBC

The arrangement and chemical composition of the SARS-CoV-2 SP glycans have been determined, with those at its 22 N-glycosylation sites having a total of nine SA terminal residues [31,48,49,56–63] and its four O-glycans having a total of three SA terminal residues [63]. This provides a basis for exploring these viral SP attachments to host cells, notably red blood cells (RBCs), platelets, leukocytes and endothelial cells [31]. RBCs and platelets have densely distributed sialoglycoproteins but no ACE2 receptors on their surfaces [64,65]; the same holds for leukocytes and most other blood cells [66–68]. Endothelial cells likewise have a heavily sialylated surface coating (glycocalyx), with about 28,000 SA-tipped CD147 receptors but only about 175 ACE2 receptors per cell [69,70].

Of particular interest are attachments of SARS-CoV-2 SP to the RBC, the latter coated with one million SA-tipped glycophorin A (GPA) molecules and a total of 35 million SA monosaccharides per cell [71–73]. The heavily sialylated GPA strands are spaced about 14 nm apart on the RBC surface and extend out 5 nm [71]. Band 3 protein is another molecule on the RBC surface, with 1.2 million copies per RBC, which extends >10 nm from the RBC surface [71,74] and is glycosylated by poly-N-acetyllactosamine, a sialylated branched-chain glycan [75–78]. GPA and poly-N-acetyllactosamine, the two most abundant glycans on the RBC membrane [77], have been found to mediate hemagglutination by various bacterial and viral pathogens [78–81]. The glycans attached to SARS-CoV-2 SP and those which extend from the RBC surface are depicted in Figure 1.

Hemagglutination as caused by these pathogen–glycan attachments is of particular interest in view of a primal defense mounted by RBCs along with platelets against pathogens having SA terminal moieties by attaching to them and delivering them to leukocytes or conveying them to macrophages in the liver and spleen for phagocytosis [72,82–88]. Notably, GPA, one of the two most abundant glycans on the RBC surface [77,89], has no other known physiological role other than spearheading this pathogen defense [71,72,83,84]. For severe COVID-19 infections, however, this primal defense, described as "immune adherence" [85], goes self-destructively overboard, with the total load and sizes of clumps formed exceeding the body's capacity to sequester them, as detailed below.

A clear experimental demonstration of binding between SARS-CoV-2 SP and sialylated glycans on host cells was provided using NMR spectroscopy [34]. It was found, in particular, that a site on the SP N-terminal domain (NTD) binds to α2,3 and α2,6 sialyl N-acetyllactosamine, which are components or variants thereof of the sialylated poly-N-acetyllactosamine glycans of the band 3 strands extending from the RBC surface. Intriguingly, this SP-to-glycan binding was found to be much more pronounced for α2,3 than for α2,6 SA-linked N-acetyllactosamine [34], while α2,3 vs. α2,6-linked SA is likewise much more prevalent in sialylated poly-N-acetyllactosamine of adult (vs. fetal) RBCs [76].

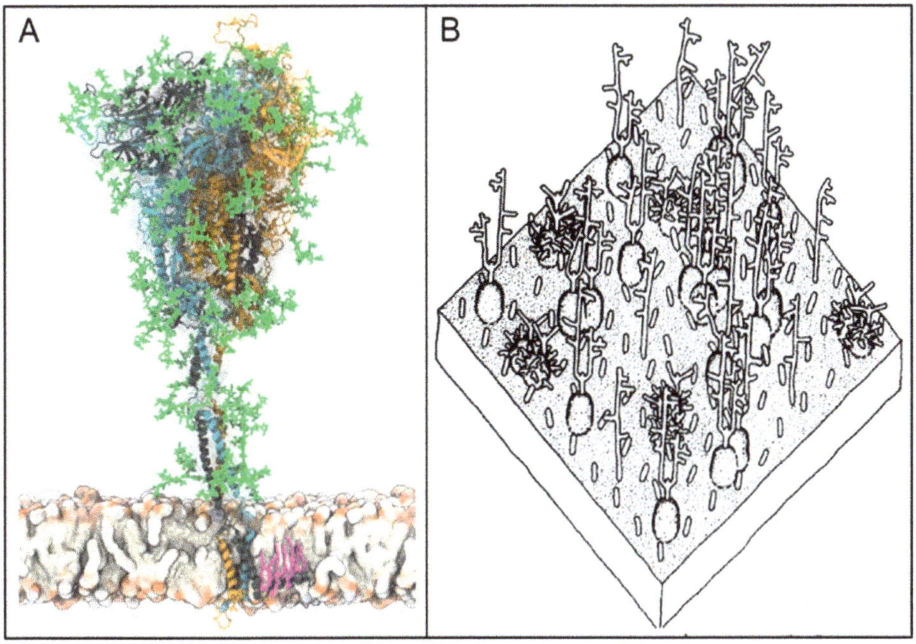

Figure 1. (**A**): Atomistic model of the full-length trimeric S protein of SARS-CoV-2 shown in cartoon representation, reproduced from Sikora et al. (2021) [90]. The three monomeric chains are differentiated by color, with glycans shown in green licorice representation, and a palmitoylated cysteine residue shown in pink, anchored into the viral envelope at the bottom. (**B**): A representation of a 35 × 35 nm area of the RBC surface depicting its sialoglycoprotein coating, reproduced from Viitala et al. (1975) [71]. Prominent among these sialylated glycans are GPA strands, which extend approximately 5 nm from the RBC surface, and band 3 protein, which extends > 10 nm from that surface and is glycosylated by poly-N-acetyllactosamine. Reproduced (**A**) under CC-BY 4.0 and (**B**) with permission from Elsevier.

Possibilities for binding are indicated as well between SARS-CoV-2 SP and/or glycans at its glycosylation sites and GPA on the RBC surface, with GPA, as noted, having no known physiological role other than this type of immune adherence. The positive electrostatic potential of SARS-CoV-2 SP [91] supports its binding to the negatively charged, densely distributed SA on the RBC surface, most on its million GPA strands [92,93]. Also, as depicted in Figure 2, SA in its predominant human form, Neu5Ac, is the most common terminal residue of GPA [71,74,94]. For the N- and O-glycans on SARS-CoV-2 SP, the most common terminal residues are galactose (Gal), with 27 total, and Neu5Ac (SA), with 12 total [61–63,90]. Through binding configurations proposed by Varki and Schnaar (2017) [95] and others [34,96–98], multivalent bonds can form via α2–3 and α2–6 linkages from Neu5Ac on GPA to Gal on glycans populating SARS-CoV-2 SP glycosylation sites.

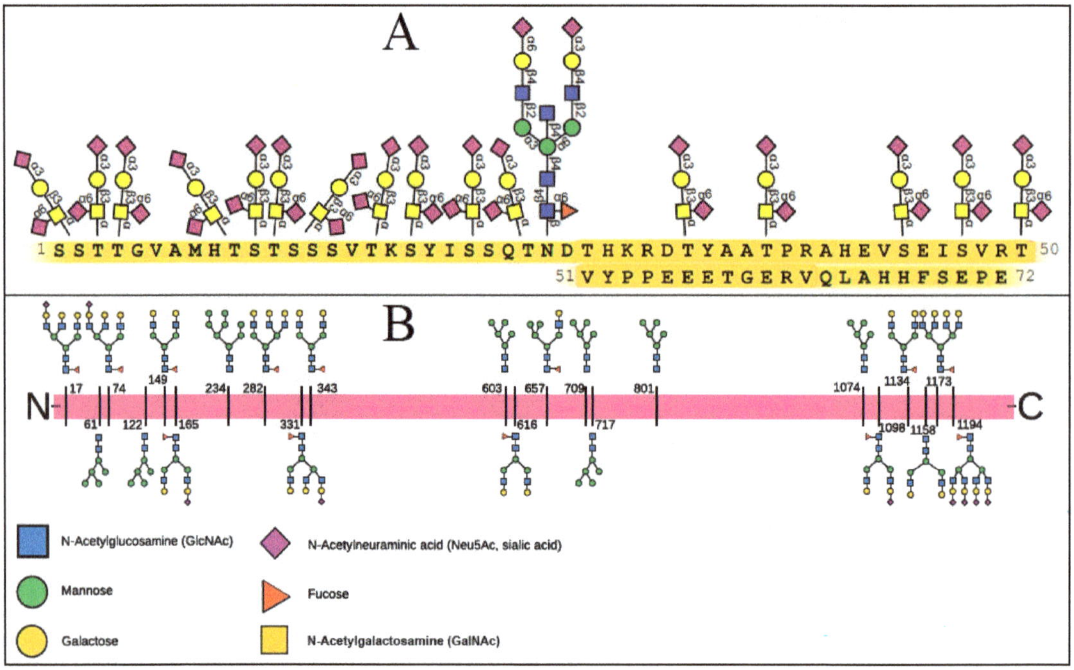

Figure 2. (**A**): Amino acid sequence of the extracellular domain (aa 1–72) of GPA with its glycan structures and attachment sites, adapted from Jaskiewicz et al. (2019) [94]. (**B**): The terminal monosaccharides for fully populated N-glycans of a SARS-CoV-2 SP monomer, with these 22 N-glycosylation sites numbered from the N-terminal end to the C-terminal end, as adapted from Sikora et al. (2021) [90]. The key to the monosaccharides shown in both (**A**) and (**B**) is at bottom of (**B**). Reproduced (**A**,**B**) under CC-BY 4.0.

2. In Vitro, In Vivo and Clinical Studies Demonstrate Induction of RBC Aggregation by SARS-CoV-2 SP

Many in vitro, in vivo and clinical studies demonstrate that SARS-CoV-2 SP attaches to RBCs and induces RBC aggregation. Boschi et al. (2022) found that SARS-CoV-2 SP from each of the Wuhan, Alpha, Delta and Omicron strains induced RBC clumping (hemagglutination) when mixed with human RBCs in phosphate-buffered saline (PBS) [91]. To explore whether bridging of adjacent RBCs by SARS-CoV-2 SP via glycan bonds might be the cause of this observed hemagglutination, an agent with indicated high-affinity binding to multiple SARS-CoV-2 SP glycan-binding sites [99], the macrocyclic lactone ivermectin (IVM), was added to the mix of SP and RBCs both before and after hemagglutination formed. IVM blocked the formation of hemagglutination when added to the initial mix and reversed hemagglutination over the course of 30 min when added after it formed [91]. In another study, SARS-CoV-2 SP added to whole blood induced clumping of RBCs, hyperactivation and clumping of platelets, and formation of anomalous fibrinogen deposits [100].

The same SP-induced RBC clumping effect as noted above was demonstrated in zebrafish embryos, which have blood cell glycosylation patterns [101] and capillary diameters [102] similar to those of humans. When SARS-CoV-2 SP was microinjected into the common cardinal vein of a zebrafish embryo at a concentration similar to that obtained in critically ill COVID-19 patients, it caused the formation of small RBC clumps and an associated reduction in blood flow velocity within 3–5 min after injection, as shown in Figure 3C, accompanied by thrombosis in capillaries, arteries and veins [103]. When SP was coinjected with a mixture of heparan sulfate and heparin (molecular mass of each $\leq$ 30 kDa), however, with both of these glycosaminoglycans having strong binding affinity to SARS-CoV-2 SP [103–105], the extent of thrombosis was markedly reduced [103].

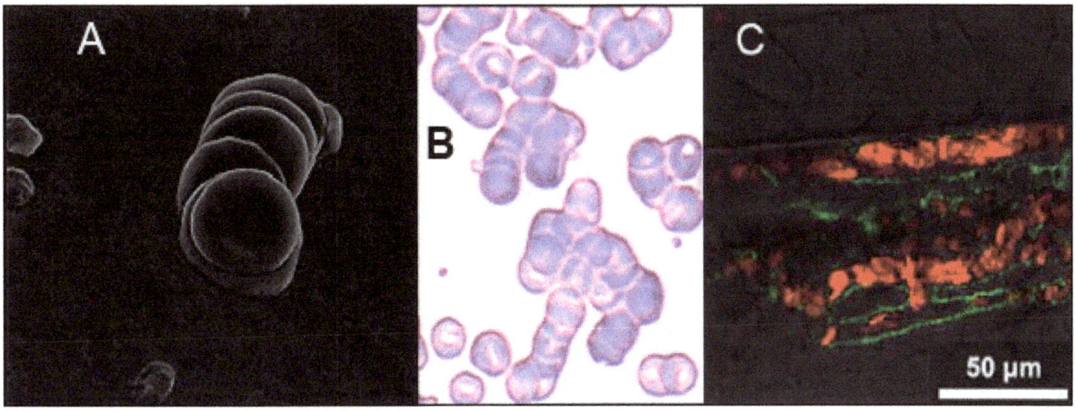

Figure 3. (**A**,**B**): Images of RBC rouleaux (stacked clumps) from the blood of COVID-19 patients, obtained using electron (magnification ×5000) [106] and light (80× objective) [107] microscopy. The first study (**A**) found RBC clumps in all 31 patients studied, all with mild COVID-19 [106], and the second (**B**) found large RBC aggregates in 85% of COVID-19 patients with anemia [107]. (**C**): A frame from a video of RBC aggregates in capillaries of zebrafish embryos that formed within 3–5 min after injection of SARS-CoV-2 SP into the common cardinal vein at a similar concentration to that obtained in critically ill COVID-19 patients [103]. The velocity of blood flow in the capillaries shown in this video frame was markedly reduced from that prior to injection of SP. Reproduced (**A**) with permission from Georg Thieme Verlag KG; (**B**) under CC-BY 4.0; (**C**) with permission from Elsevier.

In various studies, SARS-CoV-2 SP and subunits were observed in the plasma of 64% of COVID-19 patients [108], in the sera of 30% of hospitalized COVID-19 patients [109] and in the brains of all of the 13 patients who died of this disease [110]. SP and spike S1 subunits were likewise observed over periods of months in the plasma [111–113] and monocytes [114], respectively, of patients having post-acute sequelae of this disease (long COVID, or PASC). Leakage of SP outside of an infected host cell during SARS-CoV-2 replication has been documented in vitro and clinically [115–117] and may be the source of the SP in blood found in COVID-19 patients.

SARS-CoV-2 SP attachments to RBCs were demonstrated directly by Lam et al. (2021) through immunofluorescence analysis of RBCs from the blood of nine hospitalized COVID-19 patients [118]. For these patients at hospital admission, the mean percentage of RBCs having SARS-CoV-2 SP traces was 41%. This finding suggests that concentrations of SARS-CoV-2 SP in blood as typically reported in other studies using plasma or serum may significantly understate actual values due to high-affinity binding to RBCs, which are removed from plasma and serum. SARS-CoV-2 SP and pseudovirus were each found to bind to nanoparticle arrays bearing SA derivatives [59] and to SA-tipped CD147 receptors, likewise detected using nanoarrays [119]. Nanoarray methods are required to detect SARS-CoV-2 SP glycan attachments, because these methods allow bindings to form multivalently, whereas univalent bindings are weak [31] and not detectable by microarray methods [42]. Studies using the latter failed to detect SARS-CoV-2 SP bindings to either SA [120] or CD147 [121]. As noted above, binding of SARS-CoV-2 SP to sialylated glycans identical or closely related to those on the RBC surface was demonstrated directly using NMR spectroscopy [34].

The presence of SARS-CoV-2 SP in the blood of COVID-19 patients and its induction of hemagglutination in vitro and in vivo would suggest that the same would occur clinically, which is indeed the case. In three publications that used scanning electron microscopy to examine blood from the cubital vein blood of patients with mild-to-moderate cases of COVID-19, all hospitalized but none requiring intensive care, a team of investigators observed blood cell clumping and other anomalies [106,122,123]. The first study found stacked RBC aggregates (rouleaux) ranging in size from 3–12 cells, as shown in Figure 3A, in the blood of all 31 of its COVID-19 patients, with none found in 32 matched healthy controls [106]. A follow-up publication reported the mean count of RBC aggregates in the COVID-19 patients at 3.1 to 5.5 per 1000 μm^2 scanning area, while controls had no RBC aggregates [122]. Aggregates of platelets, some with leukocytes or RBCs, were likewise found in all COVID-19 patients to significant extents, but none were found in the controls [122].

Light microscopy examination of smears from the blood of 20 hospitalized COVID-19 patients with anemia detected large, stacked RBC clumps (rouleaux), as shown in Figure 3B, in 85% of those patients [107]. Another study, which examined the sublingual microcirculation of 38 COVID-19 patients in intensive care using video microscopy, found that the mean number of RBC microaggregates detected in these patients was 15 times the mean number for 33 healthy volunteers [124]. These RBC microaggregates were found in two-thirds of the COVID-19 patients vs. two of the 33 healthy volunteers. A study of the blood of 172 hospitalized COVID-19 patients found that both RBC aggregability and the strength of RBC aggregates formed were significantly greater than those values for healthy controls and that this RBC hyperaggregability correlated with enhanced blood coagulation, all of these effects highly significant ($p < 0.001$) [125]. The much greater degree and strength of RBC aggregation found in COVID-19 vs. sepsis, with both having elevated levels of inflammation-related markers, indicate that inflammation alone cannot explain these RBC aggregation effects for COVID-19 [125].

Paralleling these studies that document RBC aggregation in severe COVID-19 are many that report microvascular occlusion. Postmortem examinations of hundreds of patients who died from COVID-19 in many studies consistently found microthrombi in the pulmonary microvasculature in most patients [7–18]. Microthrombi in alveolar capillaries were nine times as prevalent in postmortem COVID-19 patients compared to influenza patients [10]. RBC clumping and microthrombi in the lungs have been regarded as likely causes of hypoxemia in severe COVID-19 patients [1,2,106,123], which in turn is closely associated with mortal outcomes [126].

Microthrombi elsewhere in the body, including in the heart, kidneys and liver, were also frequently observed in autopsy examinations of COVID-19 patients, with indications that these may have contributed to multiorgan damage and failure [7,8,20]. Another indication of the widespread distribution of microthrombi throughout the body in severe COVID-19 patients, persisting even after recovery from acute illness, was provided using video capillaroscopy to examine ocular conjunctival microvessels in 17 hospitalized COVID-19 patients within 28 days after hospital discharge and 17 healthy controls [127]. The mean percentage of occluded microvessels was found to be six times as high in the hospital-discharged COVID-19 patients vs. controls, while the mean rates of blood flow in the conjunctival capillaries and postcapillary venules were significantly lower [127]. Such widespread indications of microvascular occlusion in severe COVID-19 patients led cardiovascular researchers at the Johns Hopkins and Harvard University medical schools to conclude that "severe COVID-19 is a microvascular disease" [21].

3. Glycan Bindings from SARS-CoV-2 SP to Platelets and Endothelial Cells Cause Endothelial Damage, Inflammation and Coagulation

Attachments of SARS-CoV-2 SP to the heavily sialylated [64,65,70] surfaces of platelets and endothelial cells cause endothelial damage, platelet activation and associated coagulation which, as with the attachments to RBCs, contribute to the severe morbidities of COVID-19. Platelets, having no ACE2 receptors, like RBCs [66,67], act with RBCs in a role that was termed "immune adherence" [85], attaching to and clearing pathogens [87,88], and are found enmeshed with RBCs in blood cell clumps in COVID-19 patients [122]. The degree of sialyation of the endothelial cell surface is exemplified by the 28,000 SA-tipped CD147 receptors vs. the 175 ACE2 receptors per endothelial cell [69]. For glomerular endothelial cells from a conditionally immortalized human cell line, the enzyme neuraminidase, which hydrolyzes SA, removed more than 50% of the cells' surface coating (glycocalyx) [70]. The endothelial cell thus provides a prime target for the SARS-CoV-2 virus, and indeed, both whole virus and viral SP have been found on endothelial cells in clinical and in vivo COVID-19 infections [10,17,24,110,128–131]. Correspondingly, damaged endothelial cells have been frequently observed in severe COVID-19 patients [21,24,132,133]. Yet the importance of this direct viral attack on the endothelium in COVID-19 has been overlooked by some researchers in the belief that ACE2, which is sparse on endothelial cells, is the only host-cell binding target of interest for SARS-CoV-2 [134,135].

These SARS-CoV-2 viral or SP attachments to the endothelium can be perilous to the human host, with trillions of RBCs each flowing once per minute through the lungs and then the extrapulmonary vasculature [136] and with the cross-sectional diameter of most capillaries so small that RBCs distort their shape to squeeze through [137]. Thus, SARS-CoV-2 virus particles or SP attached to endothelial cells or RBCs could create resistance to blood flow or even potentially rip off a piece of an endothelial cell or the entire cell [31]. Indeed, one study found that serum levels of circulating endothelial cells (CECs) in mild-to-moderate COVID-19 patients were up to 100 times the levels for matched controls. The study also found that each of these CECs from the COVID-19 patients typically had several holes in their membranes approximately the size of the SARS-CoV-2 viral capsid (the viral envelope) [106]. A marker of endothelial damage, von Willebrand factor (VWF), which promotes platelet activation and, in turn, coagulation [138–140], has been found to be significantly elevated in COVID-19 patients [21,132,141,142]. These and other coagulation and proinflammatory pathways can cause blood clots or trigger a cytokine storm in the most serious cases of this infection [21,132,133].

While these pathological pathways contribute significantly to the severe morbidities of COVID-19, the role of SARS-CoV-2 SP-induced RBC aggregation in these morbidities is nevertheless central, as demonstrated below through multiple avenues of substantiation. We show below that experimentally induced RBC clumping in vivo causes the same morbidities and the same redistribution of blood flow from smaller to larger blood vessels as for COVID-19. We further demonstrate the following: (i) key risk factors for COVID-19 morbidity are associated with markedly increased RBC aggregation; (ii) SARS-CoV-2 SP in the absence of whole virus induces microvascular occlusion in vivo and clinically; (iii) three generic drugs that have aroused widespread interest as potential COVID-19 treatments all significantly inhibit RBC aggregation; and (iv) for mammalian species, the degree of clinical susceptibility to COVID-19 correlates to aggregation propensity of RBCs with $p = 0.033$.

4. Experimentally Induced RBC Clumping In Vivo: Parallels to Severe COVID-19

Studies dating back to the 1940s in dogs, rabbits, mice, hamsters and other animals closely examined the effects of IV injection of high-molecular-weight dextran (HMWD), generally of molecular weight (MW, loosely equivalent to molecular mass) $\geq$ 100 kDa or other blood cell-agglutinating agents. In several studies, blood cell aggregation was induced within minutes to hours after IV injection of HMWD [143–148], with molecular bridging of RBCs by HMWD molecules being a hypothesized mechanism for this effect [149–152]. After HMWD injection in vivo, small clumps of RBCs formed and then enlarged into longer stacked clumps (rouleaux) and, in some cases, into vast trees with branches of hundreds of stacked RBCs [144,145,153]. Also, the addition of low-MW dextran (LMWD, e.g., MW $\leq$ 40 kDa) in vivo prevented the formation of RBC aggregates when injected with HMWD [146,154] and rapidly disaggregated them with accompanying reversal of microvascular occlusion when injected after HMWD-induced clumps had formed [148,155–158].

In vitro, the addition of HMWD to blood likewise induced RBC aggregation [159,160] and did so as well when added to RBCs in PBS [161,162]. The same RBC disaggregating effect of LMWD was observed in vitro [163], possibly caused by competitive binding to RBCs that limited bridging between adjacent RBCs by larger molecules. Although we have focused on aggregation of RBCs, these same aggregating effects of HMWD and disaggregating effects of LMWD have been observed, both in vitro and in vivo, for platelets as well [147,153].

Even in healthy humans or animals, RBC clumps can transiently form under conditions of slow blood flow, e.g., in deep veins of the lower limbs, but they typically disaggregate as they move into regions of faster blood flow [164–174] and are rarely problematical in healthy subjects [148,157,175]. Yet under pathological conditions in diseases such as diabetes, malignant hypertension and malaria [154,167,175–177], these RBC aggregates can persist and grow via a positive feedback loop whereby the clumps cause decreased blood flow velocity with a concomitant reduction in shear forces that in turn causes further aggregation [164,166–171,173,175]. In mammals, a significant total mass of blood cell aggregates can lodge in a distributed network of arterioles before obstruction of blood flow reaches a critical stage [178]. Pulmonary artery tips provide a catch-trap architecture that sequesters large blood cell aggregates, which limits disseminated microvascular occlusion and mitigates resulting hypoxia and associated widespread tissue damage, including to the heart wall [167,178].

The capability of LMWD to rapidly reverse RBC aggregation and associated microvascular occlusion caused by injection of HMWD, as noted above, distinguishes blood clumping, e.g., as induced by HMWD, from clotting, in which blood cell clumps harden into fibrin-enmeshed clots via the coagulation cascade. Indeed, several mammalian diseases are associated with increased levels of RBC aggregation and microvascular occlusion which do not typically cause blood clotting, although risks of this complication are increased [154,175]. Blood cell clumping and clotting are not completely unrelated phenomena, however, given the potential of RBC aggregation to trigger deep vein thrombosis [179,180] and the role of fibrinogen, an essential promoter of blood clotting, in blood cell clumping as well [164,181–183].

4.1. Induced RBC Aggregation Causes Microvascular Occlusion, Hypoxia, Blood Clots, and Redistribution of Blood Flow from Smaller to Larger Blood Vessels

When HMWD or other agglutinating agents were injected into animals at sufficient concentrations to overwhelm the host's ability to safely sequester the RBC aggregates formed, these clumps caused microvascular occlusion as detected in a variety of host tissues [154], including the myocardium [153,184], muscle [185] and abdominal cavity [153] of rats; the conjunctival vessels of dogs, cats and rabbits [147,186]; the cheek pouch of hamsters [148,157]; and the kidney, liver, ear chamber, bone marrow and heart tissue of rabbits, including the myocardium and pericardium [144–146,155,156]. In the myocardium of rabbits and rats, the degree of myocardial tissue damage was correlated with the observed degree of intravascular aggregation of blood cells [144,146,153], with hypoxia resulting from vascular occlusion proposed to be the cause of tissue damage [144,146].

Associated with the microvascular occlusion that it triggered, experimentally induced RBC aggregation caused decreased velocity of blood flow [143,145–148,154,171,184], increased blood viscosity [143,154,186,187], increased incidence of blood clotting [144,154,167] and decreased oxygen tension in arteries, veins and tissues, with accompanying hypoxic damage to body organs [144,146,154,188,189]. Another effect caused by induced blood cell clumping as observed in the conjunctiva of cats, dogs and rabbits and bone marrow of rabbits was a reduction in blood flow in the capillaries and other small vessels having cross-sectional diameters of about 10 μm or smaller [147,155], indicative of a shift of blood flow into the larger vessels. A similar redistribution of blood flow from the smaller blood vessels of micrometer cross-sectional diameter to larger blood vessels was observed in patients with type II diabetes [177,190], a disease characterized by an increased extent of RBC aggregation and accompanying microvascular occlusion [167,177,191–194].

4.2. Corresponding Morbidities in Severe COVID-19

As considered above, SARS-CoV-2 SP, like HMWD dextran, induces RBC aggregation, and the same morbidities caused by experimentally induced RBC aggregation have been commonly observed for cases of severe COVID-19. These morbidities of severe

COVID-19 include microvascular occlusion in the lungs and other organ systems [7–20], hypoxia [1,195], arterial and venous thromboembolisms [9,15,17,18,21,196–198], disseminated intravascular coagulation [15,21,196–200] and multiorgan damage associated with these vascular aberrations and hypoxia [7,200,201]. Decreased oxygen saturation is a particularly dangerous morbidity of COVID-19, with a peripheral oxygen saturation (SpO2) of <88% associated with a 3.7-fold increased risk of death [126] and an SpO2 of ≤93% deemed to be a sufficient condition for classifying a COVID-19 infection as severe according to U.S. National Institutes of Health guidelines [202].

4.3. Redistribution of Blood Flow from Smaller to Larger Blood Microvessels in COVID-19 Patients

Another effect of experimentally induced RBC aggregation, the redistribution of blood flow from microvessels to blood vessels of larger cross-sectional diameter, as described above, is also paralleled in COVID-19 is. Osiaevi et al. (2023) compared videomicroscopic imaging of the sublingual microvasculature of 16 critically ill COVID-19 patients, 17 patients with long COVID and 15 healthy controls [203]. As shown in Figure 4, the density of functional capillaries (having flowing RBC content ≥ 50%) with cross-sectional diameter 4–10 μm was sharply reduced for active COVID-19 patients vs. controls, with values for long COVID patients roughly halfway between those for active COVID-19 patients and healthy controls. The study investigators concluded from these and other measures of microvascular health that the long COVID patients had significant microvasculature impairment, lasting even 18 months after infection for some [203].

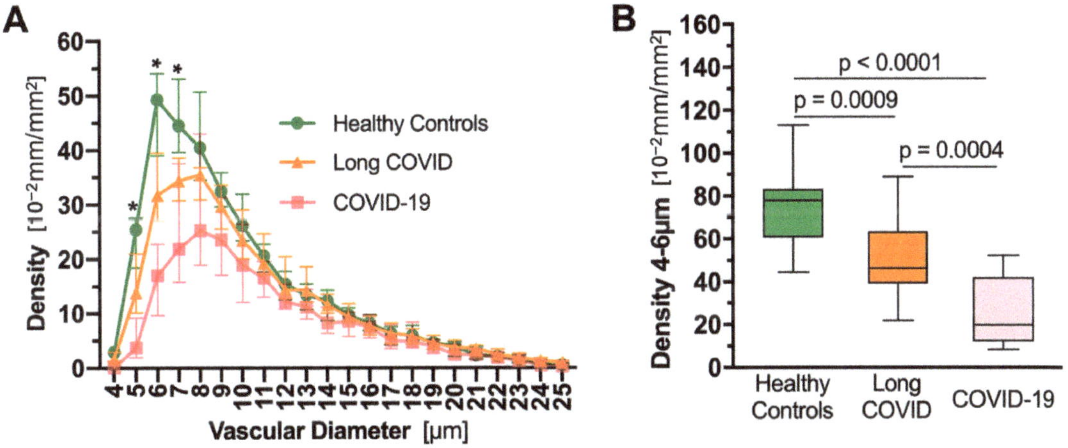

Figure 4. Density of functional capillaries (with flowing RBC content ≥ 50%) of cross-sectional diameter 4–25 μm in the sublingua of long and active, hospitalized COVID-19 patients and healthy controls. (**A**): Functional capillary density by diameter; * denotes $q < 0.05$ (q per Storey-Tibshirani). (**B**): Functional capillary density for capillaries of diameter 4–6 μm. Mean values for healthy controls and long and active COVID-19 patients were 77.9, 46.4 and 19.9, respectively, with $p < 0.001$ for comparisons between each pair of patient groups. Reproduced from Osiaevi et al. (2023) [203] (CC-BY 4.0).

Rovas et al. (2021) reported similar sharp reductions in densities of functional capillaries at the lower end of the 4–25 μm cross-sectional diameter range in the sublingual microvasculature of COVID-19 patients vs. healthy controls [201]. The extent of reduction in density of functional capillaries of diameter 4–6 μm in the COVID-19 patients correlated with their oxygenation index (PaO_2/FiO_2) and with an index of multiorgan failure and associated mortality risk. Rovas et al. concluded from these correlations that the observed reduction in sublingual small capillary density was another manifestation of the pathological clogging of capillaries as also observed in pulmonary microthrombi at autopsies of COVID-19 patients. A similar marked shift in blood flow from smaller to larger vessels in active [204–207] and long [208] COVID-19 patients was also observed in blood vessels of larger cross-sectional diameter, 1 mm and greater, using high-resolution CT scans.

Further insights into the prevalence of microvascular occlusion in both active and long COVID-19 were provided by studies that imaged the ocular conjunctiva and retina in human subjects using noninvasive techniques. As noted previously, the percentage of occluded microvessels in the conjunctiva was found to be six times as high in hospital-discharged COVID-19 patients vs. healthy controls [209], while other studies reported that RBC aggregation in the conjunctiva correlated closely with measures of that elsewhere in the body [158,175]. Three studies of perfusion density in various retinal capillary layers found small (e.g., 3–4%) but statistically significant differences (e.g., $p = 0.011$, $p = 0.04$, $p = 0.003$) for COVID-19 patients one month after recovery [210,211] and for long COVID patients [212] vs. healthy controls. Retinal capillary perfusion density was determined with optical coherence tomography angiography (OCT-A), which uses noninvasive laser imaging of RBC flow in retinal capillaries to detect perfusion aberrations.

5. Major Risk Factors of Age, Diabetes and Obesity for COVID-19 Severity Correlate with Increased Propensity to RBC Aggregation

The most significant risk factor for severe COVID-19 is age, with several studies showing a multifold increased risk of fatal outcomes with older age [195,213,214]. One multivariate analysis of 17 million subjects in the UK reported a sixfold increased mortality for ages 70 through 79 vs. 50 through 59 years [215]. A meta-analysis of 612,000 subjects in several countries conducted in 2020 found a mortality rate of 22.8% for ages 70–79 years vs. 0.3% for ages $\leq$ 29 years [216]. Note that the risk factor data considered in this section are for pre-Omicron variants of SARS-CoV-2. Since Omicron variants do not penetrate deeply into the lungs or bloodstream and cause less severe illness than prior variants, as considered in the Discussion section, risk factors for Omicron infections are not necessarily the same as those for pre-Omicron variants nor is the efficacy of various therapeutics.

This multifold increase in COVID-19 mortality with older age aligns with a much greater extent of microvascular occlusion in older vs. younger healthy subjects, linked to both a significantly greater propensity to RBC aggregation and slower blood flow with increased age. Microscopic examinations of the bulbar conjunctiva of healthy subjects found that 30% of those of ages 56–75 years had aggregation in the smaller venules and capillaries, as compared with a 3% rate of such aggregation of those of ages 16–35 years [190]. This tenfold increased rate of microvascular occlusion in the older subjects corresponds to much greater RBC aggregation and slower blood flow with increased age. One study that measured RBC aggregability by multiple detection methods found a statistically significant increase in this value in the blood of middle-aged versus young adults [217]. Another study found highly significant ($p < 0.001$) increases in RBC aggregability and average RBC aggregate size for subjects of ages 66–89 vs. those of 20–30 years [218]. Both of these studies measured RBC aggregability in vitro using drawn blood.

As noted, RBC aggregate formation in vivo depends not only on aggregability under static conditions but also on the degree of shear forces that promote disaggregation, as associated with velocity of blood flow [164,168–170]. It is, thus, noteworthy that blood flow is slower with increased age [219–225]. Mean velocity of capillary flow under fingernail and toenails for subjects of mean age 63 years was half of that for subjects of mean age 26 years [219]. Older subjects had 23% [220] and 40% [221] diminished flow velocities vs. younger subjects for capillary flow in other tissues. Arterial blood flow velocities were 26–27% lower for older vs. younger subjects in two studies [223,224]. The combined effects of increased RBC aggregability and decreased blood flow velocity would appear to account for the tenfold incidence of microvascular occlusion in smaller venules and capillaries of the bulbar conjunctiva with increased age, as noted above.

In a multivariate analysis of COVID-19 risk factors for 17 million patients in the UK, mortality was increased with hazard ratios of 1.31 for diabetics with good glucose control, 1.95 for diabetics with poor glucose control and 1.92 for obesity [215]. An umbrella review of 32 high- or moderate-quality reviews reported odds ratios for mortality of 2.09 for diabetes and 2.18 for obesity [226]. A significant degree of RBC aggregation is characteristic of diabetes [167,177,191,193,194], with this effect especially pronounced for type 1 disease [191] and for diabetics with poor glycemic control [193]. In studies of RBC attributes for subjects of varying body mass index (BMI), BMI correlated with RBC adhesiveness/aggregability at $p < 0.001$, while obese subjects had larger RBC aggregates ($p < 0.009$) that were more resistant to dispersion by flow [227,228]. In summary, three major risk factors for severe COVID-19—increased age, diabetes and obesity—were all characterized by increased RBC aggregability, with this correlation especially striking for age.

6. SARS-CoV-2 SP Unattached to Whole Virus Induces Microvascular Occlusion In Vivo

Akin to the studies noted previously demonstrating induction of RBC clumping by SARS-CoV-2 SP in vitro [91,100,229] and in vivo [103], other studies likewise demonstrate that SARS-CoV-2 SP in the absence of whole virus caused microvascular occlusion.

6.1. Myocardial Damage as a Signal of Microvascular Occlusion

A clinical window into morbidities associated with RBC aggregation is provided by the myocardium—the heart muscle—which is among the tissues most susceptible to the damaging effects of experimentally induced RBC aggregation and ensuing microvascular occlusion. Several studies found that injection of HMWD (high-MW dextran) caused myocardial damage [144,146,154,230] and/or electrocardiogram (ECG) changes [153,154,187,230] characteristic of myocarditis. In one study, 40 min after HMWD injection, ECG abnormalities were apparent, and HMWD induced lasting myocardial damage [230]. Both the degree of myocardial damage [144,146] and of ECG abnormalities [153] correlated with the extent of microvascular occlusion. Clinically, for hospitalized patients with coronary heart disease, the number of microthrombi per field of observation in the bulbar conjunctival microcirculation was found to be correlated with both the extent of ECG and symptomatic abnormalities [153].

6.2. Myocardial Damage Experimentally Induced by SARS-CoV-2 SP in the Absence of Whole Virus

Induction of myocarditis by SARS-CoV-2 SP in the absence of whole virus was evidenced in two rodent studies by IV injection of BNT162b2, the Pfizer-BioNTech mRNA vaccine, an experimental system in which SP is generated by host cells, distinct from intramuscular (IM) injection used for clinically administered COVID-19 vaccinations. Clinical cases of SARS-CoV-2 SP found in endothelial cells after IV mRNA vaccination [231–233] support the possibility that SP could be generated by nucleated endothelial cells in blood vessels post-vaccination. In mice, after a second IV vaccine dose, 67% had grossly visible white patches over the visceral pericardium and all showed changes of myopericarditis, compared with only mild degenerative changes in the myocardium in the intramuscular (IM)-injection group [234]. All of the mice in the IV-injection and the IM-injection groups had myocardial WBC infiltration and cardiomyocyte degeneration and necrosis vs. none in saline-injection controls. Rats given two IV doses of BNT162b2 vaccine two weeks apart in another study manifested marked blood hypercoagulability along with apoptotic cardiac muscle fibers, ECG changes and other abnormalities that reflected myocardial injury [235].

6.3. Clinical Signs of Microvascular Occlusion and Myocarditis after Exposure to SARS-CoV-2 SP

Further insights into microvascular occlusion caused by SARS-CoV-2 SP in the absence of whole virus in a clinical setting were provided by optical coherence tomography angiography (OCT-A) imaging of the retinal microvasculature. Determinations of the vascular density (VD) of flowing blood vessels in various retinal layers of human subjects, an indicator of microvascular occlusion, found that the CoronaVac vaccine, made from inactivated whole virus, caused no changes after vaccination [236,237]. The Pfizer-BioNTech mRNA vaccine caused small but statistically significant reductions in VD vs. controls at three days [238] and at two and four weeks [237] after vaccination. Reductions in many of these VD values at two weeks after vaccination were statistically significant at $p < 0.001$; most of these resolved by four weeks after vaccination, but seven of these VD reductions persisted at statistically significant levels at that time [237].

The significance of these findings derives not from the occasional ocular adverse effects that have been reported after mRNA COVID-19 vaccinations [239,240] but rather from indications that ocular microvascular occlusion mirrors a pathology elsewhere in the body [158,175]. Myocardial injury is another indicator of microvascular occlusion, as noted above, which opens another diagnostic window, PET-CT scanning, since fluorodeoxyglucose F18 (FDG) uptake in myocardial tissue has been found to track myocardial injury [241,242]. In one study, 700 SARS-CoV-2-vaccinated and 303 nonvaccinated subjects were given PET/CT scans either to evaluate malignancies or perform other medical screenings unrelated to COVID-19 or myocarditis. In PET/CT scans taken 1−180 days after vaccination, myocardial FDG uptake was significantly higher as compared to that for unvaccinated subjects (median of 4.8 vs. 3.3, $p < 0.0001$) [243]. Similar potential risks at a less than clinically overt level were indicated from cardiac test markers 2–10 weeks after COVID-19 mRNA vaccinations vs. pre-vaccination values in 566 patients at a cardiac clinic, with an increase in the 5-year predicted risk of acute cardiac events from 11% to 25% [244].

Whether the clinical indicator is the rare incidence of myocarditis following COVID mRNA vaccinations [245,246] or the greater incidence of cardiac irregularities following such vaccinations, e.g., 1–7% rates of chest pains and abnormal ECG readings in two post-COVID vaccination studies in adolescents [247,248], an association with the presence of SARS-CoV-2 SP in such adverse events is indicated. A study conducted in the US in Boston-area hospitals found that of 16 patients hospitalized for myocarditis after COVID-19 mRNA vaccinations, all had significant levels of SARS-CoV-2 SP unbound by antibodies in blood, whereas 45 asymptomatic, vaccinated subjects had no detectable SP [249]. Investigators at the same hospitals found indications that SARS-CoV-2 mRNA vaccines routinely persist up to 30 days following vaccination and are detectable in the heart [250]. SARS-CoV-2 SP was found on cardiomyocytes of 9 of 15 mRNA-vaccinated subjects with symptoms of myocarditis in another clinical series [251].

7. Decreased Clinical Severity of COVID-19 by Agents That Inhibit RBC Aggregation

Analogous to the activity of LWMD (MW $\leq$ 40 kDa) in limiting and reversing induced RBC aggregation, as noted above, various forms of heparin and heparan sulfate, glycosaminoglycans of MW $\leq$ 30 kDa, have shown benefits by clinical or laboratory criteria for COVID-19 in a scattering of clinical studies. The specific agents used were subcutaneous heparin plus enoxaparin (low-MW heparin) [252], enoxaparin [122] and a low-MW mixture of 80% heparan sulfate and 20% dermatan sulfate (sulodexide) [123,253]. As noted previously, both heparin and heparan sulfate bind strongly to SARS-CoV-2 SP [103–105].

Of particular interest as potential treatments for COVID-19 are three generic drugs which have been closely studied and have received wide attention.

7.1. Fluvoxamine

Fluvoxamine (FLV), a selective serotonin reuptake inhibitor (SSRI), attracted interest from prominent medical researchers [254–256] after early clinical trials indicated promising results for COVID-19 treatment [257–260]. Although rapid recovery from severe illness was not generally observed, one study showed a significant reduction in residual symptoms of COVID-19 at 14 days after start of FLV treatment vs. untreated controls [257], and another showed significant reductions in emergency room visits or hospitalizations [259]. Yet the puzzling question raised by these indications of clinical activity was by what biochemical mechanism could an SSRI used to treat depression and anxiety disorders offer therapeutic benefits against a viral disease?

A plausible biochemical mechanism is the sharp reduction by FLV in serum levels of serotonin, which is a powerful inducer of RBC and platelet aggregation. In vitro, serotonin caused marked aggregation of RBCs, platelets and leukocytes [147]. In vivo, injection of serotonin resulted in blood cell aggregates being trapped in small venules and capillaries in the ocular conjunctival vasculature [147]. In dogs, a serotonin antagonist prevented an increase in pulmonary alveolar dead space, an indication of pulmonary vascular obstruction, after hemorrhagic shock [261].

Several studies have found that SSRIs, including FLV, sharply reduce serotonin levels in blood, with reductions in plasma serotonin levels to 20–40% of baseline values over two to eight weeks being typical after the start of SSRI treatment [262–268]. All of these studies used high-performance liquid chromatography (HPLC) or enzyme-linked immunosorbent assay (ELISA) methodology for detection of serotonin plasma levels to avoid potential skewing of results from platelet uptake of serotonin [256,267]. For FLV in particular, mean plasma serotonin levels were reduced to 69% of the baseline value one hour after first dose of the drug [263]. A study of blood from humans and mice found that serotonin induced platelet aggregation [269] and platelet aggregation by arachidonic acid was decreased by 68% ($p = 0.00001$) in patients taking an SSRI vs. controls [270].

7.2. *Hydroxychloroquine (HCQ)*

The application of HCQ, an aminoquinoline, for treatment of COVID-19, as developed by an infectious disease team at Aix-Marseilles University in France [271–273], has been the subject of significant controversy, a review of which is not attempted here. However, it is of note that HCQ has been found to have pronounced activity in reducing blood cell aggregation and associated microvascular occlusion. In 44 human subjects with vascular conditions including coronary artery and cerebrovascular disease, all having initial manifestations of microvascular occlusion, ocular conjunctival microvasculature was observed over a nine-month period following the start of HCQ treatment [274]. Marked reductions in the size of blood cell aggregates and the extent of microvascular occlusion were observed for most patients. Accompanying symptomatic improvements were observed in many of these subjects beginning three days after the start of HCQ treatment for some and persisting over the nine-month follow-up period.

In another human study, HCQ was administered over a three-month period to 22 patients with rheumatoid arthritis who had signs of occlusion in the microcirculation of the ocular fundus. Twenty of the 22 patients had complete normalization of the observed vasculature occlusion [275]. In mice previously injected with an RBC clumping agent, HCQ sharply reduced thrombus size and the time that thrombi persisted as compared with untreated controls [276].

7.3. *Ivermectin (IVM)*

To identify potential therapeutics for COVID-19, four in silico studies collectively screened over 1000 molecules for binding to SARS-CoV-2 SP and other SARS-CoV-2 viral targets [105,277–279]. In each of these studies, the strongest or close-to-strongest binding affinity to SP was obtained for IVM, a macrocyclic lactone with multifaceted antiparasitic and antimicrobial activity, distributed in four billion doses for human diseases worldwide since 1987 [280–282]. Aminpour et al. (2022) found by molecular docking computations that IVM binds with high affinity (<-7.0 kcal/mol) to seven sialoside-binding sites or other glycan-binding sites on SARS-CoV-2 S1, six on the N-terminal domain (NTD) and one on the receptor-binding domain (RBD). These binding energy values of <-7.0 kcal/mol were obtained for the RBD in both the open ("up") and closed ("down") positions [99]. As a measure of significance of this binding energy value, binding energies of <-7.0 kcal/mol predicted efficacy for a large set of HIV inhibitors with 98% sensitivity and 95% specificity in another study [283]. Additional molecular modeling studies of IVM binding to

SARS-CoV-2 SP [284–288], including one by Lehrer and Rheinstein (2020) [289], likewise found strong binding affinities for IVM.

Competitive binding by IVM to SP glycan-binding sites is thus a likely biochemical mechanism for the in vitro inhibition and reversal by IVM of aggregation of human RBCs by SARS-CoV-2 SP as noted above [91]. In early 2020, two Florida physicians, Jean-Jacques and Juliana Rajter, were intrigued by an indication of a clinical parallel to this in vitro effect—observations that several COVID-19 patients with severe respiratory impairment and SpO2 deficits experienced normalized breathing function within 1–2 days after treatment with IVM [290,291]. Months later, Rajter et al. (2020) reported results of a propensity-matched case control study of COVID-19 patients treated with a low dose of IVM plus standard of care (SOC) at four Florida hospitals, which yielded a 40% reduction in mortality vs. controls given only SOC [292]. After that study was concluded, through mid-2021, more than 20 randomized controlled trials (RCTs) of IVM treatment of COVID-19 were conducted, with six of seven meta-analyses reporting notable reductions in deaths and with a mean 0.31 relative risk of mortality vs. controls (a 69% reduction) [293].

By 2022, however, several other RCTs reported that IVM yielded no statistically significant benefits for COVID-19 treatment, as summarized in an August 2022 editorial which declared that it was "time to stop using ineffective COVID-19 drugs" [294]. Curiously, however, the editorial prominently cited in support a June 2022 meta-analysis of ten RCTs for IVM treatment of COVID-19 encompassing 3472 patients [295] which actually reported as the first finding in its results section a twofold reduction in deaths in its pooled IVM treatment vs. placebo groups (pooled log odds ratio of −0.67, 95% CI = −1.20 to −0.13, with low heterogeneity). The mortality reduction was less (log OR = −0.12) for the RCTs rated as having a low risk of bias, but included in that group, weighted to account for 63% of that pooled log OR, was a study of dubious credibility.

Coauthors of the aforementioned study, the TOGETHER trial [296], have repeatedly refused to disclose four of their key outcome numbers, namely per protocol deaths and hospitalizations, treatment vs. placebo [297], which are of key importance given critiques of the primary outcome used in all arms of the TOGETHER trial by the U.S. Food and Drug Administration [298] and National Institutes of Health [299]. Instead, a TOGETHER trial coauthor directed inquiring scientists to the ICODA data repository, listed as the data source in the study's data sharing statement [297,300]. After two months of futile attempts by scientists to obtain the data from ICODA, however, on 7 June 2022, an ICODA manager reported that the TOGETHER trial data were never held by that data repository and that she had instructed its authors to stop citing it as their data source [297,301].

In another prominently cited RCT of IVM treatment of COVID-19 that reported negative conclusions [302], IVM was substituted for placebo doses for 38 patients, a mistake caught a month later, and blinding was broken by use of sugar water as the placebo for one-third of the study's patients (liquid IVM has a bitter taste). Adverse events that are distinctive to the high IVM dose used (transient and non-critical) occurred at almost identical rates in the placebo and IVM arms, while over-the-counter sales of IVM surged in the study region during the study period [303].

The RCT evidence for IVM-based treatments of COVID-19 is thus mixed; however, in rare cases, efficacy of a drug has been conclusively established without RCT findings when it has achieved consistent major clinical benefits in the face of an established baseline of null effect. For example, the 96% cure rate for peptic ulcers by a triple therapy achieved in a 1990 clinical trial [304] provided conclusive evidence of the therapy's efficacy, given a baseline of palliative but rarely curative results for that chronic condition [305,306]. The associated discovery of *H. pylori* as the underlying pathogen for peptic ulcers was honored with the Nobel prize for medicine in 2005 [307]. For penicillin, early in vitro and mouse studies provided convincing indications of marked antibacterial activity. Alexander Fleming found in 1929 that transparent regions formed around penicillin embedded in agar plates of several species of cultured bacteria, indicating inhibition of bacterial growth [308]. In a 1940 study, almost all penicillin-treated mice survived when exposed to bacterial strains that consistently caused fatal infections in untreated control mice [309]. In the absence of RCT evidence, penicillin production was then ramped up to industrial scale, saving the lives of thousands of soldiers during World War II [310].

For cases of moderate and severe COVID-19 in patients on room air, there is a consistent baseline of null effect in a 1–2 week timeframe: the magnitude of reductions in SpO2 levels correlate with the extent of pulmonary damage, and neither of these normalize in that timeframe [311–317]. With that backdrop of null effect, as shown in Figure 5, three studies of severe COVID-19 patients on room air treated with IVM-based regimens observed sharp increases in SpO2 after 1 day of treatment [318–321] while SpO2 decreased during the same 1-day period in a fourth group of such patients under standard care. The two studies that used the triple therapy of IVM, doxycycline and zinc [318,319], one of these coauthored by Thomas Borody [319], who developed the successful triple therapy for *H. pylori* [304], showed the most pronounced effect. For each of these three studies using IVM-based treatments, SpO2 changes one day after treatment differed from those values for a comparison study of COVID-19 patients on room air under standard care [321,322] with differences far outside the 95% confidence intervals for treatment vs. control values.

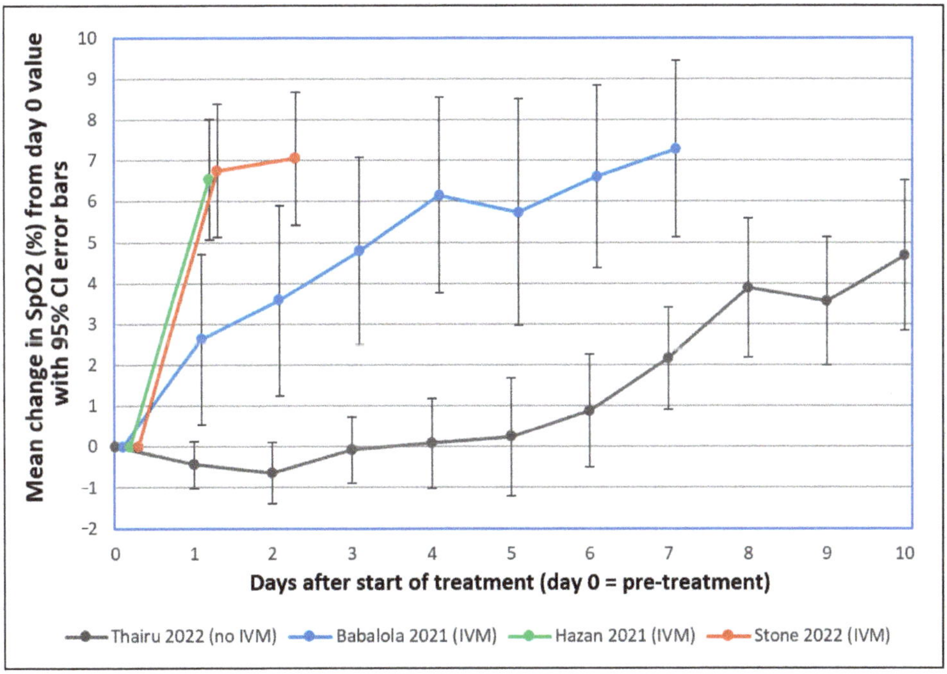

Figure 5. Mean changes in oxygen saturation (SpO2) for severe COVID-19 patients following treatments including or excluding IVM. Reproduced from Stone et al. (2022) [318] (CC-BY 4.0). Patients tracked over various time periods from each regimen were those with SpO2 values all recorded on room air, having pre-treatment (day 0) values $\leq$ 93%. The y-axis value at day n is the mean of changes in SpO2 values from day 0 to day n, with error bars designating 95% confidence intervals. • Thairu et al. (2022) [321,322]: 26 patients, median age 45 years, treated with different combinations of lopinavir/ritonavir (Alluvia), remdesivir, azithromycin and enoxaparin as well as zinc sulfate and vitamin C. • Stone et al. (2022) [318]: 34 patients, median age 56.5, treated with IVM, doxycycline and zinc. • Hazan et al. (2021) [319]: 19 patients, median age 63, treated with IVM, doxycycline and zinc. • Babalola et al. (2021) [320,321]: 19 patients, median age 33, treated with IVM, zinc and vitamin C, with some also given azithromycin and hydroxychloroquine.

For the Stone et al. (2022) study, taking into account some missing values for the 34 treated patients at <48 h post-treatment, paired t-test calculations were performed for post-treatment minus pre-treatment SpO2 values for the study patients at +12 h, +24 h and +48 h after the start of IVM administration. These paired t-test values were highly significant, with $p < 10^{-6}$ in each case. One patient in the study had an increase in SpO2 from 79% recorded at the first IVM dose to 95% three hours later, and four other patients had increases of 12 or more in SpO2% within 12 h after the first IVM dose. These sharp, rapid improvements parallel the disaggregation of RBC clumps observed in vitro over the course of 30 min by Boschi et al. (2022) and can be explained by rapid clearance of RBC aggregates in the vasculature and corresponding increases in efficiency of oxygenation in pulmonary and extrapulmonary tissues.

In 2020, Peru provided a unique setting to track clinical efficacy of IVM-based treatment for COVID-19 with close consideration of confounding factors, using excess deaths data from its national health system, which aligned with WHO monthly summary data [323]. Treatment with IVM and adjunct agents was deployed at intensive, moderate or limited levels under semi-autonomous policies in its 25 states, enabling comparisons with reductions in excess deaths at 30 days after peak values, state by state. A Kendall tau calculation yields a two-tailed p-value of 0.002 for reductions in excess deaths correlated with level of IVM use in Peru's 25 states. On a national scale, during four months of IVM use in 2020, before a new president of Peru elected on November 17 restricted its use, there was a 14-fold reduction in nationwide excess deaths, and then a 13-fold increase in the two months following the restriction of IVM use [323]. This set of real-world national health data, accompanied by extensive additional data by which potential confounding influences can be tracked, provides another significant indication of efficacy of IVM treatment of COVID-19.

8. A Comparison of Degree of Clinical Susceptibility to COVID-19 and RBC Aggregability in Various Animal Species

Susceptibility to COVID-19 and severity of this disease have been tracked for dozens of mammalian species, as reported in a summary figure by Meekins et al. (2021) [324]. RBC aggregability values and related values of blood viscosity at low shear velocity have been tracked for many mammalian species as well, as reported by Baskurt and Meiselman in 2013 [325]. A correlation calculation between these two values, by species, provides a test of whether RBC aggregability is likely associated with COVID-19 morbidity.

The COVID status of mammalian species was reported by Meekins et al. using designators for viral shedding, clinical signs, mortality and transmission. We derived a composite COVID status index from the first three of these indicators (transmission was not used) with values of 0 for none of these three, 1 for viral shedding only, 2 for clinical signs and 3 for clinical signs and mortality. For RBC aggregability, an aggregation index shown in Baskurt and Meiselman for 22 mammalian species was used. They also reported values of blood viscosity under low-shear conditions for 27 mammalian species that were closely correlated with the corresponding RBC aggregation index for species having values shown in both figures. For a species tracked in Baskurt and Meiselman that reported blood viscosity but not RBC aggregability, the latter value was interpolated from the blood viscosity value. Correspondence between RBC aggregability and blood viscosity was established using the values of each for cattle and horses; these species had the minimum and maximum values of all species tracked by Baskurt and Meiselman, respectively, for both of these indices.

Table 1 shows the COVID status index and the RBC aggregability index, as described above, for the 13 species as tracked by both Meekins et al. and Baskurt and Meiselman, with the following adjustments: For the White-Tailed Deer as listed in Meekins et al., the mean of the RBC aggregation indices as interpolated from viscosity values for H. Deer, P.D. Deer and S. Deer (21.6, 23.5 and 9.1, respectively) reported by Baskurt and Meiselman was used. The contrast between high RBC aggregability in athletic species including horse, leopard and rhinoceros vs. low RBC aggregability in sedentary species including domestic cattle, sheep and goats has been noted by several observers [326–328], including Baskurt and Meiselman [325], who furnished these values for all four species. The susceptibility of domestic sheep and goats, neither tracked by Meekins et al., is consistently reported to be the same (minimal [329,330]) as that for domestic cattle, and the COVID status index for these two species, 0—the same as the Meekins et al. value for domestic cattle—was, therefore, added.

Using the methodology described above to determine indices for COVID status index and RBC aggregation for 13 matching mammalian species, the Kendall tau two-tailed rank coefficient was calculated [331]; this statistical test was selected because COVID status was meaningful as a ranking rather than a numerical measure. This calculation demonstrated a moderately significant correlation ($p = 0.033$, $\tau b = 0.52$), which could be interpreted to indicate that RBC aggregation is a key determinant but not the exclusive causal factor for COVID-19 morbidity in mammals.

Table 1. Indices of COVID-19 status and RBC aggregability for mammalian species.

Species	COVID Index	RBC Aggregation Index
Domestic cat (Cat)	1 (V)	38.18
Malayan Tiger (Tiger)	2 (VC)	35.10
Lion (Lion)	2 (VC)	37.58 *
Snow Leopard (Leopard)	2 (C)	50.12 *
Domestic Dog (Dog)	0	28.15
White-Tailed Deer (H. Deer, P.D. Deer, S. Deer) **	1 (V)	18.06 *
Domestic Cattle (Cattle)	0	1.34
Domestic Pig (Pig)	0	30.27
House Mouse (Mouse)	0	0.18
Cottontail Rabbit (Rabbit)	0	5.20
Common Marmoset (Marmoset)	2 (C)	3.40 *
Sheep, domestic livestock (Sheep) ***	0	0.18
Goat, domestic livestock (Goat) ***	0	0.18
KENDALL TAU	$\tau b = 0.52$	$p = 0.033$

COVID index from Meekins et al. (2021) [324], with RBC aggregation index for the matching species (listed in parentheses) from Baskurt and Meiselman 2013 [325]. For COVID index, V = viral shedding, C = clinical signs; no matching species here was reported as having mortal cases. * Value was interpolated from low-shear blood viscosity. ** RBC aggregation index is the mean of those for the three deer species listed. *** COVID index values for these species were added as commonly reported in other sources [329,330].

9. Discussion

Consistent with coronavirus and RBC biochemistry established over past decades, the findings presented here demonstrate the central role of attachments from SARS-CoV-2 SP to sialylated glycans on RBCs and other blood cells in the severe morbidities of COVID-19. The glycans that decorate the SP of a coronavirus serve, metaphorically, as the virus's arms and legs, its appendages of initial attachment to a host cell. The RBC, with its million strands of GPA per cell, along with platelets, offers an "immune adherence" defense of pathogens which can bind to glycans [72,82–88]. The associated hemagglutination is observed for many strains of coronaviruses [30,32,35–39,41,42], including SARS-CoV-2 [91].

Although these hemagglutinating properties of coronaviruses have been closely studied and the only known role of the GPA molecule on the RBC, the most abundant cell in the human body [332,333], is for pathogen binding and clearance [71,72,83,84], these glycan attachments have been largely overlooked in SARS-CoV-2 research. It is well established that RBCs, platelets and endothelial cells, which play key roles in COVID-19, are densely coated with sialylated glycans [64,65,70] but have no ACE2 (or, for endothelial cells, minimal ACE2 [69]) and that the various coronavirus strains use several different host-cell receptors for replication [30], yet ACE2 has been the exclusive host-cell target of interest in much of the research on SARS-CoV-2.

One explanation for this limited focus on the RBC and its pathogen-snagging GPA strands, one million per RBC, may be the lack of consensus on a solved structure of the extracellular domain of GPA [334,335]. Obstacles to this determination have been the extensive glycosylation of GPA, hindering the formation of a stable crystal for X-ray crystallography, and its intrinsically disordered structure [336,337] which allows a set of variable, extended and unfolded conformations [338–340].

An overemphasis on the role of viral replication and associated viral load in the pathology of SARS-CoV-2 has led to questionable conclusions. As noted, for the five human betacoronaviruses, the two benign and three deadly strains are distinguished not by viral load, which is about the same for the two common cold strains and SARS-CoV-2 [55], but by the expression of the enzyme HE, which releases glycan attachments to viral SP, only in the common cold strains, not in SARS, SARS-CoV-2 and MERS [50–54]. For an agent for which competitive binding to SARS-CoV-2 SP glycan-binding sites has been indicated in silico [99], IVM, one RCT tested it at a single low dose given on day 1 together with three other prophylactic regimens, each given daily for 42 days for prevention of COVID-19 infection [341]. The study concluded that IVM was ineffective because it yielded no significant reduction in viral load vs. controls, yet IVM at that single dose reduced the incidence of symptomatic COVID-19 and acute respiratory distress syndrome (ARDS) each by half, with associated p values of 0.0034 and 0.012, respectively [341].

Among the multifaceted demonstrations that SARS-CoV-2 SP-induced RBC aggregation and associated microvascular occlusion and hypoxia are central to severe morbidities of COVID-19, particularly informative are the countervailing effects of agents that inhibit glycan bindings of SP to RBCs. A mixture of heparan sulfate and heparin, both of which have strong binding affinity to SARS-CoV-2 SP [103–105], markedly reduced SARS-CoV-2 SP-induced thrombosis in zebrafish [103]. As noted, the strongest or close-to-strongest binding affinity to SARS-CoV-2 SP in molecular modeling screenings of more than 1000 total molecules was found for IVM [105,277–279]. Just as LMWD rapidly reversed HMWD-induced RBC aggregation in vitro [163] and in vivo [148,155–158], IVM both blocked and reversed SARS-CoV-2 SP-induced hemagglutination in vitro [91]. This effect was paralleled in three clinical studies as shown in Figure 5, in which depressed SpO2 values in severe COVID-19 patients on room air were sharply increased within 1–2 days [318–320] after the first IVM dose, in many cases within hours [318], in contrast to a null effect under SOC treatment in the fourth study shown.

Neither fibrin-hardened blood clots nor the blockage of all blood flow in a small-diameter capillary by RBC clumps would be readily reversible by clump disaggregation, even if effectively achieved. Observations of the reversal of HMWD-induced blood cell clumping by LMWD, however, provide insights into how disaggregation of RBC clumps by agents that competitively bind to SARS-CoV-SP could rapidly normalize blood flow and oxygen levels in severe COVID-19 patients. In mammals, a distributed network of arterioles can hold a significant total mass of RBC clumps before obstruction of blood flow becomes critical, while a pulmonary catch-trap architecture can also sequester large blood cell aggregates [167,178]. The dynamic, reversible character of RBC clumps in vivo up to a point at which the extent of aggregation becomes critical is demonstrated in the LMWD disaggregation studies noted above. A direct in vitro parallel, as noted, is the reversal of hemagglutination induced by SARS-CoV-2 SP over the course of 30 min by IVM in vitro [91]. A similar effect is strikingly demonstrated in the hemagglutination assay for viruses that express an enzyme (HE or similar) that cleaves host cell glycans. An interlaced sheet of RBCs initially forms and then subsequently collapses as that enzyme breaks the glycan attachments between viral SP and RBCs [31,32].

Although the central role of sialylated glycan bindings between SARS-CoV-2 SP and RBCs in the severe morbidities of COVID-19 has been the focus of this paper, such SP bindings to the heavily sialylated platelets and endothelial cells (which have no ACE2 and minimal ACE2, respectively) also contribute significantly to these morbidities, as noted above. Of particular interest is extensive damage to endothelial cells in severe COVID-19 patients, with an associated presence of SARS-CoV-2 virus and SP and elevated levels of VWF. As noted, an SA-cleaving enzyme was found to remove more than 50% of the glycocalyx of human kidney endothelial cells [70].

This examination of attachments from SARS-CoV-2 SP to sialylated glycans of RBCs and other blood cells and endothelial cells was spurred in part by an examination of possible molecular mechanisms of IVM activity in COVID-19 treatment and prevention. This may seem curious, given a general perception that IVM is ineffective against COVID-19 [294], yet major irregularities in some of the best-known such studies with negative conclusions, as noted in Section 7.3, indicate that the RCT evidence is more accurately characterized as mixed. It was also noted that in rare cases, such as for the triple therapy for peptic ulcers and for penicillin, striking demonstrations of drug efficacy against a consistent baseline of null effect under standard care established drug efficacy without accompanying RCT evidence. The findings of four studies depicted in Figure 5 appear to present a similar decisive demonstration of efficacy of IVM in treatment of pre-Omicron COVID infections.

The reports of distinguished scholars of scientific integrity, including current and past editors of leading scientific journals [342–347], on the vulnerability of science to commodification [343,347] and "flagrant conflicts of interest" [342] are also useful to bear in mind as this evidence is sorted out. As one case in point, although the triple-therapy cure for *H. pylori* was rapidly deployed in Australia, preventing an estimated 18,665 deaths there between 1990 and 2015 [348], it was not widely used in the rest of the world until the late 1990s, after the patents for the two best-selling palliative drugs for that condition had expired [349].

It is important to note, in evaluating drug treatment options for evolving COVID-19 variants, that Omicron viral strains, which became predominant in early 2022 [350], replicate less efficiently in the lung alveolar epithelium as compared with prior variants, in contrast to Omicron's faster replication in the bronchi [351,352]. The disruption of the alveolar–capillary barrier is a prime route by which SARS-CoV-2 enters the blood stream [353], so limited replication of Omicron in alveolar tissue would limit viral loads in blood with associated reductions in RBC clumping and disease severity as caused by Omicron vs. prior variants. Thus, although Boschi et al. (2022) reported a tenfold greater hemagglutinating activity of Omicron as compared with prior variants [91], this would not appear to increase the severity of clinical infections, yet could possibly affect the incidence of adverse effects of COVID-19 booster vaccines for the Omicron variant, which have not been tested on human subjects [354]. Also, due to limited penetration by Omicron into the bloodstream, drugs that offer clinical benefits through reductions in RBC aggregation for pre-Omicron SARS-CoV-2 variants may not have significant efficacy against the less severe Omicron infections.

This has implications, for example, for evaluation of RCTs for FLV treatment of COVID-19, given that two recent such studies had substantial numbers of Omicron patients among their subjects [355,356]. On the other hand, IVM may maintain clinical efficacy against Omicron variants of SARS-CoV-2 though molecular mechanisms besides competitive inhibition of glycan bindings. For example, high-energy binding by IVM to the alpha-7 nicotinic acetylcholine receptor (α7nAChr), the main receptor activating the cholinergic anti-inflammatory pathway controlled by the vagus nerve [99,357], was predicted in silico [99] and was confirmed experimentally in both human and animal cells [358]. Activation of the α7nAChr by IVM has been demonstrated to trigger a marked increase in Ca++ current evoked by acetylcholine (e.g., a 20-fold shift in the affinity of acetylcholine [358]) and, accordingly, may dramatically decrease excessive macrophage inflammation and tumor necrosis factor (TNF), which play a major role during the inflammatory phase of

COVID-19 infection (i.e., the cytokine storm) [99,357,359]. IVM binding to α7nAChr could also competitively inhibit viral penetration of macrophages and neuronal, endothelial and type II alveolar epithelial cells through this receptor [99,357].

For long COVID-19 patients, the demonstrated persistent presence of SP and subunits in plasma [111–113] and monocytes [114], respectively, and microvascular occlusion as seen in their sublingual vasculature [203] indicate an active therapeutic opportunity for drugs that limit SARS-CoV-2 SP binding to RBCs. Both optical coherence tomography angiography (OCT-A) and videomicroscopic imaging of the sublingual microvasculature offer tools to track microvascular occlusion that typically occurs in long COVID patients and to track any improvements that may be provided by drugs, either those highlighted here or others, in clinical treatment as well as in research settings.

10. Conclusions

The central role of sialylated glycan attachments between SARS-CoV-2 SP and RBCs and other blood cells in the severe morbidities of COVID-19 is founded on well-established biochemistry of coronaviruses and RBCs and established here through multiple channels of substantiation. Many preclinical and clinical studies show that SARS-CoV-2 SP attaches to and aggregates RBCs. Experimentally induced RBC clumping in vivo causes the same morbidities and the same redistribution of blood flow from smaller to larger blood vessels as for severe COVID-19. The key risk factors of increased age, diabetes and obesity for COVID-19 morbidity are each associated with significantly increased RBC aggregation. SARS-CoV-2 SP in the absence of whole virus as generated experimentally by IV injection of mRNA COVID vaccines in vivo, which caused SP to be generated in the absence of whole virus, induced microvascular occlusion.

Three generic agents which attracted prominent interest as COVID-19 therapeutics all yielded significant reductions in RBC aggregation. For mammalian species, the degree of clinical susceptibility to COVID-19 correlates with the aggregation propensity of RBCs with $p = 0.033$. These in vitro, in vivo and clinical findings, together, provide a convincing demonstration that RBC aggregation induced by SARS-CoV-2 SP through sialylated glycan attachments and resulting microvascular occlusion is key to the morbidities of severe COVID-19. These insights can support therapeutic and preventative strategies for evolving variants of this disease and for long COVID, while imaging of the retinal or sublingual microvasculature of active or long COVID patients can provide important support to these efforts.

Author Contributions: Conceptualization, D.E.S. and A.D.S.; investigation, formal analysis and visualization, D.E.S.; validation, A.D.S., P.V. and A.G.H.; writing—original draft preparation, D.E.S.; writing—review and editing, D.E.S., P.V., A.D.S. and A.G.H. All authors have read and agreed to the published version of the manuscript.

Funding: This research received no external funding.

Institutional Review Board Statement: Not applicable.

Informed Consent Statement: Not applicable.

Data Availability Statement: Not applicable.

Acknowledgments: The authors are grateful to the brothers Jerome Dancis (University of Maryland) and Barry Dancis for close editing and helpful comments in developing this manuscript.

Conflicts of Interest: A.D.S. reports grants from Verastem Oncology, Puma, Gilead, Synthon, Merck, Boehringer-Ingelheim and Genentech and personal fees for consulting services from TESARO, Eisai, GSK, Merck and Gilead. A.G.H. is the CEO of CryoBioPhysica Inc. The other authors declare no conflicts of interest.

Abbreviations

The following abbreviations are used in this manuscript:

α7nAChr	alpha-7 nicotinic acetylcholine receptor
ARDS	acute respiratory distress syndrome
BMI	body mass index
CEC	circulating endothelial cell
COVID-19	coronavirus disease 2019
ECG	electrocardiogram
ELISA	enzyme-linked immunosorbent assay
FDG	fluorodeoxyglucose F18
FLV	fluvoxamine
Gal	galactose
GPA	glycophorin A
HCQ	hydroxychloroquine
HE	hemagglutinin esterase
HMWD	high-molecular-weight dextran
HPLC	high-performance liquid chromatography
IM	intramuscular
IV	intravenous
IVM	ivermectin
LMWD	low-molecular-weight dextran
long COVID	post-acute sequelae of COVID-19 or PASC
MW	molecular weight
Neu5Ac	α5-N-acetylneuraminic acid
NTD	N-terminal domain
OCT-A	optical coherence tomography angiography
PBS	phosphate-buffered saline
RBC	red blood cell
RBD	receptor-binding domain
RCT	randomized controlled trial
SA	sialic acid
SARS-CoV-2	severe acute respiratory syndrome coronavirus 2
SOC	standard of care
SP	spike protein
SpO2	peripheral oxygen saturation
SSRI	selective serotonin reuptake inhibitor
VD	vascular density
VWF	von Willebrand factor

References

1. Gattinoni, L.; Gattarello, S.; Steinberg, I.; Busana, M.; Palermo, P.; Lazzari, S.; Romitti, S.; Quintel, M.; Meissner, K.; Marini, J.J.; et al. COVID-19 pneumonia: Pathophysiology and management. *Eur. Respir. Rev.* **2021**, *30*, 210138. [CrossRef]
2. Poor, H.D. Pulmonary Thrombosis and Thromboembolism in COVID-19. *Chest* **2021**, *160*, 1471–1480. [CrossRef]
3. Selickman, J.; Vrettou, C.S.; Mentzelopoulos, S.D.; Marini, J.J. COVID-19-Related ARDS: Key Mechanistic Features and Treatments. *J. Clin. Med.* **2022**, *11*, 4896. [CrossRef]
4. Halawa, S.; Pullamsetti, S.S.; Bangham, C.R.M.; Stenmark, K.R.; Dorfmüller, P.; Frid, M.G.; Butrous, G.; Morrell, N.W.; de Jesus Perez, V.A.; Stuart, D.I.; et al. Potential long-term effects of SARS-CoV-2 infection on the pulmonary vasculature: A global perspective. *Nat. Rev. Cardiol.* **2022**, *19*, 314–331. [CrossRef]
5. Couzin-Frankel, J. The mystery of the pandemic's 'happy hypoxia'. *Science* **2020**, *368*, 455–456. [CrossRef]
6. Marini, J.J.; Gattinoni, L. Management of COVID-19 Respiratory Distress. *JAMA* **2020**, *323*, 2329–2330. [CrossRef]
7. Li, H.; Deng, Y.; Li, Z.; Dorken Gallastegi, A.; Mantzoros, C.S.; Frydman, G.H.; Karniadakis, G.E. Multiphysics and multiscale modeling of microthrombosis in COVID-19. *PLoS Comput. Biol.* **2022**, *18*, e1009892. [CrossRef]
8. Rapkiewicz, A.V.; Mai, X.; Carsons, S.E.; Pittaluga, S.; Kleiner, D.E.; Berger, J.S.; Thomas, S.; Adler, N.M.; Charytan, D.M.; Gasmi, B.; et al. Megakaryocytes and platelet-fibrin thrombi characterize multi-organ thrombosis at autopsy in COVID-19: A case series. *eClinicalMedicine* **2020**, *24*, 100434. [CrossRef]

9. Wichmann, D.; Sperhake, J.-P.; Lütgehetmann, M.; Steurer, S.; Edler, C.; Heinemann, A.; Heinrich, F.; Mushumba, H.; Kniep, I.; Schröder, A.S.; et al. Autopsy Findings and Venous Thromboembolism in Patients With COVID-19. *Ann. Intern. Med.* **2020**, *173*, 268–277. [CrossRef]
10. Ackermann, M.; Verleden, S.E.; Kuehnel, M.; Haverich, A.; Welte, T.; Laenger, F.; Vanstapel, A.; Werlein, C.; Stark, H.; Tzankov, A.; et al. Pulmonary Vascular Endothelialitis, Thrombosis, and Angiogenesis in COVID-19. *N. Engl. J. Med.* **2020**, *383*, 120–128. [CrossRef]
11. Fox, S.E.; Akmatbekov, A.; Harbert, J.L.; Li, G.; Quincy Brown, J.; Vander Heide, R.S. Pulmonary and cardiac pathology in African American patients with COVID-19: An autopsy series from New Orleans. *Lancet Respir. Med.* **2020**, *8*, 681–686. [CrossRef]
12. Hanff, T.C.; Mohareb, A.M.; Giri, J.; Cohen, J.B.; Chirinos, J.A. Thrombosis in COVID-19. *Am. J. Hematol.* **2020**, *95*, 1578–1589. [CrossRef]
13. Fahmy, O.H.; Daas, F.M.; Salunkhe, V.; Petrey, J.L.; Cosar, E.F.; Ramirez, J.; Akca, O. Is Microthrombosis the Main Pathology in Coronavirus Disease 2019 Severity?-A Systematic Review of the Postmortem Pathologic Findings. *Crit. Care Explor.* **2021**, *3*, e0427. [CrossRef] [PubMed]
14. Menter, T.; Haslbauer, J.D.; Nienhold, R.; Savic, S.; Hopfer, H.; Deigendesch, N.; Frank, S.; Turek, D.; Willi, N.; Pargger, H.; et al. Postmortem examination of COVID-19 patients reveals diffuse alveolar damage with severe capillary congestion and variegated findings in lungs and other organs suggesting vascular dysfunction. *Histopathology* **2020**, *77*, 198–209. [CrossRef] [PubMed]
15. McFadyen, J.D.; Stevens, H.; Peter, K. The Emerging Threat of (Micro)Thrombosis in COVID-19 and Its Therapeutic Implications. *Circ. Res.* **2020**, *127*, 571–587. [CrossRef]
16. Poh, K.C.; Jia Tay, V.Y.; Lin, S.H.; Chee, H.L.; Thangavelautham, S. A review of COVID-19-related thrombosis and anticoagulation strategies specific to the Asian population. *Singap. Med. J.* **2022**, *63*, 350–361. [CrossRef]
17. Bussani, R.; Schneider, E.; Zentilin, L.; Collesi, C.; Ali, H.; Braga, L.; Volpe, M.C.; Colliva, A.; Zanconati, F.; Berlot, G.; et al. Persistence of viral RNA, pneumocyte syncytia and thrombosis are hallmarks of advanced COVID-19 pathology. *eBioMedicine* **2020**, *61*, 103104. [CrossRef]
18. Overton, P.M.; Toshner, M.; Mulligan, C.; Vora, P.; Nikkho, S.; de Backer, J.; Lavon, B.R.; Klok, F.A.; the PVRI Innovative Drug Development Initiative. Pulmonary thromboembolic events in COVID-19—A systematic literature review. *Pulm. Circ.* **2022**, *12*, e12113. [CrossRef]
19. Tang, N.; Li, D.; Wang, X.; Sun, Z. Abnormal coagulation parameters are associated with poor prognosis in patients with novel coronavirus pneumonia. *J. Thromb. Haemost.* **2020**, *18*, 844–847. [CrossRef]
20. Pellegrini, D.; Kawakami, R.; Guagliumi, G.; Sakamoto, A.; Kawai, K.; Gianatti, A.; Nasr, A.; Kutys, R.; Guo, L.; Cornelissen, A.; et al. Microthrombi as a Major Cause of Cardiac Injury in COVID-19: A Pathologic Study. *Circulation* **2021**, *143*, 1031–1042. [CrossRef] [PubMed]
21. Lowenstein, C.J.; Solomon, S.D. Severe COVID-19 Is a Microvascular Disease. *Circulation* **2020**, *142*, 1609–1611. [CrossRef] [PubMed]
22. Price, L.C.; McCabe, C.; Garfield, B.; Wort, S.J. Thrombosis and COVID-19 pneumonia: The clot thickens! *Eur. Respir. J.* **2020**, *56*, 2001608. [CrossRef]
23. Lodigiani, C.; Lapichino, G.; Carenzo, L.; Cecconi, M.; Ferrazzi, P.; Sebastian, T.; Kucher, N.; Studt, J.D.; Sacco, C.; Alexia, B.; et al. Venous and arterial thromboembolic complications in COVID-19 patients admitted to an academic hospital in Milan, Italy. *Thromb. Res.* **2020**, *191*, 9–14. [CrossRef]
24. Magro, C.; Mulvey, J.J.; Berlin, D.; Nuovo, G.; Salvatore, S.; Harp, J.; Baxter-Stoltzfus, A.; Laurence, J. Complement associated microvascular injury and thrombosis in the pathogenesis of severe COVID-19 infection: A report of five cases. *Transl. Res.* **2020**, *220*, 1–13. [CrossRef] [PubMed]
25. Gómez, J.; Albaiceta, G.M.; García-Clemente, M.; López-Larrea, C.; Amado-Rodríguez, L.; Lopez-Alonso, I.; Hermida, T.; Enriquez, A.I.; Herrero, P.; Melón, S.; et al. Angiotensin-converting enzymes (ACE, ACE2) gene variants and COVID-19 outcome. *Gene* **2020**, *762*, 145102. [CrossRef] [PubMed]
26. Aung, A.K.; Aitken, T.; Teh, B.M.; Yu, C.; Ofori-Asenso, R.; Chin, K.L.; Liew, D. Angiotensin converting enzyme genotypes and mortality from COVID-19: An ecological study. *J. Infect.* **2020**, *81*, 961–965. [CrossRef]
27. Abassi, Z.; Higazi, A.A.R.; Kinaneh, S.; Armaly, Z.; Skorecki, K.; Heyman, S.N. ACE2, COVID-19 Infection, Inflammation, and Coagulopathy: Missing Pieces in the Puzzle. *Front. Physiol.* **2020**, *11*, 574753. [CrossRef]
28. Kong, W.; Montano, M.; Corley, M.J.; Helmy, E.; Kobayashi, H.; Kinisu, M.; Suryawanshi, R.; Luo, X.; Royer, L.A.; Roan, N.R.; et al. Neuropilin-1 Mediates SARS-CoV-2 Infection of Astrocytes in Brain Organoids, Inducing Inflammation Leading to Dysfunction and Death of Neurons. *mBio* **2022**, *13*, e0230822. [CrossRef]
29. Cantuti-Castelvetri, L.; Ojha, R.; Pedro, L.D.; Djannatian, M.; Franz, J.; Kuivanen, S.; van der Meer, F.; Kallio, K.; Kaya, T.; Anastasina, M.; et al. Neuropilin-1 facilitates SARS-CoV-2 cell entry and infectivity. *Science* **2020**, *370*, 856–860. [CrossRef]
30. Hulswit, R.J.G.; de Haan, C.A.M.; Bosch, B.J. Chapter Two—Coronavirus Spike Protein and Tropism Changes. In *Advances in Virus Research*; Ziebuhr, J., Ed.; Academic Press: New York, NY, USA, 2016; Volume 96, pp. 29–57.
31. Scheim, D.E. A Deadly Embrace: Hemagglutination Mediated by SARS-CoV-2 Spike Protein at its 22 N-Glycosylation Sites, Red Blood Cell Surface Sialoglycoproteins, and Antibody. *Int. J. Mol. Sci.* **2022**, *23*, 2558. [CrossRef]

32. Matrosovich, M.; Herrler, G.; Klenk, H.D. Sialic Acid Receptors of Viruses. In *SialoGlyco Chemistry and Biology II: Tools and Techniques to Identify and Capture Sialoglycans*; Gerardy-Schahn, R., Delannoy, P., von Itzstein, M., Eds.; Springer International Publishing: New York, NY, USA, 2015; pp. 1–28.
33. Tortorici, M.A.; Walls, A.C.; Lang, Y.; Wang, C.; Li, Z.; Koerhuis, D.; Boons, G.J.; Bosch, B.J.; Rey, F.A.; de Groot, R.J.; et al. Structural basis for human coronavirus attachment to sialic acid receptors. *Nat. Struct. Mol. Biol.* **2019**, *26*, 481–489. [CrossRef]
34. Unione, L.; Moure, M.J.; Lenza, M.P.; Oyenarte, I.; Ereño-Orbea, J.; Ardá, A.; Jiménez-Barbero, J. The SARS-CoV-2 Spike Glycoprotein Directly Binds Exogeneous Sialic Acids: A NMR View. *Angew. Chem. Int. Ed.* **2022**, *61*, e202201432. [CrossRef] [PubMed]
35. Kapikian, A.Z.; James, H.D., Jr.; Kelly, S.J.; King, L.M.; Vaughn, A.L.; Chanock, R.M. Hemadsorption by coronavirus strain OC43. *Proc. Soc. Exp. Biol. Med.* **1972**, *139*, 179–186. [CrossRef] [PubMed]
36. Agafonov, A.P.; Gus'kov, A.A.; Ternovoi, V.A.; Ryabchikova, E.I.; Durymanov, A.G.; Vinogradov, I.V.; Maksimov, N.L.; Ignat'ev, G.M.; Nechaeva, E.A.; Netesov, S.V. Primary characterization of SARS coronavirus strain Frankfurt 1. *Dokl. Biol. Sci.* **2004**, *394*, 58–60. [CrossRef]
37. Vlasak, R.; Luytjes, W.; Spaan, W.; Palese, P. Human and bovine coronaviruses recognize sialic acid-containing receptors similar to those of influenza C viruses. *Proc. Natl. Acad. Sci. USA* **1988**, *85*, 4526–4529. [CrossRef]
38. Storz, J.; Zhang, X.M.; Rott, R. Comparison of hemagglutinating, receptor-destroying, and acetylesterase activities of avirulent and virulent bovine coronavirus strains. *Arch. Virol.* **1992**, *125*, 193–204. [CrossRef]
39. Brian, D.A.; Hogue, B.G.; Kienzle, T.E. The Coronavirus Hemagglutinin Esterase Glycoprotein. In *The Coronaviridae. The Viruses*; Siddell, S.G., Ed.; Springer: Boston, MA, USA, 1995.
40. Qing, E.; Hantak, M.; Perlman, S.; Gallagher, T. Distinct Roles for Sialoside and Protein Receptors in Coronavirus Infection. *mBio* **2020**, *11*, e02764-19. [CrossRef]
41. Schultze, B.; Cavanagh, D.; Herrler, G. Neuraminidase treatment of avian infectious bronchitis coronavirus reveals a hemagglutinating activity that is dependent on sialic acid-containing receptors on erythrocytes. *Virology* **1992**, *189*, 792–794. [CrossRef]
42. Li, W.; Hulswit, R.J.G.; Widjaja, I.; Raj, V.S.; McBride, R.; Peng, W.; Widagdo, W.; Tortorici, M.A.; van Dieren, B.; Lang, Y.; et al. Identification of sialic acid-binding function for the Middle East respiratory syndrome coronavirus spike glycoprotein. *Proc. Natl. Acad. Sci. USA* **2017**, *114*, E8508–E8517. [CrossRef]
43. Hulswit, R.J.G.; Lang, Y.; Bakkers, M.J.G.; Li, W.; Li, Z.; Schouten, A.; Ophorst, B.; van Kuppeveld, F.J.M.; Boons, G.J.; Bosch, B.J.; et al. Human coronaviruses OC43 and HKU1 bind to 9-O-acetylated sialic acids via a conserved receptor-binding site in spike protein domain A. *Proc. Natl. Acad. Sci. USA* **2019**, *116*, 2681–2690. [CrossRef]
44. Neu, U.; Bauer, J.; Stehle, T. Viruses and sialic acids: Rules of engagement. *Curr. Opin. Struct. Biol.* **2011**, *21*, 610–618. [CrossRef]
45. Huang, X.; Dong, W.; Milewska, A.; Golda, A.; Qi, Y.; Zhu, Q.K.; Marasco, W.A.; Baric, R.S.; Sims, A.C.; Pyrc, K.; et al. Human Coronavirus HKU1 Spike Protein Uses O-Acetylated Sialic Acid as an Attachment Receptor Determinant and Employs Hemagglutinin-Esterase Protein as a Receptor Destroying Enzyme. *J. Virol.* **2015**, *89*, 7202–7213. [CrossRef]
46. Park, Y.-J.; Walls, A.C.; Wang, Z.; Sauer, M.M.; Li, W.; Tortorici, M.A.; Bosch, B.-J.; DiMaio, F.; Veesler, D. Structures of MERS-CoV spike glycoprotein in complex with sialoside attachment receptors. *Nat. Struct. Mol. Biol.* **2019**, *26*, 1151–1157. [CrossRef] [PubMed]
47. Wielgat, P.; Rogowski, K.; Godlewska, K.; Car, H. Coronaviruses: Is Sialic Acid a Gate to the Eye of Cytokine Storm? From the Entry to the Effects. *Cells* **2020**, *9*, 1963. [CrossRef]
48. Koehler, M.; Delguste, M.; Sieben, C.; Gillet, L.; Alsteens, D. Initial Step of Virus Entry: Virion Binding to Cell-Surface Glycans. *Annu. Rev. Virol.* **2020**, *7*, 143–165. [CrossRef]
49. Ströh, L.J.; Stehle, T. Glycan Engagement by Viruses: Receptor Switches and Specificity. *Annu. Rev. Virol.* **2014**, *1*, 285–306. [CrossRef]
50. Chan, J.F.-W.; Kok, K.-H.; Zhu, Z.; Chu, H.; To, K.K.-W.; Yuan, S.; Yuen, K.-Y. Genomic characterization of the 2019 novel human-pathogenic coronavirus isolated from a patient with atypical pneumonia after visiting Wuhan. *Emerg. Microbes Infect.* **2020**, *9*, 221–236. [CrossRef] [PubMed]
51. Chen, Y.; Liu, Q.; Guo, D. Emerging coronaviruses: Genome structure, replication, and pathogenesis. *J. Med. Virol.* **2020**, *92*, 418–423. [CrossRef] [PubMed]
52. Zaki, A.M.; van Boheemen, S.; Bestebroer, T.M.; Osterhaus, A.D.; Fouchier, R.A. Isolation of a novel coronavirus from a man with pneumonia in Saudi Arabia. *N. Engl. J. Med.* **2012**, *367*, 1814–1820. [CrossRef]
53. Kumar, S.; Nyodu, R.; Maurya, V.K.; Saxena, S.K. Morphology, Genome Organization, Replication, and Pathogenesis of Severe Acute Respiratory Syndrome Coronavirus 2 (SARS-CoV-2). In *Coronavirus Disease 2019 (COVID-19): Epidemiology, Pathogenesis, Diagnosis, and Therapeutics*; Saxena, S.K., Ed.; Springer: Singapore, 2020; pp. 23–31.
54. Yoshimoto, F.K. The Proteins of Severe Acute Respiratory Syndrome Coronavirus-2 (SARS-CoV-2 or n-COV19), the Cause of COVID-19. *Protein J.* **2020**, *39*, 198–216. [CrossRef]
55. Jacot, D.; Greub, G.; Jaton, K.; Opota, O. Viral load of SARS-CoV-2 across patients and compared to other respiratory viruses. *Microbes Infect.* **2020**, *22*, 617–621. [CrossRef] [PubMed]
56. Shajahan, A.; Supekar, N.T.; Gleinich, A.S.; Azadi, P. Deducing the N- and O-glycosylation profile of the spike protein of novel coronavirus SARS-CoV-2. *Glycobiology* **2020**, *30*, 981–988. [CrossRef]

57. Guo, W.; Lakshminarayanan, H.; Rodriguez-Palacios, A.; Salata, R.A.; Xu, K.; Draz, M.S. Glycan Nanostructures of Human Coronaviruses. *Int. J. Nanomed.* **2021**, *16*, 4813–4830. [CrossRef] [PubMed]
58. Choi, Y.K.; Cao, Y.; Frank, M.; Woo, H.; Park, S.-J.; Yeom, M.S.; Croll, T.I.; Seok, C.; Im, W. Structure, Dynamics, Receptor Binding, and Antibody Binding of the Fully Glycosylated Full-Length SARS-CoV-2 Spike Protein in a Viral Membrane. *J. Chem. Theory Comput.* **2021**, *17*, 2479–2487. [CrossRef] [PubMed]
59. Baker, A.N.; Richards, S.-J.; Guy, C.S.; Congdon, T.R.; Hasan, M.; Zwetsloot, A.J.; Gallo, A.; Lewandowski, J.R.; Stansfeld, P.J.; Straube, A.; et al. The SARS-CoV-2 Spike Protein Binds Sialic Acids and Enables Rapid Detection in a Lateral Flow Point of Care Diagnostic Device. *ACS Cent. Sci.* **2020**, *6*, 2046–2052. [CrossRef] [PubMed]
60. Lardone, R.D.; Garay, Y.C.; Parodi, P.; de la Fuente, S.; Angeloni, G.; Bravo, E.O.; Schmider, A.K.; Irazoqui, F.J. How glycobiology can help us treat and beat the COVID-19 pandemic. *J. Biol. Chem.* **2021**, *296*, 100375. [CrossRef]
61. Gao, C.; Zeng, J.; Jia, N.; Stavenhagen, K.; Matsumoto, Y.; Zhang, H.; Li, J.; Hume, A.J.; Mühlberger, E.; van Die, I.; et al. SARS-CoV-2 Spike Protein Interacts with Multiple Innate Immune Receptors. *bioRxiv* **2020**. [CrossRef]
62. Chen, W.; Hui, Z.; Ren, X.; Luo, Y.; Shu, J.; Yu, H.; Li, Z. The N-glycosylation sites and Glycan-binding ability of S-protein in SARS-CoV-2 Coronavirus. *bioRxiv* 2020. [CrossRef]
63. Casalino, L.; Gaieb, Z.; Goldsmith, J.A.; Hjorth, C.K.; Dommer, A.C.; Harbison, A.M.; Fogarty, C.A.; Barros, E.P.; Taylor, B.C.; McLellan, J.S.; et al. Beyond Shielding: The Roles of Glycans in the SARS-CoV-2 Spike Protein. *ACS Cent. Sci.* **2020**, *6*, 1722–1734. [CrossRef]
64. Hyvärinen, S.; Meri, S.; Jokiranta, T.S. Disturbed sialic acid recognition on endothelial cells and platelets in complement attack causes atypical hemolytic uremic syndrome. *Blood* **2016**, *127*, 2701–2710. [CrossRef]
65. Kasinrerk, W.; Tokrasinwit, N.; Phunpae, P. CD147 monoclonal antibodies induce homotypic cell aggregation of monocytic cell line U937 via LFA-1/ICAM-1 pathway. *Immunology* **1999**, *96*, 184–192. [CrossRef] [PubMed]
66. Campbell, R.A.; Boilard, E.; Rondina, M.T. Is there a role for the ACE2 receptor in SARS-CoV-2 interactions with platelets? *J. Thromb. Haemost.* **2021**, *19*, 46–50. [CrossRef] [PubMed]
67. Cosic, I.; Cosic, D.; Loncarevic, I. RRM Prediction of Erythrocyte Band3 Protein as Alternative Receptor for SARS-CoV-2 Virus. *Appl. Sci.* **2020**, *10*, 4053. [CrossRef]
68. Scheim, D.E.; From Cold to Killer: How SARS-CoV-2 Evolved without Hemagglutinin Esterase to Agglutinate, Then Clot Blood Cells in Pulmonary and Systemic Microvasculature. *OSF Preprints*. Available online: https://osf.io/sgdj2 (accessed on 30 October 2023).
69. Ahmetaj-Shala, B.; Vaja, R.; Atanur, S.; George, P.; Kirkby, N.; Mitchell, J. Systemic analysis of putative SARS-CoV-2 entry and processing genes in cardiovascular tissues identifies a positive correlation of BSG with age in endothelial cells. *bioRxiv* **2020**. [CrossRef]
70. Singh, A.; Satchell, S.C.; Neal, C.R.; McKenzie, E.A.; Tooke, J.E.; Mathieson, P.W. Glomerular endothelial glycocalyx constitutes a barrier to protein permeability. *J. Am. Soc. Nephrol.* **2007**, *18*, 2885–2893. [CrossRef]
71. Viitala, J.; Järnefelt, J. The red cell surface revisited. *Trends Biochem. Sci.* **1985**, *10*, 392–395. [CrossRef]
72. Baum, J.; Ward, R.H.; Conway, D.J. Natural selection on the erythrocyte surface. *Mol. Biol. Evol.* **2002**, *19*, 223–229. [CrossRef]
73. Levine, S.; Levine, M.; Sharp, K.A.; Brooks, D.E. Theory of the electrokinetic behavior of human erythrocytes. *Biophys. J.* **1983**, *42*, 127–135. [CrossRef]
74. Aoki, T. A Comprehensive Review of Our Current Understanding of Red Blood Cell (RBC) Glycoproteins. *Membranes* **2017**, *7*, 56. [CrossRef]
75. Zhou, D. Why are glycoproteins modified by poly-N-acetyllactosamine glyco-conjugates? *Curr. Protein Pept. Sci.* **2003**, *4*, 1–9. [CrossRef]
76. Fukuda, M.; Dell, A.; Oates, J.E.; Fukuda, M.N. Structure of branched lactosaminoglycan, the carbohydrate moiety of band 3 isolated from adult human erythrocytes. *J. Biol. Chem.* **1984**, *259*, 8260–8273. [CrossRef] [PubMed]
77. Bua, R.O.; Messina, A.; Sturiale, L.; Barone, R.; Garozzo, D.; Palmigiano, A. N-Glycomics of Human Erythrocytes. *Int. J. Mol. Sci.* **2021**, *22*, 8063. [CrossRef] [PubMed]
78. Liukkonen, J.; Haataja, S.; Tikkanen, K.; Kelm, S.; Finne, J. Identification of N-acetylneuraminyl alpha 2-->3 poly-N-acetyllactosamine glycans as the receptors of sialic acid-binding Streptococcus suis strains. *J. Biol. Chem.* **1992**, *267*, 21105–21111. [CrossRef] [PubMed]
79. Nycholat, C.M.; McBride, R.; Ekiert, D.C.; Xu, R.; Rangarajan, J.; Peng, W.; Razi, N.; Gilbert, M.; Wakarchuk, W.; Wilson, I.A.; et al. Recognition of Sialylated Poly-N-acetyllactosamine Chains on N- and O-Linked Glycans by Human and Avian Influenza I A Virus Hemagglutinins. *Angew. Chem. Int. Ed.* **2012**, *51*, 4860–4863. [CrossRef] [PubMed]
80. Paul, R.W.; Lee, P.W.K. Glycophorin is the reovirus receptor on human erythrocytes. *Virology* **1987**, *159*, 94–101. [CrossRef] [PubMed]
81. Korhonen, T.K.; Haahtela, K.; Pirkola, A.; Parkkinen, J. A N-acetyllactosamine-specific cell-binding activity in a plant pathogen, Erwinia rhapontici. *FEBS Lett.* **1988**, *236*, 163–166. [CrossRef]
82. Nelson, D.S. Immune Adherence. In *Advances in Immunology*; Dixon, F.J., Humphrey, J.H., Eds.; Academic Press: Cambridge, MA, USA, 1963; Volume 3, pp. 131–180.
83. Anderson, H.L.; Brodsky, I.E.; Mangalmurti, N.S. The Evolving Erythrocyte: Red Blood Cells as Modulators of Innate Immunity. *J. Immunol.* **2018**, *201*, 1343–1351. [CrossRef]

84. Varki, A.; Gagneux, P. Multifarious roles of sialic acids in immunity. *Ann. N. Y. Acad. Sci.* **2012**, *1253*, 16–36. [CrossRef]
85. Nelson, R.A. The Immune-Adherence Phenomenon: An Immunologically Specific Reaction Between Microorganisms and Erythrocytes Leading to Enhanced Phagocytosis. *Science* **1953**, *118*, 733–737. [CrossRef]
86. De Back, D.Z.; Kostova, E.; Klei, T.; Beuger, B.; van Zwieten, R.; Kuijpers, T.; Juffermans, N.; van den Berg, T.; Korte, D.; van Kraaij, M.; et al. RBC Adhesive Capacity Is Essential for Efficient 'Immune Adherence Clearance' and Provide a Generic Target to Deplete Pathogens from Septic Patients. *Blood* **2016**, *128*, 1031. [CrossRef]
87. Siegel, I.; Lin Liu, T.; Gleicher, N. The Red-Cell Immune System. *Lancet* **1981**, *318*, 556–559. [CrossRef]
88. Stocker, T.J.; Ishikawa-Ankerhold, H.; Massberg, S.; Schulz, C. Small but mighty: Platelets as central effectors of host defense. *Thromb. Haemost.* **2017**, *117*, 651–661. [PubMed]
89. Salinas, N.D.; Tolia, N.H. Red cell receptors as access points for malaria infection. *Curr. Opin. Hematol.* **2016**, *23*, 215–223. [CrossRef] [PubMed]
90. Sikora, M.; von Bülow, S.; Blanc, F.E.C.; Gecht, M.; Covino, R.; Hummer, G. Computational epitope map of SARS-CoV-2 spike protein. *PLoS Comput. Biol.* **2021**, *17*, e1008790. [CrossRef]
91. Boschi, C.; Scheim, D.E.; Bancod, A.; Militello, M.; Bideau, M.L.; Colson, P.; Fantini, J.; Scola, B.L. SARS-CoV-2 Spike Protein Induces Hemagglutination: Implications for COVID-19 Morbidities and Therapeutics and for Vaccine Adverse Effects. *Int. J. Mol. Sci.* **2022**, *23*, 15480. [CrossRef]
92. Reid, M.E.; Mohandas, N. Red blood cell blood group antigens: Structure and function. *Semin. Hematol.* **2004**, *41*, 93–117. [CrossRef]
93. Pretini, V.; Koenen, M.H.; Kaestner, L.; Fens, M.H.A.M.; Schiffelers, R.M.; Bartels, M.; Van Wijk, R. Red Blood Cells: Chasing Interactions. *Front. Physiol.* **2019**, *10*, 945. [CrossRef] [PubMed]
94. Jaskiewicz, E.; Jodłowska, M.; Kaczmarek, R.; Zerka, A. Erythrocyte glycophorins as receptors for Plasmodium merozoites. *Parasites Vectors* **2019**, *12*, 317. [CrossRef]
95. Varki, A.; Schnaar, R.L.; Schauer, R. Chapter 15: Sialic Acids and Other Nonulosonic Acids. In *Essentials of Glycobiology*, 3rd ed.; Varki, A., Cummings, R., Esko, J., Eds.; Cold Spring Harbor Laboratory Press: Cold Spring Harbor, NY, USA, 2017.
96. Soares, C.O.; Grosso, A.S.; Ereño-Orbea, J.; Coelho, H.; Marcelo, F. Molecular Recognition Insights of Sialic Acid Glycans by Distinct Receptors Unveiled by NMR and Molecular Modeling. *Front. Mol. Biosci.* **2021**, *8*, 727847. [CrossRef]
97. Cohen, M.; Varki, A. Chapter Three—Modulation of Glycan Recognition by Clustered Saccharide Patches. In *International Review of Cell and Molecular Biology*; Jeon, K.W., Ed.; Academic Press: Cambridge, MA, USA, 2014; Volume 308, pp. 75–125.
98. Cohen, M.; Varki, A. The sialome—Far more than the sum of its parts. *Omics* **2010**, *14*, 455–464. [CrossRef]
99. Aminpour, M.; Cannariato, M.; Safaeeardebili, M.E.; Preto, J.; Moracchiato, A.; Doria, D.; Donato, F.; Zizzi, E.A.; Deriu, M.A.; Scheim, D.E.; et al. In Silico Analysis of the Multi-Targeted Mode of Action of Ivermectin and Related Compounds. *Computation* **2022**, *10*, 51. [CrossRef]
100. Grobbelaar, L.M.; Venter, C.; Vlok, M.; Ngoepe, M.; Laubscher, G.J.; Lourens, P.J.; Steenkamp, J.; Kell, D.B.; Pretorius, E. SARS-CoV-2 spike protein S1 induces fibrin(ogen) resistant to fibrinolysis: Implications for microclot formation in COVID-19. *Biosci. Rep.* **2021**, *41*, BSR20210611. [CrossRef]
101. Yamakawa, N.; Vanbeselaere, J.; Chang, L.-Y.; Yu, S.-Y.; Ducrocq, L.; Harduin-Lepers, A.; Kurata, J.; Aoki-Kinoshita, K.F.; Sato, C.; Khoo, K.-H.; et al. Systems glycomics of adult zebrafish identifies organ-specific sialylation and glycosylation patterns. *Nat. Commun.* **2018**, *9*, 4647. [CrossRef] [PubMed]
102. Au Sam, H.; Storey Brian, D.; Moore John, C.; Tang, Q.; Chen, Y.-L.; Javaid, S.; Sarioglu, A.F.; Sullivan, R.; Madden Marissa, W.; O'Keefe, R.; et al. Clusters of circulating tumor cells traverse capillary-sized vessels. *Proc. Natl. Acad. Sci. USA* **2016**, *113*, 4947–4952. [PubMed]
103. Zheng, Y.; Zhao, J.; Li, J.; Guo, Z.; Sheng, J.; Ye, X.; Jin, G.; Wang, C.; Chai, W.; Yan, J.; et al. SARS-CoV-2 spike protein causes blood coagulation and thrombosis by competitive binding to heparan sulfate. *Int. J. Biol. Macromol.* **2021**, *193*, 1124–1129. [CrossRef] [PubMed]
104. Gupta, Y.; Maciorowski, D.; Zak, S.E.; Kulkarni, C.V.; Herbert, A.S.; Durvasula, R.; Fareed, J.; Dye, J.M.; Kempaiah, P. Heparin: A simplistic repurposing to prevent SARS-CoV-2 transmission in light of its in-vitro nanomolar efficacy. *Int. J. Biol. Macromol.* **2021**, *183*, 203–212. [CrossRef]
105. Dayer, M.R. Coronavirus (SARS-CoV-2) Deactivation via Spike Glycoprotein Shielding by Old Drugs: Molecular Docking Approach. *J. Epigenet.* **2021**, *2*, 31–38.
106. Melkumyants, A.; Buryachkovskaya, L.; Lomakin, N.; Antonova, O.; Serebruany, V. Mild COVID-19 and Impaired Blood Cell–Endothelial Crosstalk: Considering Long-Term Use of Antithrombotics? *Thromb. Haemost.* **2022**, *122*, 123–130. [CrossRef]
107. Berzuini, A.; Bianco, C.; Migliorini, A.C.; Maggioni, M.; Valenti, L.; Prati, D. Red blood cell morphology in patients with COVID-19-related anaemia. *Blood Transfus.* **2021**, *19*, 34–36.
108. Ogata, A.F.; Maley, A.M.; Wu, C.; Gilboa, T.; Norman, M.; Lazarovits, R.; Mao, C.P.; Newton, G.; Chang, M.; Nguyen, K.; et al. Ultra-sensitive Serial Profiling of SARS-CoV-2 Antigens and Antibodies in Plasma to Understand Disease Progression in COVID-19 Patients with Severe Disease. *Clin. Chem.* **2020**, *66*, 1562–1572. [CrossRef]
109. Perico, L.; Morigi, M.; Galbusera, M.; Pezzotta, A.; Gastoldi, S.; Imberti, B.; Perna, A.; Ruggenenti, P.; Donadelli, R.; Benigni, A.; et al. SARS-CoV-2 Spike Protein 1 Activates Microvascular Endothelial Cells and Complement System Leading to Platelet Aggregation. *Front. Immunol.* **2022**, *13*, 827146. [CrossRef] [PubMed]

110. Nuovo, G.J.; Magro, C.; Shaffer, T.; Awad, H.; Suster, D.; Mikhail, S.; He, B.; Michaille, J.-J.; Liechty, B.; Tili, E. Endothelial cell damage is the central part of COVID-19 and a mouse model induced by injection of the S1 subunit of the spike protein. *Ann. Diagn. Pathol.* **2021**, *51*, 151682. [CrossRef] [PubMed]
111. Swank, Z.; Senussi, Y.; Manickas-Hill, Z.; Yu, X.G.; Li, J.Z.; Alter, G.; Walt, D.R. Persistent circulating SARS-CoV-2 spike Is associated With post-acute COVID-19 sequelae. *Clin. Infect. Dis.* **2022**, *76*, e487–e490. [CrossRef] [PubMed]
112. Craddock, V.; Mahajan, A.; Spikes, L.; Krishnamachary, B.; Ram, A.K.; Kumar, A.; Chen, L.; Chalise, P.; Dhillon, N.K. Persistent circulation of soluble and extracellular vesicle-linked Spike protein in individuals with postacute sequelae of COVID-19. *J. Med. Virol.* **2023**, *95*, e28568. [CrossRef] [PubMed]
113. Schultheiß, C.; Willscher, E.; Paschold, L.; Gottschick, C.; Klee, B.; Bosurgi, L.; Dutzmann, J.; Sedding, D.; Frese, T.; Girndt, M.; et al. Liquid biomarkers of macrophage dysregulation and circulating spike protein illustrate the biological heterogeneity in patients with post-acute sequelae of COVID-19. *J. Med. Virol.* **2023**, *95*, e28364. [CrossRef]
114. Patterson, B.K.; Francisco, E.B.; Yogendra, R.; Long, E.; Pise, A.; Rodrigues, H.; Hall, E.; Herrera, M.; Parikh, P.; Guevara-Coto, J.; et al. Persistence of SARS-CoV-2 S1 Protein in CD16+ Monocytes in Post-Acute Sequelae of COVID-19 (PASC) up to 15 Months Post-Infection. *Front. Immunol.* **2022**, *12*, 5526. [CrossRef]
115. Rajah, M.M.; Bernier, A.; Buchrieser, J.; Schwartz, O. The Mechanism and Consequences of SARS-CoV-2 Spike-Mediated Fusion and Syncytia Formation. *J. Mol. Biol.* **2021**, *434*, 167280. [CrossRef] [PubMed]
116. Cattin-Ortolá, J.; Welch, L.G.; Maslen, S.L.; Papa, G.; James, L.C.; Munro, S. Sequences in the cytoplasmic tail of SARS-CoV-2 Spike facilitate expression at the cell surface and syncytia formation. *Nat. Commun.* **2021**, *12*, 5333. [CrossRef]
117. Duan, L.; Zheng, Q.; Zhang, H.; Niu, Y.; Lou, Y.; Wang, H. The SARS-CoV-2 Spike Glycoprotein Biosynthesis, Structure, Function, and Antigenicity: Implications for the Design of Spike-Based Vaccine Immunogens. *Front. Immunol.* **2020**, *11*, 576622. [CrossRef]
118. Lam, L.K.M.; Reilly, J.P.; Rux, A.H.; Murphy, S.J.; Kuri-Cervantes, L.; Weisman, A.R.; Ittner, C.A.G.; Pampena, M.B.; Betts, M.R.; Wherry, E.J.; et al. Erythrocytes identify complement activation in patients with COVID-19. *Am. J. Physiol. Lung Cell Mol. Physiol.* **2021**, *321*, L485–L489. [CrossRef]
119. Wang, K.; Chen, W.; Zhang, Z.; Deng, Y.; Lian, J.-Q.; Du, P.; Wei, D.; Zhang, Y.; Sun, X.-X.; Gong, L.; et al. CD147-spike protein is a novel route for SARS-CoV-2 infection to host cells. *Signal Transduct. Target. Ther.* **2020**, *5*, 283. [CrossRef] [PubMed]
120. Hao, W.; Ma, B.; Li, Z.; Wang, X.; Gao, X.; Li, Y.; Qin, B.; Shang, S.; Cui, S.; Tan, Z. Binding of the SARS-CoV-2 spike protein to glycans. *Sci. Bull. (Beijing)* **2021**, *66*, 1205–1214. [CrossRef] [PubMed]
121. Shilts, J.; Crozier, T.W.M.; Greenwood, E.J.D.; Lehner, P.J.; Wright, G.J. No evidence for basigin/CD147 as a direct SARS-CoV-2 spike binding receptor. *Sci. Rep.* **2021**, *11*, 413. [CrossRef] [PubMed]
122. Buryachkovskaya, L.; Lomakin, N.; Melkumyants, A.; Docenko, J.; Ermishkin, V.; Serebruany, V. Enoxaparin dose impacts blood cell phenotypes during mild SARS-CoV-2 infection: The observational single-center study. *Rev. Cardiovasc. Med.* **2021**, *22*, 1685–1691. [CrossRef] [PubMed]
123. Melkumyants, A.; Buryachkovskaya, L.; Lomakin, N.; Antonova, O.; Docenko, J.; Ermishkin, V.; Serebruany, V. Effect of Sulodexide on Circulating Blood Cells in Patients with Mild COVID-19. *J. Clin. Med.* **2022**, *11*, 1995. [CrossRef]
124. Favaron, E.; Ince, C.; Hilty, M.P.; Ergin, B.; van der Zee, P.; Uz, Z.; Wendel Garcia, P.D.; Hofmaenner, D.A.; Acevedo, C.T.; van Boven, W.J.; et al. Capillary Leukocytes, Microaggregates, and the Response to Hypoxemia in the Microcirculation of Coronavirus Disease 2019 Patients. *Crit. Care Med.* **2021**, *49*, 661–670. [CrossRef]
125. Nader, E.; Nougier, C.; Boisson, C.; Poutrel, S.; Catella, J.; Martin, F.; Charvet, J.; Girard, S.; Havard-Guibert, S.; Martin, M.; et al. Increased blood viscosity and red blood cell aggregation in patients with COVID-19. *Am. J. Hematol.* **2022**, *97*, 283–292. [CrossRef]
126. Petrilli, C.M.; Jones, S.A.; Yang, J.; Rajagopalan, H.; O'Donnell, L.; Chernyak, Y.; Tobin, K.A.; Cerfolio, R.J.; Francois, F.; Horwitz, L.I. Factors associated with hospital admission and critical illness among 5279 people with coronavirus disease 2019 in New York City: Prospective cohort study. *BMJ* **2020**, *369*, m1966. [CrossRef]
127. Koutsiaris, A.G.; Riri, K.; Boutlas, S.; Panagiotou, T.N.; Kotoula, M.; Daniil, Z.; Tsironi, E.E. COVID-19 hemodynamic and thrombotic effect on the eye microcirculation after hospitalization: A quantitative case-control study. *Clin. Hemorheol. Microcirc.* **2022**, *82*, 379–390. [CrossRef]
128. Ko, C.J.; Harigopal, M.; Gehlhausen, J.R.; Bosenberg, M.; McNiff, J.M.; Damsky, W. Discordant anti-SARS-CoV-2 spike protein and RNA staining in cutaneous perniotic lesions suggests endothelial deposition of cleaved spike protein. *J. Cutan. Pathol.* **2021**, *48*, 47–52. [CrossRef]
129. Liu, F.; Han, K.; Blair, R.; Kenst, K.; Qin, Z.; Upcin, B.; Wörsdörfer, P.; Midkiff, C.C.; Mudd, J.; Belyaeva, E.; et al. SARS-CoV-2 Infects Endothelial Cells In Vivo and In Vitro. *Front. Cell. Infect. Microbiol.* **2021**, *11*, 701278. [CrossRef]
130. Magro, C.M.; Mulvey, J.J.; Laurence, J.; Seshan, S.; Crowson, A.N.; Dannenberg, A.J.; Salvatore, S.; Harp, J.; Nuovo, G.J. Docked severe acute respiratory syndrome coronavirus 2 proteins within the cutaneous and subcutaneous microvasculature and their role in the pathogenesis of severe coronavirus disease 2019. *Hum. Pathol.* **2020**, *106*, 106–116. [CrossRef] [PubMed]
131. Perico, L.; Benigni, A.; Remuzzi, G. SARS-CoV-2 and the spike protein in endotheliopathy. *Trends Microbiol.* **2023**. [CrossRef] [PubMed]
132. Goshua, G.; Pine, A.B.; Meizlish, M.L.; Chang, C.H.; Zhang, H.; Bahel, P.; Baluha, A.; Bar, N.; Bona, R.D.; Burns, A.J.; et al. Endotheliopathy in COVID-19-associated coagulopathy: Evidence from a single-centre, cross-sectional study. *Lancet Haematol.* **2020**, *7*, e575–e582. [CrossRef]

133. Huertas, A.; Montani, D.; Savale, L.; Pichon, J.; Tu, L.; Parent, F.; Guignabert, C.; Humbert, M. Endothelial cell dysfunction: A major player in SARS-CoV-2 infection (COVID-19)? *Eur. Respir. J.* **2020**, *56*, 2001634. [CrossRef]
134. Muhl, L.; He, L.; Sun, Y.; Andaloussi Mäe, M.; Pietilä, R.; Liu, J.; Genové, G.; Zhang, L.; Xie, Y.; Leptidis, S.; et al. The SARS-CoV-2 receptor ACE2 is expressed in mouse pericytes but not endothelial cells: Implications for COVID-19 vascular research. *Stem Cell Rep.* **2022**, *17*, 1089–1104. [CrossRef]
135. Nicosia, R.F.; Ligresti, G.; Caporarello, N.; Akilesh, S.; Ribatti, D. COVID-19 Vasculopathy: Mounting Evidence for an Indirect Mechanism of Endothelial Injury. *Am. J. Pathol.* **2021**, *191*, 1374–1384. [CrossRef] [PubMed]
136. Blom, J.A. *Monitoring of Respiration and Circulation*; CRC Press: Boca Raton, FL, USA, 2003; p. 27.
137. Guest, M.M.; Bond, T.P.; Cooper, R.G.; Derrick, J.R. Red Blood Cells: Change in Shape in Capillaries. *Science* **1963**, *142*, 1319–1321. [CrossRef]
138. Becker, R.C.; Sexton, T.; Smyth, S.S. Translational Implications of Platelets as Vascular First Responders. *Circ. Res.* **2018**, *122*, 506–522. [CrossRef]
139. O'Sullivan, J.M.; Gonagle, D.M.; Ward, S.E.; Preston, R.J.S.; O'Donnell, J.S. Endothelial cells orchestrate COVID-19 coagulopathy. *Lancet Haematol.* **2020**, *7*, e553–e555. [CrossRef]
140. Turner, S.; Khan, M.A.; Putrino, D.; Woodcock, A.; Kell, D.B.; Pretorius, E. Long COVID: Pathophysiological factors and abnormalities of coagulation. *Trends Endocrinol. Metab.* **2023**, *34*, 321–344. [CrossRef]
141. Helms, J.; Tacquard, C.; Severac, F.; Leonard-Lorant, I.; Ohana, M.; Delabranche, X.; Merdji, H.; Clere-Jehl, R.; Schenck, M.; Fagot Gandet, F.; et al. High risk of thrombosis in patients with severe SARS-CoV-2 infection: A multicenter prospective cohort study. *Intensive Care Med.* **2020**, *46*, 1089–1098. [CrossRef] [PubMed]
142. Mei, Z.W.; van Wijk, X.M.R.; Pham, H.P.; Marin, M.J. Role of von Willebrand Factor in COVID-19 Associated Coagulopathy. *J. Appl. Lab. Med.* **2021**, *6*, 1305–1315. [CrossRef] [PubMed]
143. Shoemaker, W.C.; Brunius, U.; Gelin, L.-E. Hemodynamic and microcirculatory effects of high and low viscosity dextrans. *Surgery* **1965**, *58*, 518–523. [PubMed]
144. Stalker, A.L. Histological changes produced by experimental erythrocyte aggregation. *J. Pathol. Bacteriol.* **1967**, *93*, 203–212. [CrossRef] [PubMed]
145. Stalker, A.L. The microcirculatory effects of dextran. *J. Pathol. Bacteriol.* **1967**, *93*, 191–201. [CrossRef] [PubMed]
146. Fajers, C.M.; Gelin, L.E. Kidney-, liver- and heart-damages from trauma and from induced intravascular aggregation of blood-cells: An experimental study. *Acta Pathol. Microbiol. Scand.* **1959**, *46*, 97–104. [CrossRef]
147. Swank, R.L.; Fellman, J.H.; Hissen, W.W. Aggregation of Blood Cells by 5-Hydroxytryptamine (Serotonin). *Circ. Res.* **1963**, *13*, 392–400. [CrossRef]
148. Cullen, C.F.; Swank, R.L. Intravascular Aggregation and Adhesiveness of the Blood Elements Associated with Alimentary Lipemia and Injections of Large Molecular Substances. *Circulation* **1954**, *9*, 335–346. [CrossRef]
149. Pribush, A.; Zilberman-Kravits, D.; Meyerstein, N. The mechanism of the dextran-induced red blood cell aggregation. *Eur. Biophys. J.* **2007**, *36*, 85–94. [CrossRef]
150. Zhu, R.; Avsievich, T.; Bykov, A.; Popov, A.; Meglinski, I. Influence of Pulsed He–Ne Laser Irradiation on the Red Blood Cell Interaction Studied by Optical Tweezers. *Micromachines* **2019**, *10*, 853. [CrossRef]
151. Lee, K.; Shirshin, E.; Rovnyagina, N.; Yaya, F.; Boujja, Z.; Priezzhev, A.; Wagner, C. Dextran adsorption onto red blood cells revisited: Single cell quantification by laser tweezers combined with microfluidics. *Biomed. Opt. Express* **2018**, *9*, 2755–2764. [CrossRef] [PubMed]
152. Chien, S.; Jan, K.-m. Ultrastructural basis of the mechanism of rouleaux formation. *Microvasc. Res.* **1973**, *5*, 155–166. [CrossRef] [PubMed]
153. Zhen, Z.-Y.; Guo, Y.-C.; Zhang, Z.-G.; Liang, Y.; Ge, P.-J.; Jin, H.-M. Experimental Study on Microthrombi and Myocardial Injuries. *Microvasc. Res.* **1996**, *51*, 99–107. [CrossRef] [PubMed]
154. Bicher, H.I. Chapter II: Pathological significance of intravascular red cell aggregation. In *Blood Cell Aggregation in Thrombotic Processes*; C. C. Thomas: Springfield, IL, USA, 1972; pp. 19–46.
155. Brånemark, P.-I. Experimental Investigation of Microcirculation in Bone Marrow. *Angiology* **1961**, *12*, 293–305. [CrossRef]
156. Engeset, J.; Stalker, A.L.; Matheson, N.A. Effects of Dextran 40 on Red Cell Aggregation in Rabbits. *Cardiovasc. Res.* **1967**, *1*, 379–384. [CrossRef] [PubMed]
157. Swank, R.L.; Cullen, C.F. Circulatory Changes in the Hamster's Cheek Pouch Associated with Alimentary Lipemia. *Proc. Soc. Exp. Biol. Med.* **1953**, *82*, 381–384. [CrossRef] [PubMed]
158. Bjoerk, V.O.; Intonti, F.; Nordlund, S. Correlation between sludge in the bulbar conjunctiva and the mesentery. *Ann. Surg.* **1964**, *159*, 428–431.
159. Reinke, W.; Gaehtgens, P.; Johnson, P.C. Blood viscosity in small tubes: Effect of shear rate, aggregation, and sedimentation. *Am. J. Physiol.-Heart Circ. Physiol.* **1987**, *253*, H540–H547. [CrossRef]
160. Volger, E.; Schmid-Schönbein, H.; Gosen, J.v.; Klose, H.J.; Kline, K.A. Microrheology and light transmission of blood. *Pflügers Arch.* **1975**, *354*, 319–337. [CrossRef]
161. Bosek, M.; Ziomkowska, B.; Pyskir, J.; Wybranowski, T.; Pyskir, M.; Cyrankiewicz, M.; Napiórkowska, M.; Durmowicz, M.; Kruszewski, S. Relationship between red blood cell aggregation and dextran molecular mass. *Sci. Rep.* **2022**, *12*, 19751. [CrossRef] [PubMed]

162. Neu, B.; Wenby, R.; Meiselman, H.J. Effects of dextran molecular weight on red blood cell aggregation. *Biophys. J.* **2008**, *95*, 3059–3065. [CrossRef] [PubMed]
163. Engeset, J.; Stalker, A.L.; Matheson, N.A. Objective measurement of the dispersing effect of dextran 40 on red cells from man, dog, and rabbit. *Cardiovasc. Res.* **1967**, *1*, 385–388. [CrossRef]
164. Baskurt, O.K.; Meiselman, H.J. Erythrocyte aggregation: Basic aspects and clinical importance. *Clin. Hemorheol. Microcirc.* **2013**, *53*, 23–37. [CrossRef]
165. Barshtein, G.; Wajnblum, D.; Yedgar, S. Kinetics of linear rouleaux formation studied by visual monitoring of red cell dynamic organization. *Biophys. J.* **2000**, *78*, 2470–2474. [CrossRef] [PubMed]
166. Fung, Y.-C. Chapter 3: The flow properties of blood. In *Biomechanics: Mechanical Properties of Living Tissues*; Springer: New York, NY, USA, 1993; pp. 66–108. [CrossRef]
167. Bicher, H.I. Chapter I: Red cell aggregation in thrombotic disease, trauma and shock. In *Blood Cell Aggregation in Thrombotic Processes*; C. C. Thomas: Springfield, IL, USA, 1972; Volume I, pp. 5–18.
168. Bicher, H.I. Chapter III: Mechanism of red cell aggregation. In *Blood Cell Aggregation in Thrombotic Processes*; C. C. Thomas: Springfield, IL, USA, 1972; Volume III, pp. 47–61.
169. Brooks, D.E.; Evans, E.A. Rheology of blood cells. In *Clinical Hemorheology: Applications in Cardiovascular and Hematological Disease, Diabetes, Surgery and Gynecology*; Chien, S., Dormandy, J., Ernst, E., Matrai, A., Eds.; Springer: Dordrecht, The Netherlands, 1987; pp. 73–96.
170. Lowe, G.D.O. Thrombosis and hemorheology. In *Clinical Hemorheology: Applications in Cardiovascular and Hematological Disease, Diabetes, Surgery and Gynecology*; Chien, S., Dormandy, J., Ernst, E., Matrai, A., Eds.; Springer: Dordrecht, The Netherlands, 1987; pp. 195–226.
171. Bishop, J.J.; Nance, P.R.; Popel, A.S.; Intaglietta, M.; Johnson, P.C. Effect of erythrocyte aggregation on velocity profiles in venules. *Am. J. Physiol.-Heart Circ. Physiol.* **2001**, *280*, H222–H236. [CrossRef]
172. Chien, S.; Sung, L.A. Physicochemical basis and clinical implications of red cell aggregation. *Clin. Hemorheol. Microcirc.* **1987**, *7*, 71–91. [CrossRef]
173. Maeda, N.; Seike, M.; Kon, K.; Shiga, T. Erythrocyte Aggregation as a Determinant of Blood Flow: Effect of pH, Temperature and Osmotic Pressure. In *Oxygen Transport to Tissue X*; Mochizuki, M., Honig, C.R., Koyama, T., Goldstick, T.K., Bruley, D.F., Eds.; Springer US: New York, NY, USA, 1988; pp. 563–570.
174. Sakariassen, K.S.; Orning, L.; Turitto, V.T. The impact of blood shear rate on arterial thrombus formation. *Future Sci. OA* **2015**, *1*, FSO30. [CrossRef]
175. Knisely, M.H.; Bloch, E.H.; Eliot, T.S.; Warner, L. Sludged Blood. *Science* **1947**, *106*, 431–440. [CrossRef]
176. Barshtein, G.; Ben-Ami, R.; Yedgar, S. Role of red blood cell flow behavior in hemodynamics and hemostasis. *Expert Rev. Cardiovasc. Ther.* **2007**, *5*, 743–752. [CrossRef]
177. Ditzel, J.; Sagild, U. Morphologic and hemodynamic changes in the smaller blood vessels in diabetes mellitus. II. The degenerative and hemodynamic changes in the bulbar conjunctiva of normotensive diabetic patients. *N. Engl. J. Med.* **1954**, *250*, 587–594. [CrossRef]
178. Vernon Jeffords, J.; Knisely, M.H. Concerning the Geometric Shapes of Arteries and Arterioles: A Contribution to the Biophysics of Health, Disease, and Death. *Angiology* **1956**, *7*, 105–136. [CrossRef]
179. Yu, F.T.; Armstrong, J.K.; Tripette, J.; Meiselman, H.J.; Cloutier, G. A local increase in red blood cell aggregation can trigger deep vein thrombosis: Evidence based on quantitative cellular ultrasound imaging. *J. Thromb. Haemost.* **2011**, *9*, 481–488. [CrossRef] [PubMed]
180. Byrnes, J.R.; Wolberg, A.S. Red blood cells in thrombosis. *Blood* **2017**, *130*, 1795–1799. [CrossRef] [PubMed]
181. Ami, R.B.; Barshtein, G.; Zeltser, D.; Goldberg, Y.; Shapira, I.; Roth, A.; Keren, G.; Miller, H.; Prochorov, V.; Eldor, A.; et al. Parameters of red blood cell aggregation as correlates of the inflammatory state. *Am. J. Physiol.-Heart Circ. Physiol.* **2001**, *280*, H1982–H1988. [CrossRef] [PubMed]
182. Wagner, C.; Steffen, P.; Svetina, S. Aggregation of red blood cells: From rouleaux to clot formation. *C. R. Phys.* **2013**, *14*, 459–469. [CrossRef]
183. Meiselman, H.J. Red blood cell aggregation: 45 years being curious. *Biorheology* **2009**, *46*, 1–19. [CrossRef]
184. Junxiu, Z.; Yu, F.; Shaodan, L.; Yi, L.; Yin, Z.; Yunxia, G.; Minghui, Y. Microvascular pathological features and changes in related injury factors in a rat acute blood stasis model. *J. Tradit. Chin. Med.* **2017**, *37*, 108–115. [CrossRef]
185. Kim, S.; Popel, A.S.; Intaglietta, M.; Johnson, P.C. Aggregate formation of erythrocytes in postcapillary venules. *Am. J. Physiol.-Heart Circ. Physiol.* **2005**, *288*, H584–H590. [CrossRef]
186. Swank, R.L. Suspension Stability of the Blood After Injections of Dextran. *J. Appl. Physiol.* **1958**, *12*, 125–128. [CrossRef]
187. Swank, R.L.; Escobar, A. Effects of Dextran Injections on Blood Viscosity in Dogs. *J. Appl. Physiol.* **1957**, *10*, 45–50. [CrossRef]
188. Bicher, H.I.; Bruley, D.; Knisely, M.H.; Reneau, D.D. Effect of microcirculation changes on brain tissue oxygenation. *J. Physiol.* **1971**, *217*, 689–707. [CrossRef]
189. Hysi, E.; Saha, R.K.; Kolios, M.C. Photoacoustic ultrasound spectroscopy for assessing red blood cell aggregation and oxygenation. *J. Biomed. Opt.* **2012**, *17*, 125006. [CrossRef] [PubMed]
190. Ditzel, J. Angioscopic Changes in the Smaller Blood Vessels in Diabetes Mellitus and their Relationship to Aging. *Circulation* **1956**, *14*, 386–397. [CrossRef] [PubMed]

191. Ziegler, O.; Guerci, B.; Muller, S.; Candiloros, H.; Mejean, L.; Donner, M.; Stoltz, J.F.; Drouin, P. Increased erythrocyte aggregation in insulin-dependent diabetes mellitus and its relationship to plasma factors: A multivariate analysis. *Metabolism* **1994**, *43*, 1182–1186. [CrossRef] [PubMed]
192. Chazan, B.I. Intravascular Red Cell Aggregation and the Chylomicron Count in Diabetes. *Angiology* **1963**, *14*, 426–429. [CrossRef]
193. Cho, Y.I.; Mooney, M.P.; Cho, D.J. Hemorheological Disorders in Diabetes Mellitus. *J. Diabetes Sci. Technol.* **2008**, *2*, 1130–1138. [CrossRef]
194. Wautier, J.L.; Paton, R.C.; Wautier, M.P.; Pintigny, D.; Abadie, E.; Passa, P.; Caen, J.P. Increased adhesion of erythrocytes to endothelial cells in diabetes mellitus and its relation to vascular complications. *N. Engl. J. Med.* **1981**, *305*, 237–242. [CrossRef]
195. Mikami, T.; Miyashita, H.; Yamada, T.; Harrington, M.; Steinberg, D.; Dunn, A.; Siau, E. Risk Factors for Mortality in Patients with COVID-19 in New York City. *J. Gen. Intern. Med.* **2020**, *36*, 17–26. [CrossRef]
196. Sastry, S.; Cuomo, F.; Muthusamy, J. COVID-19 and thrombosis: The role of hemodynamics. *Thromb. Res.* **2022**, *212*, 51–57. [CrossRef]
197. Avila, J.; Long, B.; Holladay, D.; Gottlieb, M. Thrombotic complications of COVID-19. *Am. J. Emerg. Med.* **2021**, *39*, 213–218. [CrossRef] [PubMed]
198. Al-Samkari, H.; Karp Leaf, R.S.; Dzik, W.H.; Carlson, J.C.T.; Fogerty, A.E.; Waheed, A.; Goodarzi, K.; Bendapudi, P.K.; Bornikova, L.; Gupta, S.; et al. COVID-19 and coagulation: Bleeding and thrombotic manifestations of SARS-CoV-2 infection. *Blood* **2020**, *136*, 489–500. [CrossRef] [PubMed]
199. Dolhnikoff, M.; Duarte-Neto, A.N.; de Almeida Monteiro, R.A.; da Silva, L.F.F.; de Oliveira, E.P.; Saldiva, P.H.N.; Mauad, T.; Negri, E.M. Pathological evidence of pulmonary thrombotic phenomena in severe COVID-19. *J. Thromb. Haemost.* **2020**, *18*, 1517–1519. [CrossRef] [PubMed]
200. Maier, C.L.; Truong, A.D.; Auld, S.C.; Polly, D.M.; Tanksley, C.-L.; Duncan, A. COVID-19-associated hyperviscosity: A link between inflammation and thrombophilia? *Lancet* **2020**, *395*, 1758–1759. [CrossRef]
201. Rovas, A.; Osiaevi, I.; Buscher, K.; Sackarnd, J.; Tepasse, P.-R.; Fobker, M.; Kühn, J.; Braune, S.; Göbel, U.; Thölking, G.; et al. Microvascular dysfunction in COVID-19: The MYSTIC study. *Angiogenesis* **2021**, *24*, 145–157. [CrossRef]
202. US National Institutes of Health (NIH). Clinical Spectrum of SARS-CoV-2 Infection, Updated 6 March 2023. Available online: https://www.covid19treatmentguidelines.nih.gov/overview/clinical-spectrum/ (accessed on 30 October 2023).
203. Osiaevi, I.; Schulze, A.; Evers, G.; Harmening, K.; Vink, H.; Kümpers, P.; Mohr, M.; Rovas, A. Persistent capillary rarefication in long COVID syndrome. *Angiogenesis* **2023**, *26*, 53–61. [CrossRef]
204. Lins, M.; Vandevenne, J.; Thillai, M.; Lavon, B.R.; Lanclus, M.; Bonte, S.; Godon, R.; Kendall, I.; De Backer, J.; De Backer, W. Assessment of Small Pulmonary Blood Vessels in COVID-19 Patients Using HRCT. *Acad. Radiol.* **2020**, *27*, 1449–1455. [CrossRef]
205. Thillai, M.; Patvardhan, C.; Swietlik, E.M.; McLellan, T.; De Backer, J.; Lanclus, M.; De Backer, W.; Ruggiero, A. Functional respiratory imaging identifies redistribution of pulmonary blood flow in patients with COVID-19. *Thorax* **2021**, *76*, 182–184. [CrossRef]
206. Morris, M.F.; Pershad, Y.; Kang, P.; Ridenour, L.; Lavon, B.; Lanclus, M.; Godon, R.; De Backer, J.; Glassberg, M.K. Altered pulmonary blood volume distribution as a biomarker for predicting outcomes in COVID-19 disease. *Eur. Respir. J.* **2021**, *58*, 2004133. [CrossRef]
207. Dierckx, W.; De Backer, W.; Lins, M.; De Meyer, Y.; Ides, K.; Vandevenne, J.; De Backer, J.; Franck, E.; Lavon, B.R.; Lanclus, M.; et al. CT-derived measurements of pulmonary blood volume in small vessels and the need for supplemental oxygen in COVID-19 patients. *J. Appl. Physiol. (1985)* **2022**, *133*, 1295–1299. [CrossRef]
208. Tipre, D.N.; Cidon, M.; Moats, R.A. Imaging Pulmonary Blood Vessels and Ventilation-Perfusion Mismatch in COVID-19. *Mol. Imaging Biol.* **2022**, *24*, 526–536. [CrossRef]
209. Atilgan, C.U.; Goker, Y.S.; Hondur, G.; Kosekahya, P.; Kocer, A.M.; Citirik, M. Evaluation of the radial peripapillary capillary density in unilateral branch retinal vein occlusion and the unaffected fellow eyes. *Ther. Adv. Ophthalmol.* **2022**, *14*. [CrossRef] [PubMed]
210. Erogul, O.; Gobeka, H.H.; Dogan, M.; Akdogan, M.; Balci, A.; Kasikci, M. Retinal microvascular morphology versus COVID-19: What to anticipate? *Photodiagn. Photodyn. Ther.* **2022**, *39*, 102920. [CrossRef] [PubMed]
211. Savastano, A.; Crincoli, E.; Savastano, M.C.; Younis, S.; Gambini, G.; De Vico, U.; Cozzupoli, G.M.; Culiersi, C.; Rizzo, S. Peripapillary Retinal Vascular Involvement in Early Post-COVID-19 Patients. *J. Clin. Med.* **2020**, *9*, 2895. [CrossRef] [PubMed]
212. Schlick, S.; Lucio, M.; Wallukat, G.; Bartsch, A.; Skornia, A.; Hoffmanns, J.; Szewczykowski, C.; Schröder, T.; Raith, F.; Rogge, L.; et al. Post-COVID-19 Syndrome: Retinal Microcirculation as a Potential Marker for Chronic Fatigue. *Int. J. Mol. Sci.* **2022**, *23*, 13683. [CrossRef]
213. Wu, R.; Ai, S.; Cai, J.; Zhang, S.; Qian, Z.M.; Zhang, Y.; Wu, Y.; Chen, L.; Tian, F.; Li, H.; et al. Predictive Model and Risk Factors for Case Fatality of COVID-19: A Cohort of 21,392 Cases in Hubei, China. *Innovation* **2020**, *1*, 100022. [CrossRef]
214. Zhou, F.; Yu, T.; Du, R.; Fan, G.; Liu, Y.; Liu, Z.; Xiang, J.; Wang, Y.; Song, B.; Gu, X.; et al. Clinical course and risk factors for mortality of adult inpatients with COVID-19 in Wuhan, China: A retrospective cohort study. *Lancet* **2020**, *395*, 1054–1062. [CrossRef]
215. Williamson, E.J.; Walker, A.J.; Bhaskaran, K.; Bacon, S.; Bates, C.; Morton, C.E.; Curtis, H.J.; Mehrkar, A.; Evans, D.; Inglesby, P.; et al. OpenSAFELY: Factors associated with COVID-19 death in 17 million patients. *Nature* **2020**, *584*, 430–436. [CrossRef]

216. Bonanad, C.; García-Blas, S.; Tarazona-Santabalbina, F.; Sanchis, J.; Bertomeu-González, V.; Fácila, L.; Ariza, A.; Núñez, J.; Cordero, A. The Effect of Age on Mortality in Patients With COVID-19: A Meta-Analysis With 611,583 Subjects. *J. Am. Med. Dir. Assoc.* **2020**, *21*, 915–918. [CrossRef]
217. Manetta, J.; Aloulou, I.; Varlet-Marie, E.; Mercier, J.; Brun, J.F. Partially opposite hemorheological effects of aging and training at middle age. *Clin. Hemorheol. Microcirc.* **2006**, *35*, 239–244.
218. Hammi, H.; Perrotin, P.; Guillet, R.; Boynard, M. Determination of red blood cell aggregation in young and elderly subjects evaluated by ultrasound. *Clin. Hemorheol. Microcirc.* **1994**, *14*, 117–126. [CrossRef]
219. Richardson, D.; Schwartz, R. Comparison of capillary blood flow in the nailfold circulations of young and elderly men. *AGE* **1985**, *8*, 70. [CrossRef]
220. Richardson, D.; Shepherd, S. The cutaneous microcirculation of the forearm in young and old subjects. *Microvasc. Res.* **1991**, *41*, 84–91. [CrossRef]
221. Tsuchida, Y. The effect of aging and arteriosclerosis on human skin blood flow. *J. Dermatol. Sci.* **1993**, *5*, 175–181. [CrossRef] [PubMed]
222. Ajmani, R.S.; Rifkind, J.M. Hemorheological changes during human aging. *Gerontology* **1998**, *44*, 111–120. [CrossRef] [PubMed]
223. Dinenno, F.A.; Jones, P.P.; Seals, D.R.; Tanaka, H. Limb Blood Flow and Vascular Conductance Are Reduced With Age in Healthy Humans. *Circulation* **1999**, *100*, 164–170. [CrossRef] [PubMed]
224. Krejza, J.; Mariak, Z.; Walecki, J.; Szydlik, P.; Lewko, J.; Ustymowicz, A. Transcranial color Doppler sonography of basal cerebral arteries in 182 healthy subjects: Age and sex variability and normal reference values for blood flow parameters. *AJR Am. J. Roentgenol.* **1999**, *172*, 213–218. [CrossRef] [PubMed]
225. Ackerstaff, R.G.A.; Keunen, R.W.M.; Pelt, W.v.; Swijndregt, A.D.M.v.; Stijnen, T. Influence of biological factors on changes in mean cerebral blood flow velocity in normal ageing: A transcranial Doppler study. *Neurol. Res.* **1990**, *12*, 187–191. [CrossRef]
226. Harrison, S.L.; Buckley, B.J.R.; Rivera-Caravaca, J.M.; Zhang, J.; Lip, G.Y.H. Cardiovascular risk factors, cardiovascular disease, and COVID-19: An umbrella review of systematic reviews. *Eur. Heart J.-Qual. Care Clin. Outcomes* **2021**, *7*, 330–339.
227. Samocha-Bonet, D.; Ben-Ami, R.; Shapira, I.; Shenkerman, G.; Abu-Abeid, S.; Stern, N.; Mardi, T.; Tulchinski, T.; Deutsch, V.; Yedgar, S.; et al. Flow-resistant red blood cell aggregation in morbid obesity. *Int. J. Obes.* **2004**, *28*, 1528–1534. [CrossRef]
228. Samocha-Bonet, D.; Lichtenberg, D.; Tomer, A.; Deutsch, V.; Mardi, T.; Goldin, Y.; Abu-Abeid, S.; Shenkerman, G.; Patshornik, H.; Shapira, I.; et al. Enhanced erythrocyte adhesiveness/aggregation in obesity corresponds to low-grade inflammation. *Obes. Res.* **2003**, *11*, 403–407. [CrossRef] [PubMed]
229. López-Farfán, D.; Irigoyen, N.; Gómez-Díaz, E. Exploring SARS-CoV-2 and Plasmodium falciparum coinfection in human erythrocytes. *Front. Immunol.* **2023**, *14*, 1120298. [CrossRef]
230. Bicher, H.I.; Beemer, A.M. Induction of ischemic myocardial damage by red blood cell aggregation (sludge) in the rabbit. *J. Atheroscler Res.* **1967**, *7*, 409–414. [CrossRef]
231. Yamamoto, M.; Kase, M.; Sano, H.; Kamijima, R.; Sano, S. Persistent varicella zoster virus infection following mRNA COVID-19 vaccination was associated with the presence of encoded spike protein in the lesion. *J. Cutan. Immunol. Allergy* **2023**, *6*, 18–23. [CrossRef]
232. Sano, H.; Kase, M.; Aoyama, Y.; Sano, S. A case of persistent, confluent maculopapular erythema following a COVID-19 mRNA vaccination is possibly associated with the intralesional spike protein expressed by vascular endothelial cells and eccrine glands in the deep dermis. *J. Dermatol.* **2023**, *50*, 1208–1212. [CrossRef]
233. Morz, M. A Case Report: Multifocal Necrotizing Encephalitis and Myocarditis after BNT162b2 mRNA Vaccination against COVID-19. *Vaccines* **2022**, *10*, 1651. [CrossRef] [PubMed]
234. Li, C.; Chen, Y.; Zhao, Y.; Lung, D.C.; Ye, Z.; Song, W.; Liu, F.-F.; Cai, J.-P.; Wong, W.-M.; Yip, C.C.-Y.; et al. Intravenous Injection of Coronavirus Disease 2019 (COVID-19) mRNA Vaccine Can Induce Acute Myopericarditis in Mouse Model. *Clin. Infect. Dis.* **2022**, *74*, 1933–1950. [CrossRef] [PubMed]
235. Hassan, G.M.; Tarek, M. COVID 19 m-RNA (Pfizer) vaccination impairs cardiac functions in adult male rats. *Bull. Egypt. Soc. Physiol. Sci.* **2023**, *43*, 211–228. [CrossRef]
236. Gedik, B.; Bozdogan, Y.C.; Yavuz, S.; Durmaz, D.; Erol, M.K. The assesment of retina and optic disc vascular structures in people who received CoronaVac vaccine. *Photodiagn. Photodyn. Ther.* **2022**, *38*, 102742. [CrossRef]
237. Saritas, O.; Yorgun, M.A.; Gokpinar, E. Effects of Sinovac-Coronavac and Pfizer-BioNTech mRNA vaccines on choroidal and retinal vascular system. *Photodiagn. Photodyn. Ther.* **2023**, *43*, 103702. [CrossRef] [PubMed]
238. Gedik, B.; Erol, M.K.; Suren, E.; Yavuz, S.; Kucuk, M.F.; Bozdogan, Y.C.; Ekinci, R.; Akidan, M. Evaluation of retinal and optic disc vascular structures in individuals before and after Pfizer-BioNTech vaccination. *Microvasc. Res.* **2023**, *147*, 104500. [CrossRef]
239. Da Silva, L.S.C.; Finamor, L.P.S.; Andrade, G.C.; Lima, L.H.; Zett, C.; Muccioli, C.; Sarraf, E.P. Vascular retinal findings after COVID-19 vaccination in 11 cases: A coincidence or consequence? *Arq. Bras. Oftalmol.* **2022**, *85*, 158–165.
240. Haseeb, A.A.; Solyman, O.; Abushanab, M.M.; Abo Obaia, A.S.; Elhusseiny, A.M. Ocular Complications Following Vaccination for COVID-19: A One-Year Retrospective. *Vaccines* **2022**, *10*, 342. [CrossRef] [PubMed]
241. Haider, A.; Bengs, S.; Schade, K.; Wijnen, W.J.; Portmann, A.; Etter, D.; Fröhlich, S.; Warnock, G.I.; Treyer, V.; Burger, I.A.; et al. Myocardial 18F-FDG Uptake Pattern for Cardiovascular Risk Stratification in Patients Undergoing Oncologic PET/CT. *J. Clin. Med.* **2020**, *9*, 2279. [CrossRef] [PubMed]

242. Yao, Y.; Li, Y.-M.; He, Z.-X.; Civelek, A.C.; Li, X.-F. Likely Common Role of Hypoxia in Driving 18F-FDG Uptake in Cancer, Myocardial Ischemia, Inflammation and Infection. *Cancer Biother. Radiopharm.* **2021**, *36*, 624–631.
243. Nakahara, T.; Iwabuchi, Y.; Miyazawa, R.; Tonda, K.; Shiga, T.; Strauss, H.W.; Antoniades, C.; Narula, J.; Jinzaki, M. Assessment of Myocardial (18)F-FDG Uptake at PET/CT in Asymptomatic SARS-CoV-2-vaccinated and Nonvaccinated Patients. *Radiology* **2023**, *308*, e230743. [CrossRef]
244. Gundry, S.R. Abstract 10712: Observational Findings of PULS Cardiac Test Findings for Inflammatory Markers in Patients Receiving mRNA Vaccines. *Circulation* **2021**, *144*, A10712. [CrossRef]
245. U.S. Centers for Disease Control and Prevention, Vaccines and Related Biological Products Advisory Committee (VRBPAC). Update on Myocarditis following mRNA COVID-19 Vaccination. 7 June 2022. Available online: https://www.fda.gov/media/159007/download (accessed on 30 October 2023).
246. Truong, D.T.; Dionne, A.; Muniz, J.C.; McHugh, K.E.; Portman, M.A.; Lambert, L.M.; Thacker, D.; Elias, M.D.; Li, J.S.; Toro-Salazar, O.H.; et al. Clinically Suspected Myocarditis Temporally Related to COVID-19 Vaccination in Adolescents and Young Adults. *Circulation* **2022**, *145*, 345–356. [CrossRef]
247. Chiu, S.N.; Chen, Y.S.; Hsu, C.C.; Hua, Y.C.; Tseng, W.C.; Lu, C.W.; Lin, M.T.; Chen, C.A.; Wu, M.H.; Chen, Y.T.; et al. Changes of ECG parameters after BNT162b2 vaccine in the senior high school students. *Eur. J. Pediatr.* **2023**, *182*, 1155–1162. [CrossRef]
248. Mansanguan, S.; Charunwatthana, P.; Piyaphanee, W.; Dechkhajorn, W.; Poolcharoen, A.; Mansanguan, C. Cardiovascular Manifestation of the BNT162b2 mRNA COVID-19 Vaccine in Adolescents. *Trop. Med. Infect. Dis.* **2022**, *7*, 196. [CrossRef]
249. Yonker, L.M.; Swank, Z.; Bartsch, Y.C.; Burns, M.D.; Kane, A.; Boribong, B.P.; Davis, J.P.; Loiselle, M.; Novak, T.; Senussi, Y.; et al. Circulating Spike Protein Detected in Post–COVID-19 mRNA Vaccine Myocarditis. *Circulation* **2023**, *147*, 867–876. [CrossRef]
250. Krauson, A.J.; Casimero, F.V.C.; Siddiquee, Z.; Stone, J.R. Duration of SARS-CoV-2 mRNA vaccine persistence and factors associated with cardiac involvement in recently vaccinated patients. *NPJ Vaccines* **2023**, *8*, 141. [CrossRef] [PubMed]
251. Baumeier, C.; Aleshcheva, G.; Harms, D.; Gross, U.; Hamm, C.; Assmus, B.; Westenfeld, R.; Kelm, M.; Rammos, S.; Wenzel, P.; et al. Intramyocardial Inflammation after COVID-19 Vaccination: An Endomyocardial Biopsy-Proven Case Series. *Int. J. Mol. Sci.* **2022**, *23*, 6940. [CrossRef] [PubMed]
252. Negri, E.M.; Piloto, B.M.; Morinaga, L.K.; Jardim, C.V.P.; Lamy, S.A.E.-D.; Ferreira, M.A.; D'Amico, E.A.; Deheinzelin, D. Heparin Therapy Improving Hypoxia in COVID-19 Patients—A Case Series. *Front. Physiol.* **2020**, *11*, 1341. [CrossRef] [PubMed]
253. Charfeddine, S.; Ibnhadjamor, H.; Jdidi, J.; Torjmen, S.; Kraiem, S.; Bahloul, A.; Makni, A.; Kallel, N.; Moussa, N.; Boudaya, M.; et al. Sulodexide Significantly Improves Endothelial Dysfunction and Alleviates Chest Pain and Palpitations in Patients With Long-COVID-19: Insights From TUN-EndCOV Study. *Front. Cardiovasc. Med.* **2022**, *9*, 866113. [CrossRef] [PubMed]
254. Prominent Researchers Look Deeper into Fluvoxamine and See Potential as COVID-19 Treatment. *Trialsite News*. 25 April 2021. Available online: https://trialsitenews.com/prominent-researchers-look-deeper-into-fluvoxamine-see-potential-as-covid-19-treatment/ (accessed on 30 October 2023).
255. Johnson, C.K. Cheap Antidepressant Shows Promise Treating Early COVID-19. *Yahoo News*. 27 October 2021. Available online: News.yahoo.com/cheap-antidepressant-shows-promise-treating-223735055.html (accessed on 30 October 2023).
256. Sukhatme, V.P.; Reiersen, A.M.; Vayttaden, S.J.; Sukhatme, V.V. Fluvoxamine: A Review of Its Mechanism of Action and Its Role in COVID-19. *Front. Pharmacol.* **2021**, *12*, 763. [CrossRef] [PubMed]
257. Seftel, D.; Boulware, D.R. Prospective Cohort of Fluvoxamine for Early Treatment of Coronavirus Disease 19. *Open Forum Infect. Dis.* **2021**, *8*, ofab050. [CrossRef] [PubMed]
258. Facente, S.N.; Reiersen, A.M.; Lenze, E.J.; Boulware, D.R.; Klausner, J.D. Fluvoxamine for the Early Treatment of SARS-CoV-2 Infection: A Review of Current Evidence. *Drugs* **2021**, *81*, 2081–2089. [CrossRef]
259. Reis, G.; Moreira Silva, E.A.; Medeiros Silva, D.C.; Thabane, L.; Milagres, A.C.; Ferreira, T.S.; dos Santos, C.V.Q.; de Souza Campos, V.H.; Nogueira, A.M.R.; de Almeida, A.P.F.G.; et al. Effect of early treatment with fluvoxamine on risk of emergency care and hospitalisation among patients with COVID-19: The TOGETHER randomised, platform clinical trial. *Lancet Glob. Health* **2022**, *10*, e42–e51. [CrossRef]
260. Lenze, E.J.; Mattar, C.; Zorumski, C.F.; Stevens, A.; Schweiger, J.; Nicol, G.E.; Miller, J.P.; Yang, L.; Yingling, M.; Avidan, M.S.; et al. Fluvoxamine vs Placebo and Clinical Deterioration in Outpatients With Symptomatic COVID-19: A Randomized Clinical Trial. *JAMA* **2020**, *324*, 2292–2300. [CrossRef]
261. Swank, R.L.; Edwards, M.J. Microvascular occlusion by platelet emboli after transfusion and shock. *Microvasc. Res.* **1968**, *1*, 15–22. [CrossRef]
262. Alvarez, J.C.; Gluck, N.; Fallet, A.; Grégoire, A.; Chevalier, J.F.; Advenier, C.; Spreux-Varoquaux, O. Plasma serotonin level after 1 day of fluoxetine treatment: A biological predictor for antidepressant response? *Psychopharmacology* **1999**, *143*, 97–101. [CrossRef] [PubMed]
263. Celada, P.; Dolera, M.; Alvarez, E.; Artigas, F. Effects of acute and chronic treatment with fluvoxamine on extracellular and platelet serotonin in the blood of major depressive patients. Relationship to clinical improvement. *J. Affect. Disord.* **1992**, *25*, 243–249. [CrossRef] [PubMed]
264. Duerschmied, D.; Suidan, G.L.; Demers, M.; Herr, N.; Carbo, C.; Brill, A.; Cifuni, S.M.; Mauler, M.; Cicko, S.; Bader, M.; et al. Platelet serotonin promotes the recruitment of neutrophils to sites of acute inflammation in mice. *Blood* **2013**, *121*, 1008–1015. [CrossRef]

265. Gupta, M.; Neavin, D.; Liu, D.; Biernacka, J.; Hall-Flavin, D.; Bobo, W.V.; Frye, M.A.; Skime, M.; Jenkins, G.D.; Batzler, A.; et al. TSPAN5, ERICH3 and selective serotonin reuptake inhibitors in major depressive disorder: Pharmacometabolomics-informed pharmacogenomics. *Mol. Psychiatry* **2016**, *21*, 1717–1725. [CrossRef]
266. Holck, A.; Wolkowitz, O.M.; Mellon, S.H.; Reus, V.I.; Nelson, J.C.; Westrin, Å.; Lindqvist, D. Plasma serotonin levels are associated with antidepressant response to SSRIs. *J. Affect. Disord.* **2019**, *250*, 65–70. [CrossRef]
267. Kristjansdottir, H.L.; Lewerin, C.; Lerner, U.H.; Waern, E.; Johansson, H.; Sundh, D.; Karlsson, M.; Cummings, S.R.; Zetterberg, H.; Lorentzon, M.; et al. High Serum Serotonin Predicts Increased Risk for Hip Fracture and Nonvertebral Osteoporotic Fractures: The MrOS Sweden Study. *J. Bone Miner. Res.* **2018**, *33*, 1560–1567. [CrossRef]
268. Urbina, M.; Pineda, S.; Piñango, L.; Carreira, I.; Lima, L. [3H]Paroxetine binding to human peripheral lymphocyte membranes of patients with major depression before and after treatment with fluoxetine. *Int. J. Immunopharmacol.* **1999**, *21*, 631–646. [CrossRef]
269. Carneiro, A.M.; Cook, E.H.; Murphy, D.L.; Blakely, R.D. Interactions between integrin alphaIIbbeta3 and the serotonin transporter regulate serotonin transport and platelet aggregation in mice and humans. *J. Clin. Investig.* **2008**, *118*, 1544–1552. [CrossRef]
270. McCloskey, D.J.; Postolache, T.T.; Vittone, B.J.; Nghiem, K.L.; Monsale, J.L.; Wesley, R.A.; Rick, M.E. Selective serotonin reuptake inhibitors: Measurement of effect on platelet function. *Transl. Res.* **2008**, *151*, 168–172. [CrossRef]
271. Gautret, P.; Lagier, J.-C.; Parola, P.; Hoang, V.T.; Meddeb, L.; Mailhe, M.; Doudier, B.; Courjon, J.; Giordanengo, V.; Vieira, V.E.; et al. Hydroxychloroquine and azithromycin as a treatment of COVID-19: Results of an open-label non-randomized clinical trial. *Int. J. Antimicrob. Agents* **2020**, *56*, 105949. [CrossRef] [PubMed]
272. Gendrot, M.; Andreani, J.; Jardot, P.; Hutter, S.; Delandre, O.; Boxberger, M.; Mosnier, J.; Le Bideau, M.; Duflot, I.; Fonta, I.; et al. In Vitro Antiviral Activity of Doxycycline against SARS-CoV-2. *Molecules* **2020**, *25*, 5064. [CrossRef]
273. Million, M.; Cortaredona, S.; Delorme, L.; Colson, P.; Levasseur, A.; Hervé, T.-D.; Karim, B.; Salima, L.; Bernard La, S.; Laurence, C.-J.; et al. Early Treatment with Hydroxychloroquine and Azithromycin: A 'Real-Life' Monocentric Retrospective Cohort Study of 30,423 COVID-19 Patients. *medRxiv* **2023**. [CrossRef]
274. Madow, B.P. Use of antimalarial drugs as "desludging" agents in vascular disease processes: Preliminary report. *JAMA* **1960**, *172*, 1630–1633. [CrossRef] [PubMed]
275. Cecchi, E.; Ferraris, F. Desludging Action of Hydroxychloroquine in R.A. *Acta Rheumatol. Scand.* **1962**, *8*, 214–221.
276. Edwards, M.H.; Pierangeli, S.; Liu, X.; Barker, J.H.; Anderson, G.; Harris, E.N. Hydroxychloroquine Reverses Thrombogenic Properties of Antiphospholipid Antibodies in Mice. *Circulation* **1997**, *96*, 4380–4384. [CrossRef]
277. Nallusamy, S.; Mannu, J.; Ravikumar, C.; Angamuthu, K.; Nathan, B.; Nachimuthu, K.; Ramasamy, G.; Muthurajan, R.; Subbarayalu, M.; Neelakandan, K. Exploring Phytochemicals of Traditional Medicinal Plants Exhibiting Inhibitory Activity Against Main Protease, Spike Glycoprotein, RNA-dependent RNA Polymerase and Non-Structural Proteins of SARS-CoV-2 Through Virtual Screening. *Front. Pharmacol.* **2021**, *12*, 667704. [CrossRef]
278. Kalhor, H.; Sadeghi, S.; Abolhasani, H.; Kalhor, R.; Rahimi, H. Repurposing of the approved small molecule drugs in order to inhibit SARS-CoV-2 S protein and human ACE2 interaction through virtual screening approaches. *J. Biomol. Struct. Dyn.* **2020**, *40*, 1299–1315. [CrossRef]
279. Suravajhala, R.; Parashar, A.; Malik, B.; Nagaraj, V.A.; Padmanaban, G.; Kavi Kishor, P.B.; Polavarapu, R.; Suravajhala, P. Comparative Docking Studies on Curcumin with COVID-19 Proteins. *Preprints.Org* **2020**. [CrossRef]
280. Yagisawa, M.; Foster, P.J.; Hanaki, H.; Omura, S. Global Trends in Clinical Studies of Ivermectin in COVID-19. *Jpn. J. Antibiot.* **2021**, *74*, 44–95.
281. Juarez, M.; Schcolnik-Cabrera, A.; Dueñas-Gonzalez, A. The multitargeted drug ivermectin: From an antiparasitic agent to a repositioned cancer drug. *Am. J. Cancer Res.* **2018**, *8*, 317–331. [PubMed]
282. Campbell, W.C. History of avermectin and ivermectin, with notes on the history of other macrocyclic lactone antiparasitic agents. *Curr. Pharm. Biotechnol.* **2012**, *13*, 853–865. [CrossRef]
283. Chang, M.W.; Lindstrom, W.; Olson, A.J.; Belew, R.K. Analysis of HIV Wild-Type and Mutant Structures via in Silico Docking against Diverse Ligand Libraries. *J. Chem. Inf. Model.* **2007**, *47*, 1258–1262. [CrossRef] [PubMed]
284. Dasgupta, J.; Sen, U.; Bakashi, A.; Dasgupta, A. Nsp7 and Spike Glycoprotein of SARS-CoV-2 Are Envisaged as Potential Targets of Vitamin D and Ivermectin. *Preprints.Org* **2020**. [CrossRef]
285. Hussien, M.A.; Abdelaziz, A.E.M. Molecular docking suggests repurposing of brincidofovir as a potential drug targeting SARS-CoV-2 ACE2 receptor and main protease. *Netw. Model. Anal. Health Inform. Bioinform.* **2020**, *9*, 56. [CrossRef]
286. Kaur, H.; Shekhar, N.; Sharma, S.; Sarma, P.; Prakash, A.; Medhi, B. Ivermectin as a potential drug for treatment of COVID-19: An in-sync review with clinical and computational attributes. *Pharmacol. Rep.* **2021**, *73*, 736–749. [CrossRef] [PubMed]
287. Maurya, D. A Combination of Ivermectin and Doxycycline Possibly Blocks the Viral Entry and Modulate the Innate Immune Response in COVID-19 Patients. *ChemRxiv* **2020**. [CrossRef]
288. Saha, J.K.; Raihan, J. The Binding mechanism of Ivermectin and levosalbutamol with spike protein of SARS-CoV-2. *Struct. Chem.* **2021**, *32*, 1985–1992. [CrossRef]
289. Lehrer, S.; Rheinstein, P.H. Ivermectin Docks to the SARS-CoV-2 Spike Receptor-binding Domain Attached to ACE2. *In Vivo* **2020**, *34*, 3023–3026. [CrossRef]
290. Rajter, J.J.; (Broward Health Medical Center, Fort Lauderdale, FL, USA). Personal communication, 28 May 2020.
291. Local Doctor Tries New Coronavirus Drug Treatment. *NBC Miami News*. 14 April 2020. Available online: https://www.nbcmiami.com/news/local/local-doctor-tries-new-coronavirus-drug-treatment/2219465/ (accessed on 30 October 2023).

292. Rajter, J.C.; Sherman, M.S.; Fatteh, N.; Vogel, F.; Sacks, J.; Rajter, J.-J. Use of Ivermectin is Associated with Lower Mortality in Hospitalized Patients with COVID-19 (ICON study). *Chest* **2020**, *159*, 85–92. [CrossRef]
293. Santin, A.D.; Scheim, D.E.; McCullough, P.A.; Yagisawa, M.; Borody, T.J. Ivermectin: A multifaceted drug of Nobel prize-honored distinction with indicated efficacy against a new global scourge, COVID-19. *New Microbes New Infect.* **2021**, *43*, 100924. [CrossRef] [PubMed]
294. Abdool Karim, S.S.; Devnarain, N. Time to Stop Using Ineffective COVID-19 Drugs. *N. Engl. J. Med.* **2022**, *387*, 654–655. [CrossRef] [PubMed]
295. Shafiee, A.; Teymouri Athar, M.M.; Kohandel Gargari, O.; Jafarabady, K.; Siahvoshi, S.; Mozhgani, S.-H. Ivermectin under scrutiny: A systematic review and meta-analysis of efficacy and possible sources of controversies in COVID-19 patients. *Virol. J.* **2022**, *19*, 102. [CrossRef] [PubMed]
296. Reis, G.; Moreira Silva, E.A.; Medeiros Silva, D.C.; Thabane, L.; Milagres, A.C.; Ferreira, T.S.; dos Santos, C.V.Q.; Campos, V.H.S.; Nogueira, A.M.R.; de Almeida, A.P.F.G.; et al. Effect of Early Treatment with Ivermectin among Patients with COVID-19. *N. Engl. J. Med.* **2022**, *386*, 1721–1731. [CrossRef] [PubMed]
297. Scheim, D.E.; Aldous, C.; Osimani, B.; Fordham, E.J.; Hoy, W.E. When Characteristics of Clinical Trials Require Per-Protocol as Well as Intention-to-Treat Outcomes to Draw Reliable Conclusions: Three Examples. *J. Clin. Med.* **2023**, *12*, 3625. [CrossRef] [PubMed]
298. U.S. Food & Drug Administration. Memorandum Explaining Basis for Declining Request for Emergency Use Authorization of Fluvoxamine Maleate. Available online: https://www.accessdata.fda.gov/drugsatfda_docs/nda/2020/EUA%2520110%2520Fluvoxamine%2520Decisional%2520Memo_Redacted.pdf (accessed on 30 October 2023).
299. NIH COVID-19 Treatment Guidelines. Fluvoxamine: Selected Clinical Data, Limitations and Interpretation. Table 4c. 16 December 2021. Available online: https://www.covid19treatmentguidelines.nih.gov/tables/fluvoxamine-data/ (accessed on 30 October 2023).
300. TOGETHER Trial DSS and Data Repository Screenshots. Date-Time Stamped Screenshots from Publications of the TOGETHER trial (NCT04727424). Available online: https://drive.google.com/file/d/1pBZ1GihxW_ROB3Aid6tFMplqAyMYOGDl/preview (accessed on 30 October 2023).
301. Email from Sarah Fullegar, Sent 7 June 2022 to Edmund Fordham, Screenshot, Email Addresses Redacted. Available online: https://drive.google.com/file/d/1lUsSRf1KX-pa9T5EX4HbegdK8mYNQ_Ty/preview (accessed on 30 October 2023).
302. López-Medina, E.; López, P.; Hurtado, I.C.; Dávalos, D.M.; Ramirez, O.; Martínez, E.; Díazgranados, J.A.; Oñate, J.M.; Chavarriaga, H.; Herrera, S.; et al. Effect of Ivermectin on Time to Resolution of Symptoms Among Adults With Mild COVID-19: A Randomized Clinical Trial. *JAMA* **2021**, *325*, 1426–1435. [CrossRef]
303. Scheim, D.E.; Hibberd, J.A.; Chamie-Quintero, J.J. Protocol Violations in López-Medina et al.: 38 Switched Ivermectin (IVM) and Placebo Doses, Failure of Blinding, Ubiquitous IVM use OTC in Cali, and Nearly Identical AEs for the IVM and Control Groups. *OSF Preprints*. 2021. [CrossRef]
304. George, L.L.; Borody, T.J.; Andrews, P.; Devine, M.; Moore-Jones, D.; Walton, M.; Brandl, S. Cure of duodenal ulcer after eradication of *Helicobacter pylori*. *Med. J. Aust.* **1990**, *153*, 145–149. [CrossRef]
305. Coghlan, J.G.; Gilligan, D.; Humphries, H.; McKenna, D.; Dooley, C.; Sweeney, E.; Keane, C.; O'Morain, C. Campylobacter pylori and recurrence of duodenal ulcers—A 12-month follow-up study. *Lancet* **1987**, *2*, 1109–1111. [CrossRef]
306. Graham, D.Y.; Lew, G.M.; Klein, P.D.; Evans, D.G.; Evans, D.J., Jr.; Saeed, Z.A.; Malaty, H.M. Effect of treatment of Helicobacter pylori infection on the long-term recurrence of gastric or duodenal ulcer. A randomized, controlled study. *Ann. Intern. Med.* **1992**, *116*, 705–708. [CrossRef]
307. Watts, G. Nobel prize is awarded to doctors who discovered H pylori. *BMJ* **2005**, *331*, 795. [CrossRef]
308. Fleming, A. On the Antibacterial Action of Cultures of a Penicillium, with Special Reference to their Use in the Isolation of B. influenzæ. *Br. J. Exp. Pathol.* **1929**, *10*, 226–236. [CrossRef]
309. Chain, E.; Florey, H.W.; Gardner, A.D.; Heatley, N.G.; Jennings, M.A.; Orr-Ewing, J.; Sanders, A.G. Penicillin as a chemotherapeutic agent. *Lancet* **1940**, *236*, 226–228. [CrossRef]
310. Lobanovska, M.; Pilla, G. Penicillin's Discovery and Antibiotic Resistance: Lessons for the Future? *Yale J. Biol. Med.* **2017**, *90*, 135–145.
311. Annunziata, A.; Coppola, A.; Carannante, N.; Simioli, F.; Lanza, M.; Di Micco, P.; Fiorentino, G. Home Management of Patients with Moderate or Severe Respiratory Failure Secondary to COVID-19, Using Remote Monitoring and Oxygen with or without HFNC. *Pathogens* **2021**, *10*, 413. [CrossRef]
312. Aoki, R.; Iwasawa, T.; Hagiwara, E.; Komatsu, S.; Utsunomiya, D.; Ogura, T. Pulmonary vascular enlargement and lesion extent on computed tomography are correlated with COVID-19 disease severity. *Jpn. J. Radiol.* **2021**, *39*, 451–458. [CrossRef] [PubMed]
313. Ding, X.; Xu, J.; Zhou, J.; Long, Q. Chest CT findings of COVID-19 pneumonia by duration of symptoms. *Eur. J. Radiol.* **2020**, *127*, 109009. [CrossRef] [PubMed]
314. Metwally, M.I.; Basha, M.A.A.; Zaitoun, M.M.A.; Abdalla, H.M.; Nofal, H.A.E.; Hendawy, H.; Manajrah, E.; Hijazy, R.f.; Akbazli, L.; Negida, A.; et al. Clinical and radiological imaging as prognostic predictors in COVID-19 patients. *Egypt. J. Radiol. Nucl. Med.* **2021**, *52*, 100. [CrossRef]
315. Osman, A.M.; Farouk, S.; Osman, N.M.; Abdrabou, A.M. Longitudinal assessment of chest computerized tomography and oxygen saturation for patients with COVID-19. *Egypt. J. Radiol. Nucl. Med.* **2020**, *51*, 255. [CrossRef]

316. Quispe-Cholan, A.; Anticona-De-La-Cruz, Y.; Cornejo-Cruz, M.; Quispe-Chirinos, O.; Moreno-Lazaro, V.; Chavez-Cruzado, E. Tomographic findings in patients with COVID-19 according to evolution of the disease. *Egypt. J. Radiol. Nucl. Med.* **2020**, *51*, 215. [CrossRef]
317. Wang, Y.; Dong, C.; Hu, Y.; Li, C.; Ren, Q.; Zhang, X.; Shi, H.; Zhou, M. Temporal Changes of CT Findings in 90 Patients with COVID-19 Pneumonia: A Longitudinal Study. *Radiology* **2020**, *296*, e55–e64. [CrossRef]
318. Stone, J.C.; Ndarukwa, P.; Scheim, D.E.; Dancis, B.M.; Dancis, J.; Gill, M.G.; Aldous, C. Changes in SpO2 on Room Air for 34 Severe COVID-19 Patients after Ivermectin-Based Combination Treatment: 62% Normalization within 24 Hours. *Biologics* **2022**, *2*, 196–210. [CrossRef]
319. Hazan, S.; Dave, S.; Gunaratne, A.W.; Dolai, S.; Clancy, R.L.; McCullough, P.A.; Borody, T.J. Effectiveness of ivermectin-based multidrug therapy in severely hypoxic, ambulatory COVID-19 patients. *Future Microbiol.* **2022**, *17*, 339–350. [CrossRef] [PubMed]
320. Babalola, O.E.; Ndanusa, Y.; Adesuyi, A.; Ogedengbe, O.J.; Thairu, Y.; Ogu, O. A Randomized Controlled Trial of Ivermectin Monotherapy Versus HCQ, IVM, and AZ Combination Therapy in COVID-19 Patients in Nigeria. *J. Infect. Dis. Epidemiol.* **2021**, *7*, 233. [CrossRef]
321. Babalola, O.E.; (Bingham University, New Karu, Nigeria). Personal communication, 28 February 2022.
322. Thairu, Y.; Babalola, O.E.; Ajayi, A.A.; Ndanusa, Y.; Ogedengbe, J.O.; Omede, O. A comparison of Ivermectin and Non Ivermectin based regimen for COVID-19 in Abuja: Effects on virus clearance, Days-to-Discharge and Mortality. *Res. Sq.* **2022**, *34*, 1–19. [CrossRef]
323. Chamie, J.J.; Hibberd, J.A.; Scheim, D.E. COVID-19 Excess Deaths in Peru's 25 States in 2020: Nationwide Trends, Confounding Factors, and Correlations With the Extent of Ivermectin Treatment by State. *Cureus* **2023**, *15*, e43168. [CrossRef] [PubMed]
324. Meekins, D.A.; Gaudreault, N.N.; Richt, J.A. Natural and Experimental SARS-CoV-2 Infection in Domestic and Wild Animals. *Viruses* **2021**, *13*, 1993. [CrossRef] [PubMed]
325. Baskurt, O.K.; Meiselman, H.J. Comparative hemorheology. *Clin. Hemorheol. Microcirc.* **2013**, *53*, 61–70. [CrossRef]
326. Rampling, M.W.; Meiselman, H.J.; Neu, B.; Baskurt, O.K. Influence of cell-specific factors on red blood cell aggregation. *Biorheology* **2004**, *41*, 91–112.
327. Popel, A.S.; Johnson, P.C.; Kameneva, M.V.; Wild, M.A. Capacity for red blood cell aggregation is higher in athletic mammalian species than in sedentary species. *J. Appl. Physiol. (1985)* **1994**, *77*, 1790–1794. [CrossRef]
328. Weng, X.; Cloutier, G.; Pibarot, P.; Durand, L.G. Comparison and simulation of different levels of erythrocyte aggregation with pig, horse, sheep, calf, and normal human blood. *Biorheology* **1996**, *33*, 365–377. [CrossRef]
329. Wernike, K.; Böttcher, J.; Amelung, S.; Albrecht, K.; Gärtner, T.; Donat, K.; Beer, M. Antibodies against SARS-CoV-2 Suggestive of Single Events of Spillover to Cattle, Germany. *Emerg. Infect. Dis. J.* **2022**, *28*, 1916. [CrossRef] [PubMed]
330. Bosco-Lauth, A.M.; Walker, A.; Guilbert, L.; Porter, S.; Hartwig, A.; McVicker, E.; Bielefeldt-Ohmann, H.; Bowen, R.A. Susceptibility of livestock to SARS-CoV-2 infection. *Emerg. Microbes Infect.* **2021**, *10*, 2199–2201. [CrossRef] [PubMed]
331. Wessa.net Free Statistics Software, Office for Research Development and Education, Version 1.2.1. Available online: https://www.wessa.net/ (accessed on 30 October 2023).
332. Nemkov, T.; Reisz, J.A.; Xia, Y.; Zimring, J.C.; D'Alessandro, A. Red blood cells as an organ? How deep omics characterization of the most abundant cell in the human body highlights other systemic metabolic functions beyond oxygen transport. *Expert Rev. Proteom.* **2018**, *15*, 855–864. [CrossRef] [PubMed]
333. Sender, R.; Fuchs, S.; Milo, R. Revised Estimates for the Number of Human and Bacteria Cells in the Body. *PLoS Biol.* **2016**, *14*, e1002533. [CrossRef] [PubMed]
334. Chang, V.T.; Crispin, M.; Aricescu, A.R.; Harvey, D.J.; Nettleship, J.E.; Fennelly, J.A.; Yu, C.; Boles, K.S.; Evans, E.J.; Stuart, D.I.; et al. Glycoprotein structural genomics: Solving the glycosylation problem. *Structure* **2007**, *15*, 267–273. [CrossRef] [PubMed]
335. Lee, J.E.; Fusco, M.L.; Saphire, E.O. An efficient platform for screening expression and crystallization of glycoproteins produced in human cells. *Nat. Protoc.* **2009**, *4*, 592–604. [CrossRef]
336. Dill, K.; Hu, S.H.; Berman, E.; Pavia, A.A.; Lacombe, J.M. One- and two-dimensional NMR studies of the N-terminal portion of glycophorin A at 11.7 Tesla. *J. Protein Chem.* **1990**, *9*, 129–136. [CrossRef]
337. Ekman, S.; Flower, R.; Mahler, S.; Gould, A.; Barnard, R.T.; Hyland, C.; Jones, M.; Malde, A.K.; Bui, X.T. In silico molecular dynamics of human glycophorin A (GPA) extracellular structure. *Ann. Blood* **2021**, *6*, 1–17. [CrossRef]
338. Trivedi, R.; Nagarajaram, H.A. Intrinsically disordered proteins: An overview. *Int. J. Mol. Sci.* **2022**, *23*, 14050. [CrossRef]
339. Uversky, V.N.; Dunker, A.K. Understanding protein non-folding. *Biochim. Biophys. Acta (BBA)-Proteins Proteom.* **2010**, *1804*, 1231–1264. [CrossRef]
340. Uversky, V.N.; Gillespie, J.R.; Fink, A.L. Why are "natively unfolded" proteins unstructured under physiologic conditions? *Proteins* **2000**, *41*, 415–427. [CrossRef] [PubMed]
341. Seet, R.C.S.; Quek, A.M.L.; Ooi, D.S.Q.; Sengupta, S.; Lakshminarasappa, S.R.; Koo, C.Y.; So, J.B.Y.; Goh, B.C.; Loh, K.S.; Fisher, D.; et al. Positive impact of oral hydroxychloroquine and povidone-iodine throat spray for COVID-19 prophylaxis: An open-label randomized trial. *Int. J. Infect. Dis.* **2021**, *106*, 314–322. [CrossRef]
342. Horton, R. Offline: What is medicine's 5 sigma? *Lancet* **2015**, *385*, 1380. [CrossRef]
343. Ioannidis, J.P. Evidence-based medicine has been hijacked: A report to David Sackett. *J. Clin. Epidemiol.* **2016**, *73*, 82–86. [CrossRef] [PubMed]

344. Steinbrook, R.; Kassirer, J.P.; Angell, M. Justifying conflicts of interest in medical journals: A very bad idea. *BMJ* **2015**, *350*, h2942. [CrossRef] [PubMed]
345. Carlisle, J.B. False individual patient data and zombie randomised controlled trials submitted to Anaesthesia. *Anaesthesia* **2021**, *76*, 472–479. [CrossRef] [PubMed]
346. Gotzsche, P. *Deadly Medicines and Organised Crime: How Big Pharma Has Corrupted Healthcare*, 1st ed.; CRC Press: London, UK, 2013.
347. Saltelli, A.; Dankel, D.J.; Di Fiore, M.; Holland, N.; Pigeon, M. Science, the endless frontier of regulatory capture. *Futures* **2022**, *135*, 102860. [CrossRef]
348. Eslick, G.D.; Tilden, D.; Arora, N.; Torres, M.; Clancy, R.L. Clinical and economic impact of "triple therapy" for *Helicobacter pylori* eradication on peptic ulcer disease in Australia. *Helicobacter* **2020**, *25*, e12751. [CrossRef]
349. Berndt, E.R.; Kyle, M.; Ling, D. The Long Shadow of Patent Expiration: Generic Entry and Rx-to-OTC Switches. In *Scanner Data and Price Indexes*; Feenstra, R.C., Shapiro, M.D., Eds.; University of Chicago Press: Chicago, IL, USA, 2003; pp. 229–274.
350. Chatterjee, S.; Bhattacharya, M.; Nag, S.; Dhama, K.; Chakraborty, C. A Detailed Overview of SARS-CoV-2 Omicron: Its Sub-Variants, Mutations and Pathophysiology, Clinical Characteristics, Immunological Landscape, Immune Escape, and Therapies. *Viruses* **2023**, *15*, 167. [CrossRef]
351. Hui, K.P.Y.; Ho, J.C.W.; Cheung, M.-c.; Ng, K.-c.; Ching, R.H.H.; Lai, K.-l.; Kam, T.T.; Gu, H.; Sit, K.-Y.; Hsin, M.K.Y.; et al. SARS-CoV-2 Omicron variant replication in human bronchus and lung ex vivo. *Nature* **2022**, *603*, 715–720. [CrossRef]
352. Peacock, T.P.; Brown, J.C.; Zhou, J.; Thakur, N.; Sukhova, K.; Newman, J.; Kugathasan, R.; Yan, A.W.C.; Furnon, W.; De Lorenzo, G.; et al. The altered entry pathway and antigenic distance of the SARS-CoV-2 Omicron variant map to separate domains of spike protein. *bioRxiv* **2022**. [CrossRef]
353. D'Agnillo, F.; Walters, K.-A.; Xiao, Y.; Sheng, Z.-M.; Scherler, K.; Park, J.; Gygli, S.; Rosas, L.A.; Sadtler, K.; Kalish, H.; et al. Lung epithelial and endothelial damage, loss of tissue repair, inhibition of fibrinolysis, and cellular senescence in fatal COVID-19. *Sci. Transl. Med.* **2021**, *13*, eabj7790. [CrossRef] [PubMed]
354. Makary, M. The Real Data Behind the New COVID Vaccines the White Houseis Pushing. *New York Post*. 14 September 2023. Available online: https://nypost.com/2023/09/14/the-real-data-behind-the-new-covid-vaccines-the-white-house-is-pushing/ (accessed on 30 October 2023).
355. Bramante, C.T.; Buse, J.B.; Liebovitz, D.M.; Nicklas, J.M.; Puskarich, M.A.; Cohen, K.; Belani, H.K.; Anderson, B.J.; Huling, J.D.; Tignanelli, C.J.; et al. Outpatient treatment of COVID-19 and incidence of post-COVID-19 condition over 10 months (COVID-OUT): A multicentre, randomised, quadruple-blind, parallel-group, phase 3 trial. *Lancet Infect. Dis.* **2023**, *23*, 1119–1129. [CrossRef] [PubMed]
356. McCarthy, M.W.; Naggie, S.; Boulware, D.R.; Lindsell, C.J.; Stewart, T.G.; Felker, G.M.; Jayaweera, D.; Sulkowski, M.; Gentile, N.; Bramante, C.; et al. Effect of Fluvoxamine vs Placebo on Time to Sustained Recovery in Outpatients With Mild to Moderate COVID-19: A Randomized Clinical Trial. *JAMA* **2023**, *329*, 296–305. [CrossRef] [PubMed]
357. Wang, H.; Yu, M.; Ochani, M.; Amella, C.A.; Tanovic, M.; Susarla, S.; Li, J.H.; Wang, H.; Yang, H.; Ulloa, L.; et al. Nicotinic acetylcholine receptor α7 subunit is an essential regulator of inflammation. *Nature* **2003**, *421*, 384–388. [CrossRef]
358. Krause, R.M.; Buisson, B.; Bertrand, S.; Corringer, P.J.; Galzi, J.L.; Changeux, J.P.; Bertrand, D. Ivermectin: A positive allosteric effector of the alpha7 neuronal nicotinic acetylcholine receptor. *Mol. Pharmacol.* **1998**, *53*, 283–294. [CrossRef]
359. Fajgenbaum, D.C.; June, C.H. Cytokine Storm. *N. Engl. J. Med.* **2020**, *383*, 2255–2273. [CrossRef]

International Journal of
Molecular Sciences

MDPI

Article

IL-6 and Neutrophil/Lymphocyte Ratio as Markers of ICU Admittance in SARS-CoV-2 Patients with Diabetes

Iulia Făgărășan [1], Adriana Rusu [2,*], Horațiu Comșa [3], Tudor-Dan Simu [4], Damiana-Maria Vulturar [1] and Doina-Adina Todea [1]

1 Department of Pneumology, "Iuliu Hațieganu" University of Medicine and Pharmacy, 400332 Cluj-Napoca, Romania; fagarasan_iulia@elearn.umfcluj.ro (I.F.); vulturar.damianamaria@elearn.umfcluj.ro (D.-M.V.); dtodea@umfcluj.ro (D.-A.T.)

2 Department of Diabetes and Nutrition Diseases, "Iuliu Hațieganu" University of Medicine and Pharmacy, 400006 Cluj-Napoca, Romania

3 Cardiology Department, Clinical Rehabilitation Hospital, "Iuliu Hațieganu" University of Medicine and Pharmacy, 400012 Cluj-Napoca, Romania; dh.comsa@gmail.com

4 Intensive Care Department, "Leon Daniello" Pulmonology Hospital, 400332 Cluj-Napoca, Romania; tudor.simu@gmail.com

* Correspondence: adriana.rusu@umfcluj.ro

Abstract: Inflammation along with coagulation disturbances has an essential role in the evolution towards a severe disease in patients with the coronavirus disease 2019 (COVID-19). This study aimed to evaluate inflammatory and coagulation biomarkers when predicting the need to visit an intensive care unit (ICU) in diabetes mellitus (DM) patients. In a retrospective study, laboratory parameters were examined for 366 participants: ICU = 90, of which 44 patients had DM and no ICU admittance = 276. The ability of inflammatory and coagulation markers to distinguish the severity of COVID-19 was determined using univariate and multivariate regression analysis. In all patients, lactate dehydrogenase was the only predictor for ICU admittance in the multivariate analysis. In the DM group, the results showed that the interleukin (IL)-6 and neutrophil/lymphocyte ratio (NLR) values at admission could predict the need for ICU admittance. Even though there were significant differences between the ICU and no ICU admittance groups regarding the coagulation markers, they could not predict the severity of the disease in DM patients. The present study showed for the first time that the IL-6 and NLR admission values could predict ICU admittance in DM patients. This finding could help clinicians manage the infection more easily if the COVID-19 pandemic strikes again.

Keywords: COVID-19; inflammation; coagulopathy; diabetes mellitus; severity

Citation: Făgărășan, I.; Rusu, A.; Comșa, H.; Simu, T.-D.; Vulturar, D.-M.; Todea, D.-A. IL-6 and Neutrophil/Lymphocyte Ratio as Markers of ICU Admittance in SARS-CoV-2 Patients with Diabetes. *Int. J. Mol. Sci.* **2023**, *24*, 14908. https://doi.org/10.3390/ijms241914908

Academic Editor: Eleni Gavriilaki

Received: 31 August 2023
Revised: 18 September 2023
Accepted: 28 September 2023
Published: 5 October 2023

1. Introduction

The severe acute respiratory syndrome coronavirus-2 (SARS-CoV-2) has been identified as the etiology of an outbreak that occurred in 2020 in Wuhan, China. Although the majority of patients developed mild to moderate symptoms with favorable evolution, a minority of patients with the coronavirus disease 2019 (COVID-19) had severe pneumonia, pulmonary edema, coagulation abnormalities with disseminated intravascular coagulation, acute respiratory distress syndrome (ARDS), septic shock, or even multiple organ failures, requiring hospitalization in the intensive care unit (ICU) or even leading to death [1]. All ages are prone to becoming infected but accumulating evidence has demonstrated that elderly individuals with comorbidities, such as hypertension, diabetes mellitus (DM), and cardio-vascular diseases (CVDs), are especially at a high risk of developing the severe disease, with a poor evolution and prognosis [2–4].

DM is a chronic metabolic disease with associated low-grade chronic inflammation [5]. Diabetes itself leads to increased cytokine production, including interleukin (IL)-1, IL-6, IL-8, and tumor necrosis factor-α (TNF-α) [6]. Also, is known to be involved in the dysregulation of the glycosylation of the fragment crystallizable region of immunoglobulin G (IgG Fc) [7]. Given these disturbances in the immune system, patients with DM are more susceptible to viral and bacterial infectious diseases [5,8].

During COVID-19, it has been shown that hyperglycemia along with a pre-existing chronic inflammation in DM patients increases the risk of an abnormal immune response and a hyperinflammatory status followed by a cytokine storm [9]. These changes are associated with an increased risk of ICU hospitalization and high mortality [4]. Inflammation has been linked to a prothrombotic status, expressed by a high level of coagulation markers: D-dimer, fibrinogen, and prothrombin time [10]. A high incidence of venous thromboembolism, pulmonary thromboembolism, stroke, or acute coronary syndrome was observed with COVID-19 [11]. In patients with DM, coagulation disorder [12] and endothelial dysfunction are essential risk factors that aggravate the infection.

Considering that during the SARS-CoV-2 infection, the morbidity and mortality among patients with diabetes were higher compared to the general population (especially for unvaccinated patients), establishing biomarkers that could be used as predictors of severity would be useful from a clinical point of view. Given the broad-spectrum clinical presentation and the potential variability of disease evolution, early recognition of a hyperinflammatory and hypercoagulation state would allow the timely application of preventive measures for a fulminant evolution.

Therefore, this study aimed to evaluate the predictive value of routinely determined inflammatory biomarkers to differentiate severe—with need of ICU—from non-severe cases in patients with DM. Secondary objectives included the evaluation of coagulation markers as predictors of disease severity.

2. Results

2.1. Demographic and Baseline Characteristics of ICU Patients and Those Who Did Not Require ICU Admittance

During this study, 588 patients were hospitalized for the SARS-CoV2 infection. After applying the inclusion and exclusion criteria, 366 were included in this study. Of the total number of participants, 90 were transferred to the ICU during hospitalization (44 with diabetes and 46 without diabetes). Figure 1 presents the flowchart of the participants' selection criteria and the distribution of the study population.

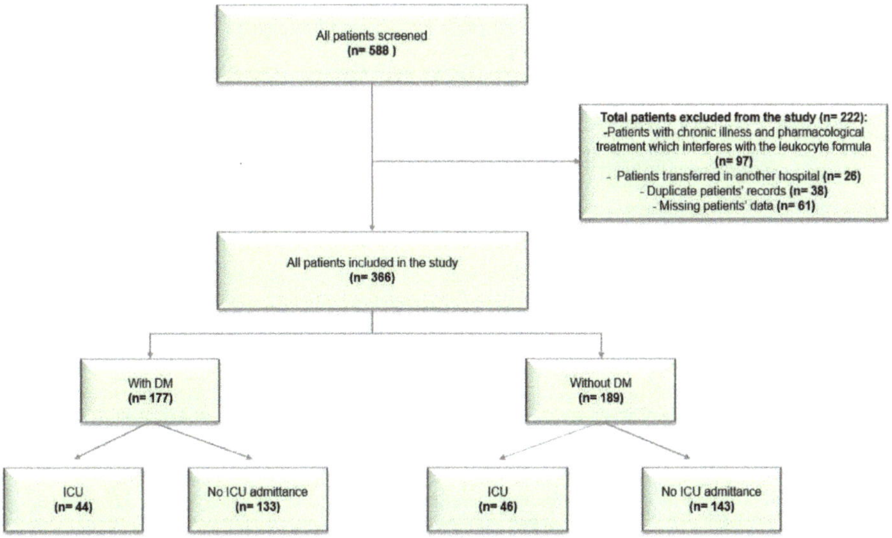

Figure 1. Flow chart of screening and enrolment of the participants.

The baseline characteristics of patients are summarized in Table 1. The median age was 68.5 (IQR 23-99) years and 228 (62.29%) were men. Of all patients, 177 were known to have type 2 diabetes. Of the total number of participants, 90 patients were admitted to the ICU department (ICU group), of which 44 had diabetes. Patients admitted to the ICU had more frequent obesity (92.22% vs. 82.24%, $p = 0.001$) or advanced-stage abnormalities on chest CT (ground-glass opacities—$p < 0.001$, and total severity score—$p < 0.001$), with a higher rate of mortality in the hospital—62.2% vs. 15.2%, $p < 0.0001$.

Table 1. Demographic and radiologic characteristics of the participants.

Characteristics		Total Patients n = 366		ICU n = 90		No ICU Admittance n = 276		
		No.	%	No.	%	No.	%	*p*-Value
Age, years (median; Q1, Q3)		68.5	[23–99]	69	[63–75]	68	[60–77]	0.627
Men, n %		228	62.29	51	56.66	177	64.13	0.205
Comorbidities, n (%)	**Obesity ($BMI \geq 30$ kg/m^2)**	153	41.8	83	92.22	227	82.24	**0.001**
	Hypertension	133	75.4	70	77.8	206	74.6	0.548
	Cardiovascular disease	24	56.6	54	60	153	55.4	0.448
	Diabetes mellitus	177	48.4	44	48.9	133	48.2	0.908
	Respiratory disease	135	18.6	19	21.1	49	17.8	0.477
Disease severity								
-mild		36	9.8	2	2.2	34	12.3	**<0.0001**
-moderate		63	17.2	4	4.4	59	21.4	
-severe		266	72.7	84	93.4	182	65.6	
Ground-glass opacity (n, %)		198	54.1	63	70.0	135	48.9	**<0.0001**
TSS								
1		181	49.6	31	34.4	150	54.5	**<0.0001**
2		82	22.5	11	12.2	71	25.8	
3		60	16.4	23	25.6	37	13.5	
4		42	11.5	25	27.8	17	6.2	
Vaccinated		34	9.3	7	7.8	27	9.8	0.569
Mechanical ventilation		52	14.2	49	54.4	3	1.1	**<0.0001**
Mortality		98	26.8	56	62.2	42	15.2	**<0.0001**

Data are expressed by median (minimum value–maximum value) or n%. *p* values comparing ICU patients and patients with no ICU admittance; BMI—body mass index; disease severity: mild: clinical symptoms without abnormal radiological findings; moderate: pneumonia on chest computed tomography (CT) without fulfilling any criterion for severe disease; severe: respiratory distress, a respiratory rate $\geq$30 per minute, $SpO_2 \leq 93\%$, or partial pressure of arterial oxygen/concentration of oxygen inhaled (PaO_2/FiO_2 ratio) $\leq$300 mmHg; TSS—total severity score; the sum of acute inflammatory lung lesions involving each lobe was scored as follows: 1—0–25%; 2-mild involvement: 26–50%; 3-moderate involvement: 51–75%; severe involvement—76–100%.

The routine blood parameters recorded on the first day of admission were further compared between the ICU and non-ICU admittance groups, as shown in Table 2. Compared to those without ICU admittance, subjects in the ICU group had a significantly higher white blood cell (WBC) count and neutrophilia but lower lymphocyte and platelet counts. Those without ICU admittance had significantly higher lymphocyte levels. Concerning coagulation markers, D-dimers were higher in the ICU group than in the group without ICU admittance, with $p = 0.001$. Thrombocytopenia was more frequently encountered in patients requiring ICU—$p = 0.049$. The platelet-to-albumin ratio (P/Alb) was lower in ICU patients. No significant difference was observed for other tested parameters.

Table 2. Laboratory findings at admission.

Parameters	Total Patients n = 366		ICU n = 90		No ICU Admittance n = 276		p Value
White blood cells ×10³/L	8.24	[1.81–39.69]	8.62	[5.39–11.24]	7.06	[5.29–10.01]	**0.023**
Neutrophil count, ×10³/L	6.87	[0.18–102.3]	6.79	[4.47–9.65]	5.43	[3.73–8.12]	**0.007**
Monocyte count ×10³/L	0.42	[0.01–1.37]	0.35	[0.21–0.51]	0.37	[0.26–0.59]	0.084
Lymphocyte count, ×10³/L	1.35	[0.1–54]	0.84	[0.64–1.15]	1.02	[0.74–1.51]	**0.001**
Eosinophil count, ×10³/L	0.17	[0–1.98]	0	[0–0.01]	0.005	[0–0.107]	**0.001**
Platelets count, ×10³/L	245.7	[34.7–634]	205	[159.75–282.25]	230.50	[174.25–308.25]	**0.049**
D-dimer, µg/mL	1429.79	[0.08–39698]	807	[434.5–1852.5]	539.5	[321–940]	**0.001**
Fibrinogen, mg/dL	412.65	[317.77–507.95]	415	[314.5–496.25]	412.65	[318.05–513.07]	0.323
Albumin, g/mL	3.30	[3.06–3.69]	3.27	[3.14–3.72]	3.33	[2.96–3.67]	0.262
Troponin, ng/mL	0.85	[0.05–5.70]	0.50	[0.05–1.20]	1.03	[0.06–1.30]	**0.011**
NT-proBNP	2148.36	[50–12931]	941	[50–4253]	742	[112.25–3082.75]	0.945
INR	1.06	[0.82–1.65]	1.01	[0.93–1.14]	1.01	[0.91–1.16]	0.613
aPTT (s)	24.02	[17.2–34.9]	27	[22.1–29.2]	22.1	[18.85–25.25]	0.110
Prothrombin time (s)	11.4	[8.1–17.2P]	11.8	[9.3–17.1]	11.3	[8.1–17.2]	0.842
PLR	281.58	[4.82–1754.54]	253.9	[164.05–345.1]	214.96	[143.26–356.78]	0.098
Fbg/Alb	131.17	[48.23–342.58]	120.08	[90.29–149.44]	123.36	[96.51–163.51]	0.265
P/Alb	66.66	[50.33–98.05]	60.99	[47.98–85.24]	67.77	[51.81–103.09]	**0.031**

INR—international normalized ratio; aPTT—activated partial thromboplastin time; PLR—platelet/lymphocyte ratio; Fbg/Alb—fibrinogen/albumin ratio; P/Alb—platelet/albumin ratio; s- second.

The results for inflammatory biomarkers at admittance are presented in Figure 2. The analysis revealed that patients admitted to the ICU department had statistically significant values, with $p < 0.05$, for C-reactive protein (CRP)—71.7 (range; 20.89–120.37) mg/L vs. 33.55 (10.53–86.15) mg/L, IL-6—35.03 (range; 16.9–82.62) pg/mL vs. 21.9 (range; 8.83–48.85) pg/mL, ferritin—842.5 (range; 353.5–1655.5) ng/mL vs. 569.9 (range; 278.9–1203) ng/mL, and lactate dehydrogenase (LDH)—529 (range; 395–755.5) U/L vs. 393 (range; 270.75–550.25) U/L. Also, the ratio value for the systemic inflammation index (SII), systemic inflammation response index (SIRI), neutrophil/lymphocyte ratio (NLR), and CRP to albumin ratio (CRP/Alb) was significantly higher in patients who required ICU admittance, as follows: SII–1830.28 (range; 810.35–3041.31) vs 1214.02 (range; 578.41–2252.46), SIRI—2.35 (range; 1.24–5.18) vs. 1.91 (range; 1.00–7.04), NLR—8.30 (range; 4.51–12.89) vs. 5.27 (3.23–8.98), and CRP/Alb—21.79 (6.18–37.87) vs. 9.77 (3.23–26.59).

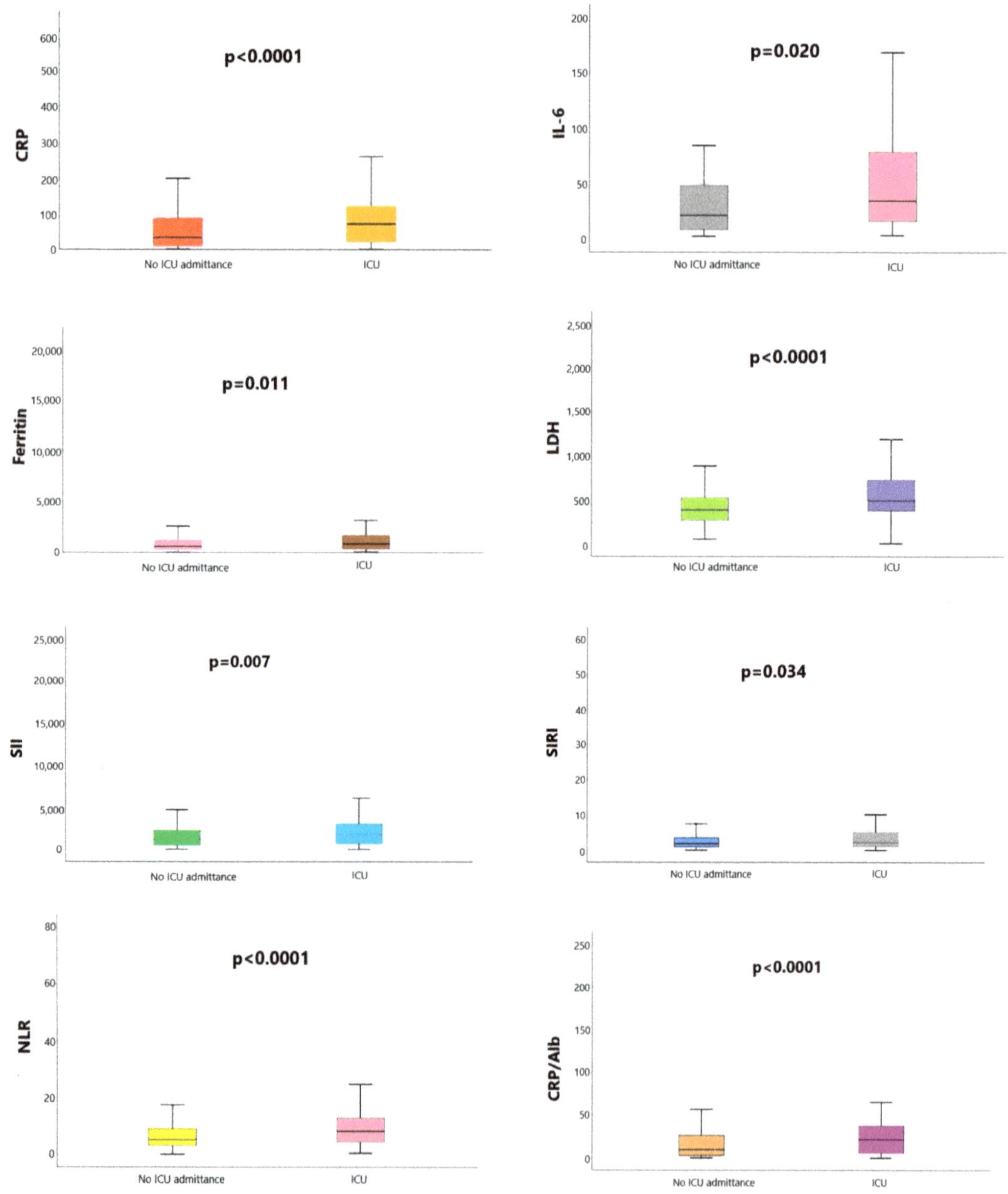

Figure 2. Inflammatory markers between groups. CRP—C-reactive protein; IL6—interleukin-6; LDH—lactate dehydrogenase; SII—systemic inflammation index; SIRI—systemic inflammation response index; NLR—neutrophil/lymphocyte ratio; CRP/Alb—C-reactive protein-to-albumin ratio; ICU—Intensive Care Unit.

2.2. Potential Markers for Identifying Severe Cases with Need of ICU Admittance

The biomarkers of interest that were statistically significantly different between the ICU patients and those not requiring ICU admittance were further included in a univariate logistic regression analysis, with the ICU need as a dependent variable. The univariate logistic regression analysis showed that the values of CRP (odds ratio [OR] = 1.006), IL-6 (OR = 1.013), ferritin (OR = 1.000), LDH (OR = 1.002), SII (OR = 1.000), SIRI (OR = 1.053), NLR (OR = 1.074), CRP/Alb (OR = 1.014), and P/Alb (OR = 0.993) were independent predictors of ICU admittance in all patients, whereas D-dimers were not. Subsequently, variables independently associated with ICU admittance in the univariate regression were used as predictors in a multivariate logistic regression model, with ICU admittance as a dependent variable. The multivariate regression model was unadjusted (Model 1[a]) and adjusted (Model 2[b]) for variables that have been shown to be associated with the severity of the disease: age, gender, body mass index, DM, cardiovascular diseases, hypertension, chronic kidney diseases, respiratory diseases, or vaccination status. The LDH level (OR = 1.002, 95% confidence interval [95%CI]: 1.000–1.005, $p = 0.044$) was the only marker associated with ICU admittance in all participants, independent of the variables correlated with the severity of the infection (Table 3).

Table 3. Univariable and multivariable logistic regression analysis for detecting the indicators for an ICU admittance in all sample analyzed.

			Model 1 [a]		**Model 2 [b]**	
Variables	**Univariable OR (95%CI)**	***p*-Value**	**Multivariable OR (95% CI)**	***p*-Value**	**Multivariable OR (95% CI)**	***p*-Value**
CRP	1.006 (1.003–1.009)	<0.0001	1.010 (0.985–1.035)	0.427	0.096 (0.965–1.027)	0.794
IL-6	1.013 (1.002–1.023)	0.017	1.014 (1.000–1.027)	0.044	1.014 (0.999–1.030)	0.070
Ferritin	1.000 (1.000–1.000)	0.006	1.000 (0.999–1.000)	0.348	1.000 (0.999–1.000)	0.328
LDH	1.002 (1.001–1.002)	<0.0001	1.002 (1.000–1.003)	0.083	1.002 (1.000–1.005)	0.044
D-dimer	1.000 (1.000–1.000)	0.091	-	-	-	-
SII	1.000 (1.000–1.000)	0.007	1.000 (1.000–1.001)	0.347	1.000 (0.999–1.001)	0.572
SIRI	1.053 (1.006–1.103)	0.028	0.950 (0.752–1.199)	0.666	1.073 (0.807–1.428)	0.628
NLR	1.074 (1.036–1.112)	<0.0001	1.052 (0.881–1.255)	0.576	1.062 (0.864–1.305)	0.569
CRP/Alb	1.014 (1.004–1.024)	0.008	0.988 (0.921–1.060)	0.735	1.035 (0.945–1.135)	0.457
P/Alb	0.993 (0.986–1.000)	0.044	0.979 (0.951–1.008)	0.161	0.973 (0.939–1.009)	0.136

a Model 1: unadjusted for age, gender, body mass index, diabetes mellitus, cardiovascular diseases, hypertension, chronic kidney diseases, respiratory diseases, vaccination status. *b* Model 2: adjusted for age, gender, body mass index, diabetes mellitus, cardiovascular diseases, hypertension, chronic kidney diseases, respiratory diseases, vaccination status. CRP—C-reactive protein; IL-6—interleukin-6; LDH—lactate dehydrogenase; SII—systemic inflammation index; SIRI—systemic inflammation response index; NLR—neutrophil/lymphocyte ratio; CRP/Alb—C-reactive protein-to-albumin ratio; P/Alb—platelet/albumin ratio.

2.3. *Predictors of Severity Correlated with Diabetic Status*

2.3.1. Predictors of ICU Admittance in DM Patients

To further investigate the predictors for ICU admittance in the DM subjects, regression analysis was performed for the DM group—Table 4. In the univariate regression, CRP, IL-6, ferritin, LDH, and NLR were significantly associated with ICU admittance, with $p < 0.05$. These were further included in the unadjusted multivariate regression model and NLR was the only variable that remained associated with the increased odds of an ICU admittance. After adjusting for age, gender, body mass index, cardiovascular diseases, hypertension, chronic kidney diseases, respiratory diseases, and vaccination status in the multivariate model, NLR and IL-6 were predictors for ICU admittance (OR 1.228 and 1.028, respectively).

Table 4. Univariable and multivariable logistic regression analysis for detecting the indicators for ICU admittance among patients with diabetes.

			Model 1 [a]		Model 2 [b]	
Variables	**Univariable OR (95%CI)**	***p*-Value**	**Multivariable OR (95%CI)**	***p*-Value**	**Multivariable OR (95% CI)**	***p*-Value**
CRP	1.007 (1.001–1.012)	0.014	1.003 (0.996–1.010)	0.376	1.000 (0.989–1.011)	0.976
IL-6	1.022 (1.004–1.041)	0.019	1.016 (0.996–1.036)	0.118	1.028 (1.002–1.055)	0.034
Ferritin	1.000 (1.000–1.001)	0.011	1.000 (0.999–1.001)	0.938	1.000 (0.999–1.001)	0.908
LDH	1.002 (1.001–1.004)	<0.0001	1.002 (0.999–1.004)	0.147	1.003 (0.999–1.006)	0.128
D-dimer	1.000 (1.000–1.000)	0.297	-	-	-	-
SII	1.000 (1.000–1.000)	0.061	-	-	-	-
SIRI	1.026 (0.968–1.088)	0.383	-	-	-	-
NLR	1.070 (1.015–1.128)	0.011	1.120 (1.011–1.241)	0.029	1.228 (1.045–1.443)	0.013
CRP/Alb	1.011 (0.998–1.024)	0.091	-	-	-	-
P/Alb	0.993 (0.984–1.002)	0.134	-	-	-	-

a Model 1: unadjusted for age, gender, body mass index, cardiovascular diseases, hypertension, chronic kidney diseases, respiratory diseases, vaccination status. *b* Model 2: adjusted for age, gender, body mass index, cardiovascular diseases, hypertension, chronic kidney diseases, respiratory diseases, vaccination status. CRP—C-reactive protein; IL6—interleukin-6; LDH—lactate dehydrogenase; SII—systemic inflammation index; SIRI—systemic inflammation response index; NLR—neutrophil/lymphocyte ratio; CRP/Alb—C-reactive protein to albumin ratio; P/Alb—platelet/albumin ratio.

2.3.2. Predictors for ICU Admittance among Patients without DM

As for patients with DM, we identified predictors of ICU admittance among those without DM using similar variables. The results are presented in Table 5. From the univariate regression analysis, predictors for ICU admittance were associated with increased CRP, D-dimers, SIRI, NLR, and CRP/Alb levels. However, neither in the unadjusted nor in the adjusted multivariate models, the parameters did not remain associated with increased odds for ICU admittance—$p > 0.05$ for all tested variables.

Table 5. Univariable and Multivariable Logistic Regression Analysis for ICU admittance among patients without diabetes.

			Model 1 [a]		Model 2 [b]	
Variables	**Univariable OR (95%CI)**	***p*-Value**	**Multivariable OR (95%CI)**	***p*-Value**	**Multivariable OR (95% CI)**	***p*-Value**
CRP	1.005 (1.001–1.010)	0.017	1.015 (0.986–1.045)	0.318	1.026 (0.987–1.067)	0.193
IL-6	1.006 (0.994–1.019)	0.323	-	-	-	-
Ferritin	1.000 (1.000–1.000)	0.059	-	-	-	-
LDH	1.001 (1.000–1.002)	0.149	-	-	-	-
D-dimer	1.000 (1.000–1.000)	0.033	1.000 (1.000–1.000)	0.246	1.000 (1.000–1.001)	0.113
SII	1.000 (1.000–1.000)	0.049	1.000 (0.999–1.000)	0.281	1.000 (0.999–1.000)	0.459
SIRI	1.092 (1.012–1.179)	0.024	1.071 (0.908–1.265)	0.414	1.088 (0.889–1.332)	0.412
NLR	1.076 (1.026–1.129)	0.003	1.090 (0.998–1.190)	0.056	1.080 (0.967–1.206)	0.172
CRP/Alb	1.017 (1.002–1.033)	0.028	0.962 (0.869–1.065)	0.457	0.932 (0.812–1.069)	0.315
P/Alb	0.991 (0.980–1.002)	0.123	-	-	-	-

a Model 1: unadjusted for age, gender, body mass index, cardiovascular diseases, hypertension, chronic kidney diseases, respiratory diseases, vaccination status. *b* Model 2: adjusted for age, gender, body mass index, cardiovascular diseases, hypertension, chronic kidney diseases, respiratory diseases, vaccination status. CRP—C-reactive protein; IL-6—interleukin-6; LDH—lactate dehydrogenase; SII—systemic inflammation index; SIRI—systemic inflammation response index; NLR—neutrophil/lymphocyte ratio; CRP/Alb—C-reactive protein-to-albumin ratio; P/Alb—platelet/albumin ratio.

3. Discussion

In the present study that evaluated inflammatory and coagulation biomarkers that may qualify as predictors for COVID-19 severity, we showed for the first time that IL-6 can predict severe cases of COVID-19 in patients with diabetes.

Studies published so far showed that IL-6 is a predictor of severity in COVID-19 patients without diabetes [13,14]. In the severe form of the disease, the immune responses induced by the coronavirus contribute to virus clearance, causing cytokine release syndrome (CRS) [15]. One of the primary inflammatory cytokines is IL-6 [16]. In critically ill patients, it has been shown that high levels of pathogenic T cells and inflammatory monocytes are secreting large amounts of IL-6. These events could trigger an inflammatory storm [17], leading to ARDS [18]. A recent report demonstrated that dehydroepiandrosterone sulfate (DHEAS) has an inhibitory role on IL-6, with a defense immune effect in the SARS-CoV-2 infection [19]. In light of the important role in predicting the severity of COVID-19, it has been proven that patients with diabetes were more likely to receive mechanical ventilation, be admitted to the ICU, and have higher mortality [20]. Moreover, IL-6 contributes to the hypercoagulability status together with TNF-α and IL-1, a phenomenon which, if accompanied by severe inflammatory syndrome, leads to disseminated intravascular coagulation [10,14]. In the SARS-CoV2 infection, there has been an "infection-induced coagulopathy" phenomenon, resulting from hyperactivation of endothelial cells (due to the increased amount of IL-6) and increased release of tissue factor [21].

In COVID-19 patients, when the cytokine storm occurs, not only the cytokines rise sharply but other inflammatory markers as well. Hyperinflammation caused by COVID-19 seems to increase NLR levels due to reactive oxygen species released from neutrophils which are causing the cell's DNA damage [22]. It has been shown that the NLR value is a more sensitive inflammatory marker than the absolute neutrophil and lymphocyte counts [23]. Both neutrophils and lymphocytes are involved in the immune response: inflammation induces neutrophilia, and lymphopenia occurs by suppressing the immune system [24]. In our study, using multivariate regression analysis, we found that NLR could predict the severity of COVID-19 in patients with DM, with results similar to those previously published [25]. The more pronounced increase in NLR in patients with diabetes is due to two mechanisms: the pre-existing chronic inflammation in diabetic patients and the acute inflammation associated with the SARS-CoV-2 infection [26]. A study published by Hussain et al. [27] showed that NLR is associated with higher values for HbA1c, FBG, and CRP in patients with DM. Considering that the COVID-19 infection triggers an important inflammatory syndrome accompanied by increased glycemic values, it can be hypothesized that NLR is also a predictor of glycemic imbalance during hospitalization for patients with diabetes.

In the present study, although the CAR ratio in ICU patients was a predictor for severe disease in the univariate regression, the multivariate regression analysis failed to show a predictive relationship between the severity of infection and CAR. A meta-analysis published by Rathore et al. [28] found that CAR is a predictor of severity in the SARS-CoV-2 infection. The differences may be due to different stages of the inflammatory period in patients analyzed, as Kuluöztürk et al. [29] showed that changes in the levels of acute phase reactants do not appear at the same time in all patients.

We also found significant differences between ICU patients and those without ICU admittance for both SII and SIRI. However, both failed as prognosis markers for the severity of the SARS-CoV2 infection, in line with previous reports [8].

The present study also showed that LDH could predict a severe disease in ICU patients, which is similar to the result published by Henry et al. [30]. In line with our findings, Wang et al. [31] reported higher LDH values (p-value < 0.001) in ICU compared to non-ICU patients. Considering that in severe/critical SARS-CoV-2 infections some patients developed ARDS, Mesa [32] proved that LDH, alongside thiol and ferritin, is a prognostic biomarker for ARDS development. LDH is an enzyme whose elevated levels indicate the lysis of cells found in different parenchymal organs: heart, liver, muscle, lung, and bone marrow. It was considered a marker of inflammation and a predictor for pneumonia in literature published so far [30]. In severe COVID-19 patients, through inflammatory lesions and cell lysis, increased values are associated with a poor prognosis [30], which is similar to the results presented in this paper. Also, high levels on the first day of admission were correlated previously with new-onset diabetes [33]. Additionally, LDH levels are higher in thrombotic microangiopathy, which is linked in previous studies to renal failure and myocardial injury [34].

Inflammation has a pivotal role in the pathophysiologic mechanism of thrombotic complications in atherosclerosis. In patients with DM, coagulation and endothelial dysfunction are essential factors that aggravate the coronavirus infection [12]. Hypercoagulation, expressed by increased levels of D-dimers, fibrinogen, and abnormalities in prothrombin time (PT), and activated partial thromboplastin time (aPTT), along with thrombocytopenia, are other causes responsible for a poor prognosis, being associated in previous studies with a more severe COVID-19 disease [35,36]. When an imbalance in coagulation pathways occurs, patients with a severe form of disease might develop disseminated intravascular coagulation, with thrombocytopenia as a key element. The hyperinflammatory state observed in COVID-19 destroys bone marrow progenitor cells, with a secondary reduction in platelet production [37]. Another proposed mechanism for thrombocytopenia results from the higher disease severity and degree of lung damage in ICU patients; the impaired lung tissue together with pulmonary endothelial cells could mobilize the lung platelets leading to aggregation and development of microthrombi, with an increase in platelet consumption [37]. High levels of D-dimers were highly correlated with blood clot formation and disseminated intravascular coagulation [36,38]. In recently published literature, a hypercoagulability state expressed by increased D-dimer levels was more frequently associated with mortality in hospitalized patients with COVID-19, as Zhang et al. showed [39]. In the present study, although lower platelet levels and higher D-dimer levels were observed in ICU patients, after adjusting for confounders in multivariate analysis, no association with ICU admittance was observed neither in the DM patients nor in the non-DM group.

This study has several limitations. Firstly, the current paper is a retrospective study, and the data were collected from electronic records; therefore, the accuracy and reliability of the data could vary from subject to subject. Secondly, although the blood laboratory tests were recorded on the first day of hospitalization, subjects could be in different stages of the disease. Thirdly, the small number of DM patients who needed ICU care could provide inaccurate results; so, the present findings should be interpreted with caution. Finally, the findings of this study were described over a considerable period, and variants of the coronavirus could interfere with the results.

4. Materials and Methods

4.1. Study Design and Participants

The present paper was designed as an observational, analytical, and retrospective study. Data were obtained from the electronic medical record system of "Leon Daniello" Pulmonology University Hospital in Cluj-Napoca, Romania. Consecutive COVID-19 patients (n = 366) admitted to a tertiary Pneumonology University Hospital in Cluj-Napoca, Romania, between 1 April 2021, and 31 January 2022 who met the inclusion criteria and without any exclusion criteria were counted in this study. The inclusion criteria were (1) age > 18 years; (2) a laboratory-confirmed diagnosis of the SARS-CoV2 infection by a real-time-polymerase chain reaction (RT-PCR) of a nasopharyngeal swab; (3) the absence of previously diagnosed chronic illness, which alters the leukocyte formula (e.g., inflammatory chronic disease, autoimmune disease, active cancer, or hematological disorders); and (4) hospitalization > 48 h. Patients excluded from this analysis were those with (1) chronic pharmacological treatment known to affect the leukocyte formula (e.g., chemotherapy or immunosuppressive therapy), (2) duplicate data records, (3) missing clinical, biochemical or radiological findings, or (4) those patients who were transferred to another hospital.

Data about age, gender, body mass index, and personal medical history of hypertension, diabetes, cardiovascular diseases, respiratory diseases, and laboratory tests were entered into a dedicated electronic database. Results of the following laboratory investigations were collected whenever available: complete blood count, including white blood cell count with leukocyte subtypes, platelet count, cardiac (troponin I, NT pro-BNP), and coagulation markers: D-dimer, fibrinogen, international normalized ratio (INR), activated partial thromboplastin time (aPTT), and prothrombin time (PT); also, inflammatory markers, such as ferritin, CRP, LDH, and outcome during hospitalization: recovery, the need of ICU, intubation, or death. The hemogram-derived ratios were calculated using a part of the complete blood count. While the NLR is calculated by dividing the neutrophil count by the lymphocyte count, the platelet-to-lymphocyte count ratio results from the division of platelets into lymphocytes. A marker that combines the previously mentioned parameters is SII, which is obtained by multiplying neutrophils with platelets and the result is divided by the number of lymphocytes. SIRI is a result of (neutrophils × monocytes)/lymphocytes. The other ratios calculated were fibrinogen divided into albumin, P/Alb, and CRP/Alb.

Also, a CT scan was performed at admission. The CT total severity score was evaluated by lobe involvement for each lung separately, as follows 1-minimal involvement: 1–25%; 2-mild involvement: 26–50%; 3-moderate involvement: 51–75%; severe involvement—76–100% [40]. The decision regarding ICU admission was made according to the Modified National Early Warning Score (Modified NEWS) for COVID-19 patients [41]. To verify the accuracy of patient data collection, two researchers independently double-checked the electronic information.

Participants were divided into two groups: ICU patients and patients without ICU admittance, and each further into DM and non-DM groups. To find the predictors for severe disease in patients with diabetes, in the first phase, we found out the predictors for ICU admittance in the entire population. All statistically significant inflammatory and coagulation markers were subsequently included in the univariate and multivariate analysis for DM and non-DM patients.

4.2. Ethics Consideration

This study was designed in accordance with the Declaration of Helsinki and authorized by the Ethics Committee of "Iuliu Hațieganu" University of Medicine and Pharmacy Cluj-Napoca, Romania (approval No 298/29.11.2022). The patient's consent was not necessary, given the retrospective, non-interventional nature of the study.

4.3. Statistical Analysis

Statistical analysis was performed using the IBM SPSS Statistics V26.0 (IBM Corp.: Armonk, NY, USA). The histograms and the Kolmogorov–Smirnov test were used to verify the normal distribution of data. The Student *t*-test and the non-parametric Mann–Whitney U test were used to test the significance of differences in continuous variables between the groups, while the chi-square test and Fisher's exact test were used for categorical variables. Continuous variables were reported as mean and standard deviation (SD) or as median (25–75% quarters), depending on the normality of the distribution for each variable. Categorical variables were expressed as frequency (percentages).

All parameters with a statistically significant difference between groups were further included in the univariate logistic regression analysis. Variables associated with the need for ICU in univariate analysis were further included in a multivariate logistic regression adjusted for variables that have been shown to be associated with the severity of COVID-19—age, gender, body mass index, cardiovascular diseases, hypertension, chronic kidney diseases, respiratory diseases, and SARS-COV-2 vaccination status. A p-value < 0.05 was considered statistically significant.

5. Conclusions

Herein we showed for the first time that IL-6 and NLR could predict the severity of the disease in COVID-19 patients with DM. Considering that patients with diabetes present a higher risk of developing a severe form of SARS-CoV2 infection, the present findings emphasize the major importance of identifying patients with an increased inflammatory status from the first day of admission. An early treatment that targets both SARS-CoV-2 infection and antihyperglycemic treatment could reduce the evolution towards a severe form, ketoacidotic coma, and mortality. Therefore, the role of IL-6 in COVID-19 deserves special attention, even if its contribution to predicting the severe case is not fully understood. Further studies are needed to elucidate its role and to determine cutoff values associated with worse outcomes.

Author Contributions: Conceptualization, I.F., T.-D.S. and D.-A.T.; methodology, I.F., A.R. and T.-D.S.; formal analysis, H.C. and A.R.; investigation, I.F. and D.-M.V.; data curation, I.F.; writing—original draft preparation, I.F.; writing—review and editing, A.R., H.C., D.-M.V. and D.-A.T. All authors have read and agreed to the published version of the manuscript.

Funding: This research was funded by "Iuliu Hațieganu" University of Medicine and Pharmacy, Cluj-Napoca, Romania; internal PhD grant number: 771/24/11.01.2023.

Institutional Review Board Statement: This study was conducted in accordance with the Declaration of Helsinki and approved by the Ethics Committee of the "Iuliu-Hațieganu" University of Medicine and Pharmacy Cluj-Napoca, Romania (approval No 298/29.11.2022).

Informed Consent Statement: Patient consent was waived due to the retrospective nature of the study.

Data Availability Statement: The data presented in this study are available on request from the corresponding author.

Conflicts of Interest: A.R. declares support from Sanofi. The other authors declare no conflict of interest.

References

1. Jesenak, M.; Brndiarova, M.; Urbancikova, I.; Rennerova, Z.; Vojtkova, J.; Bobcakova, A.; Ostro, R.; Banovcin, P. Immune Parameters and COVID-19 Infection—Associations with Clinical Severity and Disease Prognosis. *Front. Cell. Infect. Microbiol.* **2020**, *10*, 364. [CrossRef] [PubMed]
2. Chen, N.; Zhou, M.; Dong, X.; Qu, J.; Gong, F.; Han, Y.; Qiu, Y.; Wang, J.; Liu, Y.; Wei, Y.; et al. Epidemiological and Clinical Characteristics of 99 Cases of 2019 Novel Coronavirus Pneumonia in Wuhan, China: A Descriptive Study. *Lancet* **2020**, *395*, 507–513. [CrossRef] [PubMed]
3. Richardson, S.; Hirsch, J.S.; Narasimhan, M.; Crawford, J.M.; McGinn, T.; Davidson, K.W.; The Northwell COVID-19 Research Consortium; Barnaby, D.P.; Becker, L.B.; Chelico, J.D.; et al. Presenting Characteristics, Comorbidities, and Outcomes Among 5700 Patients Hospitalized With COVID-19 in the New York City Area. *JAMA* **2020**, *323*, 2052. [CrossRef] [PubMed]
4. Wu, Z.; McGoogan, J.M. Characteristics of and Important Lessons from the Coronavirus Disease 2019 (COVID-19) Outbreak in China: Summary of a Report of 72 314 Cases from the Chinese Center for Disease Control and Prevention. *JAMA* **2020**, *323*, 1239. [CrossRef] [PubMed]
5. Hodgson, K.; Morris, J.; Bridson, T.; Govan, B.; Rush, C.; Ketheesan, N. Immunological Mechanisms Contributing to the Double Burden of Diabetes and Intracellular Bacterial Infections. *Immunology* **2015**, *144*, 171–185. [CrossRef]
6. Erickson, J.R.; Pereira, L.; Wang, L.; Han, G.; Ferguson, A.; Dao, K.; Copeland, R.J.; Despa, F.; Hart, G.W.; Ripplinger, C.M.; et al. Diabetic Hyperglycaemia Activates CaMKII and Arrhythmias by O-Linked Glycosylation. *Nature* **2013**, *502*, 372–376. [CrossRef]
7. Wang, T.T. IgG Fc Glycosylation in Human Immunity. In *Fc Mediated Activity of Antibodies*; Ravetch, J.V., Nimmerjahn, F., Eds.; Current Topics in Microbiology and Immunology; Springer International Publishing: Cham, Switzerland, 2019; Volume 423, pp. 63–75. [CrossRef]
8. Muller, L.M.A.J.; Gorter, K.J.; Hak, E.; Goudzwaard, W.L.; Schellevis, F.G.; Hoepelman, A.I.M.; Rutten, G.E.H.M. Increased Risk of Common Infections in Patients with Type 1 and Type 2 Diabetes Mellitus. *Clin. Infect. Dis.* **2005**, *41*, 281–288. [CrossRef] [PubMed]
9. De Lucena, T.M.C.; Da Silva Santos, A.F.; De Lima, B.R.; De Albuquerque Borborema, M.E.; De Azevêdo Silva, J. Mechanism of Inflammatory Response in Associated Comorbidities in COVID-19. *Diabetes Metab. Syndr. Clin. Res. Rev.* **2020**, *14*, 597–600. [CrossRef]
10. Ragnoli, B.; Da Re, B.; Galantino, A.; Kette, S.; Salotti, A.; Malerba, M. Interrelationship between COVID-19 and Coagulopathy: Pathophysiological and Clinical Evidence. *Int. J. Mol. Sci.* **2023**, *24*, 8945. [CrossRef]
11. CRICS TRIGGERSEP Group (Clinical Research in Intensive Care and Sepsis Trial Group for Global Evaluation and Research in Sepsis); Helms, J.; Tacquard, C.; Severac, F.; Leonard-Lorant, I.; Ohana, M.; Delabranche, X.; Merdji, H.; Clere-Jehl, R.; Schenck, M.; et al. High Risk of Thrombosis in Patients with Severe SARS-CoV-2 Infection: A Multicenter Prospective Cohort Study. *Intensive Care Med.* **2020**, *46*, 1089–1098. [CrossRef]
12. Abou-Ismail, M.Y.; Diamond, A.; Kapoor, S.; Arafah, Y.; Nayak, L. The Hypercoagulable State in COVID-19: Incidence, Pathophysiology, and Management. *Thromb. Res.* **2020**, *194*, 101–115. [CrossRef] [PubMed]
13. Broman, N.; Rantasärkkä, K.; Feuth, T.; Valtonen, M.; Waris, M.; Hohenthal, U.; Rintala, E.; Karlsson, A.; Marttila, H.; Peltola, V.; et al. IL-6 and Other Biomarkers as Predictors of Severity in COVID-19. *Ann. Med.* **2021**, *53*, 410–412. [CrossRef] [PubMed]
14. Tomo, S.; Kiran Kumar, P.; Yadav, D.; Sankanagoudar, S.; Charan, J.; Purohit, A.; Nag, V.L.; Bhatia, P.K.; Singh, K.; Dutt, N.; et al. Association of Serum Complement C3 Levels with Severity and Mortality in COVID-19. *Indian J. Clin. Biochem.* **2023**, *38*, 447–456. [CrossRef] [PubMed]
15. Lim, Z.J.; Subramaniam, A.; Ponnapa Reddy, M.; Blecher, G.; Kadam, U.; Afroz, A.; Billah, B.; Ashwin, S.; Kubicki, M.; Bilotta, F.; et al. Case Fatality Rates for Patients with COVID-19 Requiring Invasive Mechanical Ventilation. A Meta-Analysis. *Am. J. Respir. Crit. Care Med.* **2021**, *203*, 54–66. [CrossRef] [PubMed]
16. Merad, M.; Martin, J.C. Pathological Inflammation in Patients with COVID-19: A Key Role for Monocytes and Macrophages. *Nat. Rev. Immunol.* **2020**, *20*, 355–362. [CrossRef]
17. Liu, B.; Li, M.; Zhou, Z.; Guan, X.; Xiang, Y. Can We Use Interleukin-6 (IL-6) Blockade for Coronavirus Disease 2019 (COVID-19)-Induced Cytokine Release Syndrome (CRS)? *J. Autoimmun.* **2020**, *111*, 102452. [CrossRef]
18. Fujino, M.; Ishii, M.; Taniguchi, T.; Chiba, H.; Kimata, M.; Hitosugi, M. The Value of Interleukin-6 among Several Inflammatory Markers as a Predictor of Respiratory Failure in COVID-19 Patients. *Diagnostics* **2021**, *11*, 1327. [CrossRef]
19. Tomo, S.; Banerjee, M.; Karli, S.; Purohit, P.; Mitra, P.; Sharma, P.; Garg, M.K.; Kumar, B. Assessment of DHEAS, Cortisol, and DHEAS/Cortisol Ratio in Patients with COVID-19: A Pilot Study. *Hormones* **2022**, *21*, 515–518. [CrossRef]
20. Yan, Y.; Yang, Y.; Wang, F.; Ren, H.; Zhang, S.; Shi, X.; Yu, X.; Dong, K. Clinical Characteristics and Outcomes of Patients with Severe COVID-19 with Diabetes. *BMJ Open Diabetes Res. Care* **2020**, *8*, e001343. [CrossRef]

21. Akácsos-Szász, O.-Z.; Pál, S.; Nyulas, K.-I.; Nemes-Nagy, E.; Fárr, A.-M.; Dénes, L.; Szilveszter, M.; Bán, E.-G.; Tilinca, M.C.; Simon-Szabó, Z. Pathways of Coagulopathy and Inflammatory Response in SARS-CoV-2 Infection among Type 2 Diabetic Patients. *Int. J. Mol. Sci.* **2023**, *24*, 4319. [CrossRef]
22. Yang, A.-P.; Liu, J.; Tao, W.; Li, H. The Diagnostic and Predictive Role of NLR, d-NLR and PLR in COVID-19 Patients. *Int. Immunopharmacol.* **2020**, *84*, 106504. [CrossRef] [PubMed]
23. Chan, A.S.; Rout, A. Use of Neutrophil-to-Lymphocyte and Platelet-to-Lymphocyte Ratios in COVID-19. *J. Clin. Med. Res.* **2020**, *12*, 448–453. [CrossRef] [PubMed]
24. Novida, H.; Soelistyo, S.; Cahyani, C.; Siagian, N.; Hadi, U.; Pranoto, A. Factors Associated with Disease Severity of COVID-19 in Patients with Type 2 Diabetes Mellitus. *Biomed. Rep.* **2022**, *18*, 8. [CrossRef]
25. Moghaddam Tabrizi, F.; Rasmi, Y.; Hosseinzadeh, E.; Rezaei, S.; Balvardi, M.; Kouchari, M.R.; Ebrahimi, G. Diabetes Is Associated with Increased Mortality and Disease Severity in Hospitalized Patients with COVID-19. *EXCLI J.* **2021**, *20*, 444–453. [CrossRef]
26. Guo, W.; Li, M.; Dong, Y.; Zhou, H.; Zhang, Z.; Tian, C.; Qin, R.; Wang, H.; Shen, Y.; Du, K.; et al. Diabetes Is a Risk Factor for the Progression and Prognosis of COVID-19. *Diabetes Metab. Res. Rev.* **2020**, *36*, e3319. [CrossRef] [PubMed]
27. Hussain, M.; Babar, M.Z.M.; Akhtar, L.; Hussain, M.S. Neutrophil Lymphocyte Ratio (NLR): A Well Assessment Tool of Glycemic Control in Type-2 Diabetic Patients. *Pak. J. Med. Sci.* **2017**, *33*, 1366–1370. [CrossRef]
28. Rathore, S.S.; Oberoi, S.; Iqbal, K.; Bhattar, K.; Benítez-López, G.A.; Nieto-Salazar, M.A.; Velasquez-Botero, F.; Moreno Cortes, G.A.; Hilliard, J.; Madekwe, C.C.; et al. Prognostic Value of Novel Serum Biomarkers, Including C-reactive Protein to Albumin Ratio and Fibrinogen to Albumin Ratio, in COVID-19 Disease: A Meta-analysis. *Rev. Med. Virol.* **2022**, *32*, e2390. [CrossRef]
29. Kuluöztürk, M.; Deveci, F.; Turgut, T.; Öner, Ö. The Glasgow Prognostic Score and Fibrinogen to Albumin Ratio as Prognostic Factors in Hospitalized Patients with COVID-19. *Expert Rev. Respir. Med.* **2021**, *15*, 1061–1068. [CrossRef]
30. Henry, B.M.; Aggarwal, G.; Wong, J.; Benoit, S.; Vikse, J.; Plebani, M.; Lippi, G. Lactate Dehydrogenase Levels Predict Coronavirus Disease 2019 (COVID-19) Severity and Mortality: A Pooled Analysis. *Am. J. Emerg. Med.* **2020**, *38*, 1722–1726. [CrossRef]
31. Wang, D.; Hu, B.; Hu, C.; Zhu, F.; Liu, X.; Zhang, J.; Wang, B.; Xiang, H.; Cheng, Z.; Xiong, Y.; et al. Clinical Characteristics of 138 Hospitalized Patients With 2019 Novel Coronavirus–Infected Pneumonia in Wuhan, China. *JAMA* **2020**, *323*, 1061. [CrossRef]
32. Martinez Mesa, A.; Cabrera César, E.; Martín-Montañez, E.; Sanchez Alvarez, E.; Lopez, P.M.; Romero-Zerbo, Y.; Garcia-Fernandez, M.; Velasco Garrido, J.L. Acute Lung Injury Biomarkers in the Prediction of COVID-19 Severity: Total Thiol, Ferritin and Lactate Dehydrogenase. *Antioxidants* **2021**, *10*, 1221. [CrossRef] [PubMed]
33. Făgărășan, I.; Rusu, A.; Cristea, M.; Bala, C.-G.; Vulturar, D.-M.; Cristea, C.; Todea, D.-A. Predictors of New-Onset Diabetes in Hospitalized Patients with SARS-CoV-2 Infection. *Int. J. Environ. Res. Public Health* **2022**, *19*, 13230. [CrossRef] [PubMed]
34. Moline, H.L.; Whitaker, M.; Deng, L.; Rhodes, J.C.; Milucky, J.; Pham, H.; Patel, K.; Anglin, O.; Reingold, A.; Chai, S.J.; et al. Effectiveness of COVID-19 Vaccines in Preventing Hospitalization Among Adults Aged $\geq$ 65 Years—COVID-NET, 13 States, February–April 2021. *MMWR Morb. Mortal. Wkly. Rep.* **2021**, *70*, 1088–1093. [CrossRef]
35. Usul, E.; Şan, İ.; Bekgöz, B.; Şahin, A. Role of Hematological Parameters in COVID-19 Patients in the Emergency Room. *Biomark. Med.* **2020**, *14*, 1207–1215. [CrossRef] [PubMed]
36. Tomo, S.; Kumar, K.P.; Roy, D.; Sankanagoudar, S.; Purohit, P.; Yadav, D.; Banerjee, M.; Sharma, P.; Misra, S. Complement Activation and Coagulopathy—An Ominous Duo in COVID-19. *Expert Rev. Hematol.* **2021**, *14*, 155–173. [CrossRef]
37. Xu, P.; Zhou, Q.; Xu, J. Mechanism of Thrombocytopenia in COVID-19 Patients. *Ann. Hematol.* **2020**, *99*, 1205–1208. [CrossRef]
38. Tang, N.; Li, D.; Wang, X.; Sun, Z. Abnormal Coagulation Parameters Are Associated with Poor Prognosis in Patients with Novel Coronavirus Pneumonia. *J. Thromb. Haemost.* **2020**, *18*, 844–847. [CrossRef]
39. Zhang, L.; Yan, X.; Fan, Q.; Liu, H.; Liu, X.; Liu, Z.; Zhang, Z. D-dimer Levels on Admission to Predict In-hospital Mortality in Patients with COVID-19. *J. Thromb. Haemost.* **2020**, *18*, 1324–1329. [CrossRef]
40. Bellos, I.; Tavernaraki, K.; Stefanidis, K.; Michalopoulou, O.; Lourida, G.; Korompoki, E.; Thanou, I.; Thanos, L.; Pefanis, A.; Argyraki, A. Chest CT Severity Score and Radiological Patterns as Predictors of Disease Severity, ICU Admission, and Viral Positivity in COVID-19 Patients. *Respir. Investig.* **2021**, *59*, 436–445. [CrossRef]
41. Liao, X.; Wang, B.; Kang, Y. Novel Coronavirus Infection during the 2019–2020 Epidemic: Preparing Intensive Care Units—The Experience in Sichuan Province, China. *Intensive Care Med.* **2020**, *46*, 357–360. [CrossRef]

International Journal of
Molecular Sciences

MDPI

Review

The Management of COVID-19-Related Coagulopathy: A Focus on the Challenges of Metabolic and Vascular Diseases

Mónika Szilveszter [1], Sándor Pál [2,*], Zsuzsánna Simon-Szabó [3,*], Orsolya-Zsuzsa Akácsos-Szász [4], Mihály Moldován [5], Barbara Réger [6], Lóránd Dénes [7], Zsuzsanna Faust [2], Mariana Cornelia Tilinca [8] and Enikő Nemes-Nagy [9]

1 Clinic of Plastic Surgery, Mureș County Emergency Hospital, 540136 Târgu-Mureș, Romania; monikaszilveszter@yahoo.com
2 Department of Transfusion Medicine, Medical School, University of Pécs, 7624 Pécs, Hungary; faust.zsuzsanna@pte.hu
3 Department of Pathophysiology, Faculty of Medicine, George Emil Palade University of Medicine, Pharmacy, Science, and Technology of Târgu-Mureș, 540142 Târgu-Mureș, Romania
4 Doctoral School, Faculty of Medicine, George Emil Palade University of Medicine, Pharmacy, Science, and Technology of Târgu-Mureș, 540142 Târgu-Mureș, Romania; szaszorsolya@yahoo.com
5 Klinik für Suchttherapie, ZtP Winnenden-Haus der Gesundheit, 73525 Schwäbisch Gümund, Germany; m.moldovan@zpf-winnenden.de
6 Department of Laboratory Medicine, Medical School, University of Pécs, 7624 Pécs, Hungary; reger.barbara@pte.hu
7 Department of Anatomy and Embryology, Faculty of Medicine, George Emil Palade University of Medicine, Pharmacy, Science, and Technology of Târgu-Mureș, 540142 Târgu-Mureș, Romania; lorand.denes@umfst.ro
8 Department of Internal Medicine I, Faculty of Medicine in English, George Emil Palade University of Medicine, Pharmacy, Science, and Technology of Târgu-Mureș, 540142 Târgu-Mureș, Romania; mariana.tilinca@umfst.ro
9 Department of Chemistry and Medical Biochemistry, Faculty of Medicine in English, George Emil Palade University of Medicine, Pharmacy, Science, and Technology of Târgu-Mureș, 540142 Târgu-Mureș, Romania; eniko.nemes-nagy@umfst.ro
* Correspondence: pal.sandor@pte.hu (S.P.); zsuzsanna.simon-szabo@umfst.ro (Z.S.-S.); Tel.: +36-7253600 (S.P.); +40-265215551 (Z.S.-S.)

Citation: Szilveszter, M.; Pál, S.; Simon-Szabó, Z.; Akácsos-Szász, O.-Z.; Moldován, M.; Réger, B.; Dénes, L.; Faust, Z.; Tilinca, M.C.; Nemes-Nagy, E. The Management of COVID-19-Related Coagulopathy: A Focus on the Challenges of Metabolic and Vascular Diseases. *Int. J. Mol. Sci.* **2023**, *24*, 12782. https://doi.org/10.3390/ijms241612782

Academic Editors: Alexandru Schiopu, Emil Marian Arbănași and Eliza Russu

Received: 1 July 2023
Revised: 7 August 2023
Accepted: 11 August 2023
Published: 14 August 2023

Abstract: The course of COVID-19 is highly dependent on the associated cardiometabolic comorbidities of the patient, which worsen the prognosis of coronavirus infection, mainly due to systemic inflammation, endothelium dysfunction, and thrombosis. A search on the recent medical literature was performed in five languages, using the PubMed, Embase, Cochrane, and Google Scholar databases, for the review of data regarding the management of patients with a high risk for severe COVID-19, focusing on the associated coagulopathy. Special features of COVID-19 management are presented, based on the underlying conditions (obesity, diabetes mellitus, and cardiovascular diseases), emphasizing the necessity of a modern, holistic approach to thromboembolic states. The latest findings regarding the most efficient therapeutic approaches are included in the article, offering guidance for medical professionals in severe, complicated cases of SARS-CoV-2 infection. We can conclude that severe COVID-19 is closely related to vascular inflammation and intense cytokine release leading to hemostasis disorders. Overweight, hyperglycemia, cardiovascular diseases, and old age are important risk factors for severe outcomes of coronavirus infection, involving a hypercoagulable state. Early diagnosis and proper therapy in complicated SARS-CoV-2-infected cases could reduce mortality and the need for intensive care during hospitalization in patients with cardiometabolic comorbidities.

Keywords: COVID-19; viscoelastometry; hypercoagulable state; thrombosis; coagulopathy; venous thromboembolism; obesity; diabetes mellitus; cardiovascular diseases; stroke

1. Introduction

COVID-19 is an acute respiratory infection caused by the severe acute respiratory syndrome virus SARS-CoV-2. Risk factors, such as age, male gender, associated chronic diseases, and/or altered metabolic states determine the severity of this condition, leading to a significant burden for intensive care units (ICUs) [1–4].

The continuously rising prevalence of type 2 diabetes mellitus (T2DM) worldwide, as well as obesity, further increases the burden on ICUs, due to the greater risk of these patient groups developing severe and critical COVID-19 symptoms. The clinical course of COVID-19 is aggravated even more by the presence of multiple comorbidities. Additionally, a higher prevalence of T2DM and vasculopathies has been reported in COVID-19 patients [5,6].

SARS-CoV-2 infects the host by binding to the angiotensin-converting enzyme 2 receptor (ACE2-R) expressed on different cell membranes. Some studies suggest that overexpressed ACE2-R in diabetic patients increases the risk of infection with the virus [7–9].

In chronic disease, constant and prolonged inflammation is present, with slightly increased synthesis of several cytokines, some of which have a predictive role in the development of type 2 diabetes (interleukins IL-1β, IL-6) [10,11]. Chronic low-grade inflammation also contributes significantly to the pathogenesis of atherosclerosis, due to the effects of tumor necrosis factor-alpha (TNF-α) and interleukin-10 (IL-10) [12].

Typically, COVID-19 causes a procoagulant state, through endothelial dysfunction and the malfunction of leukocytes and platelets, systemic inflammation, and the activation of several inflammatory pathways. This pattern has been termed COVID-19-associated coagulopathy (CAC), and can result in deep vein thrombosis (DVT), pulmonary embolism (PE) and stroke, further increasing the risk of mortality. SARS-CoV-2-infected patients with preexisting comorbidities are at risk of even higher mortality rates [13,14].

Hemostasis is the balanced interplay of the prothrombotic and antithrombotic processes. Conventional plasma-based hemostasis assays are mostly used for the assessment of the bleeding and coagulation risk in a surgical, traumatized, or intensive care patient. These tests carry limitations, as well, due to their ability to assess isolated diseases related to clotting factors, or the effect of an anticoagulant therapy.

Viscoelastic hemostatic tests were introduced in the 1950s, and were primarily used intraoperatively, as point-of-care methods. The utility of viscoelastic tests is to provide information about the global activity of hemostasis, including platelet aggregation effectiveness, thrombin generation, clot formation, and clot lysis. The duration of the measurements is 60 min, although, in most cases, valuable information is obtained after the first 20 min of the test, providing the possibility of early, individualized therapy for the patient [15,16]. According to Tyler et al., point-of-care viscoelastometric tests should be included for all patients requiring a massive transfusion, whether surgical or non-surgical, and whether trauma-related or not. In the USA, viscoelastometric test training is recommended for general surgery residents, and a further expansion of this method is expected in the near future [17]. Significant differences in the levels of inflammatory biomarkers and metabolic parameters in moderate or severe COVID-19 patients (with diabetes/obesity) have been described: in contrast to infected subjects without these comorbidities, the diabetic/obese patients with severe COVID-19 presented a significantly increased leukocyte count, erythrocyte sedimentation rate (ESR), C-reactive protein (CRP), D-dimers, and serum glucose concentration [18]. A comprehensive study performed in Romania revealed that elevated inflammatory markers were independent predictors of poor outcomes for all SARS-CoV-2-infected patients. In the same study, the authors observed that patients with associated cardiac and renal diseases, peripheral arteriopathy, obesity, dyslipidemia, malignancies, and tobacco use were predisposed to a higher mortality [19].

In a pilot study, eosinopenia and lymphopenia were associated with a severe outcome in COVID-19 [20].

The unfortunate coexistence of a proinflammatory and prothrombotic status in SARS-CoV-2 infection in some patients is considered a key mechanism in the progression of severe and critical cases of COVID-19, with the severity further increasing in patients with an existing proinflammatory and prothrombotic status due to recorded comorbidities. The recommended therapies for the different patient groups, based on their risk of developing serious COVID-19 conditions, aim to reduce inflammatory processes and viremia, and mitigate the thrombosis risk.

The authors aimed to synthesize the population-specific impact of comorbidities, such as diabetes, obesity, and cardiovascular disease, on COVID-19 outcomes, and to highlight the difficulties in diagnosis, and the challenges in the management of COVID-19 patients with comorbidities. Many observational studies and research reports were published during the pandemic, mostly in English, but presumably also in other languages, so the search criteria included not only papers published in English, but also in Spanish, German, Hungarian, and Romanian.

2. Materials and Methods

A literature search was conducted between 10 December 2022 and 10 June 2023, using PubMed, Embase, Cochrane Library, and Google Scholar, restricting the results to open-access articles written in English, Hungarian, Romanian, German, or Spanish, and published between 1 January 2020 and 1 June 2023. A combination of the following keywords and phrases was used in the five different languages: "COVID-19 coagulopathy therapy", "COVID-19 thrombosis therapy", "COVID-19 thrombosis treatment", "cytokines", "obesity", "type 2 diabetes", "anticoagulation", "hypercoagulable state", "SARS-CoV-2 induced hypercoagulability", "critically ill COVID-19 viscoelastometry", "critically ill COVID-19 thromboelastometry", "viscoelastic tests and COVID-19", and "vasculopathy and COVID-19".

After performing the search, the authors screened the articles based on the title and abstract, and a further selection was also performed after the full-text assessment of the remaining articles. The authors also selected secondary sources cited by recent systematic reviews or meta-analyses, including the most relevant research articles.

3. Proinflammatory and Procoagulant Effects of COVID-19

During SARS-CoV-2 infection, inflammation plays a significant role in the development of the disease. Studies have demonstrated the release of numerous inflammatory cytokines and chemokines in COVID-19. The innate immune system is instrumental in the immune response against pathogens, and while the production of proinflammatory cytokines is crucial, excessive activation of these cytokines can lead to widespread damage in certain cases of COVID-19. Several cytokines, including IL-2, IL-6, TNF-α, IFN-γ, MIP (macrophage inflammatory protein), and MCP-1 (monocyte chemoattractant protein-1), are prominently present in severely ill patients. Angiotensin II (AngII) triggers the activation of nuclear factor kappa-B (NF-κB), resulting in hyperinflammation, primarily through the increased synthesis of IL-6 and IL-1β, leading to an enhanced transcription of proinflammatory cytokines. These interleukins exhibit elevated levels in severe cases of COVID-19 [21].

IL-6, a proinflammatory cytokine, not only stimulates the release of other cytokines, but also activates immune cells, playing an important role in the systemic inflammation which is common in severe COVID-19 cases [22]. IL-6 and IL-1α play a major role in connecting the inflammatory reaction and the blood-clotting system. During inflammation, macrophages release tissue factor in response to IL-6 [23]. The overexpression of IL-6 and its receptor in COVID-19 leads to the hyperactivation of endothelial cells. This hyperactivation will release a substantial amount of tissue factor, contributing to infection-induced coagulopathy, which is involved in the mechanism of thrombocytopenia, while the cytokine storm induces thrombocytosis. IL-6 is also involved in the production of certain coagulation factors, such as fibrinogen and factor VIII. Furthermore, IL-6 acts on the endothelium to enhance the synthesis of vascular endothelial growth factor (VEGF), leading to vascular hyperpermeability and hypotension [24]. Other cytokines, including TNF-α, IFN-γ, and IL-1β, have also been involved in the intense cytokine release described in COVID-19 patients, contributing to the proinflammatory state and hypercoagulability. These cytokines are present on different cell types, such as activated platelets, monocytes, and endothelial cells during the proinflammatory phase. IL-1α not only activates the cascade of inflammation in thrombo-inflammatory pathologies, but also plays a key role in thrombogenesis, by recruiting granulocytes, prolonging the clot-lysis time, and increasing the platelet activity [25]. Conversely, together with TNF-α, IL-1 is the most important mediator of the suppression of the endogenous coagulation cascade [23].

4. Low-Grade Chronic Inflammation and Its Consequences in COVID-19 Patients with Comorbidities

The precise mechanisms and interactions between cytokines in individuals with diabetes mellitus, other chronic comorbidities, and vascular and metabolic diseases who are infected with SARS-CoV-2 are currently the subject of active research.

Adipose cells release cytokines, and prolonged high blood sugar levels have an immunomodulatory effect, contributing to the maintenance of chronic low-grade inflammation. Obese people are more prone to develop insulin resistance and type 2 diabetes, and insulin resistance is also commonly seen in diabetic patients. Type 2 diabetes mellitus leads to complications affecting both the microvascular and macrovascular systems, particularly impacting endothelial cells [26,27]. Endothelial dysfunction, in turn, induces a prothrombotic state often accompanied by chronic inflammatory processes. Obesity and cardiovascular comorbidities in patients with COVID-19 significantly increase the risk of severe and/or critical symptoms, prolonged hospitalization, the need for intensive therapy, mechanical ventilation (both non-invasive and invasive), and higher mortality rates [28–31]. Additionally, the combination of these comorbidities further escalates the risk of morbidity and mortality. Endothelial dysfunction, when exacerbated by the cytokine storm triggered by SARS-CoV-2, emerges as the primary cause of death [32–34]. Viral toxicity also contributes to the severity of COVID-19. Particularly in vulnerable patients, virus-induced pathomechanisms, such as a prothrombotic state, cytokine storm, immune system dysregulation, and inflammation are underlying factors in the critical manifestation of COVID-19. These pathomechanisms are more frequently observed in obese and diabetic patients, and in those with multiple comorbidities. Deceased COVID-19 patients exhibited significantly higher levels of D-dimers and fibrin degradation products (FDPs) compared to the surviving COVID-19 group. In addition, disseminated intravascular coagulopathy (DIC) was found to be more common in the group of deceased COVID-19 patients compared to survivors [7,35].

In elderly obese patients with COVID-19, elevated C-reactive protein (CRP), ferritin, and interleukin 6 (IL-6) levels were strongly associated with critical disease. Type 2 diabetes mellitus was more prevalent in severe-COVID-19 patients compared to less-severe cases and the general population [36]. After infection with SARS-CoV-2, some non-diabetic subjects showed hyperglycemia and significantly higher interleukin-8 (IL-8) concentrations compared to the normoglycemic COVID-19 group [37]. COVID-19 patients with diabetes mellitus (DM) had significantly higher mortality rates compared to non-diabetic COVID-19 subjects, especially those with poorly controlled glucose levels, who were at the highest risk of complications [27,38].

5. Assessment of Hemostatic Activity in COVID-19

The hemostatic activity of COVID-19 patients is frequently hindered, and the pathomechanisms triggered by the SARS-CoV-2 infection result in a prothrombotic state [39]. Performing conventional or point-of-care hemostatic assays enables clinicians to assess and correct the underlying cause of the prothrombotic state. The activated partial thromboplastin time (APTT), prothrombin time (PT), thrombin time (TT), fibrinogen, and fibrinolysis parameters (such as D-dimers), were useful in COVID-19 patients for thrombosis risk assessment, and also for therapy.

Hemostatic abnormalities of COVID-19 patients include increased D-dimer levels and hyperfibrinogenemia [40]. Several scientific papers suggest that the severity of COVID-19 is associated with prolonged PT and TT, and a trend toward a shortened APTT [13,41].

Compared to the sepsis-related DIC, the D-dimer levels of COVID-19 patients are significantly higher. Furthermore, as fibrinogen is an acute-phase protein, excessive inflammation leads to markedly increased fibrinogen levels, as well. The D-dimer concentration is in a positive correlation with poorer outcomes of COVID-19 cases. In asymptomatic COVID-19 cases, high D-dimer and fibrinogen levels were associated with a high risk of hospitalization [42,43]. Further laboratory anomalies include thrombocytopenia [44] or thrombocytosis [45].

A higher FVIII and higher Von Willebrand factor (VWF) are also specific features of COVID-19-associated coagulopathy [46]. Their elevation in patients with ongoing inflammatory processes is expected, with both being acute-phase reactants. Elevated FV concentrations were reported in severe COVID-19 cases, and these were associated with a high risk of venous thromboembolic events [47].

Conventional hemostatic assays are important elements of coagulopathy diagnosis in COVID-19, based on which the clinicians decide the patient's therapy. The measurement of procoagulant factors is often expanded with laboratory assays assessing thrombophilia, whether it is inherited or acquired. These assays most commonly include protein C (PC)-, protein S (PS)-, and antithrombin (AT)-deficiency testing [48]. Acquired thrombophilias are also often related to viral infections, and SARS-CoV-2 infection does not seem to be an exception. In severe COVID-19 cases, PS deficiency has been described in 20% of the subjects [49], while other studies reported near-threshold low levels of AT, PC, or PS [50].

Viscoelastic hemostatic tests are based on the distinctive property of blood, wherein its viscosity undergoes changes parallel to the formation of the blood clot during coagulation. Moreover, the resulting blood clot has elastic properties. The method, known as the viscoelastic test, is named after the combined assessment of two physical properties: the viscosity and elasticity. Viscoelastic tests are performed on whole-blood samples and, therefore, measure the hemostatic activity of the patient, including their cells, platelets, and plasma proteins, that can assess their hypocoagulation or hypercoagulation status.

In clinical practice, the viscoelastic method provides valuable data regarding the initiation of coagulation processes, blood clot development and firmness, clot lysis, and fibrinolysis effectiveness. The method includes several parameters, e.g., the clotting time (CT), clot formation time (CFT), maximum clot firmness (MCF), maximum lysis (ML), and lysis time (LT) [51]. The viscoelastic test is an ex vivo model of certain coagulation pathways, which analyze extrinsic (EX-test), or intrinsic (IN-test) pathways, or intrinsic and common pathways, and there are possibilities for the assessment of coagulation with the inhibition of certain elements (the FIB-test eliminates the effect of thrombocytes in the coagulation process). For more details, we refer you to Table 1.

Table 1. Short description of viscoelastic tests. EX-test, extrinsic test; IN-test, intrinsic test; FIB-test, fibrinogen-test; HI-test, heparin test; tPA-test, tissue plasminogen activator test; AP-test, aprotinin-test; RVV-test: Russel viper venom test; ECA test: ecarin (saw-scaled viper venom) test [52].

Test	Reagents Used	Assessed Mechanism	Diagnosis
EX-test	Tissue factor (TF), $CaCl_2$, polybrene (to inactivate heparin therapy)	Potential and dynamics of clot formation during tissue damage	Factor deficiencies of extrinsic pathway
IN-test	phospholipid, ellagic acid, $CaCl_2$	Potential and dynamics of clot formation during foreign-body contact	Intrinsic pathway factor deficiencies
FIB-test	TF, Ca^{2+}, polybrene, cytochalasin D, GPIIb-IIIa inhibitor	Potential and dynamics of secondary clot formation during tissue damage	Fibrinogen deficiency, factor deficiencies of extrinsic pathway
HI-test	lyophilized heparinase, phospholipid, ellagic acid, $CaCl_2$	Intrinsic pathway deficiency	Presence of heparin compared to IN-test
tPA-test	TF, $CaCl_2$, polybrene, recombinant tissue plasminogen activator (rtPA)	Potential and dynamics of extrinsic coagulation and fibrinolysis	Diagnosis of pathologic fibrinolysis

Table 1. *Cont.*

Test	Reagents Used	Assessed Mechanism	Diagnosis
AP-test	TF, $CaCl_2$, polybrene, aprotinin	Extrinsic and common pathway activation and fibrinolysis inhibition	Hyperfibrinolytic bleeding
RVV-test	Russell's viper venom, $CaCl_2$	Factor X activation, common pathway activation, potential and dynamics of clot formation	Direct-acting oral anticoagulant effect
ECA-test	Saw-scaled viper venom (ecarin)	Prothrombin–thrombin activation, dynamics of clot formation	Direct acting oral anticoagulant effect and antithrombin activity

In patients with COVID-19, the EX-test, IN-test, FIB-test, and TPA-test (EX-test with additional fibrinolysis initiation with the addition of tissue plasminogen activator—tPA) provide the most useful information on the coagulation status. In COVID-19, the EX-test and IN-test may assess the relative procoagulation (shortened CT) or hypercoagulation (increased MCF). An up-regulated platelet aggregation may also be diagnosed if, when comparing the FIB-test and EX-test, the MCF is more increased during the latter than in the case of the FIB-test. The TPA-test is useful in the assessment of antifibrinolytic dysfunction (fibrinolysis shutdown), with the test resulting in reduced ML or prolonged LT following tPA deficiency, plasminogen deficiency, or an increase in the plasminogen activator inhibitor-1 [52].

ROTEM is frequently used in polytrauma (patients with massive bleeding who require massive transfusions [53]), and can also be a valuable tool for the diagnosis of hemostatic disorders, and therapy-efficiency monitoring in antiplatelet or anticoagulant treatment. The SARS-CoV-2 pandemic further expanded the utility of the method, enabling a faster diagnosis of certain coagulation disorders in COVID-19 patients [54].

The fibrinolytic activity of a critically ill COVID-19 patient is impaired. Hypofibrinolysis occurs frequently in these cases, and it can be diagnosed using a visco-elastometric method, generally measuring a lysis time (LT) longer than 393 s. The hypofibrinolytic status of COVID-19 patients has also been named by several authors as "fibrinolysis shut down" [55,56]. This mechanism could be treated via thrombolytic therapy, using recombinant tissue plasminogen activators.

6. Management of COVID-19 Patients

6.1. The Therapeutic Approach of COVID-19

The special recommendations suggest a different therapeutic approach based on patient risk stratification, considering antiviral therapy, inhalation, or systemic corticosteroids, and thromboprophylaxis. Thus, the management of COVID-19 patients considers the individual characteristics of the cases, including the age, comorbidities, COVID-19 symptom severity, and risks for hospitalization, critical illness, and mechanical ventilation necessity. The therapeutic approach and drug recommendations are shown in Figure 1, based on the latest National Institutes of Health guidelines [57,58].

The management of outpatients infected with SARS-CoV-2 includes the revised therapy of their eventual comorbidities and chronic illnesses, with further recommendations and, in high-risk subpopulations, the available antiviral therapies should also be prescribed.

In several countries, ivermectin, an antiparasitic drug, has been prescribed for SARS-CoV-2-infected patients, based on the positive results of a research on the ability of ivermectin to inhibit the replication of SARS-CoV-2 in cell cultures [59]. However, pharmacokinetic and pharmacodynamic studies revealed that a 100-fold increase in the plasma concentration of ivermectin would be necessary to achieve this antiviral effect [60]. Furthermore, human clinical trials revealed that, compared to a placebo or standard care, ivermectin could not significantly benefit COVID-19 patients, and had minimal effect. Thus, after concluding these trials, the use of ivermectin for the therapy of COVID-19 is not recommended [61–63]. Outpatients with a high risk of developing severe COVID-19 symptoms should receive antiviral agents that include ritonavir-boosted nirmatrelvir or remdesivir [64,65]. In the case of hospitalized patients, intravenous antivirals would be appropriate (tocilizumab). These antiviral agents may be available in developed countries but, in underdeveloped areas, the patient's access to these therapies may be limited or absent. Moreover, the expensive therapy in severe COVID-19 cases may also limit the possibility of acquiring the latest medications, even in a developed country.

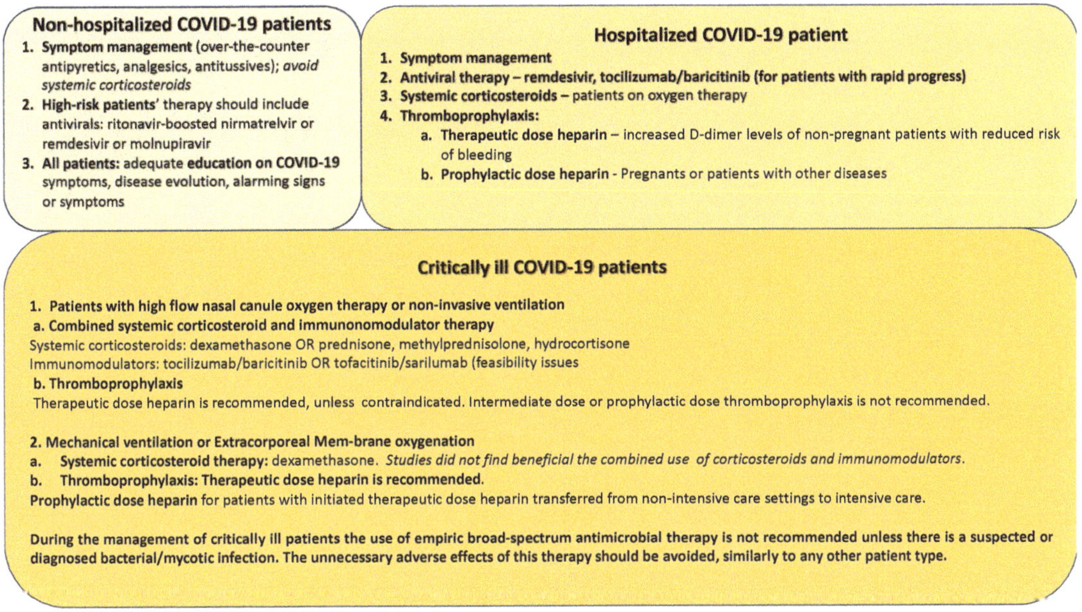
Non-hospitalized COVID-19 patients
1. Symptom management (over-the-counter antipyretics, analgesics, antitussives); avoid systemic corticosteroids
2. High-risk patients' therapy should include antivirals: ritonavir-boosted nirmatrelvir or remdesivir or molnupiravir
3. All patients: adequate education on COVID-19 symptoms, disease evolution, alarming signs or symptoms
Hospitalized COVID-19 patient
1. Symptom management
2. Antiviral therapy – remdesivir, tocilizumab/baricitinib (for patients with rapid progress)
3. Systemic corticosteroids – patients on oxygen therapy
4. Thromboprophylaxis:
a. Therapeutic dose heparin – increased D-dimer levels of non-pregnant patients with reduced risk of bleeding
b. Prophylactic dose heparin - Pregnants or patients with other diseases
Critically ill COVID-19 patients
1. Patients with high flow nasal canule oxygen therapy or non-invasive ventilation
a. Combined systemic corticosteroid and immunonomodulator therapy
Systemic corticosteroids: dexamethasone OR prednisone, methylprednisolone, hydrocortisone
Immunomodulators: tocilizumab/baricitinib OR tofacitinib/sarilumab (feasibility issues
b. Thromboprophylaxis
Therapeutic dose heparin is recommended, unless contraindicated. Intermediate dose or prophylactic dose thromboprophylaxis is not recommended.
2. Mechanical ventilation or Extracorporeal Mem-brane oxygenation
a. Systemic corticosteroid therapy: dexamethasone. Studies did not find beneficial the combined use of corticosteroids and immunomodulators.
b. Thromboprophylaxis: Therapeutic dose heparin is recommended.
Prophylactic dose heparin for patients with initiated therapeutic dose heparin transferred from non-intensive care settings to intensive care.
During the management of critically ill patients the use of empiric broad-spectrum antimicrobial therapy is not recommended unless there is a suspected or diagnosed bacterial/mycotic infection. The unnecessary adverse effects of this therapy should be avoided, similarly to any other patient type.

Figure 1. The management of COVID-19.

The combined use of the available antiviral agents is not fully understood, and the available data on the combined use of antiviral therapies is limited [66].

Antiviral therapy further includes anti-SARS-CoV-2 monoclonal antibodies (mAbs). According to the latest clinical data, the efficacy of anti-SARS-CoV-2 mAbs depends on the subvariant of the SARS-CoV-2; moreover, Omicron and its sub variants show an increased resistance to this therapy type. Thus, the use of anti-SARS-CoV-2 mAbs is not recommended [67–73].

Multisystem Inflammatory Syndrome (MIS)

A special condition in COVID-19 occurs in patients with minimal respiratory symptoms and confirmed SARS-CoV-2 infection, in association with extreme systemic inflammation, markedly elevated C-reactive protein levels, ferritin, D-dimers, cardiac enzymes, creatinine, and liver enzymes, along with various other symptoms, including fever and shock. Furthermore, neurologic, cardiac, and gastrointestinal diseases are also frequently present in these cases. The above-mentioned signs and symptoms have been referred to as multisystem inflammatory syndrome in adults (MIS-A) [74–76].

According to the Centers for Disease Control and Prevention in the United States of America, the case definition of MIS-A is as follows: patients at least 21 years old, who were hospitalized for at least 24 h or whose illness concluded with fatality, and who met the clinical and laboratory criteria included below during the first 3 days of hospitalization. Alternative diagnoses for the condition should also be excluded.

The primary criteria for MIS-A include severe cardiac disease or rash, accompanied by nonpurulent conjunctivitis. The secondary criteria include new-onset neurologic disorders (encephalopathy, seizures, etc.), shock or hypotension not related to medical therapy, thrombocytopenia, abdominal pain, or vomiting or diarrhea. The laboratory criteria are based on the presence of SARS-CoV-2 infection concomitantly with extremely high levels of inflammatory biomarkers (at least two out of CRP, ferritin, erythrocyte sedimentation rate, procalcitonin, and IL-6) [77].

The management of MIS-A involves supportive care, immunosuppression, anticoagulant therapy, and inotropes. Biologic therapies targeting IL-6 and IL-1 have also been reported as being in use for cytokine storm, but the lack of evidence and randomized control trial data on their efficacy in the management of MIS-A means that the therapy is based on the expertise and protocols for Kawasaki disease (KD). A suggested approach could be the use of colchicine, an antiinflammatory drug, which has been reported to have clear cardiovascular benefits in pericarditis and myocardial infarction, and may hasten the resolution of cardiogenic shock in MIS-A. The long-term outcome of recovered MIS-A is uncertain because of the cardiovascular sequels [78].

The United States Centers for Disease Control and Prevention (CDC) and the World Health Organization (WHO) have defined multisystem inflammatory syndrome in children (MIS-C) as an acute condition, which includes what the Royal College of Pediatrics and Child Health has termed as pediatric multisystem inflammatory syndrome temporally associated with COVID-19 (PIMS-TS), and which has symptoms similar to those of Kawasaki disease (KD) and toxic shock syndrome (TSS) [77,79]. The systemic review conducted between December 2019 and July 2021 by M.O Santos at al. summarized a total of 98 articles from 18 countries, and concluded that a differential diagnosis between KD- or TSS-related MIS-C, and MIS-C in COVID-19 was a real challenge for physicians, due to the clinical resemblance; however, there were some particularities that were characteristic only of COVID-19-related MIS-C: the mean age of 9 years; severe abdominal pain due to ascites and mesenteric lymphadenitis, which needed advanced imaging and surgical investigations; and the presence of gastrointestinal symptoms, which occurred more often than in adults. The developed cardiac dysfunction progressed rapidly, and admission into the ICU and the management of hypotension and shock was necessary in some cases, while less-severe cases developed mild and transient coronary artery dilation [79]. There were several theories regarding the development of MIS-C related to COVID-19, and some findings suggest that the hyperinflammatory syndrome most likely occurs due to a postinfectious cytokine storm, rather than as a result of direct cell injury caused by intracellular SARS-CoV-2 replication. Riollano-Cruz et al. demonstrated that an elevated IL-6 level is present in MIS-C in comparison to COVID-19, and IL-1 elevation is absent in contrast to KD, where increased IL-1 levels play an important role in hyperinflammation [80]. According to the systemic review, the management of MIS-C related to COVID-19 involved the WHO protocols of KD and shock, and were represented by intravenous immunoglobulin, antiplatelet, or anticoagulant drugs, and the administration of steroids and biological immunomodulators. Inotropic agents, fluid resuscitation, and ventilatory support were provided when indicated (in a minority of cases) and, in severe cases, extracorporeal membrane oxygenation (ECMO) was used. If applicable, the initial broad-spectrum antibiotic administration was suspended after confirmation of MIS-C related to COVID-19 [79].

The mortality of MIS-A was 5–7% overall, threefold higher than MIS-C, and the predominant cause was reported to be refractory shock, myocarditis, vasculitis, and endothelitis [78].

6.2. The Therapeutic Approach to COVID-19 Coagulopathy

According to several studies, elevated D-dimer and fibrinogen levels are important predictors of mortality; thus, anticoagulation has been proposed in these cases. Heparin can be a good option for thromboprophylaxis, except in patients with antithrombin III

(AT-III) deficiency, who use direct thrombin inhibitors, such as argatroban, which can be a better choice for systemic anticoagulation [33].

The measurement of serum albumin and AT-III activity is recommended in the algorithm of evaluating SARS-CoV-2-infected patients, and supplementation of these parameters at low levels has been shown to be beneficial. Albumin deficiency is involved in the development of edemas and circulatory failure (major mortality factors), while a low AT-III activity increases thromboembolic complications [81]. Deep vein thrombosis and pulmonary embolism are the most frequent thromboembolic conditions in COVID-19, with the affected patients showing a poor outcome and high mortality rate [19]. Medication of the most common cardiovascular disease, arterial hypertension, is an important concern during the pandemic [82].

The requirement of unusually large doses of heparin to achieve therapeutic values of APTT raises the suspicion of heparin resistance. Patients' resistance to heparin therapy may occur in different circumstances: heparin pseudo-resistance, antithrombin III (ATIII) deficiency, low heparin concentration, and COVID-19-related heparin resistance.

Heparin pseudo-resistance is characterized by the temporary inability to detect the effect of heparin after the administration of the therapeutic dose. This occurs due to higher levels of FVIII and fibrinogen, which lead to a shortened APTT and, in certain inflammatory processes, this artificially low APTT value masks the effectiveness of the administered heparin. Thus, clinicians may misinterpret the results, believing that heparin therapy is ineffective, although it is exerting the desired effect [83].

Real heparin resistance is caused by a deficiency of ATIII. Heparin acts by binding to ATIII, and the lack of the latter leads to true heparin ineffectiveness. ATIII deficiency could occur due to consumption or lack of synthesis, and may be related to numerous pathological states, including liver diseases, acute thrombosis, and DIC.

Severe systemic inflammatory processes may hinder the binding of heparin to ATIII, causing a low heparin concentration. Acute-phase proteins and systemic inflammation enhance the synthesis of proteins that can bind to heparin, such as PF-4 (platelet factor 4).

The heparin resistance observed in COVID-19 patients is based on a combination of several factors. This phenomenon occurs due to increased levels of von-Willebrand factor and antiphospholipid antibodies, or based on the mechanism described in the case of pseudo-heparin resistance or low antithrombin III, or a combination of these mechanisms [84].

The management of heparin resistance consists of increased heparin dose administration, or use of alternative therapies, such as ATIII supplementation or the administration of direct thrombin inhibitors [85].

In the case of COVID-19 patients with elevated D-dimer levels, requiring conventional oxygen therapy without an increased bleeding risk, the administration of a therapeutic dose of heparin is recommended. Those patients, with different criteria, or pregnant, should receive a prophylactic heparin dose [86–88].

Furthermore, for patients starting therapeutic heparin prophylaxis in non-intensive care settings, who are then transferred to an intensive care unit, it is recommended to up-dose to therapeutic heparin if there is an indication for the administration of heparin therapy. Therapeutic or intermediate dose venous thromboembolism (VTE) prophylaxis for critical COVID-19 patients is not recommended, apart from being included in a clinical trial [89,90].

The benefits and drawbacks of routine screening for VTE in COVID-19 patients have not been established, so healthcare professionals should determine the frequency of such examinations. Nevertheless, COVID-19 patients experiencing a rapid deterioration in their condition, or developing cardiovascular or neurological complications should undergo routine VTE screening. In suspected cases of thromboembolism, therapeutic anticoagulation should be initiated, even without diagnostic imaging confirmation. Critically ill COVID-19 patients requiring life-support therapies, such as ECMO, NIV, and hemodialysis should be managed with anticoagulants, similar to other patient groups.

Several studies investigated the incidence of VTE in COVID-19 patients, and reported variable results. Notably, clinical data demonstrated that ultrasound screening has led to more frequent VTE diagnoses, compared to laboratory and clinical screening, with the results showing a four-fold difference in favor of ultrasound screening [91–93].

Compared to critically ill septic patients, the incidence of VTE in the COVID-19 patient group was similar; after thromboprophylaxis or antithrombotic therapy, the VTE incidence declined in all patient groups [94,95].

The therapeutic or prophylactic administration of oral anticoagulants is not recommended; instead, a prophylactic dose or therapeutic dose of heparin should be administered for VTE prophylaxis or the prevention of COVID-19 progression.

The interaction between antithrombotic agents and the newly introduced ritonavir-boosted nirmatrelvir, an antiviral combination that strongly affects the cytochrome P450 (CYP450) liver enzyme, can significantly alter the effectiveness of other co-administered drugs.

It is important to continue antithrombotic therapy for COVID-19 patients with pre-existing comorbidities if it was already initiated prior to SARS-CoV-2 infection. However, in the case of a significant bleeding risk or of other hemostasis disorders, it is advisable to modify the therapy. Antiplatelet therapy prior to COVID-19 disease has been shown to reduce the overall mortality in hospitalized patient groups. However, the bias of these retrospective cohort studies cannot be fully removed from these studies [96–99].

Other clinical trials concluded that additional aspirin therapy in COVID-19-hospitalized patients did not affect mortality, and increased the bleeding risk of the patients [100]. Similar results were obtained in another trial regarding the additional use of purinergic P2Y12 receptor inhibitors [101]. According to the results of these studies, there is an inconsistency regarding the beneficial effects of these additional therapies; therefore, the initiation of antiplatelet therapies should not be used to treat patients with COVID-19 unless they are already receiving those drugs to treat pre-existing conditions.

6.3. *Therapy of Comorbidities in COVID-19 Patients*

COVID-19 has the potential to progress to severe conditions, such as hypoxemic respiratory failure, acute respiratory distress syndrome (ARDS), septic shock, cardiac dysfunction, thromboembolism, liver and/or kidney dysfunction, central nervous system disease, or the worsening of comorbidities. Furthermore, weeks or months after SARS-CoV-2 infection, adults may experience multisystem inflammatory syndrome, potentially resulting in critical illness (MIS-A or, in a child, MIS-C). Thus, the therapy for COVID-19 should also include the treatment of comorbidities. The general recommendations regarding the management of COVID-19 patients with comorbidities are shown in Table 2.

Table 2. Guidelines for the management of obese, diabetic subjects, and patients with cardiovascular disease, in the context of SARS-CoV-2 infection.

Obese Patients	Diabetic Patients	Patients with Cardiovascular Diseases
Patient information about COVID-19 symptoms and algorithms to follow in case of symptom progression—telemedicine		
Prevention of infection/reinfection through vaccination; recommendation of wearing a facial mask in crowds, especially during the outbreaks of newer variants		
Monitoring blood pressure and heart rate, with consecutive therapy initiation/modification according to the findings	Monitoring blood pressure and heart rate with consecutive therapy initiation/modification according to the findings and, additionally, dynamic monitoring of carbohydrate balance (blood glucose, HbA1c, C peptide) and, eventually, acid–base balance	Monitoring blood pressure and heart rate, with consecutive therapy modification according to the findings
Diagnosis and therapy of further comorbidities; cardiometabolic risk reduction		
Ensure the availability of hospitalization and eventual intensive care for an unfavorable course of COVID-19		
Weight-loss strategy modification/initiation including diet and physical activity	Considering treatment administration for diabetes mellitus, depending on the type of DM and the severity of COVID-19 symptoms	Treatment of hypertension and/or heart failure focusing on thromboprophylaxis and secondary prevention of complications in the context of COVID-19
Outpatient care after discharge specifically considering the comorbidities of each patient; ideally, an individualized care would be recommended		

Diabetic patients frequently use oral antidiabetic therapy. Among these, metformin has shown potential, based on several in vitro studies, to be effective in the therapy of COVID-19, due to its antiviral, antithrombotic, and antiinflammatory activities [102–105].

Observational studies concluded that COVID-19 patients on metformin therapy were at a lower risk of progressing to severe and critical illness; therefore, these patients should continue their treatment [106–108].

In the case of metformin therapy, the side effects of this drug should also be considered (nausea, vomiting, diarrhea, headache), including the rarely occurring lactic acidosis, especially in high-risk patient groups (elderly, obese, metabolic diseases, cardiac dysfunction, hepatic or renal function impairment, excessive alcohol use) [109].

Additionally, vitamin C, vitamin D, and zinc and magnesium could also be part of the COVID-19 patients' treatment, to improve the immune response in these subjects [110–113].

Currently, there is a lack of clinical data regarding the effectiveness or the utility of supplement administration. Notably, patients with comorbidities have reduced concentrations of several vitamins and trace elements; therefore, it sounds reasonable to supply COVID-19 patients with comorbidities with the vitamins and trace elements they lack [114]. Further data are needed to clarify whether the high-dose parenteral administration of certain vitamin supplements is recommended or not.

Community-based studies have revealed the efficacy of molnupiravir and paxlovid in the treatment of high-risk COVID-19-infected patients, including diabetic, obese, elderly subjects, and those suffering from cardiovascular disease. Molnupiravir proved to be highly effective in patients with an incomplete vaccination scheme [115,116].

7. Discussion

Treatment of a COVID-19 patient requires interdisciplinary management. Prompt clinical and paraclinical investigations are necessary for the best patient status assessment, enabling the possibility of more individualized care. However, uncertainties arise around the optimal timing of thromboprophylactic therapies, as well as the necessity of these pharmacological interventions, especially in the outpatient setting; some studies contradict each other regarding the clinical outcome of these patients. Chinese guidelines recommend a thrombosis risk assessment for COVID-19 outpatients with underlying vascular pathologies, while others do not recommend pharmacological prophylaxis for any COVID-19 outpatient [117–120].

A study conducted in Romania, analyzing the effects of the pandemic on the incidence and type of surgical procedures in vascular surgery cases, and providing a comparison with the pre-pandemic period, showed a 34.51% decrease in the overall procedures performed in the pandemic period in this vascular surgery unit. An 80.6% decrease in acute venous insufficiency cases, and a 67.21% increase in acute arterial ischemia were found compared to the pre-pandemic period; furthermore, all the procedures that were not emergencies were postponed, or alternative treatments were used [121]. Unfortunately, the enrollment of the subjects was based on the clinical diagnosis of the acute event, with no mention of the underlying comorbidities, so there is no information on the exact number of acute ischemia or venous insufficiency patients with T2DM as a comorbidity. However, based on another study conducted by the same authors during the pandemic, it can be estimated that this group comprised approximately 40% of all cases [122].

A retrospective study from the Central Ohio Trauma Center involving a total of 260 T2DM patients admitted to the foot and ankle surgery unit showed higher numbers of urgent surgeries and amputations of all kinds during the pandemic versus the pre-pandemic period, and the risk of major amputations increased. The severity of infections also increased in patients with diabetes-related foot problems.

Even with the adoption of telemedicine, home health visits, and reduced in-person clinic hours, medical care was significantly disrupted.

We speculate that the increased severity of diabetic foot infections and major amputations could be linked to an abrupt interruption of, and limited access to, diabetic foot-wound care and limb preservation, as well as patients' perception of the safety of care during the COVID-19 pandemic [123].

Although venous thromboembolism occurs frequently, and contributes to mortality in COVID-19 patients, arterial thrombosis has also been described (coronary arteries, brain, mesenteric and aortoiliac thrombosis). In a study conducted in the USA, the investigators reported an elevated number of cases presenting lower-extremity ischemia and severe arterial thrombosis during the period of the pandemic. This research reveals an association between lower-extremity arterial thrombosis and SARS-CoV-2 infection (mostly proximal vessels). A higher incidence of death and amputation in COVID-19 patients was described [124].

Despite the administration of anticoagulant medication, the risk of arterial thrombosis continued to rise compared to previous years. The systemic coagulopathy in COVID-19, including the release of inflammatory cytokines, thrombotic events, and microangiopathy, is considered a multifactorial manifestation. Arterial thrombosis, which is less common than venous thrombosis, affected mostly critically ill patients [125].

In a single-center study on the relationship between the coagulation profile and morbidity/mortality in COVID-19 patients performed by A. E. Abd El-Lateef et al., the D-dimer was shown to be a less powerful parameter to predict disease severity and overall survival, compared to FVIII, the von-Willebrand factor antigen, and ristocetin cofactor activity. The ristocetin cofactor activity, alongside the D-dimer and FVIII, independently predicted the disease severity. In the same study, the authors reported reduced survival (30.3%) in patients with higher FVIII levels, and the risk of mortality was extremely (16-fold) increased. Measuring these parameters would help a clinician to decide the therapeutic approach for these patients, aiding in an improvement in disease severity, and in the overall patient survival rates. However, the high costs of these assays are a powerful limitation worldwide, especially in underdeveloped countries [126].

Complications pertaining to the vascular system, such as the cytokine storm that precipitates DIC, and thrombotic microvascular injury affecting the medium- and small-size vessels (coronary heart disease, lung thromboembolism, stroke, mesenteric ischemia, renal-artery thrombosis, and limb-artery thrombosis) are characteristic of COVID-19. Cutaneous lesions associated with arterial and venous thrombotic events appear as gangrene of the limbs [127].

COVID toes or chilblain-like lesions are cutaneous manifestations of COVID-19, especially in pediatric patients, on a background of vascular lesions due to microthrombosis and endothelial inflammation, which might occur in COVID-19, but also after vaccination against SARS-CoV-2. Steroid treatment (systemic, followed by topical therapy) has been proven to be effective in this dermatological disorder [128]. Corticotherapy is also recommended in acute disseminated encephalomyelitis, a life-threatening, immune-mediated neurological complication of COVID-19 [129].

A new, promising perspective for COVID-19 therapy is a combination of anticoagulants and antidepressant drugs (selective serotonin reuptake inhibitors—SSRIs). SSRIs have proven beneficial in the treatment of SARS-CoV-2 infection, by preventing cytokine release [130].

8. Originality and Limitations of the Paper

The originality of this review lies in the fact that the authors also included articles published in Hungarian, Romanian, German, and Spanish, besides the English literature, ensuring a wide dissemination of the data obtained. As well as scholarly articles, certain recommendations from national and international guides were also included.

A limitation is the poor consensus on the management of severe COVID-19 cases in different countries, the discrepancy between the available resources of the medical units dealing with these cases, and the lack of broad worldwide experience regarding viscoelastic methods, which represent a further challenge for a comprehensive review on this subject and the formulation of recommendations.

9. Conclusions

Inflammation- and infection-induced cytokine storm, vasculopathy, overweight, hyperglycemia, and old age are important risk factors for severe outcomes of COVID-19, involving a hypercoagulable state. Early intervention and proper management could reduce the number of severe cases and the hospitalization time for coronavirus-infected patients with comorbidities.

Author Contributions: Conceptualization, M.S., S.P., O.-Z.A.-S., B.R., Z.F., M.C.T. and E.N.-N.; methodology, S.P., Z.S.-S. and M.M.; writing—original draft preparation, M.S., S.P., O.-Z.A.-S., M.M. and E.N.-N.; writing—review and editing, Z.S.-S., B.R., L.D., Z.F. and M.C.T.; visualization, L.D. All authors have read and agreed to the published version of the manuscript.

Funding: This research received no external funding.

Institutional Review Board Statement: Not applicable.

Informed Consent Statement: Not applicable.

Data Availability Statement: No new data were created or analyzed in this study. Data sharing is not applicable to this article.

Acknowledgments: This work was supported by the University of Medicine, Pharmacy, Science and Technology, "George Emil Palade" of Targu Mures, Research Grant number 294/6/14.01.2020.

Conflicts of Interest: The authors declare no conflict of interest.

References

1. Djaharuddin, I.; Munawwarah, S.; Nurulita, A.; Ilyas, M.; Tabri, N.A.; Lihawa, N. Comorbidities and mortality in COVID-19 patients. *Gac. Sanit.* **2021**, *35*, S530–S532. [CrossRef]
2. Fekete, M.; Szarvas, Z.; Fazekas-Pongor, V.; Kováts, Z.; Müller, V.; Varga, J.T. Ambuláns rehabilitációs programok COVID–19-betegek számára (Outpatient rehabilitation programs for COVID-19 patients). *Orvosi Hetil.* **2021**, *162*, 1671–1677.
3. Mureșan, A.V.; Russu, E.; Arbănași, E.M.; Kaller, R.; Hosu, I.; Arbănași, E.M.; Voidăzan, S.T. Negative Impact of the COVID-19 Pandemic on Kidney Disease Management—A Single-Center Experience in Romania. *J. Clin. Med.* **2022**, *11*, 2452.
4. Wu, Z.; McGoogan, J. Outbreak in China: Summary of a report of 72314 cases from the Chinese center for disease control and prevention. *JAMA* **2020**, *323*, 1239–1242.
5. Li, Y.; Zhang, Z.; Yang, L.; Lian, X.; Xie, Y.; Li, S.; Xin, S.; Cao, P.; Lu, J. The MERS-CoV receptor DPP4 as a candidate binding target of the SARS-CoV-2 spike. *Iscience* **2020**, *23*, 101160.
6. Onder, G.; Rezza, G.; Brusaferro, S. Case-fatality rate and characteristics of patients dying in relation to COVID-19 in Italy. *JAMA* **2020**, *323*, 1775–1776.
7. Carvalho, D.B.; Ferreira, V.L.; Assunção, C.M.; Silva, J.A.; Augusto, M.F.; da Silva, R.V.; da Silva Lacerda Filho, S.L.; de Lima Goulart, T.; Fonseca, I.F.; de Figueiredo Júnior, H.S. Uma análise acerca das características das coagulopatias na Covid-19: Revisão de literatura (Analysis on the characteristics of coagulopathy in Covid-19: A literature review). *Rev. Eletrônica Acervo Médico* **2022**, *6*, e10074.
8. Garreta, E.; Prado, P.; Stanifer, M.L.; Monteil, V.; Marco, A.; Ullate-Agote, A.; Moya-Rull, D.; Vilas-Zornoza, A.; Tarantino, C.; Romero, J.P.; et al. A diabetic milieu increases ACE2 expression and cellular susceptibility to SARS-CoV-2 infections in human kidney organoids and patient cells. *Cell Metab.* **2022**, *34*, 857–873.
9. Kazakou, P.; Lambadiari, V.; Ikonomidis, I.; Kountouri, A.; Panagopoulos, G.; Athanasopoulos, S.; Korompoki, E.; Kalomenidis, I.; Dimopoulos, M.A.; Mitrakou, A. Diabetes and COVID-19; a bidirectional interplay. *Front. Endocrinol.* **2022**, *13*, 780663.
10. Kedia-Mehta, N.; Tobin, L.; Zaiatz-Bittencourt, V.; Pisarska, M.M.; De Barra, C.; Choi, C.; Elamin, E.; O'Shea, D.; Gardiner, C.M.; Finlay, D.K.; et al. Cytokine-induced natural killer cell training is dependent on cellular metabolism and is defective in obesity. *Blood Adv.* **2021**, *5*, 4447–4455.
11. Kreiner, F.F.; Kraaijenhof, J.M.; von Herrath, M.; Hovingh, G.K.; von Scholten, B.J. Interleukin 6 in diabetes, chronic kidney disease, and cardiovascular disease: Mechanisms and therapeutic perspectives. *Expert Rev. Clin. Immunol.* **2022**, *18*, 377–389.
12. Martín-Núñez, E.; Donate-Correa, J.; Ferri, C.; López-Castillo, Á.; Delgado-Molinos, A.; Hernández-Carballo, C.; Pérez-Delgado, N.; Rodríguez-Ramos, S.; Cerro-López, P.; Tagua, V.G.; et al. Association between serum levels of Klotho and inflammatory cytokines in cardiovascular disease: A case-control study. *Aging* **2020**, *12*, 1952.
13. Huang, C.; Wang, Y.; Li, X.; Ren, L.; Zhao, J.; Hu, Y.; Zhang, L.; Fan, G.; Xu, J.; Gu, X.; et al. Clinical features of patients infected with 2019 novel coronavirus in Wuhan, China. *Lancet* **2020**, *395*, 497–506.
14. Lelapi, N.; Licastro, N.; Provenzano, M.; Andreucci, M.; Franciscis, S.D.; Serra, R. Cardiovascular disease as a biomarker for an increased risk of COVID-19 infection and related poor prognosis. *Biomark. Med.* **2020**, *14*, 713–716.

15. Hartmann, J.; Ergang, A.; Mason, D.; Dias, J.D. The Role of TEG Analysis in Patients with COVID-19-Associated Coagulopathy: A Systematic Review. *Diagnostics* **2021**, *11*, 172.
16. Pavoni, V.; Gianesello, L.; Pazzi, M.; Dattolo, P.; Prisco, D. Questions about COVID-19 associated coagulopathy: Possible answers from the viscoelastic tests. *J. Clin. Monit. Comput.* **2022**, *36*, 55–69.
17. Tyler, A.; Yang, P.D.; Snider, L.M.; Lerner, S.B.; Aird, W.C.; Shapiro, N.I. New Uses for Thromboelastography and Other Forms of Viscoelastic Monitoring in the Emergency Department: A Narrative Review. *Ann. Emerg. Med.* **2021**, *77*, 357–366.
18. Giubelan, L.; Dragonu, L.; Stoian, A.C.; Dumitrescu, F. O analiză intermediară a formelor medii şi severe de Covid-19 tratate în Clinica de Boli infecţioase Craiova (An intermediate analysis on moderate and severe Covid-19 cases treated at the Infectious Disease Clinic in Craiova). *Rom. J. Infect. Dis.* **2020**, *23*, 272–277. [CrossRef]
19. Mureșan, A.V.; Hălmaciu, I.; Arbănași, E.M.; Kaller, R.; Arbănași, E.M.; Budișcă, O.A.; Melinte, R.M.; Vunvulea, V.; Filep, R.C.; Mărginean, L.; et al. Prognostic Nutritional Index, Controlling Nutritional Status (CONUT) Score, and Inflammatory Biomarkers as Predictors of Deep Vein Thrombosis, Acute Pulmonary Embolism, and Mortality in COVID-19 Patients. *Diagnostics* **2022**, *12*, 2757.
20. Sun, D.W.; Zhang, D.; Tian, R.H.; Li, Y.; Wang, Y.S.; Cao, J.; Tang, Y.; Zhang, N.; Zan, T.; Gao, L.; et al. The underlying changes and predicting role of peripheral blood inflammatory cells in severe COVID-19 patients: A sentinel? *Clin. Chim. Acta* **2020**, *508*, 122–129.
21. Zhang, H.; Penninger, J.M.; Li, Y.; Zhong, N.; Slutsky, A.S. Angiotensin-converting enzyme 2 (ACE2) as a SARS-CoV-2 receptor: Molecular mechanisms and potential therapeutic target. *Intensive Care Med.* **2020**, *46*, 586–590.
22. Ragab, D.; Salah Eldin, H.; Taeimah, M.; Khattab, R.; Salem, R. The COVID-19 Cytokine Storm; What We Know So Far. *Front. Immunol.* **2020**, *11*, 1446.
23. Gómez-Mesa, J.E.; Galindo-Coral, S.; Montes, M.C.; Martin, A.J.M. Thrombosis and Coagulopathy in COVID-19. *Curr. Probl. Cardiol.* **2021**, *46*, 100742.
24. Tomerak, S.; Khan, S.; Almasri, M.; Hussein, R.; Abdelati, A.; Aly, A.; Salameh, M.A.; Saed Aldien, A.; Naveed, H.; Elshazly, M.B.; et al. Systemic inflammation in COVID-19 patients may induce various types of venous and arterial thrombosis: A systematic review. *Scand. J. Immunol.* **2021**, *94*, e13097.
25. Savla, S.R.; Prabhavalkar, K.S.; Bhatt, L.K. Cytokine storm associated coagulation complications in COVID-19 patients: Pathogenesis and Management. *Expert Rev. Anti-Infect. Ther.* **2021**, *19*, 1397–1413.
26. Lima-Martínez, M.M.; Boada, C.C.; Madera-Silva, M.D.; Marín, W.; Contreras, M. Covid-19 y diabetes mellitus: Una relación bidireccional (Covid-19 and diabetes: A bidirectional relationship). *Clin. Investig. Arterioscler.* **2021**, *33*, 151–157.
27. Vudu, S.; Cazac, N.; Munteanu, D.; Vudu, L. Impactul COVID-19 la pacienţii cu diabet zaharat şi alte maladii endocrine (The impact of COVID-19 in patients with diabetes mellitus and other endocrine diseases). *MJHS* **2020**, *2*, 49–58.
28. Lighter, J.; Phillips, M.; Hochman, S.; Sterling, S.; Johnson, D.; Francois, F.; Stachel, A. Obesity in patients younger than 60 years is a risk factor for COVID-19 hospital admission. *Clin. Infect. Dis.* **2020**, *71*, 896–897.
29. García, L.F.; Gutiérrez, A.B.; Bascones, M.G. Relación entre obesidad, diabetes e ingreso en UCI en pacientes COVID-19 (Relationship between obesity, diabetes and ICU admission in COVID-19 patients). *Med. Clin.* **2020**, *155*, 314–315.
30. Arentz, C.; Wild, F. *Vergleich Europäischer Gesundheitssysteme in der COVID-19-Pandemie (Comparison of European Healthcare Systems in the COVID-19 Pandemic)*; WIP-Wissenschaftliches Institut der PKV: Köln, Germany, 2020; Volume 3.
31. Simonnet, A.; Chetboun, M.; Poissy, J.; Raverdy, V.; Noulette, J.; Duhamel, A.; Labreuche, J.; Mathieu, D.; Pattou, F.; Jourdain, M.; et al. High prevalence of obesity in severe acute respiratory syndrome coronavirus-2 (SARS-CoV-2) requiring invasive mechanical ventilation. *Obesity* **2020**, *28*, 1195–1199.
32. Ruan, Q.; Yang, K.; Wang, W.; Jiang, L.; Song, J. Clinical predictors of mortality due to COVID-19 based on an analysis of data of 150 patients from Wuhan, China. *Intensive Care Med.* **2020**, *46*, 846–848.
33. Gardner, A.J.; Kirkin, D.J.; Rodriguez-Villar, S.; Abellanas, G.L.; Tee, A.; Valentin, A. Antithrombin III deficiency-induced coagulopathy in the context of COVID-19: A case series. *Br. J. Haematol.* **2021**, *194*, 1007–1009.
34. Jonigk, D.; Werlein, C.; Lee, P.D.; Kauczor, H.U.; Länger, F.; Ackermann, M. Pulmonale und systemische Pathologie bei COVID-19 (Pulmonary and systemic pathology in COVID-19). *Dtsch. Ärztebl. Int.* **2022**, *119*, 429–435.
35. Tang, N.; Li, D.; Wang, X.; Sun, Z. Abnormal coagulation parameters are associated with poor prognosis in patients with novel coronavirus pneumonia. *J. Thromb. Haemost.* **2020**, *18*, 844–847.
36. Tilinca, M.C.; Merlan, I.; Salcudean, A.; Tilea, I.; Nemes-Nagy, E. Oxidative stress and cytokines' involvement in the occurence and progression of diabetic complications in the COVID-19 pandemic context. *Farmacia* **2021**, *69*, 635–641.
37. Zhang, Y.; Li, H.; Zhang, J.; Cao, Y.; Zhao, X.; Yu, N.; Gao, Y.; Ma, J.; Zhang, H.; Zhang, J.; et al. The clinical characteristics and outcomes of patients with diabetes and secondary hyperglycaemia with coronavirus disease 2019: A single-centre, retrospective, observational study in Wuhan. *Diabetes Obes. Metab.* **2020**, *22*, 1443–1454.
38. Zhu, L.; She, Z.G.; Cheng, X.; Qin, J.J.; Zhang, X.J.; Cai, J.; Lei, F.; Wang, H.; Xie, J.; Wang, W.; et al. Association of blood glucose control and outcomes in patients with COVID-19 and pre-existing type 2 diabetes. *Cell Metab.* **2020**, *31*, 1068–1077.
39. Iba, T.; Levy, J.H.; Levi, M.; Connors, J.M.; Thachil, J. Coagulopathy of coronavirus disease 2019. *Crit. Care Med.* **2020**, *48*, 1358–1364.
40. Connors, J.M.; Levy, J.H. COVID-19 and its implications for thrombosis and anticoagulation. *Blood* **2020**, *135*, 2033–2040.

41. Christensen, B.; Favaloro, E.J.; Lippi, G.; Van Cott, E.M. Hematology laboratory abnormalities in patients with coronavirus disease 2019 (COVID-19). *Semin. Thromb. Hemost.* **2020**, *46*, 845–849.
42. Zhou, F.; Yu, T.; Du, R.; Fan, G.; Liu, Y.; Liu, Z.; Xiang, J.; Wang, Y.; Song, B.; Gu, X.; et al. Clinical course and risk factors for mortality of adult inpatients with COVID-19 in Wuhan, China: A retrospective cohort study. *Lancet* **2020**, *395*, 1054–1062.
43. Iba, T.; Levy, J.H.; Levi, M.; Thachil, J. Coagulopathy in COVID-19. *J. Thromb. Haemost.* **2020**, *18*, 2103–2109.
44. Zhao, X.; Wang, K. Early decrease in blood platelet count is associated with poor prognosis in COVID-19 patients—Indications for predictive, preventive, and personalized medical approach. *EPMA J.* **2020**, *11*, 139–145.
45. Tchachil, J. What do monitoring platelet counts in COVID-19 teach us? *J. Thromb. Haemost.* **2020**, *18*, 2071–2072. [CrossRef]
46. Peyvandi, F.; Artoni, A.; Novembrino, C.; Aliberti, S.; Panigada, M.; Boscarino, M.; Gualtierotti, R.; Rossi, F.; Palla, R.; Martinelli, I.; et al. Hemostatic alterations in COVID-19. *Haematologica* **2021**, *106*, 1472–1475.
47. Stefely, J.A.; Christensen, B.B.; Gogakos, T.; Cone Sullivan, J.K.; Montgomery, G.G.; Barranco, J.P.; Van Cott, E.M. Marked factor V activity elevation in severe COVID-19 is associated with venous thromboembolism. *Am. J. Hematol.* **2020**, *95*, 1522–1530.
48. Asmis, L.; Hellstern, P. Thrombophilia Testing—A Systematic Review. *Clin. Lab.* **2023**, *69*, 670–691. [CrossRef]
49. Ferrari, E.; Sartre, B.; Squara, F.; Contenti, J.; Occelli, C.; Lemoel, F.; Levraut, J.; Doyen, D.; Dellamonica, J.; Mondain, V.; et al. High Prevalence of Acquired Thrombophilia Without Prognosis Value in Patients with Coronavirus Disease 2019. *J. Am. Heart Assoc.* **2020**, *9*, e017773.
50. Zhang, Y.; Cao, W.; Jiang, W.; Xiao, M.; Li, Y.; Tang, N.; Liu, Z.; Yan, X.; Zhao, Y.; Li, T.; et al. Profile of natural anticoagulant, coagulant factor and anti-phospholipid antibody in critically ill COVID-19 patients. *J. Thromb. Thrombolysis* **2020**, *50*, 580–586.
51. Mitrovic, M.; Sabljic, N.; Cvetkovic, Z.; Pantic, N.; Zivkovic Dakic, A.; Bukumiric, Z.; Libek, V.; Savic, N.; Milenkovic, B.; Virijevic, M.; et al. Rotational Thromboelastometry (ROTEM) Profiling of COVID–19 Patients. *Platelets* **2021**, *32*, 690–696. [CrossRef]
52. Zátroch, I.; Smudla, A.; Babik, B.; Tánczos, K.; Kóbori, L.; Szabó, Z.; Fazakas, J. Procoagulation, hypercoagulatio és fibrinolysis "shut down" kimutatása ClotPro® viszkoelasztikus tesztek segítségével COVID-19 betegekben (Procoagulation, hypercoagulation and fibrinolytic "shut down" detected with ClotPro® viscoelastic tests in COVID-19 patients). *Orvosi Hetil.* **2020**, *161*, 899–907.
53. Volod, O.; Bunch, C.M.; Zackariya, N.; Moore, E.E.; Moore, H.B.; Kwaan, H.C.; Neal, M.D.; Al-Fadhl, M.D.; Patel, S.S.; Wiarda, G.; et al. Viscoelastic Hemostatic Assays: A Primer on Legacy and New Generation Devices. *J. Clin. Med.* **2022**, *11*, 860.
54. Gergi, M.; Goodwin, A.; Freeman, K.; Colovos, C.; Volod, O. Viscoelastic hemostasis assays in septic, critically ill coronavirus disease 2019 patients: A practical guide for clinicians. *Blood Coagul. Fibrinolysis* **2021**, *32*, 225–228. [CrossRef]
55. Bachler, M.; Bosch, J. Impaired fibrinolysis in critically ill COVID-19 patients. *Br. J. Anaesth.* **2021**, *126*, 590–598.
56. Schrick, D.; Tőkés-Füzesi, M.; Réger, B.; Molnár, T. Plasma Fibrinogen Independently Predicts Hypofibrinolysis in Severe COVID-19. *Metabolites* **2021**, *11*, 826.
57. Centers for Disease Control and Prevention. Underlying Medical Conditions Associated with HIGHER risk for Severe COVID-19: Information for Healthcare Professionals. 2023. Available online: https://www.cdc.gov/coronavirus/2019-ncov/hcp/clinical-care/underlyingconditions.html (accessed on 20 June 2023).
58. RECOVERY Collaborative Group. Dexamethasone in hospitalized patients with COVID-19. *N. Engl. J. Med.* **2021**, *384*, 693–704. [CrossRef]
59. Caly, L.; Druce, J.D.; Catton, M.G.; Jans, D.A.; Wagstaff, K.M. The FDA-approved drug ivermectin inhibits the replication of SARS-CoV-2 in vitro. *Antivir. Res.* **2020**, *178*, 104787. [CrossRef]
60. Chaccour, C.; Hammann, F.; Ramón-García, S.; Rabinovich, N.R. Ivermectin and COVID-19: Keeping rigor in times of urgency. *Am. J. Trop. Med. Hyg.* **2020**, *102*, 1156–1157. [CrossRef]
61. TOGETHER Investigators. Effect of early treatment with ivermectin among patients with COVID-19. *N. Engl. J. Med.* **2022**, *40*, 1721–1731.
62. Naggie, S.; Boulware, D.R.; Lindsell, C.J.; Stewart, T.G.; Gentile, N.; Collins, S.; McCarthy, M.W.; Jayaweera, D.; Castro, M.; Sulkowski, M.; et al. Effect of ivermectin vs placebo on time to sustained recovery in outpatients with mild to moderate COVID-19: A randomized controlled trial. *JAMA* **2022**, *328*, 1595–1603.
63. Lim, S.C.L.; Hor, C.P.; Tay, K.H.; Jelani, A.M.; Tan, W.H.; Ker, H.B.; Chow, T.S.; Zaid, M.; Cheah, W.K.; Lim, H.H.; et al. Efficacy of ivermectin treatment on disease progression among adults with mild to moderate COVID-19 and comorbidities: The I-TECH randomized clinical trial. *JAMA Intern. Med.* **2022**, *182*, 426–435. [CrossRef] [PubMed]
64. Food and Drug Administration. *Fact Sheet for Healthcare Providers: Emergency Use Authorization for Paxlovid*; Food and Drug Administration: Silver Spring, MD, USA, 2023.
65. Toussi, S.S.; Neutel, J.M.; Navarro, J.; Preston, R.A.; Shi, H.; Kavetska, O.; LaBadie, R.R.; Binks, M.; Chan, P.L.; Demers, N.; et al. Pharmacokinetics of oral nirmatrelvir/ritonavir, a protease inhibitor for treatment of COVID-19, in subjects with renal impairment. *Clin. Pharmacol. Ther.* **2022**, *112*, 892–900. [CrossRef]
66. Gliga, S.; Lübke, N.; Killer, A.; Gruell, H.; Walker, A.; Dilthey, A.T.; Thielen, A.; Lohr, C.; Flaßhove, C.; Krieg, S.; et al. Rapid selection of sotrovimab escape variants in severe acute respiratory syndrome coronavirus 2 Omicron-infected immunocompromised patients. *Clin. Infect. Dis.* **2023**, *76*, 408–415. [CrossRef] [PubMed]
67. Food and Drug Administration. Fact Sheet for Healthcare Providers: Emergency Use Authorization (EUA) of Sotrovimab. 2022. Available online: https://www.fda.gov/media/149534/download (accessed on 13 May 2023).
68. Food and Drug Administration. Fact Sheet for Healthcare Providers: Emergency Use Authorization for Evusheld (Tixagevimab Co-Packaged with Cilgavimab). 2023. Available online: https://www.fda.gov/media/154701/download (accessed on 13 May 2023).

69. Food and Drug Administration. Fact Sheet for Healthcare Providers: Emergency Use Authorization for Bebtelovimab. 2022. Available online: https://www.fda.gov/media/156152/download (accessed on 13 May 2023).
70. Imai, M.; Ito, M.; Kiso, M.; Yamayoshi, S.; Uraki, R.; Fukushi, S.; Watanabe, S.; Suzuki, T.; Maeda, K.; Sakai-Tagawa, Y.; et al. Efficacy of antiviral agents against Omicron subvariants BQ.1.1 and XBB. *N. Engl. J. Med.* **2023**, *388*, 89–91. [CrossRef] [PubMed]
71. Wang, Q.; Iketani, S.; Li, Z.; Liu, L.; Guo, Y.; Huang, Y.; Bowen, A.D.; Liu, M.; Wang, M.; Yu, J.; et al. Alarming antibody evasion properties of rising SARS-CoV-2 BQ and XBB subvariants. *Cell* **2023**, *186*, 279–286.e8. [CrossRef]
72. Wang, Q.; Li, Z.; Ho, J.; Guo, Y.; Yeh, A.Y.; Mohri, H.; Liu, M.; Wang, M.; Yu, J.; Shah, J.G.; et al. Resistance of SARS-CoV-2 Omicron subvariant BA.4.6. to antibody neutralisation. *Lancet Infect. Dis.* **2022**, *22*, 1666–1668. [CrossRef] [PubMed]
73. Takashita, E.; Yamayoshi, S.; Simon, V.; Van Bakel, H.; Sordillo, E.M.; Pekosz, A.; Fukushi, S.; Suzuki, T.; Maeda, K.; Halfmann, P.; et al. Efficacy of antibodies and antiviral drugs against Omicron BA.2.12.1, BA.4, and BA.5 subvariants. *N. Engl. J. Med.* **2022**, *387*, 468–470. [CrossRef]
74. Morris, S.B.; Schwartz, N.G.; Patel, P.; Abbo, L.; Beauchamps, L.; Balan, S.; Lee, E.H.; Paneth-Pollak, R.; Geevarughese, A.; Lash, M.K.; et al. Case series of multisystem inflammatory syndrome in adults associated with SARS-CoV-2 infection—United Kingdom and United States, March-August 2020. *Morb. Mortal. Wkly. Rep.* **2020**, *69*, 1450–1456. [CrossRef]
75. Sansone, M.; Studahl, M.; Berg, S.; Gisslen, M.; Sundell, N. Severe multisystem inflammatory syndrome (MIS-C/A) after confirmed SARS-CoV-2 infection: A report of four adult cases. *Infect. Dis.* **2022**, *54*, 378–383. [CrossRef]
76. Martins, A.; Policarpo, S.; Silva-Pinto, A.; Santos, A.S.; Figueiredo, P.; Sarmento, A.; Santos, L. SARS-CoV-2-related multisystem inflammatory syndrome in adults. *Eur. J. Case Rep. Intern. Med.* **2021**, *8*, 003025. [CrossRef]
77. Available online: https://www.cdc.gov/mis/mis-a/hcp.html (accessed on 2 May 2023).
78. Worku, D. Multisystem Inflammatory Syndrome in Adults (MIS-A) and SARS-CoV2: An Evolving Relationship. *BioMed* **2023**, *3*, 195–201. [CrossRef]
79. Santos, M.O.; Gonçalves, L.C.; Silva, P.A.N.; Moreira, A.L.E.; Ito, C.R.M.; Peixoto, F.A.O.; Wastowski, I.J.; Carneiro, L.C.; Avelino, M.A.G. Multisystem inflammatory syndrome (MIS-C): A systematic review and meta-analysis of clinical characteristics, treatment, and outcomes. *J. Pediatr.* **2022**, *98*, 338–349. [CrossRef]
80. Riollano-Cruz, M.; Akkoyun, E.; Briceno-Brito, E.; Kowalsky, S.; Reed, J.; Posada, R.; Sordillo, E.M.; Tosi, M.; Trachtman, R.; Paniz-Mondolfi, A. Multisystem inflammatory syndrome in children related to COVID-19: A New York City experience. *J. Med. Virol.* **2021**, *93*, 424–433. [CrossRef] [PubMed]
81. Gross, O.; Moerer, O.; Rauen, T.; Boeckhaus, J.; Hoxha, E.; Joerres, A.; Kamm, M.; Elfanish, A.; Windisch, W.; Dreher, M.; et al. Validation of a Prospective Urinalysis-Based Prediction Model for ICU Resources and Outcome of COVID-19 Disease: A Multicenter Cohort Study. *J. Clin. Med.* **2021**, *10*, 3049. [CrossRef]
82. ESC guidance for the diagnosis and management of cardiovascular disease during the COVID-19 pandemic: Part 2—Care pathways, treatment, and follow-up. *Cardiovasc. Res.* **2022**, *118*, 1618–1666. [CrossRef]
83. Nykänen, A.I.; Selby, R.; McRae, K.M.; Zhao, Y.; Asghar, U.M.; Donahoe, L.; Granton, J.; de Perrot, M. Pseudo heparin resistance after pulmonary endarterectomy: Role of thrombus production of Factor VIII. *Semin. Thorac. Cardiovasc. Surg.* **2022**, *34*, 315–323. [CrossRef] [PubMed]
84. White, D.; MacDonald, S.; Bull, T.; Hayman, M.; de Monteverde-Robb, R.; Sapsford, D.; Lavinio, A.; Varley, J.; Johnston, A.; Besser, M.; et al. Heparin resistance in COVID-19 patients in the intensive care unit. *J. Thromb. Thrombolysis* **2020**, *50*, 287–291. [CrossRef] [PubMed]
85. Levy, J.H.; Connors, J.M. Heparin resistance—Clinical perspectives and management strategies. *N. Engl. J. Med.* **2021**, *385*, 826–832. [CrossRef] [PubMed]
86. ATTACC Investigators; ACTIV-4a Investigators; REMAP-CAP Investigators. Therapeutic anticoagulation with heparin in noncritically ill patients with COVID-19. *N. Engl. J. Med.* **2021**, *385*, 790–802. [CrossRef] [PubMed]
87. Sholzberg, M.; Tang, G.H.; Rahhal, H.; AlHamzah, M.; Kreuziger, L.B.; Áinle, F.N.; Alomran, F.; Alayed, K.; Alsheef, M.; AlSumait, F.; et al. Effectiveness of therapeutic heparin versus prophylactic heparin on death, mechanical ventilation, or intensive care unit admission in moderately ill patients with COVID-19 admitted to hospital: RAPID randomised clinical trial. *BMJ* **2021**, *375*, n2400. [CrossRef]
88. Spyropoulos, A.C.; Goldin, M.; Giannis, D.; Diab, W.; Wang, J.; Khanijo, S.; Mignatti, A.; Gianos, E.; Cohen, M.; Sharifova, G.; et al. Efficacy and safety of therapeutic-dose heparin vs standard prophylactic or intermediate-dose heparins for thromboprophylaxis in high-risk hospitalized patients with COVID-19: The HEP-COVID randomized clinical trial. *JAMA Int. Med.* **2021**, *181*, 1612–1620. [CrossRef]
89. INSPIRATION Investigators. Effect of Intermediate-Dose vs Standard-Dose Prophylactic Anticoagulation on Thrombotic Events, Extracorporeal Membrane Oxygenation Treatment, or Mortality Among Patients With COVID-19 Admitted to the Intensive Care Unit: The INSPIRATION Randomized Clinical Trial. *JAMA* **2021**, *325*, 1620–1630.
90. REMAP-CAP Investigators; ACTIV-4a Investigators; ATTACC Investigators. Therapeutic anticoagulation with heparin in critically ill patients with COVID-19. *N. Engl. J. Med.* **2021**, *385*, 777–789. [CrossRef]
91. Nopp, S.; Moik, F.; Jilma, B.; Pabinger, I.; Ay, C. Risk of venous thromboembolism in patients with COVID-19: A systematic review and meta-analysis. *Res. Pract. Thromb. Haemost.* **2020**, *4*, 1178–1191. [CrossRef]

92. Cohen, A.T.; Davidson, B.L.; Gallus, A.S.; Lassen, M.R.; Prins, M.H.; Tomkowski, W.; Turpie, A.G.; Egberts, J.F.; Lensing, A.W. Efficacy and safety of fondaparinux for the prevention of venous thromboembolism in older acute medical patients: Randomised placebo controlled trial. *BMJ* **2006**, *332*, 325–329. [CrossRef] [PubMed]
93. Leizorovicz, A.; Cohen, A.T.; Turpie, A.G.; Olsson, C.G.; Vaitkus, P.T.; Goldhaber, S.Z. Randomized, placebo-controlled trial of dalteparin for the prevention of venous thromboembolism in acutely ill medical patients. *Circulation* **2004**, *110*, 874–879. [CrossRef]
94. PROTECT Investigators for the Canadian Critical Care Trials Group; Australian and New Zealand Intensive Care Society Clinical Trials Group. Dalteparin versus unfractionated heparin in critically ill patients. *N. Engl. J. Med.* **2011**, *364*, 1305–1314. [CrossRef] [PubMed]
95. Kaplan, D.; Casper, T.C.; Elliott, C.G.; Men, S.; Pendleton, R.C.; Kraiss, L.W.; Weyrich, A.S.; Grissom, C.K.; Zimmerman, G.A.; Rondina, M.T. VTE incidence and risk factors in patients with severe sepsis and septic shock. *Chest* **2015**, *148*, 1224–1230. [CrossRef]
96. Chow, J.H.; Yin, Y.; Yamane, D.P.; Davison, D.; Keneally, R.J.; Hawkins, K.; Parr, K.G.; Al-Mashat, M.; Berger, J.S.; Bushardt, R.L.; et al. Association of prehospital antiplatelet therapy with survival in patients hospitalized with COVID-19: A propensity score-matched analysis. *J. Thromb. Haemost.* **2021**, *19*, 2814–2824. [CrossRef]
97. Chow, J.H.; Khanna, A.K.; Kethireddy, S.; Yamane, D.; Levine, A.; Jackson, A.M.; McCurdy, M.T.; Tabatabai, A.; Kumar, G.; Park, P.; et al. Aspirin use is associated with decreased mechanical ventilation, intensive care unit admission, and in-hospital mortality in hospitalized patients with coronavirus disease 2019. *Anesth. Analg.* **2021**, *132*, 930–941. [CrossRef] [PubMed]
98. Chow, J.H.; Rahnavard, A.; Gomberg-Maitland, M.; Chatterjee, R.; Patodi, P.; Yamane, D.P.; Levine, A.R.; Davison, D.; Hawkins, K.; Jackson, A.M.; et al. Association of early aspirin use with in-hospital mortality in patients with moderate COVID-19. *JAMA Netw. Open* **2022**, *5*, e223890. [CrossRef] [PubMed]
99. Abdi, M.; Hosseini, Z.; Shirjan, F.; Mohammadi, L.; Abadi, S.S.; Massoudi, N.; Zangiabadian, M.; Nasiri, M.J. The effect of aspirin on the prevention of pro-thrombotic states in hospitalized COVID-19 patients: Systematic review. *Cardiovasc. Hematol. Agents Med. Chem.* **2022**, *20*, 189–196. [PubMed]
100. RECOVERY Collaborative Group. Aspirin in patients admitted to hospital with COVID-19 (RECOVERY): A randomised, controlled, open-label, platform trial. *Lancet* **2022**, *399*, 143–151. [CrossRef] [PubMed]
101. Berger, J.S.; Kornblith, L.Z.; Gong, M.N.; Reynolds, H.R.; Cushman, M.; Cheng, Y.; McVerry, B.J.; Kim, K.S.; Lopes, R.D.; Atassi, B.; et al. Effect of P2Y12 inhibitors on survival free of organ support among non-critically ill hospitalized patients with COVID-19: A randomized clinical trial. *JAMA* **2022**, *327*, 227–236. [CrossRef]
102. Karam, B.S.; Morris, R.S.; Bramante, C.T.; Puskarich, M.; Zolfaghari, E.J.; Lotfi-Emran, S.; Ingraham, N.E.; Charles, A.; Odde, D.J.; Tignanelli, C.J. mTOR inhibition in COVID-19: A commentary and review of efficacy in RNA viruses. *J. Med. Virol.* **2021**, *93*, 1843–1846. [CrossRef] [PubMed]
103. Del Campo, J.A.; García-Valdecasas, M.; Gil-Gómez, A.; Rojas, Á.; Gallego, P.; Ampuero, J.; Gallego-Durán, R.; Pastor, H.; Grande, L.; Padillo, F.J.; et al. Simvastatin and metformin inhibit cell growth in hepatitis C virus infected cells via mTOR increasing PTEN and autophagy. *PLoS ONE* **2018**, *13*, e0191805. [CrossRef]
104. Postler, T.S.; Peng, V.; Bhatt, D.M.; Ghosh, S. Metformin selectively dampens the acute inflammatory response through an AMPK-dependent mechanism. *Sci. Rep.* **2021**, *11*, 18721. [CrossRef]
105. Xin, G.; Wei, Z.; Ji, C.; Zheng, H.; Gu, J.; Ma, L.; Huang, W.; Morris-Natschke, S.L.; Yeh, J.L.; Zhang, R.; et al. Metformin uniquely prevents thrombosis by inhibiting platelet activation and mtDNA release. *Sci. Rep.* **2016**, *6*, 36222. [CrossRef]
106. Li, Y.; Yang, X.; Yan, P.; Sun, T.; Zeng, Z.; Li, S. Metformin in patients with COVID-19: A systematic review and meta-analysis. *Front. Med.* **2021**, *8*, 704666. [CrossRef] [PubMed]
107. Bramante, C.T.; Buse, J.; Tamaritz, L.; Palacio, A.; Cohen, K.; Vojta, D.; Liebovitz, D.; Mitchell, N.; Nicklas, J.; Lingvay, I.; et al. Outpatient metformin use is associated with reduced severity of COVID-19 disease in adults with overweight or obesity. *J. Med. Virol.* **2021**, *93*, 4273–4279. [CrossRef]
108. Luo, P.; Qiu, L.; Liu, Y.; Liu, X.L.; Zheng, J.L.; Xue, H.Y.; Liu, W.H.; Liu, D.; Li, J. Metformin treatment was associated with decreased mortality in COVID-19 patients with diabetes in a retrospective analysis. *Am. J. Trop. Med. Hyg.* **2020**, *103*, 69–72. [CrossRef] [PubMed]
109. Reis, G.; Silva, E.A.D.S.M.; Silva, D.C.M.; Thabane, L.; Milagres, A.C.; Ferreira, T.S.; Dos Santos, C.V.; de Figueiredo Neto, A.D.; Callegari, E.D.; Savassi, L.C.; et al. Effect of early treatment with metformin on risk of emergency care and hospitalization among patients with COVID-19: The TOGETHER randomized platform clinical trial. *Lancet Reg. Health–Am.* **2022**, *6*, 100142. [CrossRef] [PubMed]
110. Thomas, S.; Patel, D.; Bittel, B.; Wolski, K.; Wang, Q.; Kumar, A.; Il'Giovine, Z.J.; Mehra, R.; McWilliams, C.; Nissen, S.E.; et al. Effect of high-dose zinc and ascorbic acid supplementation vs usual care on symptom length and reduction among ambulatory patients with SARS-CoV-2 infection: The COVID A to Z randomized clinical trial. *JAMA Netw. Open* **2021**, *4*, e210369. [CrossRef] [PubMed]
111. Chen, J.; Mei, K.; Xie, L.; Yuan, P.; Ma, J.; Yu, P.; Zhu, W.; Zheng, C.; Liu, X. Low vitamin D levels do not aggravate COVID-19 risk or death, and vitamin D supplementation does not improve outcomes in hospitalized patients with COVID-19: A meta-analysis and GRADE assessment of cohort studies and RCTs. *Nutr. J.* **2021**, *20*, 89. [CrossRef]
112. National Institutes of Health (NIH). COVID-19 Treatment Guidelines 3 Office of Dietary Supplements, National Institutes of Health. In *Zinc Fact Sheet for Health Professionals*; National Institutes of Health (NIH): Bethesda, MD, USA, 2022.

113. Moscatelli, F.; Sessa, F.; Valenzano, A.; Polito, R.; Monda, V.; Cibelli, G.; Villano, I.; Pisanelli, D.; Perrella, M.; Daniele, A.; et al. COVID-19: Role of nutrition and supplementation. *Nutrients* **2021**, *13*, 976. [CrossRef]
114. Zhang, J.; Rao, X.; Li, Y.; Zhu, Y.; Liu, F.; Guo, G.; Luo, G.; Meng, Z.; De Backer, D.; Xiang, H.; et al. Pilot trial of high-dose vitamin C in critically ill COVID-19 patients. *Ann. Intensive Care* **2021**, *11*, 5. [CrossRef]
115. Najjar-Debbiny, R.; Gronich, N.; Weber, G.; Khoury, J.; Amar, M.; Stein, N.; Goldstein, L.H.; Saliba, W. Effectiveness of Paxlovid in reducing severe coronavirus 2019 and mortality in high-risk patients. *Clin. Infect. Dis.* **2023**, *76*, 342–349. [CrossRef]
116. Najjar-Debbiny, R.; Gronich, N.; Weber, G.; Khoury, J.; Amar, M.; Stein, N.; Goldstein, L.H.; Saliba, W. Efectiveness of molnupiravir in high-risk patients: A propensity score matched analysis. *Clin. Infect. Dis.* **2023**, *76*, 453–460. [CrossRef]
117. Long, B.; Chavez, S.; Carius, B.M.; Brady, W.J.; Liang, S.Y.; Koyfman, A.; Gottlieb, M. Clinical update on COVID-19 for the emergency and critical care clinician: Medical management. *Am. J. Emerg. Med.* **2022**, *56*, 158–170. [CrossRef]
118. Moores, L.K.; Tritschler, T.; Brosnahan, S.; Carrier, M.; Collen, J.F.; Doerschug, K.; Holley, A.B.; Jimenez, D.; Le Gal, G.; Rali, P.; et al. Prevention, Diagnosis, and Treatment of VTE in Patients with Coronavirus Disease 2019: CHEST Guideline and Expert Panel Report. *Chest* **2020**, *158*, 1143–1163. [CrossRef]
119. Thachil, J.; Juffermans, N.P.; Ranucci, M.; Connors, J.M.; Warkentin, T.E.; Ortel, T.L.; Levi, M.; Iba, T.; Levy, J.H. ISTH DIC subcommittee communication on anticoagulation in COVID-19. *J. Thromb. Haemost.* **2020**, *18*, 2138–2144. [CrossRef] [PubMed]
120. Thachil, J.; Tang, N.; Gando, S.; Falanga, A.; Cattaneo, M.; Levi, M.; Clark, C.; Iba, T. ISTH interim guidance on recognition and management of coagulopathy in COVID-19. *J. Thromb. Haemost.* **2020**, *18*, 1023–1026. [CrossRef] [PubMed]
121. Arbănași, E.M.; Kaller, R.; Mureșan, V.A.; Voidăzan, S.; Arbănași, E.M.; Russu, E. Impact of COVID-19 Pandemic on Vascular Surgery Unit Activity in Central Romania. *Front. Surg.* **2022**, *9*, 883935.
122. Arbănași, E.M.; Halmaciu, I.; Kaller, R.; Mureșan, V.A.; Arbănași, E.M.; Suciu, B.A.; Coșarcă, C.M.; Cojocaru, I.I.; Melinte, R.M.; Russu, E. Systemic Inflammatory Biomarkers and Chest CT Findings as Predictors of Acute Limb Ischemia Risk, Intensive Care Unit Admission, and Mortality in COVID-19 Patients. *Diagnostics* **2022**, *12*, 2379. [CrossRef] [PubMed]
123. Casciato, D.J.; Yancovitz, S.; Thompson, J.; Anderson, S.; Bischoff, A.; Ayres, S.; Barron, I. Diabetes-related major and minor amputation risk increased during the Covid-19 pandemic. *J. Am. Podiatr. Med. Assoc.* **2020**, *113*, 202–224. [CrossRef]
124. Goldman, I.A.; Ye, K.; Scheinfeld, M.H. Lower extremity arterial thrombosis associated with COVID-19 is characterized by greater thrombus burden and increased rate of amputation and death. *Radiology* **2020**, *297*, E263–E269. [CrossRef]
125. Nana, P.; Dakis, K.; Spanos, K.; Tsolaki, V.; Karavidas, N.; Zakynthinos, G.; Kouvelos, G.; Giannoukas, A.; Matsagkas, M. COVID-19 related peripheral arterial thrombotic events in intensive care unit and non-intensive care unit patients: A retrospective case series. *Vascular* **2022**, 17085381221140159. [CrossRef]
126. Abd El-Lateef, A.E.; Alghamdi, S.; Ebid, G.; Khalil, K.; Kabrah, S.; Abdel Ghafar, M.T. Coagulation profile in COVID-19 patients and its relation to disease severity and overall survival: A single-center study. *Br. J. Biomed. Sci.* **2022**, *79*, 10098. [CrossRef]
127. Rastogi, A.; Dogra, H.; Jude, E.B. Covid-19 and peripheral arterial complications in people with diabetes and hypertension: A systemic review. *Diabetes Metab. Syndr. Clin. Res. Rev.* **2021**, *15*, 102204. [CrossRef]
128. Paparella, R.; Tarani, L.; Properzi, E.; Costantino, F.; Saburri, C.; Lucibello, R.; Richetta, A.; Spalice, A.; Leonardi, L. Chilblain-like lesions onset during SARS-CoV-2 infection in a COVID-19-vaccinated adolescent: Case report and review of literature. *Ital. J. Pediatr.* **2022**, *48*, 93. [CrossRef]
129. Stoian, A.; Bajko, Z.; Stoian, M.; Cioflinc, R.A.; Niculescu, R.; Arbănași, E.M.; Russu, E.; Botoncea, M.; Bălașa, R. The Occurrence of Acute Disseminated Encephalomyelitis in SARS-CoV-2 Infection/Vaccination: Our Experience and a Systematic Review of the Literature. *Vaccines* **2023**, *11*, 1225. [CrossRef] [PubMed]
130. Anar, M.A.; Foroughi, E.; Sohrabi, E.; Peiravi, S.; Tavakoli, Y.; Khouzani, M.K.; Behshood, P.; Shamshiri, M.; Faridzadeh, A.; Keylani, K.; et al. Selective serotonin reuptake inhibitors: New hope in the fight against COVID-19. *Front. Pharmacol.* **2022**, *13*, 1036093. [CrossRef] [PubMed]

International Journal of
Molecular Sciences

MDPI

Article

SARS-CoV-2 Spike Proteins and Cell–Cell Communication Induce P-Selectin and Markers of Endothelial Injury, NETosis, and Inflammation in Human Lung Microvascular Endothelial Cells and Neutrophils: Implications for the Pathogenesis of COVID-19 Coagulopathy

Biju Bhargavan and Georgette D. Kanmogne *

Department of Pharmacology and Experimental Neuroscience, College of Medicine, University of Nebraska Medical Center, Omaha, NE 68198-5800, USA; bbhargavan@unmc.edu
* Correspondence: gkanmogne@unmc.edu

Abstract: COVID-19 progression often involves severe lung injury, inflammation, coagulopathy, and leukocyte infiltration into pulmonary tissues. The pathogenesis of these complications is unknown. Because vascular endothelium and neutrophils express angiotensin-converting enzyme-2 and spike (S)-proteins, which are present in bodily fluids and tissues of SARS-CoV-2-infected patients, we investigated the effect of S-proteins and cell–cell communication on human lung microvascular endothelial cells and neutrophils expression of P-selectin, markers of coagulopathy, NETosis, and inflammation. Exposure of endothelial cells or neutrophils to S-proteins and endothelial–neutrophils co-culture induced P-selectin transcription and expression, significantly increased expression/secretion of IL-6, von Willebrand factor (vWF, pro-coagulant), and citrullinated histone H3 (cit-H3, NETosis marker). Compared to the SARS-CoV-2 Wuhan variant, Delta variant S-proteins induced 1.4–15-fold higher P-selectin and higher IL-6 and vWF. Recombinant tissue factor pathway inhibitor (rTFPI), 5,5′-dithio-bis-(2-nitrobenzoic acid) (thiol blocker), and thrombomodulin (anticoagulant) blocked S-protein induced vWF, IL-6, and cit-H3. This suggests that following SARS-CoV-2 contact with the pulmonary endothelium or neutrophils and endothelial–neutrophil interactions, S-proteins increase adhesion molecules, induce endothelial injury, inflammation, NETosis and coagulopathy via the tissue factor pathway, mechanisms involving functional thiol groups, and/or the fibrinolysis system. Using rTFPI, effectors of the fibrinolysis system and/or thiol-based drugs could be viable therapeutic strategies against SARS-CoV-2-induced endothelial injury, inflammation, NETosis, and coagulopathy.

Keywords: SARS-CoV-2 spike proteins; human lung endothelial cells; neutrophils; P-selectin; von willebrand factor; IL-6; citrullinated histone H3; neutrophils extracellular traps; TFPI; DTNB; thrombomodulin

Citation: Bhargavan, B.; Kanmogne, G.D. SARS-CoV-2 Spike Proteins and Cell–Cell Communication Induce P-Selectin and Markers of Endothelial Injury, NETosis, and Inflammation in Human Lung Microvascular Endothelial Cells and Neutrophils: Implications for the Pathogenesis of COVID-19 Coagulopathy. *Int. J. Mol. Sci.* **2023**, *24*, 12585. https://doi.org/10.3390/ijms241612585

Academic Editors: Eliza Russu, Alexandru Schiopu and Emil Marian Arbănaşi

Received: 28 April 2023
Revised: 31 July 2023
Accepted: 3 August 2023
Published: 9 August 2023

1. Introduction

Severe acute respiratory syndrome coronavirus-2 (SARS-CoV-2), the causative agent of coronavirus disease 2019 (COVID-19), has so far infected over 686 million people worldwide, resulting in over 6.88 million deaths and counting [1–3]. Although SARS-CoV2-induced immunopathology can affect several organs, postmortem examination shows that for most COVID-19 patients, the primary cause of death was acute lung injury associated with the presence of virions and spike (S) proteins in lung blood vessels, endothelial injury, increases in leukocyte infiltration in lung tissues, circulating prothrombotic factors, inflammation, and thrombosis [4–7]. Endothelial injury is also associated with the release of von Willebrand factor (vWF) from endothelial granules, upregulation of adhesion molecules, increased neutrophil activation, adhesion and transmigration into vascular walls [8,9]. The pathogenesis of these pulmonary complications in COVID-19 patients is unknown.

Coronaviruses enter and infect target cells by binding their S-protein to cellular angiotensin-converting enzyme-2 (ACE2) [10,11], and human neutrophils [12,13] and endothelial cells [14–16] express ACE2. Because SARS-CoV-2 and its S-proteins are present in tissues and bodily fluids of infected patients and COVID-19 pathology includes endotheliopathy and leukocyte infiltration into the lungs [7,17,18], it is important to determine whether viral S-proteins directly contribute to these lung pathologies and whether leukocyte interactions with the vascular endothelium influence SARS-CoV-2-induced pathologies. In the present study, we investigate the direct and indirect effects of S-protein exposure on the expression and secretion of adhesion molecules, markers of endothelial injury, and inflammation. Because increased levels of neutrophil extracellular traps (NETs) are associated with COVID-19 pathology and disease severity [19–22], we also investigated the direct and indirect effects of S-protein exposure on markers of NET activation and release (NETosis). We demonstrate that exposure of primary human lung microvascular endothelial cells (HLMEC) or neutrophils to S-proteins and endothelial–neutrophil interactions induced transcription and expression of P-selectin and significantly increased the expression and secretion of vWF, interleukin (IL)-6, and citrullinated histone H3 (cit-H3), a marker of NETosis. A trend toward higher P-selectin and vWF levels and significantly higher IL-6 levels was observed with SARS-CoV-2 Delta variant S-proteins (SD) compared to Wuhan variant S-proteins (SW). Recombinant tissue factor pathway inhibitor (rTFPI; the primary physiological inhibitor of the extrinsic pathway of blood coagulation [23–26]), as well as 5,5′-dithio-bis-(2-nitrobenzoic acid) (DTNB; a thiol blocker) and thrombomodulin (TM; a high affinity thrombin receptor [27]), blocked S-protein-induced expression of vWF, IL-6, and cit-H3.

These data suggest that when the lung endothelium or neutrophils are exposed to SARS-CoV-2, viral S-proteins increase adhesion molecules and induce endothelial injury, inflammation, and NETosis via the TF pathway and mechanisms involving functional thiol groups and the fibrinolysis system. Furthermore, any of these two cell populations exposed to SARS-CoV-2 or viral S-proteins can induce injury, inflammation, and NETosis in non-exposed neighboring cells. These findings suggest that viable therapeutic strategies against SARS-CoV-2-induced cellular injury, NETosis, and inflammation could include rTFPI, effectors of the fibrinolysis system, and/or thiol-based drugs.

2. Results

2.1. Exposure of HLMEC or Neutrophils to S-Proteins and Endothelial–Neutrophil Interactions Increased P-Selectin Transcription

Compared to controls (untreated cells, cells treated with heat-inactivated S-proteins, or cells pretreated with recombinant human (rh) ACE2), exposure (6–24 h) of HLMEC to SW or SD increased P-selectin mRNA by 12- to 20-fold and 10- to 67-fold, respectively; with the largest increase (51.7- to 67-fold) observed at 12 h (Figure 1A). Co-culture of SW- or SD-treated HLMEC with neutrophils increased P-selectin mRNA in HLMEC by 64.7- to 258-fold and 138- to 650-fold, respectively (Figure 1B), and increased P-selectin mRNA in neutrophils by 17- to 92-fold and 148- to 652-fold, respectively (Figure 1C). Co-culture of SW- or SD-treated neutrophils with HLMEC increased P-selectin mRNA in HLMEC by 2.8- to 62-fold and 4- to 262-fold, respectively (Figure 1D), and increased P-selectin mRNA in neutrophils by 11- to 136-fold and 77- to 228-fold, respectively (Figure 1E).

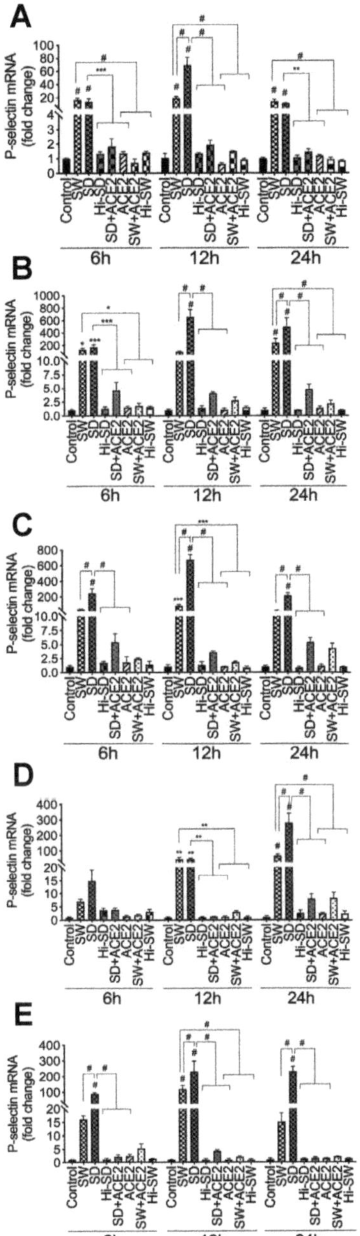

Figure 1. S-proteins and endothelial–neutrophil interactions induce P-selectin transcriptional upregulation in HLMEC and neutrophils. (**A**): HLMEC treated (for 6–24 h) with 1 nM S-protein Wuhan (SW) or Delta (SD) variants. (**B**,**C**): HLMEC were treated (6 h) with SW or SD, washed, and co-cultured (6–24 h) with neutrophils. (**D**,**E**): neutrophils treated (6 h) with SW or SD, washed, and co-cultured (6–24 h) with HLMEC. P-selectin mRNA in endothelial cells (**A**,**B**,**D**) and neutrophils (**C**,**E**) was quantified by real-time PCR. Data presented as mean ± standard deviation. Control: untreated cells; ACE2: cells treated with recombinant human (rh) ACE2 (1 μg/mL). Hi: cells treated with heat-inactivated S-proteins. * $p < 0.015$; ** $p < 0.007$; *** $p < 0.0007$; # $p < 0.0001$.

2.2. Exposure of HLMEC to S-Proteins Induced P-Selectin Expression

Immunofluorescence imaging showed that, compared to controls, exposure (12 h) of HLMEC to SW or SD increased P-selectin expression by 7- to 9-fold and by 8.9- to 11.3-fold, respectively (Figure 2A,B). Western blot analysis further confirmed these findings; compared to controls, SW and SD, respectively, increased P-selectin levels by 4.5- to 63-fold and by 6.4- to 110-fold (Figure 2C,D).

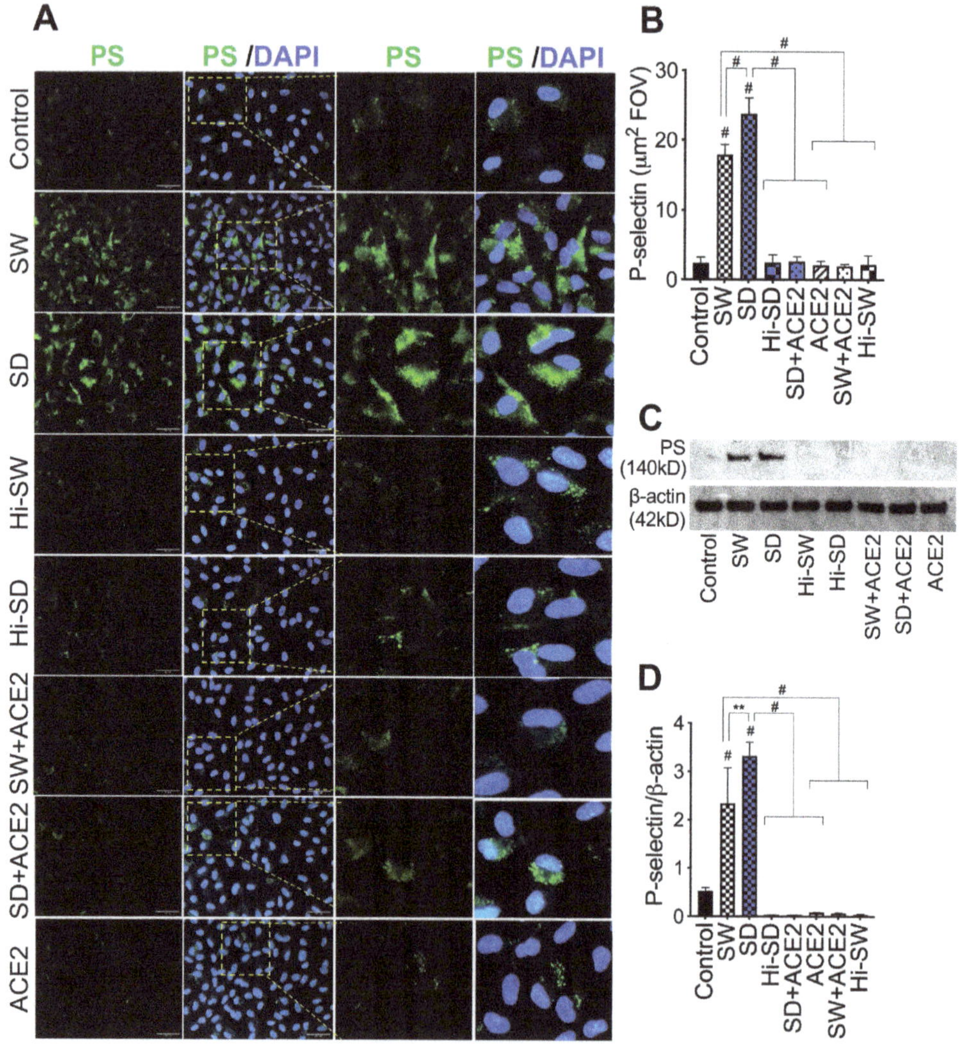

Figure 2. S-proteins induce P-selectin expression in HLMEC. HLMEC were treated with 1 nM S-proteins (SW or SD) for 12 h and P-selectin expression was quantified by immunofluorescence (**A**,**B**) and Western blot (**C**,**D**) analysis. DAPI (blue) was used for nuclear counterstaining. ImageJ software was used for densitometry quantification. For immunofluorescence images, five fields of view (FOV) were analyzed for each sample (**B**). For Western blot analysis, densitometry values were normalized to the sample's β-actin levels (**D**). For panel (**A**), all images were at 20×. PS: P-selectin; control: untreated cells; ACE2: cells treated with rhACE2; Hi: cells treated with heat-inactivated S-proteins ** $p = 0.01$; # $p < 0.0001$.

2.3. Delta Variant S-Proteins Induced Higher P-Selectin Transcription and Expression Than the Wuhan Variant

At 12 h, compared to SW, SD induced significantly higher P-selectin mRNA in HLMEC following direct exposure (3.7-fold, Figure 1A) or co-culture with neutrophils (2- to 6.8-fold, Figure 1B); and induced higher P-selectin mRNA in neutrophils (7.6- to 12.4-fold, Figure 1C). For neutrophils treated with S-proteins and co-cultured with HLMEC, SD induced 4-fold higher P-selectin transcription in HLMEC at 24 h (Figure 1D) and 2- to 15-fold higher P-selectin mRNA in neutrophils (Figure 1E), compared to SW. Immunofluorescence and Western blot analyses also showed that SD increased P-selectin expression in HLMEC by 1.3- to 1.4-fold compared to SW (Figure 2). No significant increase in P-selectin transcription (Figure 1) or expression (Figure 2) was observed in cells treated with Hi-SW or Hi-SD; recombinant human (rh) ACE2 blocked or significantly abrogated SW- and SD-induced P-selectin.

2.4. Exposure of Human Neutrophils and HLMEC to S-Proteins and Neutrophil–Endothelial Interactions Induces Histone H3 Citrullination

Hallmarks of NETosis include increased citrullination of histone proteins, including H3 [28–30]. Therefore, we assessed whether S-proteins and/or endothelial–neutrophil interactions affect the production of cit-H3. Compared to controls, SW and SD significantly increased cit-H3 levels in neutrophil culture supernatants following direct exposure (6–24 h) (1.6- to 3.3-fold, Figure 3A), co-culture of S-proteins-treated neutrophils with untreated HLMEC (2- to 4.3-fold, Figure 3B), or co-culture of S-proteins-treated endothelial cells with untreated neutrophils (1.7- to 3.3-fold, Figure 3C).

2.5. Exposure of HLMEC and Neutrophils to S-Proteins and Neutrophil–Endothelial Interactions Increased vWF Expression

Compared to controls, SW and SD significantly increased vWF levels in HLMEC culture supernatants (by 1.2- to 7.2-fold, Figure 4A) and cell lysates (2.2- to 5.2-fold, Figure 4B) following direct exposure (Figure 4A,B), co-culture of S-proteins-treated endothelial cells with untreated neutrophils (2- to 8.8-fold, Figure 4C), and co-culture of S-proteins-treated neutrophils with untreated HLMEC (1.5- to 4.6-fold, Figure 4D). Data showed a trend toward increased vWF following SD treatments and co-cultures, compared to SW (Figure 4).

2.6. Exposure of HLMEC and Neutrophils to S-Proteins and Endothelial-Neutrophil Interactions Increased IL-6 Expression

Compared to untreated cells, cells treated with Hi-SW, Hi-SD, or cells pretreated with rhACE2, exposure of HLMEC to SW or SD (6–24 h) increased IL-6 levels in culture supernatants by 1.2 to 4.6-fold (Figure 5A). Co-culture of SW- or SD-treated HLMEC with neutrophils increased IL-6 levels by 1.4 to 3.8-fold (Figure 5B). Compared to SW, SD induced significantly (1.3- to 1.6-fold) higher IL-6 expression following exposure to endothelial cells (Figure 5A) and co-culture of exposed endothelial cells with neutrophils (Figure 5B). Co-culture of SW- or SD-treated neutrophils with HLMEC increased IL-6 levels in culture supernatants by 1.4 to 4.7-fold (Figure 5C); rhACE2 blocked SW- and SD-induced IL-6. IL-6 levels in culture supernatants of cells treated with Hi-SW, Hi-SD, or rhACE2 were similar to untreated controls (Figure 5).

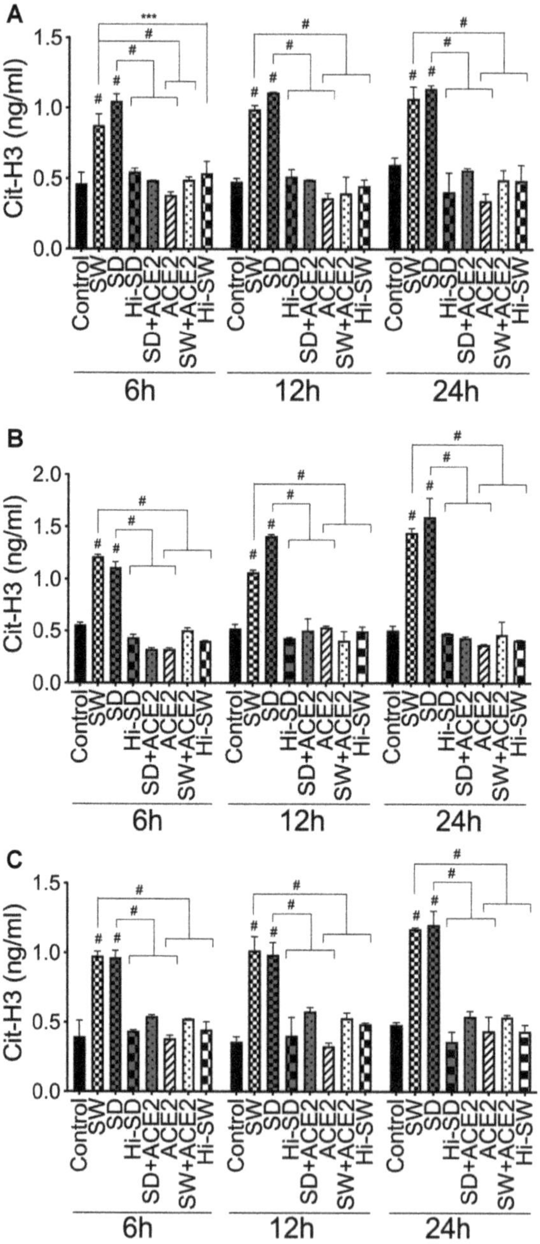

Figure 3. S-proteins and endothelial–neutrophil interactions induce/increase the expression and secretion of cit-H3. Human neutrophils were treated with 1 nM S-proteins (SW or SD) for 6–24 h (**A**). In separate experiments, neutrophils (**B**) and HLMEC (**C**) were treated with S-proteins for 6 h, washed, and co-cultured (for 6–24 h) with HLMEC (**B**) or neutrophils (**C**). Levels of cit-H3 in culture supernatants were quantified by ELISA. Data presented as mean ± standard deviation. Control: untreated cells; ACE2: cells treated with rhACE2; Hi: cells treated with heat-inactivated S-proteins. *** $p = 0.0003$; # $p < 0.0001$.

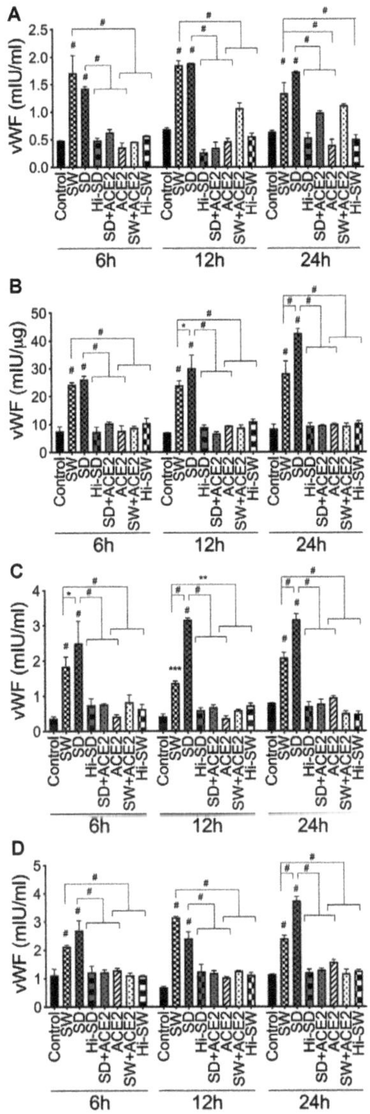

Figure 4. S-proteins and endothelial–neutrophil interactions induce vWF expression and release in HLMEC. (**A**,**B**) HLMEC were treated (for 6–24 h) with SW or SD (1 nM). HLMEC (**C**) and neutrophils (**D**) were treated (for 6 h) with SW or SD, washed, and co-cultured (for 6–24 h) with neutrophils (**C**) or endothelial cells (**D**). vWF levels in culture supernatants (**A**,**C**,**D**) and endothelial cell lysates (**B**) were quantified by ELISA. Data presented as mean ± standard deviation. Control: untreated cells; Hi: cells treated with heat-inactivated S-proteins; ACE2: cells treated with rhACE2. * $p < 0.03$; ** $p < 0.01$; *** $p = 0.0002$; # $p < 0.0001$.

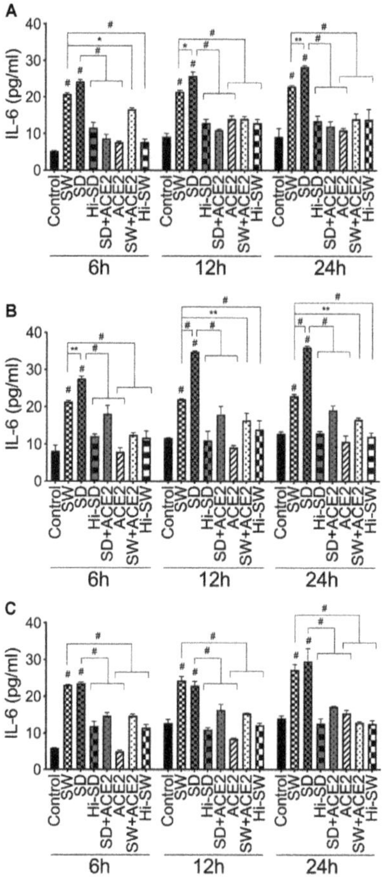

Figure 5. S-proteins and endothelial–neutrophil interactions increased IL-6 expression. (**A**) HLMEC treated (6–24 h) with SW or SD. HLMEC (**B**) and neutrophils (**C**) were treated (for 6 h) with SW or SD and co-cultured (for 6–24 h) with untreated neutrophils (**B**) or endothelial cells (**C**). IL-6 levels in culture supernatants were quantified by ELISA. Data presented as mean ± standard deviation. Control: untreated cells; ACE2: cells treated with rhACE2. Hi: cells treated with heat-inactivated S-proteins. * $p < 0.02$; ** $p < 0.005$; # $p < 0.0001$.

2.7. *rTFPI Blocked S-Protein-Induced Citrullination of Histone H3, Expression and Secretion of vWF and IL-6*

H3 citrullination: Compared to controls, exposure (24 h) of neutrophils to SW or SD increased cit-H3 levels in culture supernatants by 2.2- to 3.5-fold (Figure 6A); co-culture of SW- and SD-treated neutrophils with HLMEC increased cit-H3 levels by 2.3- to 3.5-fold (Figure 6B), and co-culture of SW- and SD-treated HLMEC with neutrophils increased cit-H3 levels by 2.8- to 3.7-fold (Figure 6C). rTFPI blocked SW- and SD-induced H3 citrullination. Pretreatment with rTFPI reduced SW- and SD-induced H3 citrullination in neutrophils (by 3-fold, Figure 5A); reduced H3 citrullination induced by co-culture of SW- and SD-treated neutrophils with HLMEC (by 3.2- to 3.7-fold; Figure 6B); and reduced H3 citrullination induced by co-culture of SW- and SD-treated HLMEC with neutrophils (by 3.2- to 3.6-fold; Figure 6C).

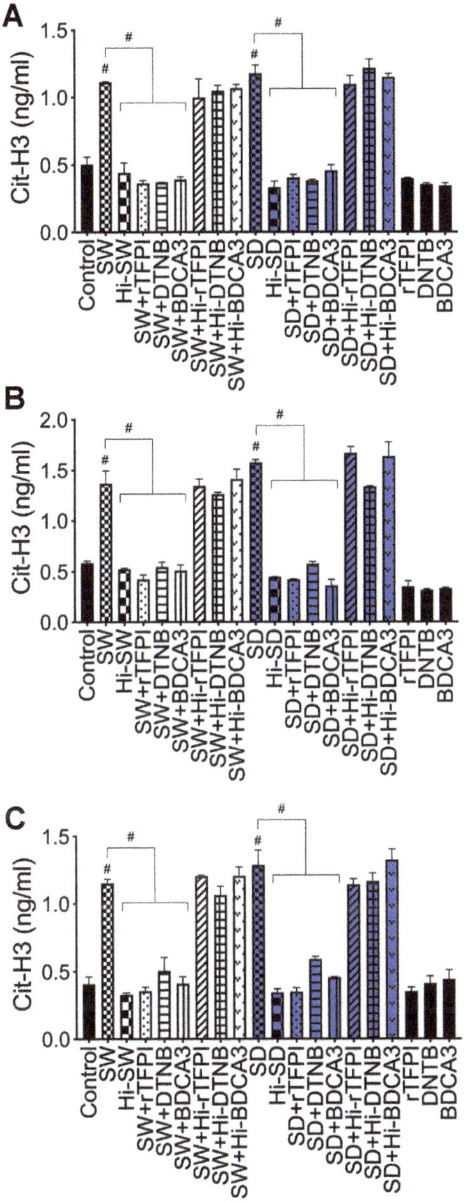

Figure 6. rTFPI, thrombomodulin (BDCA3), and thiol blockers (DTNB) prevent S-protein-induced H3 citrullination. (**A**): human neutrophils treated for 24 h with SW or SD, with or without rTFPI, DTNB, and BDCA3 (200 ng/mL). Neutrophils (**B**) and HLMEC (**C**) were treated (6 h) with SW or SD, with or without rTFPI, DTNB, and BDCA3, washed, and co-cultured (for 24 h) with HLMEC (**B**) or neutrophils (**C**). cit-H3 levels in culture supernatants quantified by ELISA. Data presented as mean ± standard deviation. Control: untreated cells; Hi: heat-inactivated (SW, SD, rTFPI, DTNB, BDCA3). # $p < 0.0001$.

vWF: Compared to controls, 24 h exposure of HLMEC to SW or SD increased vWF levels in culture supernatants (by 6.3- to 9.4-fold; Figure 7A) and cell lysates (by 8.7 to 14.6-fold; Figure 7B). Co-culture of SW- and SD-treated HLMEC with neutrophils increased vWF in culture supernatants by 6.5- to 9.8-fold (Figure 7C), and co-culture of SW- and SD-treated neutrophils with HLMEC increased vWF in culture supernatants by 5.8- to 8.7-fold (Figure 7D). rTFPI blocked SW- and SD-induced vWF expression and secretion. Pretreatment with rTFPI reduced SW- and SD-induced vWF in HLMEC culture supernatants (by 4.7- to 8-fold, Figure 7A) and cell lysates (by 11.4- to 17-fold, Figure 7B); reduced vWF induced by co-culture of SW- and SD-treated HLMEC with neutrophils (by 7.4-fold; Figure 7C); and reduced vWF induced by co-culture of SW- and SD-treated neutrophils with endothelial cells (by 6.3- to 8.5-fold; Figure 7D).

IL-6: Compared to controls, 24 h exposure of HLMEC to SW or SD increased IL-6 levels in culture supernatants by 1.8- to 2.6-fold (Figure 8A). Co-culture of SW- and SD-treated HLMEC with untreated neutrophils increased IL-6 expression by 2-fold (Figure 8B), and co-culture of SW- and SD-treated neutrophils with untreated HLMEC increased IL-6 expression by 1.8- to 2-fold (Figure 8C). rTFPI blocked SW- and SD-induced IL-6 expression. Pretreatment with rTFPI reduced SW- and SD-induced IL-6 in HLMEC culture supernatants (by 1.6 to 1.9-fold, Figure 8A); reduced IL-6 induced by co-culture of SW- and SD-treated HLMEC with neutrophils (by 2-fold; Figure 8B); and reduced IL-6 induced by co-culture of SW- and SD-treated neutrophils with endothelial cells (by 1.8-fold; Figure 8C).

2.8. DTNB Blocked S-Protein-Induced Citrullination of Histone H3, Expression and Secretion of vWF and IL-6

H3 citrullination. DTNB blocked SW- and SD-induced H3 citrullination. Pretreatment with DTNB reduced SW- and SD-induced H3 citrullination in neutrophils (by 3-fold, Figure 6A); reduced H3 citrullination induced by co-culture of SW- and SD-treated neutrophils with HLMEC (by 2.5- to 2.7-fold; Figure 6B); and reduced H3 citrullination induced by co-culture of SW- and SD-treated HLMEC with neutrophils (by 2.2- to 2.3-fold, Figure 6C).

vWF. DTNB blocked SW- and SD-induced vWF expression: reduced SW- and SD-induced vWF in HLMEC culture supernatants (by 6.5- to 9-fold, Figure 6A) and cell lysates (by 10- to 13-fold, Figure 7B); reduced vWF induced by co-culture of SW- and SD-treated HLMEC with neutrophils (by 8- to 10-fold; Figure 7C); and reduced vWF induced by co-culture of SW- and SD-treated neutrophils with EC (by 5- to 8-fold; Figure 7D).

IL-6. DTNB blocked SW- and SD-induced IL-6 expression and secretion: reduced SW- and SD-induced IL-6 in HLMEC culture supernatants (by 1.6- to 1.9-fold, Figure 8A); reduced IL-6 induced by co-culture of SW- and SD-treated HLMEC with neutrophils (by 2-fold; Figure 8B); and reduced IL-6 induced by co-culture of SW- and SD-treated neutrophils with HLMEC (by 1.7- 1.8-fold; Figure 8C).

2.9. Thrombomodulin Blocked S-Protein-Induced Citrullination of Histone H3 and Blocked vWF and IL-6 Expression and Secretion

H3 citrullination. Thrombomodulin (TM, BDCA3) blocked SW- and SD-induced H3 citrullination. Pretreatment with TM reduced SW- and SD-induced H3 citrullination in neutrophils (by 2.6- to 2.8-fold, Figure 6A); reduced H3 citrullination induced by co-culture of SW- and SD-treated neutrophils with HLMEC (by 2.7- to 4.4-fold; Figure 6B); and reduced H3 citrullination induced by co-culture of SW- and SD-treated HLMEC with neutrophils (by 2.8-fold; Figure 6C).

vWF. TM blocked SW- and SD-induced vWF expression: reduced SW- and SD-induced vWF in HLMEC culture supernatants (by 4- to 13-fold, Figure 6A) and cell lysates (by 9- to 17-fold, Figure 7B); reduced vWF induced by co-culture of SW- and SD-treated HLMEC with neutrophils (by 7- to 8-fold; Figure 7C); and reduced vWF induced by co-culture of SW- and SD-treated neutrophils with endothelial cells (by 6.2- to 10.2-fold; Figure 7D).

IL-6. TM blocked SW- and SD-induced IL-6 expression: reduced SW- and SD-induced IL-6 in HLMEC culture supernatants (by 1.6- to 2.3-fold, Figure 8A); reduced IL-6 induced by co-culture of SW- and SD-treated HLMEC with neutrophils (by 2-fold; Figure 8B); and reduced IL-6 induced by co-culture of SW- and SD-treated neutrophils with EC (by 1.7- to 1.9-fold; Figure 8C).

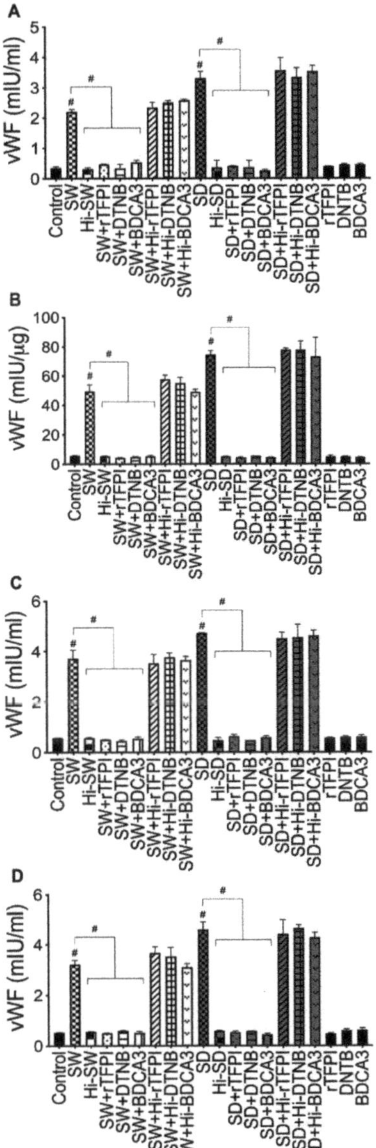

Figure 7. rTFPI, thrombomodulin, and thiol blockers prevent S-protein-induced vWF expression. (**A**,**B**) HLMEC were treated (24 h) with SW or SD, with or without rTFPI, DTNB, and BDCA3. HLMEC (**C**) and neutrophils (**D**) were treated (6 h) with SW or SD, with or without rTFPI, DTNB, and BDCA3, washed, and co-cultured (for 24 h) with neutrophils (**C**) or HLMEC (**D**). vWF levels in culture supernatants (**A**,**C**,**D**) and endothelial cell lysates (**B**) were quantified by ELISA. Data presented as mean ± standard deviation. Control: untreated cells; Hi: heat-inactivated (SW, SD, rTFPI, DTNB, BDCA3). # $p < 0.0001$.

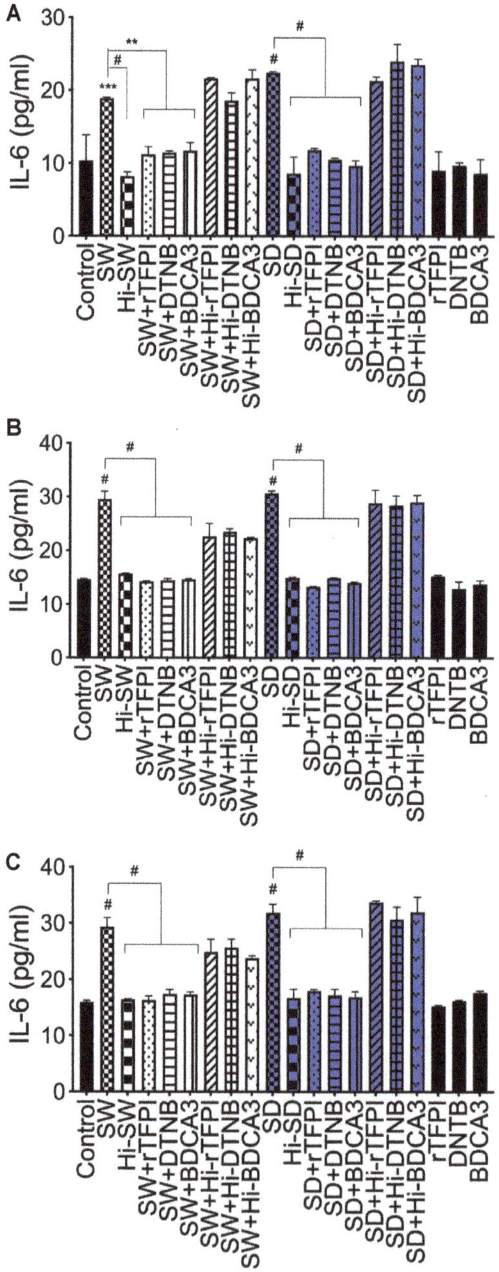

Figure 8. rTFPI, thrombomodulin, and thiol blockers prevent S-protein-induced IL-6 expression. (**A**) HLMEC were treated (24 h) with SW or SD, with or without rTFPI, DTNB, and BDCA3. HLMEC (**B**) and neutrophils (**C**) were treated (6 h) with SW or SD, with or without rTFPI, DTNB, and BDCA3, washed, and co-cultured (for 24 h) with neutrophils (**B**) or HLMEC (**C**). IL-6 levels in culture supernatants were quantified by ELISA. Data presented as mean ± standard deviation. Control: untreated cells; Hi: heat-inactivated (SW, SD, rTFPI, DTNB, BDCA3). ** $p < 0.007$; *** $p = 0.0009$; # $p < 0.0001$.

3. Discussion

The lungs are a prime target for SARS-CoV-2 infection. COVID-19 disease progression is often associated with acute respiratory distress syndrome involving severe lung injury, increased inflammation and coagulopathy [4,5,31,32], as well as increased leukocyte infiltration into tissues associated with endothelial apoptosis and microcirculatory clots [4–6]. The pathogenesis of these pulmonary complications in COVID-19 patients is unknown. Considering that neutrophils are the most abundant leukocytes in humans [33], that blood leukocytes infiltrate tissues by transmigrating through the vascular endothelium, and that S-proteins can be shed and are present in bodily fluids, microvessels, and tissues of SARS-CoV-2 infected patients [7,17], we investigated the effect of S-proteins and endothelial–neutrophils interactions on the adhesion molecule P-selectin, markers of endothelial injury and increased coagulopathy (vWF), NETosis (cit-H3) and inflammation (IL-6).

We demonstrate that exposure of HLMEC or neutrophils to S-proteins and endothelial–neutrophils interactions significantly increased IL-6 expression and secretion. S-proteins have also been shown to increase the production of IL-6 and other inflammatory cytokines and chemokines in endothelial cells from other vascular beds, including human aortic endothelial cells [34], as well as in human pulmonary epithelial cells [35,36], peripheral blood mononuclear cells and human and murine macrophages [37–39]. Studies of COVID-19 patients also showed significant increases in proinflammatory cytokines and chemokines, including IL-6, IL-1β, TNF-α, and granulocyte–macrophage colony-stimulating factor, in patients' plasma, with much higher levels in the plasma of critically ill patients [40]. Our current study suggests that following SARS-CoV-2 infection, viral S-proteins contribute to inflammation of the lung endothelium and disease pathology; and that in the presence of S-proteins, endothelial–neutrophil interactions also induce inflammation.

P-selectin is expressed on activated endothelial cells, platelets and leukocytes, and functions as an adhesion molecule. During inflammatory responses, P-selectin plays a critical role in the recruitment and aggregation of platelets and leukocytes to the vascular wall and to areas of vascular and tissue injury [41,42]. Our data show that S-proteins increase P-selectin transcription and expression in HLMEC, and co-culture of S-protein-treated endothelial cells with non-treated neutrophils or co-culture of S-protein-treated neutrophils with non-treated endothelial cells further increases P-selectin in both HLMEC and neutrophils. These results suggest that S-protein-induced P-selectin would increase leukocyte adhesion to the lung endothelium and infiltration into lung tissues and that endothelial–neutrophil interactions further potentiate leukocyte adhesion and transmigration into tissues.

Our data also showed that exposure of HLMEC to S-proteins increased vWF expression and release, and co-culture of S-protein-treated endothelial cells with non-treated neutrophils, or co-culture of S-protein-treated neutrophils with non-treated endothelial cells, further increased vWF expression and secretion. vWF are stored in endothelial granules (Weibel–Palade bodies) and are released/secreted following endothelial activation [43]; vWF released further mediates the adhesion of platelets and leukocytes to the vascular endothelium and their recruitment to sites of injury. Thus, increased vWF release is a marker of endothelial activation and vascular injury [44]. vWF is a carrier of factor (F)-VIII and both vWF and F-VIII increase fibrin generation and coagulopathy [45]. Our previous study showed that exposure of human endothelial cells or neutrophils to S-proteins and endothelial–neutrophils interactions, increased expression and release of prothrombogenic factors, including tissue factor (TF), fibrinogen, and thrombin, via the TF pathway [46]. Our current findings are in agreement with clinical data showing that COVID-19 patients have significantly increased levels of circulating P-selectin, vWF antigen, and F-VIII activity [6,47–49]. The highest levels of P-selectin, vWF antigen, and F-VIII activity were observed among critically ill patients and were associated with thrombosis, severe disease, lower rates of hospital discharge, and higher mortality [6,47–49].

Our current study also demonstrates that exposure of neutrophils to S-proteins and neutrophil–endothelial interactions significantly increased the formation and release of cit-H3. Histone citrullination is a hallmark of NETosis and is mediated by peptidyl arginine deiminase-4 following neutrophil activation [28,50–52]. This citrullination leads to a loss of charge and deamination of histone arginine residues, which alter histone DNA and protein-binding properties and enable chromatin decondensation and the release of nuclear DNA fragments [50–52]. Thus, when activated, neutrophils can release NETs, which consist of web-like structures composed of double-stranded (ds) DNA, citrullinated histones and granule proteins [28,50–52]. NETosis has been linked to coagulopathy and thrombosis. NET components have been shown to degrade TFPI, thus activating the coagulation cascade TF pathway [53]. NETs released can further serve as a scaffold for the binding of other procoagulant molecules such as vWF, fibronectin, and fibrinogen [54], thus trapping circulating blood cells and promoting their aggregation, resulting in the formation of thrombi and vessel occlusion [54,55]. NET components (histones, dsDNA) further promote thrombosis by increasing the thickness, rigidity, and stability of fibrin fibers and impeding fibrinolysis [56,57].

Our current data showing that exposure of human neutrophils to S-proteins and neutrophil–endothelial interaction increases the production and release of a NET component (cit-H3) are in agreement with clinical studies showing increased NETosis in COVID-19. Plasma, neutrophils, and lung fluids from COVID-19 patients showed increased markers of neutrophil activation and NET components, including cit-H3, myeloperoxidase (MPO), and the MPO-DNA complex [19,40]. Exposure of healthy human neutrophils to SARS-CoV-2 virions also induced the release of NET components, including the MPO, MPO-DNA complex, and cit-H3 [19]. The NETs produced can further injure the vascular endothelium. There is evidence that NETs can induce toxicity, apoptosis, and dysfunction of the vascular endothelium; induce endothelial cell expression and release of adhesion molecules and TF, thus further promoting leukocyte recruitment to the vascular endothelium and thrombosis [53,58–60]. NETs produced following SARS-CoV-2 treatment of neutrophils also induced apoptosis in lung epithelial cells [19].

Our current data showed that compared to SW, exposure of HLMEC or neutrophils to SD and endothelial–neutrophil interactions induced 2- to 15-fold higher P-selectin transcription and significantly higher expression of P-selectin, IL-6 and vWF. Our previous studies also demonstrated that, compared to SW, exposure of HLMEC or neutrophils to SD and endothelial–neutrophil interactions induced significantly higher TF levels [46]. This evidence suggests that different SARS-CoV-2 genetic variants and subvariants that have been driving waves of infection and disease epidemiology since the beginning of the COVID-19 pandemic [61–63], can influence the production of pro-thrombotic factors, inflammation, leukocyte adhesion to the vascular endothelium and infiltration into tissues. These differential effects of SARS-CoV-2 variants and genotypes would influence disease pathology in infected individuals.

We previously demonstrated that exposure of HLMEC or neutrophils to S-proteins and neutrophil–endothelial interactions induced prothrombogenic factors (TF, F-V, thrombin, and fibrinogen), inhibited TFPI, and that both rTFPI and DTNB blocked S-protein-induced upregulation of F-V, thrombin, and fibrinogen [46]. TFPI is a serine protease inhibitor that inhibits TF activity and blocks the coagulation cascade extrinsic pathway [64–66]. Disulfide bonds are essential for TF activation and increased TF activity that drives the coagulation extrinsic pathway signaling cascade [67–69]. DTNB reacts with free thiol groups to prevent the formation of disulfide bonds [70], and thiol-based drugs can decrease S-proteins binding to ACE2, inhibit viral entry and infection, and decrease SARS-CoV-2-induced inflammation of lung neutrophils [71,72]. Our current data show that rTFPI and DTNB also blocked S-protein-induced expression and secretion of IL-6, vWF, and cit-H3. These results suggest that following direct contact of SARS-CoV-2 with the pulmonary endothelium or neutrophils, and endothelial–neutrophil interactions, viral S-proteins induce endothelial degranulation (leading to the release of vWF from cellular granules), NETosis and inflammation via the TF pathway and mechanisms involving functional thiol groups.

TM is an endothelial receptor and a natural anticoagulant that binds thrombin to form a stable thrombin–TM complex that induces fibrinolysis and prevent/reduce coagulation [27]. We previously demonstrated that TM blocked S-protein-induced upregulation of fibrinogen but had no effect on S-protein-induced expression of F-V or thrombin [46]. Our current study demonstrates that TM blocks S-protein-induced increases in IL-6, vWF, and cit-H3 production. These results suggest that SARS-CoV-2-induced vWF, NETosis, and inflammation occur downstream of the coagulation TF pathway, and as TM binds thrombin and limits the intrinsic and common pathways of the coagulation cascade, it abrogates vWF production, inflammation and NETosis.

Because S-proteins are shed by infected cells in vivo and most COVID-19 vaccines encode SARS-CoV-2 S-proteins, increases in markers of inflammation, coagulopathy, and NETosis following exposure of neutrophils and lung endothelial cells to S-proteins could explain some vascular complications observed in COVID-19 patients [73] and post-COVID-19 vaccination adverse events. In fact, reported post vaccination complications include increased vasculitis, endothelial activation, increased inflammatory cytokines and chemokines, and thrombosis [74–76]. Studies in a SARS-CoV-2 mouse model showed that the S-protein S1 subunit was primarily responsible for the observed lung injury, increase in inflammatory cytokines and blood cells in lung fluids [77]. In vitro studies also showed that S1 significantly decreased trans-endothelial electric resistance and increased endothelial permeability [77]. Our future studies will determine whether a specific S-protein subunit is responsible for the increased coagulopathy, histone citrullination and inflammation observed in our current study.

In summary, our current data demonstrate that exposure of primary HLMEC or neutrophils to S-proteins and endothelial–neutrophil interactions increased the transcription and expression of P-selectin (adhesion molecule), increased the expression and secretion of markers of endothelial activation and coagulopathy (vWF), NETosis (cit-H3) and inflammation (IL-6). rTFPI, DNTB, and TM prevented these S-protein-induced effects (Figure 9), which suggests that following SARS-CoV-2 contact with the lung endothelium or neutrophils and endothelial–neutrophil interactions, viral S-proteins induce inflammation, NETosis, and coagulopathy via the TF pathway and mechanisms involving free and functional thiol groups. These findings also suggest that therapeutic strategies against SARS-CoV-2-induced inflammation, NETosis, and coagulopathy could include supplementation with rTFPI, natural anticoagulants such as TM, and/or thiol-based drugs.

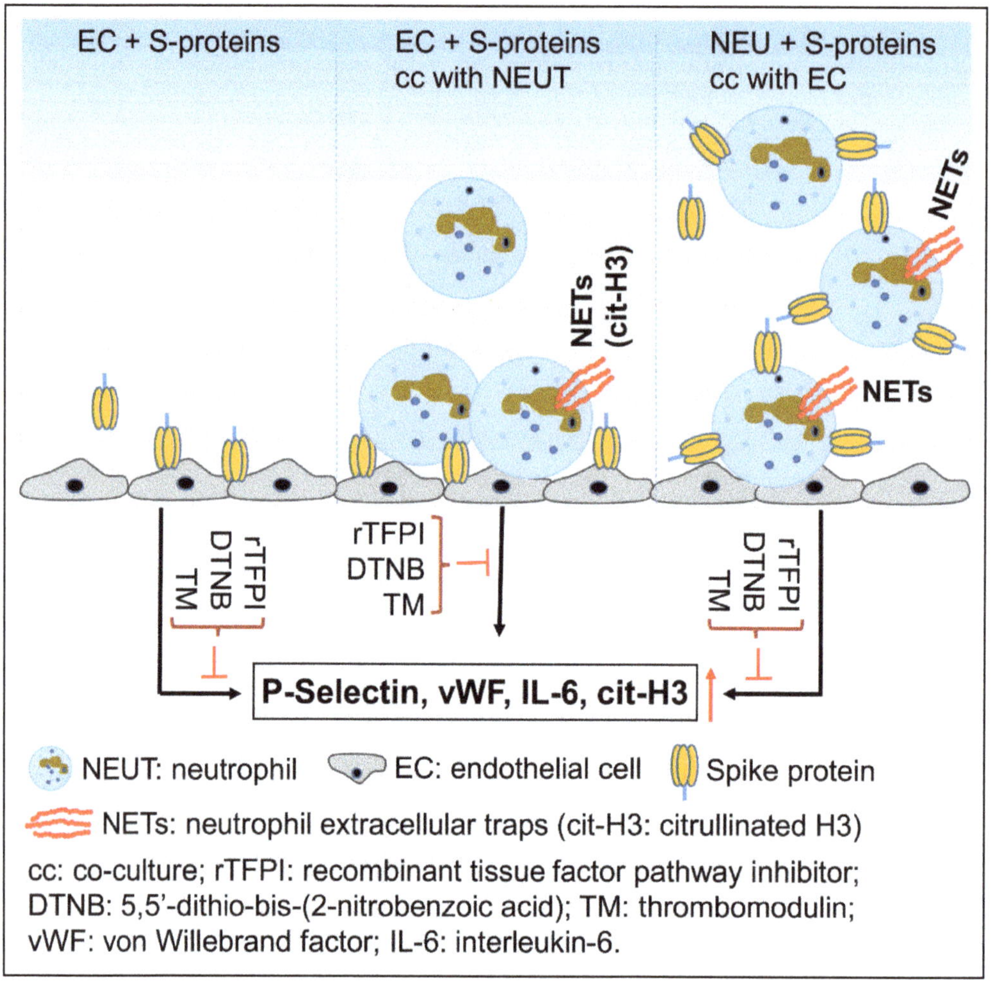

Figure 9. Model illustrating S-protein-induced P-selectin, vWF, IL-6 and cit-H3. Arrows indicate direct activation. The red arrows indicate upregulation; the red perpendicular symbol (⊥) indicates pharmacological inhibitors.

4. Materials and Methods

4.1. Reagents

Recombinant SARS-CoV-2 S-proteins, SW, SD, rhACE2, rTFPI, and TM (BDCA3), were purchased from R&D Systems (Minneapolis, MN, USA). DTNB was from Sigma-Aldrich (St. Louis, MO, USA). Anti-human CD66b and anti-human CD45 antibodies were from Stemcell Technologies (Cambridge, MA, USA); anti-human CD16 antibodies were from Ancell Corporation (Stillwater, MN, USA). Monoclonal P-selectin antibodies and DAPI were from Thermo Fisher/Invitrogen (Waltham, MA, USA), and β-actin antibodies were from Santa Cruz Biotechnology (Dallas, TX, USA).

4.2. HLMEC and Neutrophils

Primary HLMEC was obtained from Lonza (Houston, TX, USA), cultured to confluence as previously described [78–80], and used at passages 2 to 4. Blood samples were obtained from human donors seronegative for HIV-1, HIV-2, and hepatitis-B [80,81]. Neutrophils were isolated from fresh donor blood using the EasySep direct human neutrophil isolation kit (Stemcell Technologies), and their purity was confirmed by FACS as previously described using antibodies to human CD16, CD66b, and CD45 [46].

4.3. Cell Treatment and Endothelial–Neutrophil Co-Culture

S-proteins (both SW and SD) were used at 1 nM and rTFPI, DTNB, and BDCA3 at 200 ng/mL, based on previous studies showing that these doses do not decrease cellular viability [46,82]. Treatment of HLMEC and neutrophils with SW and SD, pre-treatment with rTFPI, DTNB, and BDCA3, culture, co-culture, collection of culture supernatants and harvesting of neutrophils and endothelial cells were performed as previously described [46]. Controls included untreated cells, cells treated with heat-inactivated (Hi) S-proteins, rTFPI, DTNB, or BDCA3, and cells pretreated with rhACE2 (1 μg/mL) to block S-protein binding.

4.4. RNA Isolation and Real-Time PCR

Total RNA was extracted from cells using the Trizol reagent (Life Technologies-Ambion, Austin, TX, USA), RNA quality was checked, and reverse transcription was performed using the Verso cDNA synthesis kit (ThermoFisher) as previously described [46]. Real-time PCR was performed using the LightCycler 480 II (Roche, Basel, Switzerland) Real-Time PCR System. Experimental details and cycling conditions were as previously described, using the following Applied Biosystems (Waltham, MA, USA) primers: Selectin-P (Hs00927900_m1) and GAPDH (Hs02786624_g1). P-selectin mRNA levels were quantified using the Delta-CT method and normalized to the sample's GAPDH levels.

4.5. Human vWF, cit-H3, and IL-6 ELISA

Following treatments, culture supernatants and cells were collected; cells were lysed in mammalian cell lysis buffer (CelLytic M, Sigma) and their protein content quantified using the bicinchoninic acid assay, as previously described [83–85]. Levels of vWF, cit-H3, and IL-6 in each culture supernatant (100 μL), as well as vWF levels in cell lysates (100 μL containing 50 μg protein), were quantified by ELISA using human vWF (Abcam, Waltham, MA, USA), cit-H3 (Cayman Chemical, Ann Arbor, MI, USA), and IL-6 (Invitrogen) ELISA kits in accordance with the manufacturer's protocols. Standard curves from human vWF, cit-H3, and IL-6 reference standards (provided with each kit) were used, respectively, to quantify vWF, cit-H3, and IL-6 levels in each sample. Data were analyzed using Student's *t*-test (two-tailed) or analysis of variance, followed by Tukey's multiple-comparison tests, as previously described [46].For all figures, data are presented as mean ± standard deviation.

4.6. Immunofluorescence Analysis

Primary HLMEC were cultured to confluence on collagen-coated coverslips, treated for 12 h with S-proteins and analyzed by immunofluorescence as previously described [85] using antibodies to P-selectin (Thermo Fisher Scientific, Waltham, MA, USA) diluted 1:100 in PBS containing 0.1% Tween 20 and 1% bovine serum albumin (PBST); and fluorescein isothiocyanate-conjugated secondary antibodies (1:2000 in PBST). Coverslips were mounted using Prolong^{TM} Gold anti-fade mounting medium with DAPI (Invitrogen) and sealed as we previously described. Images were captured using an Eclipse TE20000-U fluorescent microscope (Nikon, Melville, NY, USA) and an Infinity 3–6 urfm monochrome camera (Luminera, Lod, Israel). Semi-quantitative analysis of P-selectin expression was performed using computer-assisted image analysis of the ImageJ software, and five fields of view (FOV) were analyzed for each sample. The staining intensity was normalized to surface area (μm^2) and averaged to estimate protein expression (μm^2 FOV).

4.7. Western Blot Analysis

Primary HLMEC cultured to confluence in six-well plates were treated for 12 h with S-proteins, harvested and lysed in CelLytic^{TM} M buffer (Sigma) containing protease inhibitors. The total protein concentration in each sample was quantified using the Bicinchoninic Acid assay as previously described [83,85,86]. Protein samples (30 μg each) were analyzed by sodium dodecyl sulfate-polyacrylamide gel electrophoresis as previously described [83,85,86] using monoclonal antibodies to P-selectin and β-actin (each at 1:1000 dilution). Densitometry analysis was performed using the ImageJ (V.1.54f 29) software; each sample's P-selectin level was normalized to its β-actin levels.

Author Contributions: Conceptualization, G.D.K.; investigation, B.B. and G.D.K.; data curation, B.B. and G.D.K.; formal analysis, B.B. and G.D.K.; writing—original draft, review, revision and editing, G.D.K. All authors have read and agreed to the published version of the manuscript.

Funding: This work was supported by a Faculty Diversity Award from UNMC.

Institutional Review Board Statement: Not applicable.

Informed Consent Statement: Not applicable.

Data Availability Statement: All data generated or analyzed during this study are included in this publication and/or are available from the corresponding author on reasonable request.

Acknowledgments: We thank the UNMC Elutriation Core Facility for assistance with obtaining donors' blood for neutrophils isolation.

Conflicts of Interest: The authors declare no conflict of interest.

Abbreviations

DTNB	5:5′-dithio-bis-(2-nitrobenzoic acid)
TFPI	Tissue factor pathway inhibitor
rTFPI	Recombinant tissue factor pathway inhibitor
BDCA3/TM	Thrombomodulin
vWF	von Willebrand factor
IL-6	Interleukin-6
Cit-H3	Citrulinated histone 3
dsDNA	Double strand DNA
NETs	Neutrophils extracellular traps
MPO	Myeloperoxidase
TF	Tissue factor
F-V	Factor-V
F-VIII	Factor-VIII
SARS-CoV-2	Severe acute respiratory syndrome coronavirus-2
COVID-19	Coronavirus disease 2019
ACE2	Angiotensin-converting enzyme-2
rhACE2	Recombinant human ACE2
S-proteins	Spike proteins
SW	Spike protein: Wuhan variant
SD	Spike protein: delta variant
Hi	Heat-inactivated
ELISA	Enzyme-linked immunosorbent assay
PCR	Polymerase chain reaction
cDNA	Complementary DNA
GAPDH	Glyceraldehyde-3-Phosphate Dehydrogenase

References

1. JHU. Coronavirus Resource Center: COVID-19 in the USA. 2023. Available online: https://coronavirus.jhu.edu/ (accessed on 24 April 2023).
2. CDC. *United States COVID-19 Cases and Deaths by State*; US Center for Disease Control and Prevention: Atlanta, GA, USA, 2023. Available online: https://www.cdc.gov/covid-data-tracker/#cases (accessed on 24 April 2023).
3. WHO. *Coronavirus Disease (COVID-19) Pandemic*; World Health Organization: Geneva, Switzerland, 2023; Available online: https://www.who.int/emergencies/diseases/novel-coronavirus-2019 (accessed on 24 April 2023).

4. Ackermann, M.; Verleden, S.E.; Kuehnel, M.; Haverich, A.; Welte, T.; Laenger, F.; Vanstapel, A.; Werlein, C.; Stark, H.; Tzankov, A.; et al. Pulmonary Vascular Endothelialitis, Thrombosis, and Angiogenesis in COVID-19. *N. Engl. J. Med.* **2020**, *383*, 120–128. [CrossRef]
5. Varga, Z.; Flammer, A.J.; Steiger, P.; Haberecker, M.; Andermatt, R.; Zinkernagel, A.S.; Mehra, M.R.; Schuepbach, R.A.; Ruschitzka, F.; Moch, H. Endothelial cell infection and endotheliitis in COVID-19. *Lancet* **2020**, *395*, 1417–1418. [CrossRef]
6. O'Sullivan, J.M.; Gonagle, D.M.; Ward, S.E.; Preston, R.J.S.; O'Donnell, J.S. Endothelial cells orchestrate COVID-19 coagulopathy. *Lancet Haematol.* **2020**, *7*, e553–e555. [CrossRef] [PubMed]
7. Magro, C.; Mulvey, J.J.; Berlin, D.; Nuovo, G.; Salvatore, S.; Harp, J.; Baxter-Stoltzfus, A.; Laurence, J. Complement associated microvascular injury and thrombosis in the pathogenesis of severe COVID-19 infection: A report of five cases. *Transl. Res.* **2020**, *220*, 1–13. [CrossRef] [PubMed]
8. Villanueva, E.; Yalavarthi, S.; Berthier, C.C.; Hodgin, J.B.; Khandpur, R.; Lin, A.M.; Rubin, C.J.; Zhao, W.; Olsen, S.H.; Klinker, M.; et al. Netting neutrophils induce endothelial damage, infiltrate tissues, and expose immunostimulatory molecules in systemic lupus erythematosus. *J. Immunol.* **2011**, *187*, 538–552. [CrossRef] [PubMed]
9. Schnoor, M.; Alcaide, P.; Voisin, M.B.; van Buul, J.D. Crossing the Vascular Wall: Common and Unique Mechanisms Exploited by Different Leukocyte Subsets during Extravasation. *Mediat. Inflamm.* **2015**, *2015*, 946509. [CrossRef]
10. Yan, R.; Zhang, Y.; Li, Y.; Xia, L.; Guo, Y.; Zhou, Q. Structural basis for the recognition of SARS-CoV-2 by full-length human ACE2. *Science* **2020**, *367*, 1444–1448. [CrossRef] [PubMed]
11. Chan, K.K.; Dorosky, D.; Sharma, P.; Abbasi, S.A.; Dye, J.M.; Kranz, D.M.; Herbert, A.S.; Procko, E. Engineering human ACE2 to optimize binding to the spike protein of SARS coronavirus 2. *Science* **2020**, *369*, 1261–1265. [CrossRef] [PubMed]
12. McKenna, E.; Wubben, R.; Isaza-Correa, J.M.; Melo, A.M.; Mhaonaigh, A.U.; Conlon, N.; O'Donnell, J.S.; Ni Cheallaigh, C.; Hurley, T.; Stevenson, N.J.; et al. Neutrophils in COVID-19: Not Innocent Bystanders. *Front. Immunol.* **2022**, *13*, 864387. [CrossRef]
13. Calvert, B.A.; Quiroz, E.J.; Lorenzana, Z.; Doan, N.; Kim, S.; Senger, C.N.; Anders, J.J.; Wallace, W.D.; Salomon, M.P.; Henley, J.; et al. Neutrophilic inflammation promotes SARS-CoV-2 infectivity and augments the inflammatory responses in airway epithelial cells. *Front. Immunol.* **2023**, *14*, 1112870. [CrossRef]
14. Hamming, I.; Timens, W.; Bulthuis, M.L.; Lely, A.T.; Navis, G.; van Goor, H. Tissue distribution of ACE2 protein, the functional receptor for SARS coronavirus. A first step in understanding SARS pathogenesis. *J. Pathol.* **2004**, *203*, 631–637. [CrossRef] [PubMed]
15. Iizuka, K.; Kusunoki, A.; Machida, T.; Hirafuji, M. Angiotensin II reduces membranous angiotensin-converting enzyme 2 in pressurized human aortic endothelial cells. *J. Renin Angiotensin Aldosterone Syst.* **2009**, *10*, 210–215. [CrossRef] [PubMed]
16. Zhao, Y.; Zhao, Z.; Wang, Y.; Zhou, Y.; Ma, Y.; Zuo, W. Single-Cell RNA Expression Profiling of ACE2, the Receptor of SARS-CoV-2. *Am. J. Respir. Crit. Care Med.* **2020**, *202*, 756–759. [CrossRef] [PubMed]
17. Perico, L.; Morigi, M.; Galbusera, M.; Pezzotta, A.; Gastoldi, S.; Imberti, B.; Perna, A.; Ruggenenti, P.; Donadelli, R.; Benigni, A.; et al. SARS-CoV-2 Spike Protein 1 Activates Microvascular Endothelial Cells and Complement System Leading to Platelet Aggregation. *Front. Immunol.* **2022**, *13*, 827146. [CrossRef] [PubMed]
18. George, S.; Pal, A.C.; Gagnon, J.; Timalsina, S.; Singh, P.; Vydyam, P.; Munshi, M.; Chiu, J.E.; Renard, I.; Harden, C.A.; et al. Evidence for SARS-CoV-2 Spike Protein in the Urine of COVID-19 Patients. *Kidney360* **2021**, *2*, 924–936. [CrossRef]
19. Veras, F.P.; Pontelli, M.C.; Silva, C.M.; Toller-Kawahisa, J.E.; de Lima, M.; Nascimento, D.C.; Schneider, A.H.; Caetite, D.; Tavares, L.A.; Paiva, I.M.; et al. SARS-CoV-2-triggered neutrophil extracellular traps mediate COVID-19 pathology. *J. Exp. Med.* **2020**, *217*, e20201129. [CrossRef] [PubMed]
20. Zuo, Y.; Yalavarthi, S.; Shi, H.; Gockman, K.; Zuo, M.; Madison, J.A.; Blair, C.; Weber, A.; Barnes, B.J.; Egeblad, M.; et al. Neutrophil extracellular traps in COVID-19. *JCI Insight* **2020**, *5*, e138999. [CrossRef]
21. Middleton, E.A.; He, X.Y.; Denorme, F.; Campbell, R.A.; Ng, D.; Salvatore, S.P.; Mostyka, M.; Baxter-Stoltzfus, A.; Borczuk, A.C.; Loda, M.; et al. Neutrophil extracellular traps contribute to immunothrombosis in COVID-19 acute respiratory distress syndrome. *Blood* **2020**, *136*, 1169–1179. [CrossRef]
22. Zuo, Y.; Zuo, M.; Yalavarthi, S.; Gockman, K.; Madison, J.A.; Shi, H.; Woodard, W.; Lezak, S.P.; Lugogo, N.L.; Knight, J.S.; et al. Neutrophil extracellular traps and thrombosis in COVID-19. *J. Thromb. Thrombolysis* **2020**, *51*, 446–453. [CrossRef]
23. Baugh, R.J.; Broze, G.J., Jr.; Krishnaswamy, S. Regulation of extrinsic pathway factor Xa formation by tissue factor pathway inhibitor. *J. Biol. Chem.* **1998**, *273*, 4378–4386. [CrossRef]
24. Bajaj, M.S.; Birktoft, J.J.; Steer, S.A.; Bajaj, S.P. Structure and biology of tissue factor pathway inhibitor. *Thromb. Haemost.* **2001**, *86*, 959–972. [PubMed]
25. Lwaleed, B.A.; Bass, P.S. Tissue factor pathway inhibitor: Structure, biology and involvement in disease. *J. Pathol.* **2006**, *208*, 327–339. [CrossRef] [PubMed]
26. Maroney, S.A.; Hansen, K.G.; Mast, A.E. Cellular expression and biological activities of alternatively spliced forms of tissue factor pathway inhibitor. *Curr. Opin. Hematol.* **2013**, *20*, 403–409. [CrossRef]
27. Loghmani, H.; Conway, E.M. Exploring traditional and nontraditional roles for thrombomodulin. *Blood* **2018**, *132*, 148–158. [CrossRef] [PubMed]
28. Wang, Y.; Li, M.; Stadler, S.; Correll, S.; Li, P.; Wang, D.; Hayama, R.; Leonelli, L.; Han, H.; Grigoryev, S.A.; et al. Histone hypercitrullination mediates chromatin decondensation and neutrophil extracellular trap formation. *J. Cell Biol.* **2009**, *184*, 205–213. [CrossRef] [PubMed]

29. Mauracher, L.M.; Posch, F.; Martinod, K.; Grilz, E.; Daullary, T.; Hell, L.; Brostjan, C.; Zielinski, C.; Ay, C.; Wagner, D.D.; et al. Citrullinated histone H3, a biomarker of neutrophil extracellular trap formation, predicts the risk of venous thromboembolism in cancer patients. *J. Thromb. Haemost.* **2018**, *16*, 508–518. [CrossRef]
30. Li, T.; Zhang, Z.; Li, X.; Dong, G.; Zhang, M.; Xu, Z.; Yang, J. Neutrophil Extracellular Traps: Signaling Properties and Disease Relevance. *Mediat. Inflamm.* **2020**, *2020*, 9254087. [CrossRef]
31. Fox, S.E.; Akmatbekov, A.; Harbert, J.L.; Li, G.; Quincy Brown, J.; Vander Heide, R.S. Pulmonary and cardiac pathology in African American patients with COVID-19: An autopsy series from New Orleans. *Lancet Respir. Med.* **2020**, *8*, 681–686. [CrossRef]
32. Barton, L.M.; Duval, E.J.; Stroberg, E.; Ghosh, S.; Mukhopadhyay, S. COVID-19 Autopsies, Oklahoma, USA. *Am. J. Clin. Pathol.* **2020**, *153*, 725–733. [CrossRef]
33. Hong, C.W. Current Understanding in Neutrophil Differentiation and Heterogeneity. *Immune Netw.* **2017**, *17*, 298–306. [CrossRef]
34. Jover, E.; Matilla, L.; Garaikoetxea, M.; Fernandez-Celis, A.; Muntendam, P.; Jaisser, F.; Rossignol, P.; Lopez-Andres, N. Beneficial Effects of Mineralocorticoid Receptor Pathway Blockade against Endothelial Inflammation Induced by SARS-CoV-2 Spike Protein. *Biomedicines* **2021**, *9*, 639. [CrossRef] [PubMed]
35. Patra, T.; Meyer, K.; Geerling, L.; Isbell, T.S.; Hoft, D.F.; Brien, J.; Pinto, A.K.; Ray, R.B.; Ray, R. SARS-CoV-2 spike protein promotes IL-6 trans-signaling by activation of angiotensin II receptor signaling in epithelial cells. *PLoS Pathog.* **2020**, *16*, e1009128. [CrossRef] [PubMed]
36. Khan, S.; Shafiei, M.S.; Longoria, C.; Schoggins, J.W.; Savani, R.C.; Zaki, H. SARS-CoV-2 spike protein induces inflammation via TLR2-dependent activation of the NF-kappaB pathway. *Elife* **2021**, *10*, e68563. [CrossRef]
37. Pantazi, I.; Al-Qahtani, A.A.; Alhamlan, F.S.; Alothaid, H.; Matou-Nasri, S.; Sourvinos, G.; Vergadi, E.; Tsatsanis, C. SARS-CoV-2/ACE2 Interaction Suppresses IRAK-M Expression and Promotes Pro-Inflammatory Cytokine Production in Macrophages. *Front. Immunol.* **2021**, *12*, 683800. [CrossRef]
38. Cao, X.; Tian, Y.; Nguyen, V.; Zhang, Y.; Gao, C.; Yin, R.; Carver, W.; Fan, D.; Albrecht, H.; Cui, T.; et al. Spike protein of SARS-CoV-2 activates macrophages and contributes to induction of acute lung inflammation in male mice. *FASEB J.* **2021**, *35*, e21801. [CrossRef] [PubMed]
39. Shirato, K.; Kizaki, T. SARS-CoV-2 spike protein S1 subunit induces pro-inflammatory responses via toll-like receptor 4 signaling in murine and human macrophages. *Heliyon* **2021**, *7*, e06187. [CrossRef]
40. Masso-Silva, J.A.; Moshensky, A.; Lam, M.T.Y.; Odish, M.F.; Patel, A.; Xu, L.; Hansen, E.; Trescott, S.; Nguyen, C.; Kim, R.; et al. Increased Peripheral Blood Neutrophil Activation Phenotypes and Neutrophil Extracellular Trap Formation in Critically Ill Coronavirus Disease 2019 (COVID-19) Patients: A Case Series and Review of the Literature. *Clin. Infect. Dis.* **2022**, *74*, 479–489. [CrossRef]
41. Patel, K.D.; Cuvelier, S.L.; Wiehler, S. Selectins: Critical mediators of leukocyte recruitment. *Semin. Immunol.* **2002**, *14*, 73–81. [CrossRef]
42. McEver, R.P. Selectins: Initiators of leucocyte adhesion and signalling at the vascular wall. *Cardiovasc. Res.* **2015**, *107*, 331–339. [CrossRef]
43. Lenting, P.J.; Christophe, O.D.; Denis, C.V. von Willebrand factor biosynthesis, secretion, and clearance: Connecting the far ends. *Blood* **2015**, *125*, 2019–2028. [CrossRef]
44. Vischer, U.M. von Willebrand factor, endothelial dysfunction, and cardiovascular disease. *J. Thromb. Haemost.* **2006**, *4*, 1186–1193. [CrossRef]
45. Chauhan, A.K.; Kisucka, J.; Lamb, C.B.; Bergmeier, W.; Wagner, D.D. von Willebrand factor and factor VIII are independently required to form stable occlusive thrombi in injured veins. *Blood* **2007**, *109*, 2424–2429. [CrossRef]
46. Bhargavan, B.; Kanmogne, G.D. SARS-CoV-2 Spike Proteins and Cell-Cell Communication Inhibits TFPI and Induces Thrombogenic Factors in Human Lung Microvascular Endothelial Cells and Neutrophils: Implications for COVID-19 Coagulopathy Pathogenesis. *Int. J. Mol. Sci.* **2022**, *23*, 10436. [CrossRef] [PubMed]
47. Goshua, G.; Pine, A.B.; Meizlish, M.L.; Chang, C.H.; Zhang, H.; Bahel, P.; Baluha, A.; Bar, N.; Bona, R.D.; Burns, A.J.; et al. Endotheliopathy in COVID-19-associated coagulopathy: Evidence from a single-centre, cross-sectional study. *Lancet Haematol.* **2020**, *7*, e575–e582. [CrossRef] [PubMed]
48. Pine, A.B.; Meizlish, M.L.; Goshua, G.; Chang, C.H.; Zhang, H.; Bishai, J.; Bahel, P.; Patel, A.; Gbyli, R.; Kwan, J.M.; et al. Circulating markers of angiogenesis and endotheliopathy in COVID-19. *Pulm. Circ.* **2020**, *10*, 2045894020966547. [CrossRef] [PubMed]
49. Iba, T.; Connors, J.M.; Levy, J.H. The coagulopathy, endotheliopathy, and vasculitis of COVID-19. *Inflamm. Res.* **2020**, *69*, 1181–1189. [CrossRef]
50. Kusunoki, Y.; Nakazawa, D.; Shida, H.; Hattanda, F.; Miyoshi, A.; Masuda, S.; Nishio, S.; Tomaru, U.; Atsumi, T.; Ishizu, A. Peptidylarginine Deiminase Inhibitor Suppresses Neutrophil Extracellular Trap Formation and MPO-ANCA Production. *Front. Immunol.* **2016**, *7*, 227. [CrossRef]
51. Rohrbach, A.S.; Slade, D.J.; Thompson, P.R.; Mowen, K.A. Activation of PAD4 in NET formation. *Front. Immunol.* **2012**, *3*, 360. [CrossRef]
52. Wong, S.L.; Wagner, D.D. Peptidylarginine deiminase 4: A nuclear button triggering neutrophil extracellular traps in inflammatory diseases and aging. *FASEB J.* **2018**, *32*, 6358–6370. [CrossRef]

53. Folco, E.J.; Mawson, T.L.; Vromman, A.; Bernardes-Souza, B.; Franck, G.; Persson, O.; Nakamura, M.; Newton, G.; Luscinskas, F.W.; Libby, P. Neutrophil Extracellular Traps Induce Endothelial Cell Activation and Tissue Factor Production Through Interleukin-1alpha and Cathepsin G. *Arterioscler. Thromb. Vasc. Biol.* **2018**, *38*, 1901–1912. [CrossRef]
54. Fuchs, T.A.; Brill, A.; Duerschmied, D.; Schatzberg, D.; Monestier, M.; Myers, D.D., Jr.; Wrobleski, S.K.; Wakefield, T.W.; Hartwig, J.H.; Wagner, D.D. Extracellular DNA traps promote thrombosis. *Proc. Natl. Acad. Sci. USA* **2010**, *107*, 15880–15885. [CrossRef] [PubMed]
55. Thalin, C.; Hisada, Y.; Lundstrom, S.; Mackman, N.; Wallen, H. Neutrophil Extracellular Traps: Villains and Targets in Arterial, Venous, and Cancer-Associated Thrombosis. *Arterioscler. Thromb. Vasc. Biol.* **2019**, *39*, 1724–1738. [CrossRef] [PubMed]
56. Longstaff, C.; Varju, I.; Sotonyi, P.; Szabo, L.; Krumrey, M.; Hoell, A.; Bota, A.; Varga, Z.; Komorowicz, E.; Kolev, K. Mechanical stability and fibrinolytic resistance of clots containing fibrin, DNA, and histones. *J. Biol. Chem.* **2013**, *288*, 6946–6956. [CrossRef] [PubMed]
57. Varju, I.; Longstaff, C.; Szabo, L.; Farkas, A.Z.; Varga-Szabo, V.J.; Tanka-Salamon, A.; Machovich, R.; Kolev, K. DNA, histones and neutrophil extracellular traps exert anti-fibrinolytic effects in a plasma environment. *Thromb. Haemost.* **2015**, *113*, 1289–1298. [CrossRef]
58. Saffarzadeh, M.; Juenemann, C.; Queisser, M.A.; Lochnit, G.; Barreto, G.; Galuska, S.P.; Lohmeyer, J.; Preissner, K.T. Neutrophil extracellular traps directly induce epithelial and endothelial cell death: A predominant role of histones. *PLoS ONE* **2012**, *7*, e32366. [CrossRef]
59. Carmona-Rivera, C.; Zhao, W.; Yalavarthi, S.; Kaplan, M.J. Neutrophil extracellular traps induce endothelial dysfunction in systemic lupus erythematosus through the activation of matrix metalloproteinase-2. *Ann. Rheum. Dis.* **2015**, *74*, 1417–1424. [CrossRef] [PubMed]
60. Rabinovitch, M. NETs Activate Pulmonary Arterial Endothelial Cells. *Arterioscler. Thromb. Vasc. Biol.* **2016**, *36*, 2035–2037. [CrossRef]
61. Dubey, A.; Choudhary, S.; Kumar, P.; Tomar, S. Emerging SARS-CoV-2 Variants: Genetic Variability and Clinical Implications. *Curr. Microbiol.* **2021**, *79*, 20. [CrossRef]
62. Boehm, E.; Kronig, I.; Neher, R.A.; Eckerle, I.; Vetter, P.; Kaiser, L.; Geneva Centre for Emerging Viral, D. Novel SARS-CoV-2 variants: The pandemics within the pandemic. *Clin. Microbiol. Infect.* **2021**, *27*, 1109–1117. [CrossRef]
63. Singh, J.; Pandit, P.; McArthur, A.G.; Banerjee, A.; Mossman, K. Evolutionary trajectory of SARS-CoV-2 and emerging variants. *Virol. J.* **2021**, *18*, 166. [CrossRef]
64. Broze, G.J., Jr.; Girard, T.J. Tissue factor pathway inhibitor: Structure-function. *Front. Biosci.* **2012**, *17*, 262–280. [CrossRef] [PubMed]
65. Ellery, P.E.; Adams, M.J. Tissue factor pathway inhibitor: Then and now. *Semin. Thromb. Hemost.* **2014**, *40*, 881–886. [CrossRef] [PubMed]
66. Mast, A.E. Tissue Factor Pathway Inhibitor: Multiple Anticoagulant Activities for a Single Protein. *Arterioscler. Thromb. Vasc. Biol.* **2016**, *36*, 9–14. [CrossRef] [PubMed]
67. Chen, V.M. Tissue factor de-encryption, thrombus formation, and thiol-disulfide exchange. *Semin. Thromb. Hemost.* **2013**, *39*, 40–47. [CrossRef]
68. Chen, V.M.; Ahamed, J.; Versteeg, H.H.; Berndt, M.C.; Ruf, W.; Hogg, P.J. Evidence for activation of tissue factor by an allosteric disulfide bond. *Biochemistry* **2006**, *45*, 12020–12028. [CrossRef]
69. Prasad, R.; Banerjee, S.; Sen, P. Contribution of allosteric disulfide in the structural regulation of membrane-bound tissue factor-factor VIIa binary complex. *J. Biomol. Struct. Dyn.* **2019**, *37*, 3707–3720. [CrossRef]
70. Winther, J.R.; Thorpe, C. Quantification of thiols and disulfides. *Biochim. Biophys. Acta* **2014**, *1840*, 838–846. [CrossRef]
71. Khanna, K.; Raymond, W.; Jin, J.; Charbit, A.R.; Gitlin, I.; Tang, M.; Werts, A.D.; Barrett, E.G.; Cox, J.M.; Birch, S.M.; et al. Thiol drugs decrease SARS-CoV-2 lung injury in vivo and disrupt SARS-CoV-2 spike complex binding to ACE2 in vitro. *bioRxiv* **2021**. [CrossRef]
72. Khanna, K.; Raymond, W.W.; Jin, J.; Charbit, A.R.; Gitlin, I.; Tang, M.; Werts, A.D.; Barrett, E.G.; Cox, J.M.; Birch, S.M.; et al. Exploring antiviral and anti-inflammatory effects of thiol drugs in COVID-19. *Am. J. Physiol. Lung Cell. Mol. Physiol.* **2022**, *323*, L372–L389. [CrossRef]
73. Wu, X.; Xiang, M.; Jing, H.; Wang, C.; Novakovic, V.A.; Shi, J. Damage to endothelial barriers and its contribution to long COVID. *Angiogenesis* **2023**, 1–18. [CrossRef]
74. Liu, R.; Pan, J.; Zhang, C.; Sun, X. Cardiovascular Complications of COVID-19 Vaccines. *Front. Cardiovasc. Med.* **2022**, *9*, 840929. [CrossRef] [PubMed]
75. Ostrowski, S.R.; Sogaard, O.S.; Tolstrup, M.; Staerke, N.B.; Lundgren, J.; Ostergaard, L.; Hvas, A.M. Inflammation and Platelet Activation After COVID-19 Vaccines—Possible Mechanisms Behind Vaccine-Induced Immune Thrombocytopenia and Thrombosis. *Front. Immunol.* **2021**, *12*, 779453. [CrossRef] [PubMed]
76. Chang, J.C.; Hawley, H.B. Vaccine-Associated Thrombocytopenia and Thrombosis: Venous Endotheliopathy Leading to Venous Combined Micro-Macrothrombosis. *Medicina* **2021**, *57*, 1163. [CrossRef]
77. Colunga Biancatelli, R.M.L.; Solopov, P.A.; Sharlow, E.R.; Lazo, J.S.; Marik, P.E.; Catravas, J.D. The SARS-CoV-2 spike protein subunit S1 induces COVID-19-like acute lung injury in Kappa18-hACE2 transgenic mice and barrier dysfunction in human endothelial cells. *Am. J. Physiol. Lung Cell. Mol. Physiol.* **2021**, *321*, L477–L484. [CrossRef] [PubMed]

78. Kanmogne, G.D.; Kennedy, R.C.; Grammas, P. Analysis of human lung endothelial cells for susceptibility to HIV type 1 infection, coreceptor expression, and cytotoxicity of gp120 protein. *AIDS Res. Hum. Retroviruses* **2001**, *17*, 45–53. [CrossRef] [PubMed]
79. Kanmogne, G.D.; Primeaux, C.; Grammas, P. Induction of apoptosis and endothelin-1 secretion in primary human lung endothelial cells by HIV-1 gp120 proteins. *Biochem. Biophys. Res. Commun.* **2005**, *333*, 1107–1115. [CrossRef]
80. Li, H.; Singh, S.; Potula, R.; Persidsky, Y.; Kanmogne, G.D. Dysregulation of claudin-5 in HIV-induced interstitial pneumonitis and lung vascular injury. Protective role of peroxisome proliferator-activated receptor-gamma. *Am. J. Respir. Crit. Care Med.* **2014**, *190*, 85–97. [CrossRef]
81. Woollard, S.M.; Li, H.; Singh, S.; Yu, F.; Kanmogne, G.D. HIV-1 induces cytoskeletal alterations and Rac1 activation during monocyte-blood-brain barrier interactions: Modulatory role of CCR5. *Retrovirology* **2014**, *11*, 20. [CrossRef]
82. Cui, X.Y.; Tjonnfjord, G.E.; Kanse, S.M.; Dahm, A.E.A.; Iversen, N.; Myklebust, C.F.; Sun, L.; Jiang, Z.X.; Ueland, T.; Campbell, J.J.; et al. Tissue factor pathway inhibitor upregulates CXCR7 expression and enhances CXCL12-mediated migration in chronic lymphocytic leukemia. *Sci. Rep.* **2021**, *11*, 5127. [CrossRef]
83. Chaudhuri, A.; Yang, B.; Gendelman, H.E.; Persidsky, Y.; Kanmogne, G.D. STAT1 signaling modulates HIV-1-induced inflammatory responses and leukocyte transmigration across the blood-brain barrier. *Blood* **2008**, *111*, 2062–2072. [CrossRef]
84. Bhargavan, B.; Kanmogne, G.D. Toll-Like Receptor-3 Mediates HIV-1-Induced Interleukin-6 Expression in the Human Brain Endothelium via TAK1 and JNK Pathways: Implications for Viral Neuropathogenesis. *Mol. Neurobiol.* **2018**, *55*, 5976–5992. [CrossRef] [PubMed]
85. Bhargavan, B.; Woollard, S.M.; McMillan, J.E.; Kanmogne, G.D. CCR5 antagonist reduces HIV-induced amyloidogenesis, tau pathology, neurodegeneration, and blood-brain barrier alterations in HIV-infected hu-PBL-NSG mice. *Mol. Neurodegener.* **2021**, *16*, 78. [CrossRef] [PubMed]
86. Bhargavan, B.; Woollard, S.M.; Kanmogne, G.D. Toll-like receptor-3 mediates HIV-1 transactivation via NFκB and JNK pathways and histone acetylation, but prolonged activation suppresses Tat and HIV-1 replication. *Cell. Signal.* **2016**, *28*, 7–22. [CrossRef] [PubMed]

International Journal of
Molecular Sciences

MDPI

Article

A Potential Association between Ribonuclease 1 Dynamics in the Blood and the Outcome in COVID-19 Patients

Elisabeth Zechendorf [1,*], Christian Beckers [1], Nadine Frank [1], Sandra Kraemer [1], Carolina Neu [1], Thomas Breuer [1], Michael Dreher [2], Edgar Dahl [3], Gernot Marx [1], Lukas Martin [1,†] and Tim-Philipp Simon [1,†]

[1] Department of Intensive Care and Intermediate Care, University Hospital RWTH Aachen, 52074 Aachen, Germany; tsimon@ukaachen.de (T.-P.S.)
[2] Department of Pneumology and Intensive Care Medicine, University Hospital RWTH Aachen, 52074 Aachen, Germany
[3] RWTH Centralized Biomaterial Bank (RWTH cBMB) at the Institute of Pathology, University Hospital RWTH Aachen, 52074 Aachen, Germany
* Correspondence: ezechendorf@ukaachen.de; Tel.: +49-(0)241-8035484
† These authors contributed equally to this work.

Abstract: The COVID-19 pandemic caused by the new SARS-CoV-2 coronavirus is the most recent and well-known outbreak of a coronavirus. RNase 1 is a small endogenous antimicrobial polypeptide that possesses antiviral activity against viral diseases. In this study, we investigated a potential association between ribonuclease 1 and the outcome in COVID-19 patients and the impact of increased and decreased RNase 1 levels serum during the course of the disease. Therefore, two patient populations, Cohort A (n = 35) and B (n = 80), were subclassified into two groups, in which the RNase 1 concentration increased or decreased from time point one to time point two. We show that the RNase 1 serum levels significantly increased in the increasing group of both cohorts ($p = 0.0171$; $p < 0.0001$). We detect that patients in the increasing group who died had significantly higher RNase 1 serum levels at both time points in Cohort A ($p = 0.0170$; $p = 0.0393$) and Cohort B ($p = 0.0253$; $p = 0.0034$) than patients who survived. Additionally, we measured a significant correlation of RNase 1 serum levels with serum creatinine as well as creatinine clearance in the increasing and decreasing group at both time points of Cohort A. Based on these results, there is now good evidence that RNase 1 may play a role in renal dysfunction associated with ICU COVID-19 patients and that increasing RNase 1 serum level may be a potential biomarker to predict outcome in COVID-19 patients.

Keywords: COVID-19; SARS-CoV-2; RNase 1; kidney injury; biomarker

Citation: Zechendorf, E.; Beckers, C.; Frank, N.; Kraemer, S.; Neu, C.; Breuer, T.; Dreher, M.; Dahl, E.; Marx, G.; Martin, L.; et al. A Potential Association between Ribonuclease 1 Dynamics in the Blood and the Outcome in COVID-19 Patients. *Int. J. Mol. Sci.* **2023**, *24*, 12428. https://doi.org/10.3390/ijms241512428

Academic Editors: Alexandru Schiopu, Emil Marian Arbănași and Eliza Russu

Received: 4 July 2023
Revised: 31 July 2023
Accepted: 1 August 2023
Published: 4 August 2023

1. Introduction

Coronaviruses are a family of seven known single-stranded RNA viruses that can cause a range of illnesses, from mild upper respiratory disease to more severe respiratory illnesses [1,2]. The most recent and well-known outbreak of a coronavirus is the COVID-19 pandemic caused by the new SARS-CoV-2 coronavirus. SARS-CoV-2 has caused a severe health crisis with millions of confirmed cases and hundreds of thousands of deaths worldwide, so the World Health Organization (WHO) declared it a Public Health Emergency of International Concern on 30 January 2020 [1]. Since the emergence of COVID-19, research on coronaviruses has been strongly promoted and grown, and scientists and clinicians are working to better understand the virus and to develop effective treatments. However, there is still much to learn about coronaviruses and their general potential to cause further outbreaks in the future. In addition, new strains of the virus have emerged in the meantime, underscoring the need for continued research on the virus and its variants.

Ribonucleases are small endogenous antimicrobial polypeptides that possess antiviral activity against viral diseases. Several studies have demonstrated that RNase 1 and 2 possess antiviral properties against human immunodeficiency virus (HIV)-1 [3,4]. In addition to its antiviral activity, RNase 1 has high ribonucleolytic activity and thus plays a potential role in regulating the immune response by recognizing and degrading single- and double-stranded RNA molecules [5]. As a result of an inflammatory response and associated cell death, extracellular RNA (eRNA) is released. The eRNA binds to Toll-like receptors (TLRs) 3 and 7 and induces various signaling pathways involved in the initiation of the innate immune response [6–8]. Due to its ribonucleolytic activity, RNase 1 is thought to have the ability to recognize and degrade viral RNA, thus preventing its replication in host cells [9]. This could contribute to preventing an excessive or dysregulated immune response that can lead to severe disease progression. Ireland and colleagues showed in a study that RNase L has a protective role on a murine coronavirus mouse hepatitis beta CoV strain (MHV-JHM) [10].

COVID-19 has been shown to be associated with renal dysfunction [11–13]. In a previous study, we showed that patients with renal dysfunction had significantly higher RNase 1 levels after thoracoabdominal aortic aneurysm (TAAA) repair than patients without renal dysfunction [14]. However, the role of RNase 1 and its association with renal function in patients infected by SARS-CoV-2 is unknown.

In this study, we therefore measured the RNase 1 dynamics in the blood of patients with SARS-CoV-2 infection in two different cohorts. To determine the prognostic value of RNase 1 as a potential new biomarker in diseases induced by SARS-CoV-2 and its potential as a possible therapeutic target, we also investigated whether RNase 1 levels decrease or increase during disease progression. Furthermore, we correlate RNase 1 serum levels with 28-day mortality and other clinical parameters such as C-reactive protein (CRP), interleukin-6 (IL-6), and procalcitonin (PCT) of patients with increasing or decreasing RNase 1 serum levels. To investigate the role of RNase in SARS-CoV-2-induced renal dysfunction, we also investigated the correlation of RNase 1 levels with serum creatinine and creatinine clearance of patients with SARS-CoV-2 and the impact of increased and decreased RNase 1 levels during the course of the disease.

2. Results

2.1. Patient Characteristics

In the first cohort, 35 patients with SARS-CoV-2 infection were included (Table 1). Patients in whom the RNase 1 serum levels increased or decreased from day 2 to day 4 were categorized in one of two groups, the increasing (n = 22) and decreasing (n = 13) RNase 1 level groups. On average, the patients were 61 years old, and 74.29% were male. Only eight patients were diagnosed with diabetes mellitus, and all eight patients belonged to the increasing RNase 1 group (p = 0.0124). While the average time in ICU was 19 days, patients belonging in the increasing RNase 1 group were in the ICU for a mean of 23.5 days and those in the decreasing group were in the ICU only for a mean of 17 days (p = 0.0443). Further details of the patient characteristics of Cohort A can be found in Table 1.

In the second cohort (Cohort B), 80 patients with SARS-CoV-2 infection were included (Table 2). The patients of this group were also categorized in two groups, where the RNase 1 serum levels increased (n = 48) or decreased (n = 32) from day 1 to week 1. On average, the patients were 64 years old, and 63.75% were male. Forty-four patients were in the ICU, 31 patients belonged to the increasing RNase 1 group, and only 13 of these patients belonged to the decreasing group (p = 0.0351). The ICU patients of the increasing group were in the ICU for an average of 18 days, whereas the patients of the decreasing RNase 1 group were in the ICU for a mean of 21 days. Further details of the patient characteristics of Cohort B can be found in Table 2.

Table 1. Patient characteristics of Cohort A.

	All (n = 35)	Increasing RNase 1 Levels (n = 22)	Decreasing RNase 1 Levels (n = 13)	p-Value
Age (year) (IQR)	61.00 (56.00–67.00)	60.50 (56.75–72.25)	62.00 (54.00–66.00)	0.4467
Male sex (%)	26 (74.29)	18 (81.82)	8 (61.54)	0.1954
BMI (kg/m^2) (IQR)	29.40 (26.30–32.30)	30.15 (26.53–33.03)	29.30 (24.25–30.80)	0.7779
Diabetes mellitus (%)	8 (22.86)	8 (36.36)	0 (0)	* 0.0124
Chronic renal failure (%)	5 (14.29)	2 (9.09)	3 (23.08)	0.2663
Smoker (%)	2 (5.71)	2 (9.09)	0 (0)	0.2762
Ex-smoker (%)	3 (8.57)	2 (9.09)	1 (7.69)	0.8905
LOS (days) (IQR)	38.00 (26.00–55.00)	38.50 (27.50–52.75)	30.00 (18.00–56.00)	0.5713
LOS ICU (days) (IQR)	19.00 (16.00–35.00)	23.50 (17.50–46.25)	17.00 (12.50–23.00)	* 0.0443
28-day mortality (%)	12 (34.29)	9 (40.91)	3 (23.08)	0.2967

Data are presented as n (%) or median (IQR). An unpaired t-test (two-tailed) was used for statistical analysis with * $p < 0.05$. IQR: interquartile ranges (Q1–Q3); BMI: body mass index; LOS: length of stay; ICU: intensive care unit.

Table 2. Patient characteristics of Cohort B.

	All (n = 80)	Increasing RNase 1 Levels (n = 48)	Decreasing RNase 1 Levels (n = 32)	p-Value
Age (year) (IQR)	64.00 (52.00–75.00)	63.00 (55.00–71.75)	68.00 (51.00–78.25)	0.5802
Male sex (%)	51 (63.75)	30 (62.5)	21 (65.63)	0.7791
BMI (kg/m^2) (IQR)	28.49 (26.10–31.95)	27.73 (25.45–31.22)	29.40 (26.64–32.89)	0.5656
LOS (days) (IQR)	18.00 (12.25–34.00)	18.50 (12.25–38.50)	16.50 (10.75–27.00)	0.5515
LOS ICU (days) (IQR)	19.00 (12.00–38.75)	18.00 (12.00–35.00)	21.00 (12.50–44.50)	0.9218
ICU patients (%)	44 (55.00)	31 (64.58)	13 (40.63)	* 0.0351
28-day mortality (%)	22 (27.50)	18 (37.50)	4 (12.5)	* 0.0138

Data are presented as n (%) or median (IQR). An unpaired t-test (two-tailed) was used for statistical analysis with * $p < 0.05$. IQR: interquartile ranges (Q1–Q3); BMI: body mass index; LOS: length of stay; ICU: intensive care unit.

2.2. RNase 1 Serum Levels

First, we wanted to analyze whether the RNase 1 serum levels increased or decreased in COVID-19 patients over two days (Figure 1A) or a week (Figure 1B). We could not detect a significant increase in RNase 1 serum levels in the different cohorts (Figure 1A,B). Therefore, we grouped the patients into two groups based on their increasing or decreasing RNase 1 serum levels. In Cohort A, 22 patients were detected in whom RNase serum levels increased (increasing group) from day 2 (564.4 ± 289.9 ng/mL) to day 4 (871.9 ± 431.7 ng/mL), whereas 13 patients in Cohort A had a decrease in RNase 1 serum levels (decreasing group) from day 2 (549.0 ± 207.7 ng/mL) to day 4 (462.4 ± 173.7 ng/mL). In Cohort B, an increase in RNase 1 serum levels (increasing group) from day 1 (260.3 ± 141.3 ng/mL) to week 1 (517.9 ± 352.9 ng/mL) was detected in 48 patients. In 32 patients of Cohort B, a decrease in RNase 1 serum levels (decreasing group) from day 1 (465.6 ± 268.2 ng/mL) to week 1 (294.9 ± 206.5 ng/mL) was measured. We showed that the RNase 1 serum levels significantly increased in the increasing group from day 2 to day 4 ($p = 0.0171$; Figure 1C). In Cohort B, we detected a significant increase in RNase 1 serum levels from day 1 to week 1, as well as a significant decrease in the decreasing group ($p < 0.0001$ and $p = 0.0077$; Figure 1D).

2.3. Correlation of RNase 1 Serum Levels with 28-Day Mortality

Next, we investigated the correlation between RNase 1 serum levels and 28-day mortality in COVID-19 patients. We show that in Cohort A, 40.9% of the patients died within 28 days in the increasing RNase 1 group, and only 23.1% of the patients were included in the deceasing group (Figure 2A). In Cohort B, we found that there were significantly more patients who died in the increasing group than in the decreasing group ($p = 0.0138$; Figure 2B). Furthermore, we analyzed the RNase 1 serum levels of the different groups and showed that patients in Cohort A of the increasing group who died had significantly higher RNase 1 serum levels on day 2 than patients who survived ($p = 0.0170$; Figure 2C). On day 4, we measured significantly higher RNase 1 serum levels in patients who died later in the increasing group compared with surviving patients in the increasing group ($p = 0.0393$) and dying patients in the decreasing group ($p = 0.0471$; Figure 2D). In the decreasing group, no significant difference between the RNase 1 concentrations in surviving or dying patients was detected in Cohort A on day 2 and 4 (Figure 2C,D). In Cohort B, we also measured significantly higher RNase 1 serum levels in dying patients of the increasing group compared with surviving patients of the increasing group on day 1 and week 1 ($p = 0.0253$ and $p = 0.0034$; Figure 2E,F). In contrast to Cohort A, we detected significantly higher RNase 1 concentrations in the serum of surviving patients in the decreasing group compared to surviving patients in the increasing group on both days in Cohort B ($p = 0.0006$; Figure 2E).

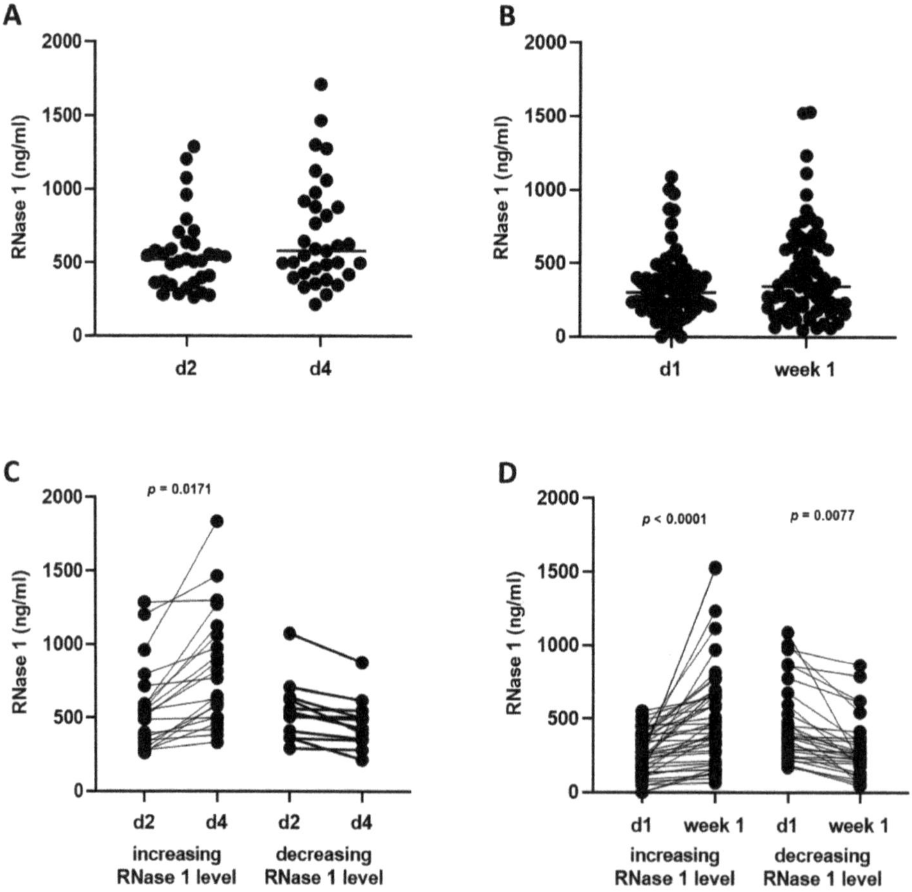

Figure 1. RNase 1 serum levels in Cohorts A and B. (**A**) RNase 1 serum levels of all patients in Cohort A on day 2 (d2) and day 4 (d4) and (**B**) Cohort B on day 1 (d1) and week 1 are presented. (**C,D**) The patients in the cohorts were grouped into two groups. In the first group, patients were included in which the RNase 1 serum levels increased (increasing RNase 1 levels), and in the second group, patients with decreasing RNase 1 serum levels (decreasing RNase 1 levels) were included. An unpaired *t*-test (two-tailed) was used for statistical analysis.

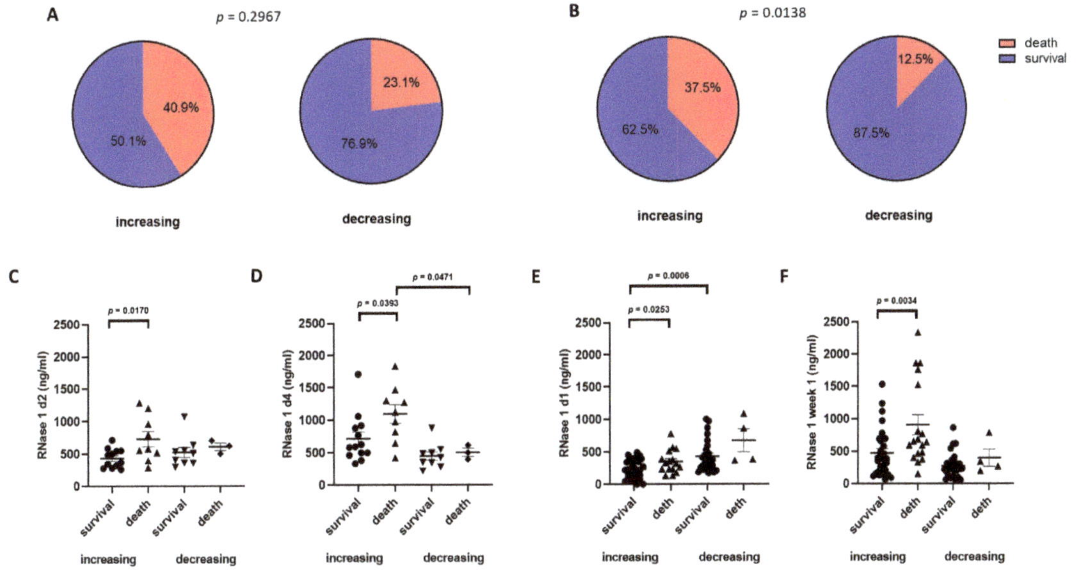

Figure 2. Association between RNase 1 serum levels and 28-day mortality. (**A**) Survival rate of all patients in Cohort A and (**B**) Cohort B grouped by increasing and decreasing RNase 1 serum levels in percentage. The correlation of RNase 1 serum levels with the mortality rate in COVID-19 patients in Cohort A on (**C**) day 2 and (**D**) day 4 as well as (**E**) in Cohort B on day 1 and (**F**) week 1 grouped in increasing and decreasing RNase 1 levels. Unpaired t-test (two-tailed) or one-way ANOVA was used for statistical analysis.

2.4. RNase 1 Serum Levels Correlate with Creatinine Serum Levels and Creatinine Clearance in COVID-19 Patients

To investigate the role of RNase 1 in kidney function/injury in patients with SARS-CoV-2 infection, we explored correlation of serum creatinine levels with RNase 1 serum levels in the different groups and time points. We measured a significant correlation between the creatinine and RNase 1 serum levels in all patients on day two ($p = 0.0007$) and day four ($p = 0.0004$) after COVID-19 diagnosis (Figure 3A,D). Next, we grouped the patients according to increasing and decreasing RNase 1 serum levels and correlated the creatinine serum levels again with the RNase 1 levels. We also detected a significant correlation on day two and day four in the increasing group ($p = 0.0254$ and $p = 0.0333$; Figure 3B,E). Interestingly, in the decreasing group, we detected a higher significance in the correlation between creatinine and RNase 1 serum levels on both days ($p < 0.0001$ and $p = 0.0002$; Figure 3C,F).

We also investigated the correlation between serum creatinine levels and RNase 1 serum levels in the second cohort on day one. We measured a significant correlation between the creatinine and RNase 1 serum levels in all patients on day one ($p = 0.0073$; Figure 4A). After grouping the patients of the second cohort into an increasing and decreasing group, we detected, in contrast to the first cohort, only a significant correlation between the creatinine and RNase 1 serum levels in the increasing group ($p = 0.0344$; Figure 4B).

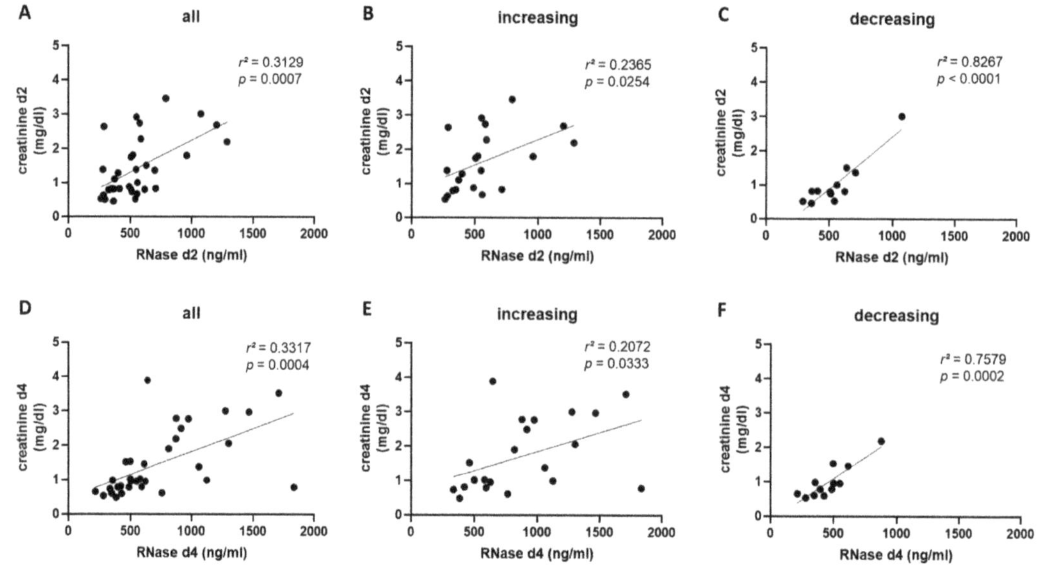

Figure 3. Correlation of RNase 1 and creatinine serum levels in Cohort A. (**A**) Correlation of RNase 1 and creatinine serum levels of all COVID-19 patients in Cohort A on day two is presented. The correlation of RNase 1 and creatinine serum levels two days after COVID-19 diagnosis in patients with (**B**) increasing or (**C**) decreasing RNase 1 serum levels from day 2 to day 4 is shown. (**D**) The correlation of RNase 1 and creatinine serum levels of all COVID-19 patients in Cohort A four days after COVID-19 infection is presented. The correlation of RNase 1 and creatinine serum levels four days after COVID-19 diagnosis in patients with (**E**) increasing or (**F**) decreasing RNase 1 serum levels from day 2 to day 4 is shown. Simple linear regression was used for statistical analysis.

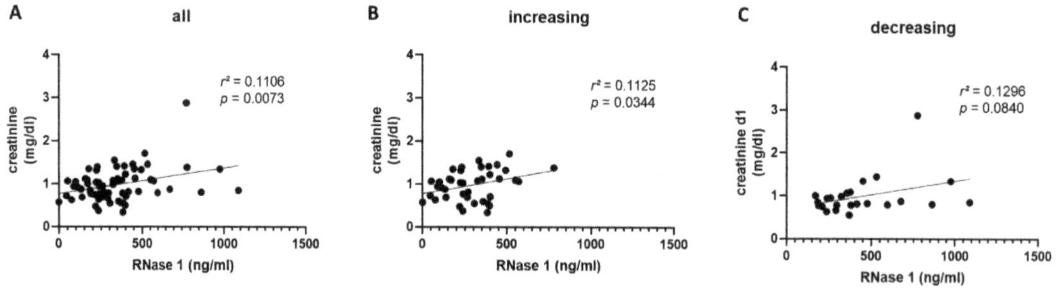

Figure 4. The correlation of RNase 1 and creatinine serum levels in Cohort B. (**A**) The correlation of RNase 1 and creatinine serum levels of all COVID-19 patients in Cohort B on the day of COVID-19 infection is shown. The correlation of RNase 1 and creatinine serum levels in patients with (**B**) increasing or (**C**) decreasing RNase 1 serum levels from day 1 to week 1 is presented. Simple linear regression was used for statistical analysis.

Furthermore, we explored the correlation of creatinine clearance with RNase 1 serum levels in the different groups and time points. In Cohort A, we measured a significant negative correlation between creatinine clearance and RNase 1 serum levels in all patients on day two ($p = 0.0016$) and day four ($p = 0.0006$) after COVID-19 diagnosis (Figure 5A,D). After grouping patients according to increasing and decreasing RNase 1 serum levels, we detected a higher significant correlation between creatinine clearance and RNase 1 serum levels on both days in the increasing group ($p = 0.0008$ and $p = 0.0012$; Figure 5C,F) than in the decreasing group ($p = 0.0409$ and $p = 0.0341$; Figure 5B,E).

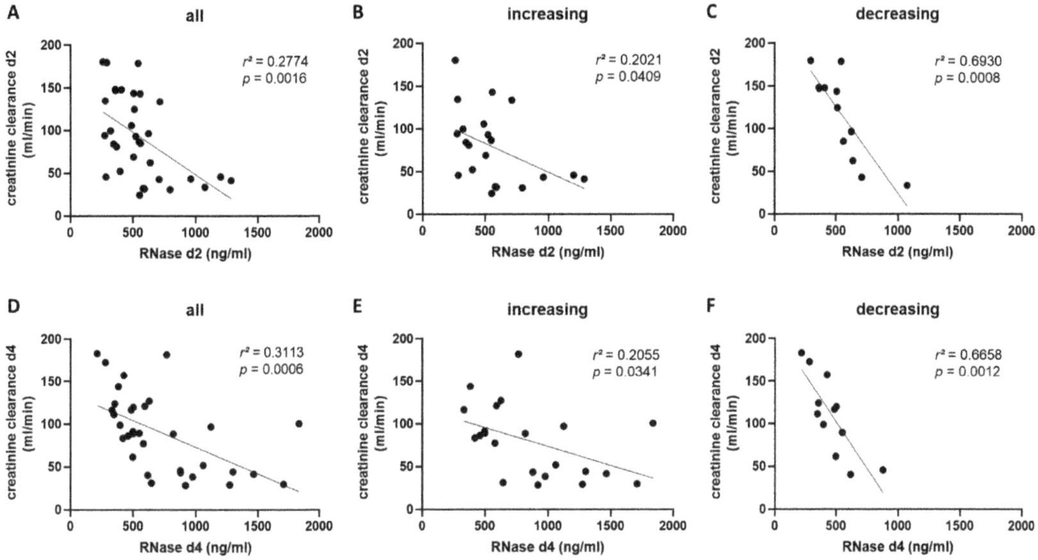

Figure 5. Correlation of RNase 1 serum levels and creatinine clearance on day 2 and 4 in Cohort A. (**A**) The correlation of RNase 1 and creatinine clearance of all COVID-19 patients in Cohort A on day two is presented. The correlation of RNase 1 and creatinine clearance two days after COVID-19 diagnosis in patients with (**B**) increasing or (**C**) decreasing RNase 1 serum levels from day 2 to day 4 is shown. (**D**) The correlation of RNase 1 and creatinine clearance of all COVID-19 patients in Cohort A four days after COVID-19 infection is presented. The correlation of RNase 1 and creatinine clearance four days after COVID-19 diagnosis in patients with (**E**) increasing or (**F**) decreasing RNase 1 serum levels from day 2 to day 4 is shown. Simple linear regression was used for statistical analysis.

In Cohort B, we did not detect a correlation between creatinine clearance and serum RNase 1 levels, neither in all patients nor in different subgroups and time points (Figure 6).

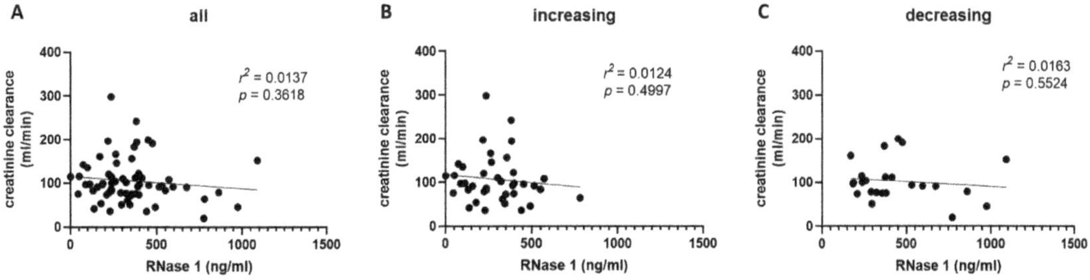

Figure 6. Correlation of RNase 1 and creatinine clearance on the day of diagnosis in Cohort B. (**A**) The correlation of RNase 1 and creatinine clearance of all COVID-19 patients in Cohort B on the day of COVID-19 infection is shown. The correlation of RNase 1 and creatinine clearance in patients with (**B**) increasing or (**C**) decreasing RNase 1 serum levels from day 1 to week 1 is presented. Simple linear regression was used for statistical analysis.

2.5. Time Course of Biomarkers and Scores over 14 Days and the Correlations of RNase 1 Levels with Clinical Parameters of ICU Patients with SARS-CoV-2 Infection

ICU patients with SARS-CoV-2 infection (Cohort A), grouped into increasing and decreasing RNase 1 serum levels, were evaluated for various biomarkers and scores (lactate, IL-6, PCT, CRP, sepsis-related organ failure assessment (SOFA) score, and Horowitz score) over a 14-day period. No relevant differences could be detected between the groups (Figure 7).

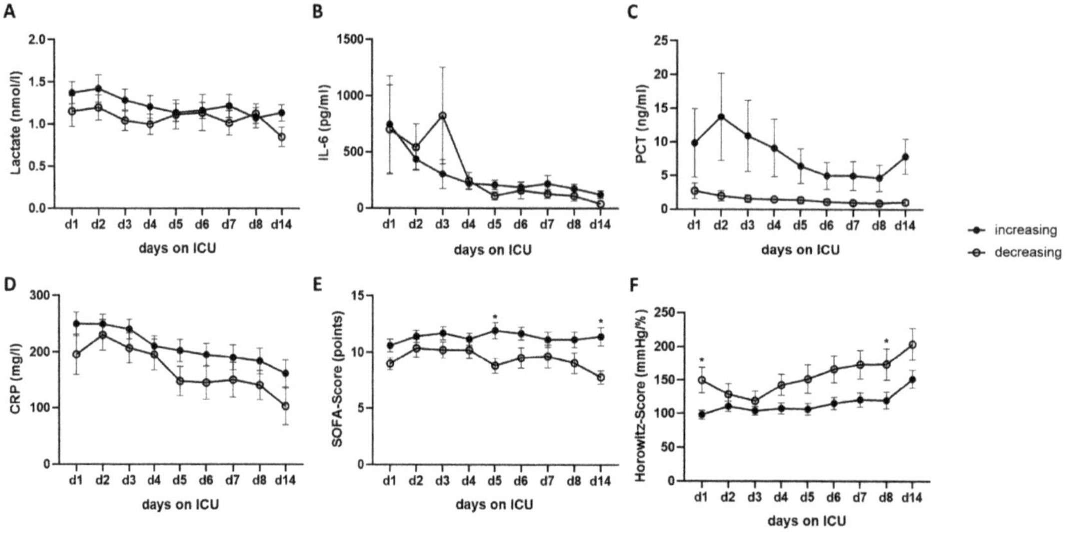

Figure 7. The time course of different biomarkers over 14 days in COVID-19 patients in Cohort A. Presented are (**A**) lactate, (**B**) IL-6, (**C**) PCT, (**D**) CRP, (**E**) the SOFA score, and (**F**) the Horowitz score over 14 days in COVID-19 patients grouped into increasing and decreasing RNase 1 serum levels. Ordinary two-way ANOVA was used for multiple comparisons (* $p < 0.05$).

To investigate the impact of increased and decreased RNase 1 levels serum during the course of the disease, we correlated RNase 1 serum level with various clinical parameters (Table 3). We detected, that RNase 1 level on day 2 of the increasing group correlate positive with PCT ($p = 0.0132$). Furthermore, we also measured a positive correlation with the days of dialysis and a negative correlation with diuresis ($p = 0.0199$; $p = 0.0044$) in the increasing group on day 2. On day 4, we detected a negative correlation with CRP and diuresis in the increasing group ($p = 0.0200$; $p = 0.0013$). A significant positive correlation with leucocytes and days of dialysis was also measured in the increasing group on day 4 ($p = 0.0167$; $p = 0.0046$). In the decreasing group, no significant correlations were detected (Table 3).

Table 3. Correlations of RNase 1 with various clinical parameters.

	Increasing RNase 1 d2		Decreasing RNase 1 d2	
Variable	Pearson *r*	*p*-Value	Pearson *r*	*p*-Value
CRP	0.0360	0.8909	−0.5112	0.1080
PCT	0.5570	* 0.0132	0.1131	0.7263
IL-6	−0.2412	0.3197	−0.2364	0.4839

Table 3. *Cont.*

Leucocytes	0.3793	0.0899	−0.3282	0.2977
days of dialysis **Diuresis**	0.5038 −0.6085	* 0.0199 * 0.0044	0.2462 −0.2475	0.4406 0.4379
	Increasing RNase 1 d4		**Decreasing RNase 1 d4**	
Variable	**Pearson *r***	***p*-value**	**Pearson *r***	***p*-value**
CRP	−0.5576	* 0.0200	0.1304	0.7023
PCT	0.3239	0.1414	0.1752	0.5859
IL-6	0.1298	0.5855	0.3544	0.2849
Leucocytes	0.5044	* 0.0167	−0.0142	0.9650
days of dialysis **Diuresis**	0.5812 −0.6414	* 0.0046 * 0.0013	0.1999 −0.3839	0.5334 0.2179

Shown are correlations of RNase 1 serum level of the increasing and decreasing groups at days 2 and 4 with various clinical parameters and correlation coefficient *r* with 95% confidence interval CI. *: significant correlations; CRP: C-reactive protein; IL-6: interleukin-6; PCT: procalcitonin.

3. Discussion

Several studies have demonstrated that RNase 1 possesses antiviral properties against HIV-1 [3,4]. Therefore, it has been postulated that RNases may be candidate drugs for host defense and could provide an alternative means to combat viral infections [9,15]. In this study, we demonstrated for the first time that RNase 1 serum levels play a potential role in patients with SARS-CoV-2 infection.

We could not detect changes in RNase 1 serum levels over time in both cohorts when all patients were analyzed together. However, after grouping patients in the two cohorts into an increasing and a decreasing group, we found that RNase 1 serum levels significantly increased in Cohort A from day 2 to day 4 and in Cohort B from day 1 to week 1. In Cohort A, a decrease in RNase 1 levels was observed in the decreasing group. The decrease in RNase 1 serum levels was even significant in Cohort B in the decreasing group from day 1 to week 1. It is possible that RNase 1 levels in Cohort A would also decrease significantly from the first to the second time point if the second measurement had been performed at a later time point, as in Cohort B. Because the patients in Cohort A were only ICU patients, whereas Cohort B also included patients who were not in the ICU, the two patient cohorts were different in the time points.

We showed that patients in the increasing group of Cohort A stayed in the ICU significantly longer than patients in the decreasing group. Similarly, patients in the increasing group of the second cohort were in the ICU significantly more often than patients in the decreasing group. In both cohorts, a higher mortality rate was observed in patients of the increasing group compared with patients with decreasing RNase 1 levels from time point 1 to 2. These data are in line with a previous study showing that patients with significantly higher serum RNase 1 levels 12 h after TAAA repair had a higher mortality rate than patients with lower RNase 1 levels [14].

In previous studies, it was shown that serum RNase 1 serum levels are associated with the development of renal failure and positively correlated with serum creatinine in patients with leukemia [16]. Consistent with this study, we also measured a significant positive correlation of RNase 1 serum levels with serum creatinine in all groups of Cohort A in the present study. In addition, we measured a positive correlation with the days of dialysis and a negative correlation with diuresis ($p = 0.0199$; $p = 0.0044$) in the increasing group on day 2. On day 4, we also detected a significant positive correlation with days of dialysis and a negative correlation diuresis in the increasing group ($p = 0.0046$; $p = 0.0013$). This suggests that increasing RNase 1 levels in patients with SARS-CoV-2 infection are associated with renal injury.

Although more patients died in the increasing group and no significant correlations with other clinical parameters were observed, a stronger positive correlation between creatinine levels and RNase 1 levels was measured in the decreasing group at both day 2 and day 4. Consistently, we showed that higher RNase 1 levels were associated with lower creatinine clearance. Moreover, there was a stronger correlation between RNase 1 levels and creatinine clearance in the decreasing group than in the increasing group. Consistent with this, our research group showed in a previous study that patients with renal dysfunction had significantly higher RNase 1 levels after TAAA repair than patients without renal dysfunction [14]. In addition, patients with higher serum RNase 1 levels were more likely to develop stage 3 acute kidney injury 48 h after surgery [14]. Furthermore, sepsis patients with renal dysfunction were found to have significantly higher RNase 1 levels than patients without renal dysfunction [17]. Additionally, Martin et al. showed that patients with sepsis have significantly higher serum RNase 1 levels than healthy volunteers [17]. Indeed, at days 5 and 14, we measured significantly higher SOFA scores in the increasing group than in the decreasing group.

SARS-CoV-2 infection can cause ARDS, which is defined according to the 2012 Berlin ARDS diagnostic criteria [18–20]. The severity of ARDS depends on the Horowitz quotient (PaO2/FiO2) [20]. Interestingly, a significant difference in Horowitz score was observed at days 1 and 8, which may suggest that increasing RNase 1 levels over time in COVID-19 patients are associated with lung injury. However, this could not be confirmed using other clinical parameters and biomarkers, where no differences were found. It could only be shown that the values of the increasing group were higher compared with the decreasing group in all biomarkers. This suggests that increasing RNase 1 levels may be associated with worse outcomes in SARS-CoV-2 patients.

Several studies have described that males with SARS-CoV-2 infection have a worse outcome than female patients [21–23]. However, in this study, we did not detect any association between RNase 1 concentration and worse outcome in relation to biological sex.

4. Materials and Methods

4.1. Study Design/Population

In this study, two different patient populations were analyzed. All serum samples were collected, based on approval by the Ethics Committee of the University Hospital RWTH Aachen (EK 100/20, proofed on the 7 April 2020 and EK 080/20, proofed on the 27 March 2020). All patients or their legal representatives provided written informed consent. The serum samples of the first cohort (Cohort A) were collected between March and April 2020. Thirty-five patients with positive SARS-CoV-2 PCR results and intensive care admission were included in this study. This patient population has been described in previous studies by our research group [24–26]. The serum samples of patients with COVID-19 infection in the second study population were collected between April 2020 and May 2021. In this cohort, 80 patients were included (Cohort B). Patients who were younger than 18 years of age, pregnant, or under palliative care were excluded. Identification of infection was carried out using real-time reverse transcription PCR (RT-PCR). All parameters, including demographics, vital signs, laboratory values, blood gas analyses, and organ support, were extracted from the patient data management system (Intellispace Critical Care and Anesthesia (ICCA) system, Philips, Amsterdam, Netherlands).

The patient populations were subclassified into an "increasing group", in which the RNase 1 concentration increased over the two time points, and a "decreasing group", in which the RNase 1 concentration decreased from time point one to time point two, similar to those in Bleilevens et al. [24].

4.2. Serum Sampling

Serum samples of Cohort A were collected one and three days (d2 and d4) after SARS-CoV-2 infection was confirmed via PCR. In Cohort B, serum samples were collected on the day when the positive PCR result was available (d1) and one week (week 1) after

SARS-CoV-2 infection was confirmed. After 10 min of coagulation, serum samples were centrifuged at 3000 rpm for 10 min at room temperature and stored at −80 °C until RNase 1 serum levels were measured.

4.3. Human Enzyme-Linked Immunosorbent Assay

Levels of RNase 1 in human serum were determined using a commercial ELISA kit (#SEK13468; Sino Biological Inc., Beijing, China) according to the manufacturer's instructions. Briefly, a 96-well microplate was coated with capture antibody and incubated overnight at 4 °C. The antibody solution was discarded, and the microplate was washed with at least 300 µL of wash buffer three times. Next, the plate was blocked by adding 300 µL of blocking buffer to each well, incubated at room temperature for 1 h, and washed. Afterward, the standard and samples were added in duplicate. After 2 h of incubation at room temperature, the washing step was repeated, and 100 µL of a detection antibody was added to each well and incubated for 1 h at room temperature. The microplate was washed three times, and 200 µL of a substrate solution was added to each well and incubated for 20 min at room temperature; 50 µL of stop solution was added to stop the reaction. For analysis, the optical density was measured at 450 nm and 570 nm as a reference using a microplate reader (Tecan Group, Männedorf, Switzerland).

4.4. Statistics

Individual values are presented as scatter plots. Lines represent the mean with SEM. To compare patient characteristics of the decreasing and increasing RNase 1 level groups, as well as RNase 1 serum levels on day two/one and day four/week one, unpaired *t*-tests were used. To assess the association between 28-day mortality (death/survival) and RNase 1 serum levels in the increasing and decreasing groups at each time point, one-way ANOVA was used. For each point in time, a simple linear regression was applied to assess the association between the outcome variables serum creatinine level and creatinine clearance with RNase 1 serum levels.

5. Limitation/Conclusions

Our study is limited by the different time points at which RNase 1 levels were determined in the two cohorts. In Cohort A, the RNase 1 levels were measured on days 2 and 4, and in Cohort B, the RNase levels were measured on day 1 and week 1, making it difficult to compare the two cohorts. Further investigation in a larger cohort in which RNase 1 serum levels are measured at multiple time points over a week should be performed to confirm our data. In addition, our measurements were limited to serum RNase 1 levels; measurement of RNase activity and determination of serum eRNA concentration would strengthen the results reported here.

In conclusion, we showed that a higher mortality rate was observed in patients with SARS-CoV-2 infection in patients with increasing RNase 1 levels from time point one to two. Moreover, in this study, we found significant positive correlations of serum RNase 1 levels with several biomarkers associated with renal injury in the increasing group of Cohort A. Additionally, at days 5 and 14, we measured significantly higher SOFA scores in the increasing group. Based on these results, there is now good evidence that increasing RNase 1 serum levels may play a role in renal dysfunction associated with COVID-19 and that increasing RNase 1 serum levels may be a potential biomarker to predict outcome in ICU patients with SARS-Cov-2 infection. However, more studies are needed to identify the underlying mechanisms.

Author Contributions: Conceptualization, E.Z., T.-P.S. and L.M.; methodology, E.Z., N.F., C.B., C.N., T.-P.S. and L.M.; validation, E.Z., T.-P.S. and L.M.; formal analysis E.Z., S.K., T.-P.S., T.B., M.D. and L.M.; resources, E.Z., T.-P.S., L.M., T.B., M.D., E.D. and G.M.; data curation, N.F., T.-P.S., C.B., E.Z. and L.M.; writing, E.Z.; review and editing, E.Z., T.-P.S., S.K., E.D. and L.M.; supervision, G.M.; project administration, E.Z., T.-P.S. and L.M.; funding acquisition, G.M. and E.Z. All authors have read and agreed to the published version of the manuscript.

Funding: This research was funded by an intramural grant to E.Z. (RWTH Aachen University, START 131/19).

Institutional Review Board Statement: The study was conducted according to the guidelines of the Declaration of Helsinki and approved by the local Ethical Committee of RWTH University (EK 100/20, proofed on the 7 April 2020 and EK 080/20, proofed on the 27 March 2020).

Informed Consent Statement: Informed consent was obtained from all subjects involved in the study.

Data Availability Statement: Not applicable.

Acknowledgments: The authors thank the whole team of the RWTH centralized Biomaterial Bank (RWTH cBMB). RWTH cBMB is an operational unit of and financed by the Medical Faculty, RWTH Aachen University.

Conflicts of Interest: The authors declare no conflict of interest. The funders had no role in the design of the study; in the collection, analyses, or interpretation of data; in the writing of the manuscript; or in the decision to publish the results.

References

1. World Health Organisation. WHO Coronavirus Disease (COVID-19) Dashboard. Available online: https://covid19.who.int/ (accessed on 12 October 2021).
2. Hasöksüz, M.; Kiliç, S.; Saraç, F. Coronaviruses and SARS-CoV-2. *Turk. J. Med. Sci.* **2020**, *50*, 549–556. [CrossRef] [PubMed]
3. Lee-Huang, S.; Huang, P.L.; Sun, Y.; Huang, P.L.; Kung, H.F.; Blithe, D.L.; Chen, H.C. Lysozyme and RNases as anti-HIV components in beta-core preparations of human chorionic gonadotropin. *Proc. Natl. Acad. Sci. USA* **1999**, *96*, 2678–2681. [CrossRef]
4. Rugeles, M.T.; Trubey, C.M.; Bedoya, V.I.; Pinto, L.A.; Oppenheim, J.J.; Rybak, S.M.; Shearer, G.M. Ribonuclease is partly responsible for the HIV-1 inhibitory effect activated by HLA alloantigen recognition. *AIDS* **2003**, *17*, 481–486. [CrossRef] [PubMed]
5. Koczera, P.; Martin, L.; Marx, G.; Schuerholz, T. The Ribonuclease A Superfamily in Humans: Canonical RNases as the Buttress of Innate Immunity. *Int. J. Mol. Sci.* **2016**, *17*, 1278. [CrossRef] [PubMed]
6. Chen, C.; Feng, Y.; Zou, L.; Wang, L.; Chen, H.H.; Cai, J.Y.; Xu, J.M.; Sosnovik, D.E.; Chao, W. Role of extracellular RNA and TLR3-Trif signaling in myocardial ischemia-reperfusion injury. *J. Am. Heart Assoc.* **2014**, *3*, e000683. [CrossRef] [PubMed]
7. Feng, Y.; Chen, H.; Cai, J.; Zou, L.; Yan, D.; Xu, G.; Li, D.; Chao, W. Cardiac RNA induces inflammatory responses in cardiomyocytes and immune cells via Toll-like receptor 7 signaling. *J. Biol. Chem.* **2015**, *290*, 26688–26698. [CrossRef] [PubMed]
8. Zechendorf, E.; O'Riordan, C.E.; Stiehler, L.; Wischmeyer, N.; Chiazza, F.; Collotta, D.; Denecke, B.; Ernst, S.; Muller-Newen, G.; Coldewey, S.M.; et al. Ribonuclease 1 attenuates septic cardiomyopathy and cardiac apoptosis in a murine model of polymicrobial sepsis. *JCI Insight* **2020**, *5*, e131571. [CrossRef]
9. Li, J.; Boix, E. Host Defence RNases as Antiviral Agents against Enveloped Single Stranded RNA Viruses. *Virulence* **2021**, *12*, 444–469. [CrossRef]
10. Ireland, D.D.; Stohlman, S.A.; Hinton, D.R.; Kapil, P.; Silverman, R.H.; Atkinson, R.A.; Bergmann, C.C. RNase L mediated protection from virus induced demyelination. *PLoS Pathog.* **2009**, *5*, e1000602. [CrossRef]
11. Legrand, M.; Bell, S.; Forni, L.; Joannidis, M.; Koyner, J.L.; Liu, K.; Cantaluppi, V. Pathophysiology of COVID-19-associated acute kidney injury. *Nat. Rev. Nephrol.* **2021**, *17*, 751–764. [CrossRef]
12. Kaye, A.D.; Okeagu, C.N.; Tortorich, G.; Pham, A.D.; Ly, E.I.; Brondeel, K.C.; Eng, M.R.; Luedi, M.M.; Urman, R.D.; Cornett, E.M. COVID-19 impact on the renal system: Pathophysiology and clinical outcomes. *Best Pract. Res. Clin. Anaesthesiol.* **2021**, *35*, 449–459. [CrossRef] [PubMed]
13. Copur, S.; Berkkan, M.; Basile, C.; Tuttle, K.; Kanbay, M. Post-acute COVID-19 syndrome and kidney diseases: What do we know? *J. Nephrol.* **2022**, *35*, 795–805. [CrossRef] [PubMed]
14. Zechendorf, E.; Gombert, A.; Bülow, T.; Frank, N.; Beckers, C.; Peine, A.; Kotelis, D.; Jacobs, M.J.; Marx, G.; Martin, L. The Role of Ribonuclease 1 and Ribonuclease Inhibitor 1 in Acute Kidney Injury after Open and Endovascular Thoracoabdominal Aortic Aneurysm Repair. *J. Clin. Med.* **2020**, *9*, 3292. [CrossRef] [PubMed]
15. Ilinskaya, O.N.; Mahmud, R.S. Ribonucleases as antiviral agents. *Mol. Biol.* **2014**, *48*, 615–623. [CrossRef]
16. Humphrey, R.L.; Karpetsky, T.P.; Neuwelt, E.A.; Levy, C.C. Levels of serum ribonuclease as an indicator of renal insufficiency in patients with leukemia. *Cancer Res.* **1977**, *37*, 2015–2022.
17. Martin, L.; Koczera, P.; Simons, N.; Zechendorf, E.; Hoeger, J.; Marx, G.; Schuerholz, T. The Human Host Defense Ribonucleases 1, 3 and 7 Are Elevated in Patients with Sepsis after Major Surgery—A Pilot Study. *Int. J. Mol. Sci.* **2016**, *17*, 294. [CrossRef]
18. Ackermann, M.; Verleden, S.E.; Kuehnel, M.; Haverich, A.; Welte, T.; Laenger, F.; Vanstapel, A.; Werlein, C.; Stark, H.; Tzankov, A.; et al. Pulmonary Vascular Endothelialitis, Thrombosis, and Angiogenesis in Covid-19. *N. Engl. J. Med.* **2020**, *383*, 120–128. [CrossRef]

19. Wu, C.; Chen, X.; Cai, Y.; Xia, J.; Zhou, X.; Xu, S.; Huang, H.; Zhang, L.; Zhou, X.; Du, C.; et al. Risk Factors Associated With Acute Respiratory Distress Syndrome and Death in Patients With Coronavirus Disease 2019 Pneumonia in Wuhan, China. *JAMA Intern. Med.* **2020**, *180*, 934–943. [CrossRef]
20. Ards Definition Task Force; Ranieri, V.M.; Rubenfeld, G.D.; Thompson, B.T.; Ferguson, N.D.; Caldwell, E.; Fan, E.; Camporota, L.; Slutsky, A.S. Acute respiratory distress syndrome: The Berlin Definition. *JAMA* **2012**, *307*, 2526–2533. [CrossRef]
21. Takahashi, T.; Ellingson, M.K.; Wong, P.; Israelow, B.; Lucas, C.; Klein, J.; Silva, J.; Mao, T.; Oh, J.E.; Tokuyama, M.; et al. Sex differences in immune responses that underlie COVID-19 disease outcomes. *Nature* **2020**, *588*, 315–320. [CrossRef]
22. Meng, Y.; Wu, P.; Lu, W.; Liu, K.; Ma, K.; Huang, L.; Cai, J.; Zhang, H.; Qin, Y.; Sun, H.; et al. Sex-specific clinical characteristics and prognosis of coronavirus disease-19 infection in Wuhan, China: A retrospective study of 168 severe patients. *PLoS Pathog.* **2020**, *16*, e1008520. [CrossRef] [PubMed]
23. Shoeb, F.; Mahdi, F.; Hussain, I. Gender Differences Associated with Hyper-Inflammatory Conditions in COVID-19 Patients. *Aging Dis.* **2023**, *14*, 299–308. [CrossRef]
24. Bleilevens, C.; Soppert, J.; Hoffmann, A.; Breuer, T.; Bernhagen, J.; Martin, L.; Stiehler, L.; Marx, G.; Dreher, M.; Stoppe, C.; et al. Macrophage Migration Inhibitory Factor (MIF) Plasma Concentration in Critically Ill COVID-19 Patients: A Prospective Observational Study. *Diagnostics* **2021**, *11*, 332. [CrossRef]
25. Zechendorf, E.; Schröder, K.; Stiehler, L.; Frank, N.; Beckers, C.; Kraemer, S.; Dreher, M.; Kersten, A.; Thiemermann, C.; Marx, G.; et al. The Potential Impact of Heparanase Activity and Endothelial Damage in COVID-19 Disease. *J. Clin. Med.* **2022**, *11*, 5261. [CrossRef] [PubMed]
26. Simon, T.P.; Stoppe, C.; Breuer, T.; Stiehler, L.; Dreher, M.; Kersten, A.; Kluge, S.; Karakas, M.; Zechendorf, E.; Marx, G.; et al. Prognostic Value of Bioactive Adrenomedullin in Critically Ill Patients with COVID-19 in Germany: An Observational Cohort Study. *J. Clin. Med.* **2021**, *10*, 1667. [CrossRef] [PubMed]

International Journal of
Molecular Sciences

MDPI

Review

Interrelationship between COVID-19 and Coagulopathy: Pathophysiological and Clinical Evidence

Beatrice Ragnoli [1,*], Beatrice Da Re [1], Alessandra Galantino [1], Stefano Kette [1], Andrea Salotti [1] and Mario Malerba [1,2]

1 Respiratory Unit, Sant'Andrea Hospital, 13100 Vercelli, Italy; beatricedare95@gmail.com (B.D.R.); alessandragalantino@gmail.com (A.G.); stefano.kette@libero.it (S.K.); salottiandrea@gmail.com (A.S.); mario.malerba@uniupo.it (M.M.)
2 Department of Traslational Medicine, University of Eastern Piedmont (UPO), 28100 Novara, Italy
* Correspondence: beatrice.ragnoli@aslvc.piemonte.it

Abstract: Since the first description of COVID-19 infection, among clinical manifestations of the disease, including fever, dyspnea, cough, and fatigue, it was observed a high incidence of thromboembolic events potentially evolving towards acute respiratory distress syndrome (ARDS) and COVID-19-associated-coagulopathy (CAC). The hypercoagulation state is based on an interaction between thrombosis and inflammation. The so-called CAC represents a key aspect in the genesis of organ damage from SARS-CoV-2. The prothrombotic status of COVID-19 can be explained by the increase in coagulation levels of D-dimer, lymphocytes, fibrinogen, interleukin 6 (IL-6), and prothrombin time. Several mechanisms have been hypothesized to explain this hypercoagulable process such as inflammatory cytokine storm, platelet activation, endothelial dysfunction, and stasis for a long time. The purpose of this narrative review is to provide an overview of the current knowledge on the pathogenic mechanisms of coagulopathy that may characterize COVID-19 infection and inform on new areas of research. New vascular therapeutic strategies are also reviewed.

Keywords: COVID-19 infection; coagulopathy; endothelial dysfunction; platelet activation; citokine storm; anticoagulant therapy

Citation: Ragnoli, B.; Da Re, B.; Galantino, A.; Kette, S.; Salotti, A.; Malerba, M. Interrelationship between COVID-19 and Coagulopathy: Pathophysiological and Clinical Evidence. *Int. J. Mol. Sci.* **2023**, *24*, 8945. https://doi.org/10.3390/ijms24108945

Academic Editors: Eliza Russu, Alexandru Schiopu and Emil Marian Arbănași

Received: 25 April 2023
Revised: 14 May 2023
Accepted: 16 May 2023
Published: 18 May 2023

1. Background

At the end of December 2019, a novel coronavirus, denominated SARS-CoV-2 according to the similarity with the previous SARS viral epidemy, was described for the first time in China, and in March 2020, it was declared a global pandemic by the WORLD Health Organization (WHO) due to high morbidity and mortality. Italy was one of the most affected countries at the beginning of the infection spreading [1]. The disease caused by this virus was denominated Coronavirus disease 2019 (COVID-19) which still represents a critical challenge for the worldwide health community despite the reduction in mortality following the global vaccination campaign. To date, there have been more than 762 million confirmed cases of COVID-19 infection, including almost 6.8 million deaths reported to WHO, while a total of 13,340,275,493 vaccine doses have been administered [2]. Among the wide range of SARS-CoV-2 clinical manifestations (cough, fever, pharyngodynia, myoarthralgia, fatigue), a respiratory tract involvement has been observed, potentially evolving with pneumonia, acute respiratory distress syndrome (ARDS), hyperinflammation, and COVID-19-associated-coagulopathy [3–5]. The hypercoagulable state is strongly associated with COVID-19 infection and may explain several phenomena observed in clinical practice. Since the beginning of the pandemic, a very high incidence of thrombo-embolic events was observed including arterial and venous thrombosis, cerebral and myocardial infarction, limb arterial thrombosis, and venous thrombosis leading to a higher incidence of stroke, acute coronary syndrome and myocardial infarction, venous thromboembolism (VTE) and pulmonary thromboembolism (PTE) [6–11]. Pathophysiological characteristics of acute pulmonary thromboembolism [12] and abnormal coagulation status [13] have been reported in these patients. Additional important laboratory findings such as high levels of D-dimer, as well as fibrinogen (FIB) and its related degradation products (FDP), have been correlated with a poorer outcome [13–15]. In patients who died from COVID-19 infection, microthrombosis of alveolar capillaries was more prevalent (nine times) than in patients who died from influenza, and about 15.2% to 79% of patients with severe COVID-19 infection have shown thrombotic events [16]. The involvement of the coagulation cascade and its abnormalities were previously identified in experimental investigations on mice infected with SARS-CoV-1 and in human autopsies. These findings suggested the hypothesis of a diffuse thrombotic microangiopathic mechanism involved in the pathogenesis of acute pulmonary interstitial disease caused by SARS-CoV-2 infection [17,18]. The prothrombotic status seems to be caused by immune cell activation, excessive coagulation, and endothelial dysfunction [19]. Immuno-thrombosis appears to be involved in the pathological mechanism of SARS-CoV-2, and it is characterized by the interaction between the hemostatic system and the innate immune system, especially between monocytes, macrophages, and neutrophils. After the endocytosis of SARS-CoV-2 in the host cells, vascular damage is induced, leading to a proinflammatory form of programmed cell death with cell lysis named "pyroptosis" and the release of various substances, the so-called damage-associated molecular patterns (DAMPs) such as adenosine triphosphate (ATP), nucleic acids, and inflammasomes [20], thus intensifying the inflammatory environment. Several mechanisms have been hypothesized to be involved in this hypercoagulable process such as inflammatory cytokine storm, platelet activation, endothelial dysfunction, and stasis for a long time [11,21,22]. The purpose of this narrative review is to provide an overview of the current knowledge on the pathogenic mechanisms of coagulopathy that may characterize COVID-19 infection and inform on new areas of research. New vascular therapeutic strategies are also reviewed.

2. Role of Platelets and Complement as Prothrombotic Factors in COVID-19 Infection

Platelets have a pivotal role in the innate immune system by activating the complement, thus playing a key role in COVID-19 "immune-thrombosis" [23]. The aggregation of PLT activated by endothelium damage and its interaction with other cells increase their potential for pathologic thrombosis; their activation is essential to the structural remodeling of the pulmonary vasculature, inflammation, and cardiovascular disease [24,25]. The mechanism of platelet activation may include different and multiple pathways even more complex in COVID-19 infection, as the virus is able to infect cells using several entry mechanisms such as TLRs and/or the ACE2-AngII axis [26]. The activated endothelial cells express P-selectin and other adhesion molecules with the recruitment of platelets and leukocytes. Bioactive molecules (e.g., adenosine diphosphate [ADP], polyphosphates, coagulation factors) and immunological mediators (e.g., complement factors) are released from activated platelets, activating the immune system through positive feedback [23]. P-selectin, a platelet activation marker, is increased in patients with COVID-19 and can lead to a procoagulant phenotype by inducing tissue factor (TF) expression in monocytes. Moreover, Von Willebrand factor (VWF) is a glycoprotein derived from activated endothelial cells, platelets, or sub-endothelial cells mediating the adhesion and aggregation of platelets. In patients affected by COVID-19, VWF is significantly increased and may suggest a tendency for thrombosis [27]. The activation of the complement system was documented in COVID-19 with the formation of the terminal membrane attack complex (MAC) that, in turn, can activate platelets with subsequent endothelial damage and the secretion of VWF [28]. For this reason, the complement activation is associated with an amplification of the prothrombotic phenotype in COVID-19. In fact, C5a can stimulate the release of TF and plasminogen activator inhibitor-1 (PAI-1) expression and activate neutrophils, which are responsible for the increased release of cytokines and the formation of neutrophil extracellular traps (NETs) [29].

3. Role of Hypoxia, Blood Viscosity, and Vasoconstriction as Prothrombotic Factors in COVID-19 Infection

Hypoxia may represent itself as a factor inducing a prothrombotic status in patients with SARS-CoV-2 infection with the production of a hypoxia-inducible transcription factor (HIF-1α), which promotes the secretion of PAI-1 (plasminogen activator inhibitor) and macrophages by the endothelium. On the other hand, the mechanisms of altered coagulation are responsible for hypoxia that, in turn, favors the thrombo-inflammatory loop. Furthermore, hypoxia causes a release of cytokines such as tumor necrosis factor-α (TNF-α) IL-6 [30], critical inflammatory cytokines with prothrombotic effects. Positive correlations have been found between IL-6 and D-dimer, especially during the exacerbation of the disease [31]. Consequently, increased blood viscosity and the release of procoagulant antibodies develop [32]. Recent studies showed that the appearance of antiphospholipid antibodies and lupus anticoagulant immunoglobulins may also play a role in the pathogenesis of coagulopathy. Indeed, the presence of IgA anti-cardiolipin antibodies and IgA and IgG anti-2-glycoprotein I antibodies have been found in association with coagulopathy, thrombocytopenia, and the development of peripheral and cerebral ischemic events. Harzallah and coworkers [33] investigated 56 patients with confirmed or suspected SARS-CoV-2 infection. Among these, 25 were found to be lupus anticoagulant immunoglobulin, while 5 were found positive for IgM or IgG anti-cardiolipin or anti-2-glycoprotein I antibodies. Endothelial dysfunction is characterized by the loss of characteristics of endothelial native cells such as the ability to regulate vascular tonus which may conduce to vasoconstriction and, subsequently, a prothrombotic status. Moreover, the down-regulation of the endothelial ACE2 receptor as a consequence of SARS-CoV-2 infection gives a pro-inflammatory, pro-coagulant, and pro-apoptotic phenotype to endothelial cells [34].

4. Interlink between Coagulation and Inflammation in COVID-19

The so-called COVID-19-associated CAC represents a key aspect in the genesis of organ damage from SARS-CoV-2 and the hypercoagulation state is based on an interaction between thrombosis and inflammation. A close relationship between inflammation and coagulation has been widely demonstrated in previous research [35,36]. The coagulation system consists of a finely regulated balance between procoagulant and anticoagulant mechanisms and inflammation can compromise this equilibrium, leading to impaired coagulation. As a result, the final clinical consequence of inflammatory conditions may consist of bleeding, thrombosis, or both of them [37]. Pathogens, inflammatory mediators such as IL-6, IL-8, and TNF-α, as well as DAMPs from injured host tissue can activate monocytes and induce the expression of tissue factors on monocytes and endothelial cell surfaces [38] (Figure 1).

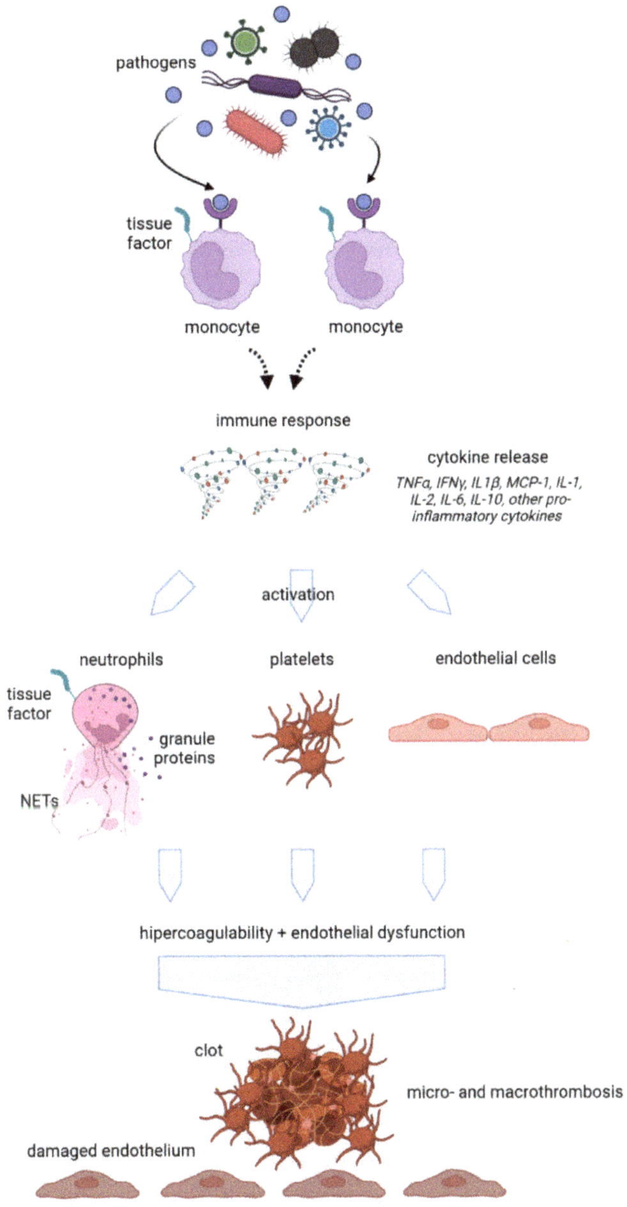

Figure 1. Schematic representation of endothelium activation towards a pro-thrombotic status. Pathogens and inflammatory mediators from injured host tissue activate monocytes and induce the expression of tissue factors on monocytes and endothelial cell surfaces. Subsequently, activated monocytes release inflammatory cytokines and chemokines amplifying the inflammatory response and stimulating vascular endothelial cells changing their properties to a procoagulant state. NETs: neutrophil extracellular traps; TNFα: tumor necrosis factor-alpha; IFNγ: interferon-gamma; MCP-1: monocyte chemotactic protein-1; IL: interleukin.

Subsequently, activated monocytes release inflammatory cytokines and chemokines that enlarge the inflammatory response and stimulate neutrophils, lymphocytes, platelets, and vascular endothelial cells. Healthy endothelial cells have an anti-thrombogenic attitude due to the expression of glycocalyx and its binding protein, antithrombin. When endothelial cells go through injury, the glycocalyx is disrupted, the anticoagulant factors are lost, and, consequently, these cells change their properties to procoagulant [39]. Furthermore, neutrophils are also involved in an important defense mechanism that may lead to a procoagulant status by means of NETs. NETs are structures of DNA, histones, and neutrophil antimicrobial proteins that bind and kill pathogens. The excessive production of NETs can facilitate microthrombosis by creating a scaffold for platelet aggregation [40]. When an infection occurs, the first leukocytes recruited are neutrophils that, producing and releasing NETs, stimulate the formation and deposition of fibrin to trap and destroy invading microorganisms. It has been previously demonstrated that NETs increase in sepsis and inflammatory conditions [41]. NETs also cause platelet adhesion, and, in some experimental models, their connection with deep vein thrombosis has been demonstrated [40]. They stimulate both the extrinsic and intrinsic coagulation pathways playing a major role in a coagulative pattern during infection-mediated inflammation. Patients with severe COVID-19 have been shown to present elevated levels of circulating histones and myeloperoxidase DNA (MPO-DNA) which are two specific markers of NETs [42]. As a consequence of the described mechanisms, an extreme inflammatory response may also occur, causing disseminated intravascular coagulation (DIC), which leads to multiple organ failure. This life-threatening acquired syndrome is characterized by the disseminated and often uncontrolled activation of coagulation and is associated with a high risk of macro- and microvascular thrombosis. In this setting, natural coagulation inhibitors also become inefficient in downregulating thrombin generation. Moreover, progressive consumption coagulopathy can be observed which leads to an increased bleeding risk [43]. Other clinical manifestations of the altered coagulation system are hemolytic uremic syndrome, idiopathic thrombocytopenic purpura, thrombotic thrombocytopenic purpura [44], and hemophagocytic lymphohistiocytosis (sHLH). Globally, all of this evidence suggests that the hypercoagulative state described in patients with COVID-19 is likely to be caused by a deep and complex inflammatory response to the virus, based on an interaction between thrombosis and inflammation as shown in Figure 2. Another important interlink between inflammation and pro-thrombotic status is represented by underlying clinical conditions such as chronic comorbidities that are linked to mortality in COVID-19 infection. In particular, obesity has been shown to increase the risk of hospitalization and COVID-19 complications [45] suggesting an interplay between obesity and inflammation. The adipose tissue, in fact, expresses higher ACE2 levels than lung tissue, being a powerful inflammatory reservoir for the replication of SARS-CoV-2 [46]. In addition, obese people are characterized by low-grade inflammation, associated with the over-expression of pro-inflammatory cytokines and chemokines such as TNF-α, IL-6, and MCP-1, high leptin levels with known pro-inflammatory effects, low adiponectin levels with anti-inflammatory effects, and, consequently, a procoagulant status. It has been calculated that one-third of total circulating concentrations of IL-6 originate from adipose tissue [47]. In addition, obese patients show higher blood IL-6 and TNF-α levels and a polarization of natural killer (NK) cells to non-cytotoxic NK cells. As both obesity and COVID-19 seem to share common metabolic and inflammatory pathways, it has been recommended by many authors to consider and classify obese and severely obese patients as high-risk patients for COVID-19. Additionally, sleep disturbances during pandemics have been suggested to be related to a major risk of infection linked to increased inflammatory status and a reduction in the efficiency of the immune system [48]. An interesting linkage was found between sleep deprivation, inflammation, and immune response to SARS-CoV-2 that may have a role in predisposing to the infection [49].

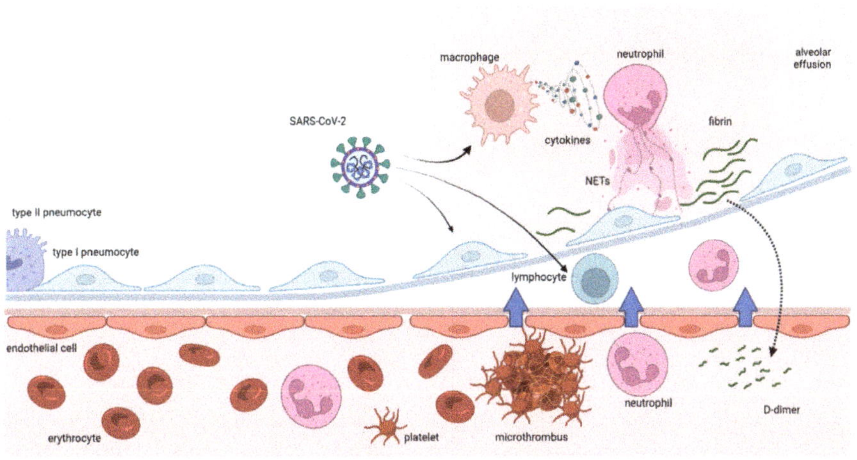

Figure 2. Schematic representation of the interlink between inflammatory and thrombotic mechanisms after COVID-19 infection.

5. Interlink between Coagulopathy in Viral Infections and in COVID-19

Since the beginning of the pandemic, a very high incidence of thrombo-embolic events (VTE) was observed. The hypercoagulative state, described in patients with COVID-19 derives from a complex inflammatory response to the virus in which hemostasis and the immune system collaborate together to limit the spread of viral infection. Physiological immune thrombosis can evolve into an excessive, dysregulated formation of immunologically mediated thrombi and spread, especially in the microcirculation. Several viral infections may share abnormal coagulation processes such as bleeding, thrombosis, or both.

5.1. Thrombosis

The increased incidence of VTE in COVID-19 patients was similar also in patients with other viral infections, i.e., severe acute respiratory syndrome (SARS) and Middle East Respiratory Syndrome (MERS-CoV) [50,51]. H1N1 influenza infection is associated with an 18-fold increased risk of developing VTE when compared to critically ill patients with ARDS with no H1N1 influenza infection [6]. A previous study by Avnon et al. found that VTE occurred in 25% of patients with severe H1N1 influenza admitted to the intensive care unit (ICU) [52]. Particular evidence for thromboembolic events was also reported during cytomegalovirus (CMV) infection in which two arterial thrombotic events were described in nine Israelitic immunocompetent CMV-infected patients (spleen and liver) [53]. The pathophysiological mechanism is yet unknown but it seems to be related to higher levels of VWF in the plasma of CMV-infected people [54]. It is likely that the SARS-CoV-2 virus does not have intrinsic procoagulant effects, while coagulopathy appears as a consequence of the intense COVID-19 inflammatory response and endothelial activation/damage [55]. Two possible mechanisms implicated in the pathogenesis of coagulation dysfunction during SARS-CoV2 infection have been proposed: the cytokine storm which seems to play a pivotal role, and virus-specific mechanisms related to the virus interaction with the renin–angiotensin system and the fibrinolytic pathway [56].

5.1.1. Cytokine Storm

Pro-inflammatory cytokines are involved in a so-called "cytokine release syndrome" responsible for the innate immune system activation and severe clinical manifestation of the disease [57]. Immune system dysfunction is a candidate risk factor for adverse outcomes in COVID-19, and the most important cause of morbidity and mortality in patients suffering from COVID-19 infection seems to be the cytokine storm causing an immune dysregulation in the peripheral tissues and in the lungs [58] (p. 2), refs. [57,59–62]. More specifically, IL-6 plays an important role in cytokine release syndrome and contributes, together with TNF-α and interleukin-1 (IL-1), to blood hyper-coagulability and to severe inflammation, sometimes evolving in disseminated intravascular coagulation (DIC) [63] Figure 3.

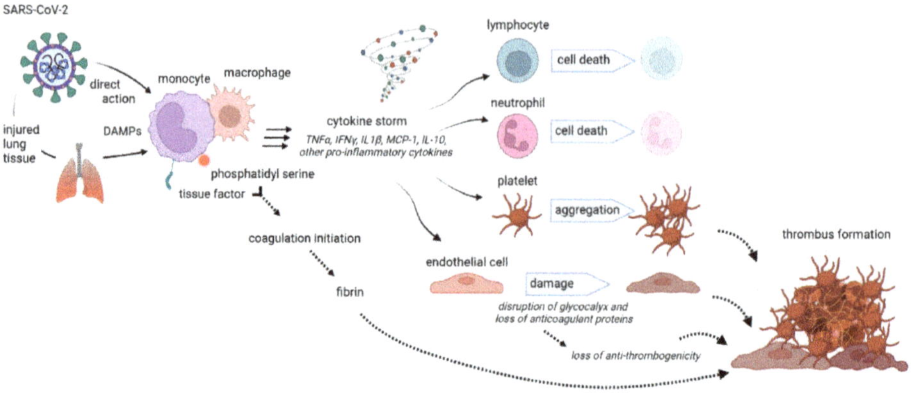

Figure 3. Effects of the inflammatory response to COVID-19 infection with cytokine release syndrome and dysregulation of the immune system with the final effect of a hyper-coagulative state. DAMPs: damage-associated molecular patterns.

Current evidence from clinical studies shows that IL-6 seems to play a prominent role in the cytokine-induced activation of coagulation. Additionally, IL-6 promotes the proliferation of megakaryocytes [64] and the release of TF, the latter detected in inflamed tissues and in particular in the lungs of patients affected by COVID-19 [65]. A postulated mechanism considers that SARS-CoV-2-infected megakaryocytes may interfere with platelet function and count, as already described in previous studies that reported thrombocytopenia during SARS-CoV infection. The virus induces the release of cytokines such as IL-6 conducting to megakaryocytic proliferation and differentiation, although the mechanism remains not completely clarified [66,67].

Furthermore, vascular permeability is mediated by IL-6 through the stimulation of vascular endothelial growth factor (VEGF) secretion and the release of other coagulation factors such as FIB and factor VIII [68]. There was a great effort during the pandemic to find inflammatory markers reflecting disease severity and eventually predicting disease prognosis. Among the most studied, increased levels of a pivotal serum cytokine, IL-1, which is a principal source of tissue damage interacting in both innate and acquired immunity, have been detected in patients suffering from severe COVID-19 infection. IL-1 stimulates the secretion of mediators stored in the granules of mast cells and macrophages, such as TNF-α, IL-6, and the release of arachidonic acid products such as prostaglandins and thromboxane A2 [69–72]. Another important marker in the cytokine network of COVID-19 infection is IL-18. The catastrophic clinical course of COVID-19 shares similar features with macrophage activation syndrome (MAS) encountered also in other conditions with a potentially rapidly fatal course without treatment. IL-1, IL-6, IL-8, IL-10, IL-18, interferon (IFN)-γ, and TNF-α are the most important elements responsible for MAS development. IL-18 is produced by macrophages at very early stages of viral infections and induces the production of IL-6 and IFN-γ which are considered critical for optimal viral host defense. A study by Satis and coworkers observed a four-fold level of IL-18 in 58 people suffering from a severe form of COVID-19. These findings contrasted with the mildly affected patients and led to the conclusion of a correlation between IL-18 and the severity of the disease [73]. An additional role is determined by TNF-α, responsible for the activation of glucuronidases, which degrades the endothelial glycocalyx, and the upregulation of hyaluronic acid synthase 2, which leads to hyaluronic acid deposition and fluid retention [74]. Due to the systemic hypoxia induced by COVID-19-related ARDS, a reduction in endothelial nitric oxide synthase activity and nitric oxide levels has been indicated as a possible pathogenic process typical of endothelial dysfunction [75].

5.1.2. Virus-Specific Mechanisms

Experiments in vitro demonstrated that SARS-CoV2 can infect primary endothelial cells [76] and there is some evidence of the infection of endothelial cells in severe cases of COVID-19 [11]. Moreover, the replication within endothelial cells is able to induce cell death causing the activation of procoagulant reactions [77]. The membrane glycoprotein (Spike) of the SARS-CoV-2 virus interacts with Angiotensin-Converting Enzyme 2 (ACE-2), an integral membrane receptor expressed in the lung but also the heart, kidney, and intestine by reducing their activity. Normally, ACE-2 reduces the availability of angiotensin II through the counter-regulated activity of ACE [78]. As a result, the virus-mediated engagement of ACE-2 decreases its expression and activates the renin-angiotensin system (RAS), promoting the activation of epithelial cells, monocytes, neutrophils, and procoagulant factors with platelet adhesion and aggregation, and consequent vasoconstriction and release of inflammatory cytokines [79], as well as a reduction in fibrinolytic activity mediated by RAS, can be observed [80] as represented in Figure 4.

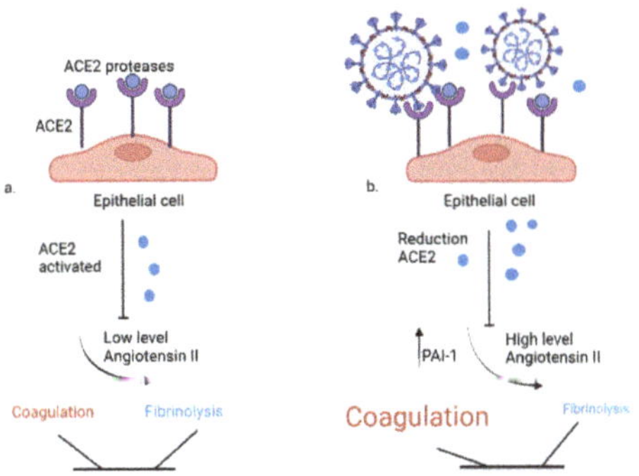

Figure 4. Imbalance between coagulation and fibrinolysis: the effects of SARS-CoV2. (**a**). Physiologically, ACE-2 reduces the availability of angiotensin II with no effects on coagulation and fibrinolysis. (**b**). SARS-CoV2 reducing ACE-2 availability, which increases the level of angiotensin II and the PAI-1 and favors the activation of the coagulation system. ACE-2: angiotensin-converting enzyme 2, PAI-1: plasminogen activator inhibitor 1.

The RAS may play a key role in SARS-CoV-2-induced COVID-19 [81]. The downregulation of ACE-2 by the virus causes an increase in angiotensin II, which, acting on the AT1 receptor, causes systemic injury [82] but also specific lung damage with pulmonary fibrosis, pulmonary inflammation, and ARDS in severe cases of COVID-19 [83]. ACE-2 is markedly expressed in pneumocytes type II, hence participating in alveolar surfactant production. The downregulation of ACE-2 receptors due to the binding of coronavirus might hinder the expression of pneumocytes type II cells, explaining the worsening of gaseous exchange [84,85]. Overall, the interaction of coronavirus with ACE-2 receptors is destructive due to increased inflammatory lesions, the downregulation of ACE-2 receptors, increased local angiotensin II effects and AT1 receptor over-activity, insufficient surfactant due to bruised pneumocytes type II causing a reduction in pulmonary compliance and amplified surface tension, and a reduction in the generation and repair of pneumocytes type I with impaired gaseous exchange along with alveolar–capillary diffusion capacity and fibrosis [86]. Moreover, a different impact of SARS-CoV-2 expression on ACE-2 may be due to gender-related dissimilarities, with the ACE-2 gene existing in the

X-chromosome [87]. The wide variances in COVID-19 death rates might be explained by significant alterations in the equilibrium of the ACE:ACE-2 system associated with gender, racial, and age differences in genetic ACE and ACE-2 polymorphism and environmental aspects manipulating ACE-2 expression [88–90]. In addition, the severity of lung injury is linked with the expression of ACE. ALI was less complicated in complete knockout (Acee/e) mice and AT1 receptor knockout mice compared to partial ACE knockout (Ace./e) mice and wild-type mice, respectively. The injection of recombinant SARS spike protein along with AT1 blockers elevated the expression of angiotensin II leading to ARDS in mice [91]. Thus, understanding the role of the ACE-2 receptor in the pathogenesis of COVID-19 may open a potential approach for therapeutic intervention [92].

Among virus-related mechanisms, high levels of PAI-1, the principal inhibitor of fibrinolysis interfering with tissue plasminogen activator (tPA) and urokinase, have been related to an increased risk of thromboembolic events [80]. Interestingly, previous studies reported high blood levels of PAI-1 in patients with SARS-CoV infection suggesting a possible direct effect of infection on the production of anti-coagulant factors [93]. One study described an important increase in another mediator of platelet adhesion, platelet-derived vitronectin (VN), in SARS-CoV pneumonia; however, it was not possible to discriminate its origin from increased expression by the liver or from lung damage [94]. Another possible virus-specific effect could be related to the induction of autoimmunity, also described in SARS patients [37]. Recent studies showed that the appearance of antiphospholipid antibodies and lupus anticoagulant immunoglobulins may have a role in the pathogenesis of coagulopathy. Indeed, the presence of IgA anti-cardiolipin antibodies and IgA and IgG anti-2-glycoprotein I antibodies have been found in association with coagulopathy, thrombocytopenia, and the development of peripheral and cerebral ischemic events. Antiphospholipid antibodies (aPL), recognized as risk factors for arterial and venous thrombosis, have been associated with different viral infections, such as parvovirus B19, herpes viruses, hepatitis viruses, and human immunodeficiency viruses. The first case report of a COVID-19 patient with aPL and arterial ischemia was described by Chinese authors [95], although, subsequently, a larger, multicentric cohort demonstrated a low rate of aPL positivity, as defined by classification criteria, suggesting that aPL found in COVID-19 patients is different from aPL found in antiphospholipid syndrome [96]. It is likely that the mechanisms of altered coagulation due to SARS-CoV-2 infection, also responsible for hypoxia, may in turn favor the thrombo-inflammatory loop and consequently increased blood viscosity and the release of procoagulant antibodies [32]. These observations were confirmed by a study by Harzallah and coworkers investigating 56 patients with confirmed or suspected SARS-CoV-2 infection. Among these, 25 were found with lupus anticoagulant immunoglobulin, whereas 5 were found positive for IgM or IgG anti-cardiolipin or anti-2-glycoprotein I antibodies [33]. Further studies are needed to address this issue.

5.2. Thrombocytopenia

COVID-19-related coagulopathy firstly determines elevated D-dimer levels that combine in turn with mildly prolonged PT, APTT, and mild thrombocytopenia. At late stages, this process evolves into a classical DIC [97]. These findings were identified in the clinical setting in a meta-analysis where 7.613 patients suffering from COVID-19 infection were examined. In this cohort, thrombocytopenia was worse in the critically ill group than in those with non-severe disease [98]. Additionally, the platelet count was lower in the elderly, in males, and in patients with higher APACHE II scores at admission [99]. This study highlights an association between low platelet counts and an increased risk of severity of the disease and mortality. As per SARS-CoV-2-infection-related thrombocytopenia, it appears that the platelets can be more rapidly removed or sequestrated by the reticuloendothelial system after the activation of antigen–antibody complexes [100,101]. Additionally, the megakaryocyte's function and the consequent platelet production can be reduced by the virus activity [102]. A possible mechanism of thrombocytopenia was described after COVID-19 vaccination. It was observed in rare cases that immune thrombotic thrombocytopenia (VITT) syndrome was induced by the vaccine, particularly the ChAdOx1 nCoV-19 vaccine. The main pathogenetic hypothesis supporting this evidence is the possible promotion of antibody synthesis against PF4 by some anti-COVID vaccines promoting the synthesis of antibodies against PF4 that provoke platelets' massive activation, inducing immune thrombotic thrombocytopenia [103]. As anti-PF4 antibodies were detected in patients with VITT, the current guidelines recommend a PF4-heparin ELISA blood test before performing a vaccine when VITT is clinically suspected [104]. The risk of clotting in the general population is estimated to be around 1:250,000, although it is higher in young people (20–29 years old) at 1.1:100,000 [105].

6. Contribution of Sepsis in Coagulopathy during COVID-19 Infection

Sepsis is a life-threatening condition as a response to a primary infection in which the body responds with extreme inflammatory reactions that create injuries in one's own tissues and organs. On the other hand, severe COVID-19 infection is commonly complicated with coagulopathy, and, in the latter stages, may evolve towards a classical DIC. These manifestations were an object of major concern during the COVID-19 pandemic. The International Society of Thrombosis and Hemostasis (ISTH) has proposed a new category to identify an early stage of DIC associated with sepsis called sepsis-induced coagulopathy (SIC). Many patients suffering from severe COVID-19 meet the Third International Consensus Definitions for Sepsis (Sepsis-3) [106] manifesting respiratory dysfunction during a viral infection. The diagnostic criteria of SIC are summarized in Table 1. A score $\geq$ 4 is diagnostic for SIC. This score can also be applied to COVID-19-affected patients to identify a coagulopathy risk induced by the virus, although it is less reliable than in other pathogen-induced infections as, in this case, especially during the initial stages of the disease, thrombocytopenia cannot be present. One study by Tang et al. studied the effects of anticoagulant treatment to validate the usefulness [107,108] of the SIC score, finding that patients who met the criteria reported in Table 1 benefit from anticoagulant therapy [12].

Table 1. Sepsis-induced coagulopathy (SIC) score. ISTH score.

Item	Value	Score
SOFA score	1 ≥2	1 2 ≥4
PT-INR	1.2–1.4 >1.4	1 2
Platelet count ($\times$mm^3)	100,000–150,000 <100,000	1 2

INR: international normalized ratio; PT: prothrombin time; SOFA: sequential organ failure assessment.

Coagulation Biomarkers in SARS-CoV-2 Infection: A Predictive Method

In the setting of the altered coagulation state, the measurements of the coagulative parameters may orient the clinicians toward the early identification of a coagulative derangement. Besides the D-dimer, as above mentioned, other parameters are of bedside interest (Table 2). Increased levels of thrombin–antithrombin complexes, plasmin-alpha-2-antiplasmin, and thrombomodulin complexes have been reported in respiratory tract infections. Increased PAI-1 serum levels were identified, suggesting impaired fibrinolysis. A study [15] highlighted an alteration of the laboratory parameters deponent for DIC (according to the diagnostic criteria of the ISTH) in 15 subjects (71.4%) who died of COVID-19-related pneumopathy. In the final stage of the disease, elevated levels of D-dimer and FIB degradation products were found. Recent contributions have reported that COVID-19 severity could be associated with some coagulopathy biomarkers, including prothrombin time (PT), activated partial thromboplastin time (APTT), and D-dimer. Nevertheless, the association between coagulopathy and COVID-19 severity still remains undefined.

Table 2. Increasing coagulation and inflammatory biomarkers.

Coagulation biomarkers	D-dimer, PLT, PT, APTT, FIB
Inflammatory biomarkers	ESR, CRP, Serum ferritin, PCT, IL-2, IL-6, IL8, IL10

Platelets (PLT), prothrombin time (PT), activated partial thromboplastin time (APTT), fibrinogen (FIB), erythrocyte sedimentation rate (ESR), C-reactive protein (CRP), procalcitonin (PCT), and interleukin (IL).

The severity of the condition is mostly associated with clinical evidence (Table 3). In particular, one study [109] demonstrated that the majority of patients developed a mild infection, and about 15% of them experienced a severe manifestation with dyspnea and hypoxia. Another 5% developed respiratory failure in conjunction with ARDS, shock, and multi-organ dysfunction. Many studies have focused on the evaluation of D-dimer, PLT, PT, APTT, and FIB. It was reported that D-dimer and PT values have been shown to be higher in patients with more severe disease [110]; moreover, several studies have shown that elevated D-dimer levels are associated with in-hospital mortality. Recent research studies have hypothesized that genetic profiles may partly explain individual differences in developing thrombotic complications during COVID-19 infection. An interesting study evaluated the genotypic distribution of targeted DNA polymorphisms in COVID-19 complicated by pulmonary embolism during hospitalization, finding significant associations between higher D-dimer levels and ACE I/D and APOE T158C polymorphism in patients with and without pulmonary embolism, suggesting a potentially useful marker of poor clinical outcomes [111]. Previous data showed a higher prevalence of ACE D/D genotype in severe COVID-19 patients compared to those with mild disease; this genotype is significantly associated with cardiometabolic diseases and obesity, known risk factors for COVID-19 [112–115]. Additionally, this genotype was associated with thrombo-embolic manifestations in patients affected by other diseases and traditional thrombophilia-related polymorphisms [116], increased venous thromboembolism risk [117,118], and endothelial damage with hypercoagulability in patients with arterial hypertension [119]. The APOE locus has been associated with increased vulnerability to severe COVID-19 mortality, especially for the APOE4 homozygous genotype [120] which is the strongest genetic risk factor for sporadic Alzheimer's disease. This appears to be very important from a clinical point of view as recent data show that dementia can predict the severity of COVID-19 infection. In fact, patients with dementia are more exposed to the severe form of the infection and are more likely to require hospitalization and to have severe sequelae or fatal outcomes compared with patients who do not [5,121]. Finally, the racial variance of ACE I/D genotype polymorphism seems to be correlated with different outcomes during COVID-19 infection; in fact, populations with higher D allele frequency (e.g., Italian) experienced higher fatality [122]. In another meta-analysis, it was demonstrated that the platelet count decreased progressively with the degree of disease severity [123]. However, a previous meta-analysis [124] demonstrated that there were no differences in PLT and APTT levels between wild and severe cases. All this is probably due to the confounding factors and biases that inevitably occur, such as age, sex, and the presence of comorbidities such as hypertension, diabetes, cardiovascular disease, and chronic kidney disease of the examined populations. As reported in another study by Wu et al., mortality from severe COVID-19 was increased 34-fold compared to a normal infection [125] and very high levels of coagulation markers were correlated with an 11-fold increase in death. These observations underline the importance of the early stratification of disease severity.

Table 3. Incidence of thrombotic events in patients with SARS-CoV-2 infections.

Study	Sample Size	Thrombotic Event Reported	Confirmatory Diagnostic Test	Incidence
Klok et al. [8]	N = 184 ICU patients	Venous arterial thrombosis	CTPA or Ultrasound	31%
Leonard-Lorant et al. [126]	N = 106 (48 ICU and 58 non-ICU)	Acute PE	CTPA	30% of all COVID-19 patients developed PE irrespective of ICU status
Helms et al. [9]	N = 150 ICU patients	Clinically significant thrombosis	CTPA	43%
Wichmann et al. [127]	N = 12 (5 ICU and 7 non-ICU)	DVT	Autopsy	58% of all COVID-19 patients autopsied had evidence of PE, irrespective of ICU status
	N = 156 non-ICU patients	DVT	Ultrasound	15%
Nahum et al. [128]	N = 34 ICU patients	DVT	Ultrasound	79%
Middeldorp et al. [129]	N = 198 (123 non-ICU and 75 ICU)	VTE in non-ICU vs. ICU	Ultrasound	9.2% in non-ICU vs. 59% in ICU
Shah et al. [130]	N = 187 (182 non-ICU and 5 ICU)	Acute PE	CTPA	23%
Cui et al. [131]	N = 81 non-ICU	DVT	Ultrasound	25%

ICU, intensive care unit; CTPA, computed tomography pulmonary angiogram; DVT, deep vein thrombosis; PE, pulmonary embolism; VTE, venous thromboembolism.

7. New Clinical Evidence of Anticoagulant Therapy in COVID-19

Data on anticoagulant therapy appear to be associated with a better outcome in moderate-to-severe COVID-19 patients with altered coagulative parameters (elevated D-dimer, elevated FIB, and low levels of anti-thrombin) [13,14,132]. A retrospective study by Shi et al. showed that these treatments can mitigate cytokine storm exerting an anti-inflammatory effect (reduction in IL-6 and increase in lymphocytes) and improving coagulation dysfunction [133]. A number of substances are used for COVID-19 VTE such as heparins, direct oral anticoagulants (DOAK), aggregation inhibitors, factor XII inhibitors, thrombolytic agents, anti-complement, anti-NET drugs, and IL-1 receptor antagonists.

Heparins, including unfractionated heparin (UFH) and low-molecular-weight heparin (LMWH), have several anti-coagulant and anti-inflammatory effects [134]. Among the various properties of heparin, a beneficial effect on endothelium has been observed. Dysfunctional endothelium leads to an inflammatory status through the production of vasoconstrictor factors and the recruitment of immune cells [135]. Histones released from damaged cells may be responsible for endothelial injury [136]. Heparin exerts its action through an effect on histone methylation and MAPK and NF-κB signaling pathways [137]. In this way, heparin can antagonize histones and therefore "protect" the endothelium [29,30]. It was proved to have a beneficial effect related to its anticoagulant function on COVID-19 [138] and anti-inflammatory properties [139]. The proposed mechanisms include binding to inflammatory cytokines, the inhibition of neutrophil chemotaxis and leukocyte migration, the neutralization of complement factor C5a, the sequestration of acute-phase proteins such as P-selectin and L-selectin, and the induction of cell apoptosis through the TNF-α and NF-κB pathways [140,141]. Another potential direct antiviral role of heparin is related to its polyanionic properties allowing it to bind to various proteins thus acting as an effective inhibitor of viral adhesion [142]. This condition mechanism was also described in other viral diseases [142,143] as well as in SARS-CoV. As Mycroft-West et al. [144] demonstrated, surface plasmon resonance and circular dichroism were used, and it was demonstrated that the receptor binding domain of the Spike S1 SARS-CoV-2 protein interacts with heparin. In a report by Tang [15], a favorable outcome was highlighted with the use of LMWHs in severe patients with COVID-19 who meet the criteria of SCI (sepsis-induced coagulopathy) or with markedly elevated D-dimer. A large, retrospective multicentric study among in-hospital patients (the CORIST study) showed that heparin treatment was associated with lower mortality, particularly in severely ill COVID-19 patients and in those with strong coagulation activation [145]. Moreover, research conducted in the neurorehabilitation department of a neuroscience referral hospital following neurological damage showed, despite a small number of patients, that hospitalized, vulnerable, patients with severe neurological damage can present a completely unexpected benign disease course of SARS-CoV-2 infection after heparin treatment. The anti-inflammatory and anticoagulant effects of enoxaparin administered much earlier before and during the infection, together with possible antiviral activity, could explain the favorable disease course observed in severe neurological patients with an increased risk of poor outcomes. Further research is needed to explore the possible mechanisms of action of enoxaparin in critical neurological patients with COVID-19 and confirm these observations [146].

However, several studies could not identify this relationship. As demonstrated by C. Coligher et al. in a randomized control trial, in critically ill patients with COVID-19, an initial strategy of therapeutic-dose anticoagulation with heparin failed to show a greater probability of survival to hospital discharge or a major number of days free of cardiovascular or respiratory organ support than usual-care pharmacologic thromboprophylaxis [147]. Interim results from multiplatform RCTs on VTE prophylaxis show that in moderate COVID-19 (hospitalized, not intensive), therapeutic doses of LMWH appear to be better than prophylactic doses, with positive effects on morbidity and mortality and less than 2% severe bleeding [148]. In patients at low or intermediate risk of thrombotic phenomena, treatment with prophylactic doses of LMWH has been noticed to produce a concomitant reduction in developing severe ARDS and venous thromboembolism, which may reduce the need for mechanical ventilation and consequentially lower cardiovascular death [149]. Treatment with heparin did not improve the course of severe COVID-19 and it seems to be inferior to prophylactic doses. The first observational cohort study examined previous prophylactic anticoagulation versus no anticoagulation in hospitalized COVID-19 patients (not intensive). Early treatment with prophylactic heparin was associated with a 34% reduction in relative 30-day mortality risk and an absolute risk reduction of 4.4%. There was no increased risk of bleeding under prophylactic anticoagulation [150]. Guidelines of medical societies currently recommend VTE prophylaxis, preferably with LMWH, for every inpatient COVID-19 patient [151]. The guidelines do not recommend VTE prophylaxis for COVID-19 outpatients. Prophylactic anticoagulation for 1–2 weeks is recommended by some guidelines in patients discharged from hospitals if there are additional risk factors [152]. Globally, the use of heparin is recommended, but it needs to be titrated against the risk of bleeding and individualized, especially in patients affected by pre-existing endothelial dysfunction (diabetes, hypertension, obesity) at higher risk of adverse outcomes during COVID-19 infection [153]. Additionally, antiplatelets have been considered an antithrombotic treatment for COVID-19, even though the rationale for aspirin use in COVID-19 is still uncertain. A recent review [154] recommends a low-dose aspirin regimen for the primary prevention of arterial thromboembolism in patients aged 40–70 with intermediate or high atherosclerotic cardiovascular risk and a low risk of bleeding. This opens a perspective on aspirin's protective role in COVID-19 with associated lung injury and vascular thrombosis even in the absence of previously known cardiovascular disease.

The contact activation system, including factor XII (FXII), factor XI (FXI), high-molecular-weight kininogen, and prekallikrein, links inflammation and coagulation, triggering thrombin generation which promotes platelet activation but also upregulates the kallikrein–kinin system (KKS) which induces the renin–angiotensin system with the release of pro-inflammatory cytokines [155]. The inhibition of contact activation has been shown, especially in animal models, to prevent consumptive coagulopathy, pathologic systemic inflammatory response, and mortality [156]. Direct FXa inhibitors have been already shown to possess an inflammatory and antiviral effect in addition to their well-established anticoagulant activity, and they have been proposed to have a potential therapeutic role in coronavirus infections [157]. FXI activation by virtue of its position as an interface between contact activation and thrombin generation has been suggested as a unique and promising target to safely prevent or treat COVID-19-related inflammatory complications including cytokine response and coagulopathy, hence reducing associated mortality, and, evidence from recent research suggests that the inhibition of FXIa seems to attenuate thrombosis with little effect on hemostasis and may also have a potential role on infections [158]. Direct inhibitors of FXIa using small peptidomimetic molecules, monoclonal antibodies, aptamers, or natural inhibitors have been developed in recent years [159]. Preclinical data and rationale exist for preventing the activation of FXI and FXII preserving the hemostatic activity of FXI in COVID-19, and several inhibitors of FXII and FXI are currently under investigation [158] representing a promising therapeutic target against COVID-19 patients with severe disease.

As soon as the data from the RCTs are available, the therapy and prophylaxis recommendations will certainly be adapted and reissued.

8. Closing Remarks

COVID-19 can be considered a systemic disease characterized by the dysregulation of the immune system and a hypercoagulable status, a consequence of direct virus-induced endothelial damage, amplified by the leukocyte- and cytokine-mediated activation of the platelets, the release of TF, and NETosis and intensified by the activation of the complement system. The strong activation of the immune system by the SARS-CoV-2 infection leads to a non-regulatable thrombosis, which can present with many microthrombi in microvascularization, VTE, and arterial events. Coagulopathy is a crucial aspect of the disease, and its early identification, prevention, and treatment may limit its evolution towards potentially irreversible pulmonary and systemic conditions. Scientific evidence suggests that coagulopathy is not to be considered only as a disease complication but may be a real primitive pathogenetic element of SARS-CoV-2 infection. An important issue still to be addressed is long COVID, which is a common condition in patients who have been infected with SARS-CoV-2, regardless of the severity of the acute illness. A recent systematic review with metanalysis [160] found that most symptoms such as neurological symptoms, respiratory conditions, mobility impairment disorders with decreased exercise tolerance, heart conditions (palpitations), and general signs and symptoms, i.e., fatigue may be present with different frequencies, and the incidence is higher in females and increases with age. Among significant abnormalities identified through biochemical laboratory testing are increased levels of ferritin, C-reactive protein, and D-dimer [161]. Moreover, persistent dysfunctions of the immune response, with the chronic activation of T and B lymphocytes [162] and the presence of long-term immune system perturbations and autoimmunity [163] have been observed. The chronic low pro-inflammatory status has been related to endothelial and vascular alterations with a cytotoxic immune response towards endothelium [164]. Endothelium activation represents a significant risk of developing cardiovascular diseases for several months following infection. Recently, it was suggested the need to approach long COVID with non-pharmacological treatments, such as promoting physical activity [165]. The current knowledge of long COVID-19, though, does not allow stratifying patients into clusters that surely will benefit from exercise or have significant side effects. A better investigation of biomarkers modulated by exercise in long COVID-19 patients could be helpful to this end. Recent data from the literature also seem to suggest a favorable prognostic effect of anticoagulant treatment with low-molecular-weight heparin in patients with COVID-19 manifestations. The latter aspect is particularly pertinent in patients with cardiovascular and/or neurological diseases, obesity, or diabetes because they have a higher risk of developing vascular thrombosis. In conclusion, however, we underline that available data concerning anticoagulant treatment in COVID-19 are not completely supported by several randomized trials, and, therefore, there is an objective difficulty in choosing the most indicated therapy, which justifies a real advantage of a full-dose anticoagulant treatment in patients with severe disease, considering the potential risk of bleeding increase.

Author Contributions: Conceptualization, B.R. and M.M; writing—original draft preparation, B.R., B.D.R., A.G., S.K., A.S.; writing—review and editing, M.M. All authors have read and agreed to the published version of the manuscript.

Funding: This research received no external funding.

Institutional Review Board Statement: Not applicable.

Informed Consent Statement: Not applicable.

Data Availability Statement: No new data were created.

Conflicts of Interest: The authors declare no conflict of interest.

References

1. Malerba, M.; Ragnoli, B.; Puca, E.; Pipero, P. Supporting healthcare workers on front lines of the COVID-19 fight. *Acta Biomed. Atenei Parm.* **2020**, *91*, e2020157. [CrossRef]
2. Coronavirus Disease (COVID-19)—World Health Organization. Available online: https://www.who.int/emergencies/diseases/novel-coronavirus-2019 (accessed on 20 April 2023).
3. Harapan, H.; Itoh, N.; Yufika, A.; Winardi, W.; Keam, S.; Te, H.; Megawati, D.; Hayati, Z.; Wagner, A.L.; Mudatsir, M. Coronavirus disease 2019 (COVID-19): A literature review. *J. Infect. Public Health* **2020**, *13*, 667–673. [CrossRef] [PubMed]
4. Zhou, F.; Yu, T.; Du, R.; Fan, G.; Liu, Y.; Liu, Z.; Xiang, J.; Wang, Y.; Song, B.; Gu, X.; et al. Clinical course and risk factors for mortality of adult inpatients with COVID-19 in Wuhan, China: A retrospective cohort study. *Lancet* **2020**, *395*, 1054–1062. [CrossRef] [PubMed]
5. Ragnoli, B.; Cena, T.; Radaeli, A.; Pochetti, P.; Conti, L.; Calareso, A.; Morjaria, J.; Malerba, M. Pneumothorax in hospitalized COVID-19 patients with severe respiratory failure: Risk factors and outcome. *Respir. Med.* **2023**, *211*, 107194. [CrossRef] [PubMed]
6. Obi, A.T.; Tignanelli, C.J.; Jacobs, B.N.; Arya, S.; Park, P.K.; Wakefield, T.W.; Henke, P.K.; Napolitano, L.M. Empirical systemic anticoagulation is associated with decreased venous thromboembolism in critically ill influenza A H1N1 acute respiratory distress syndrome patients. *J. Vasc. Surg. Venous Lymphat. Disord.* **2019**, *7*, 317–324. [CrossRef]
7. Fraissé, M.; Logre, E.; Pajot, O.; Mentec, H.; Plantefève, G.; Contou, D. Thrombotic and hemorrhagic events in critically ill COVID-19 patients: A French monocenter retrospective study. *Crit. Care* **2020**, *24*, 275. [CrossRef]
8. Klok, F.A.; Kruip, M.J.H.A.; van der Meer, N.J.M.; Arbous, M.S.; Gommers, D.A.M.P.J.; Kant, K.M.; Kaptein, F.H.J.; van Paassen, J.; Stals, M.A.M.; Huisman, M.V.; et al. Incidence of thrombotic complications in critically ill ICU patients with COVID-19. *Thromb. Res.* **2020**, *191*, 145–147. [CrossRef]
9. Helms, J.; Tacquard, C.; Severac, F.; Leonard-Lorant, I.; Ohana, M.; Delabranche, X.; Merdji, H.; Clere-Jehl, R.; Schenck, M.; Fagot Gandet, F.; et al. High risk of thrombosis in patients with severe SARS-CoV-2 infection: A multicenter prospective cohort study. *Intensive Care Med.* **2020**, *46*, 1089–1098. [CrossRef]
10. Lodigiani, C.; Iapichino, G.; Carenzo, L.; Cecconi, M.; Ferrazzi, P.; Sebastian, T.; Kucher, N.; Studt, J.-D.; Sacco, C.; Bertuzzi, A.; et al. Venous and arterial thromboembolic complications in COVID-19 patients admitted to an academic hospital in Milan, Italy. *Thromb. Res.* **2020**, *191*, 9–14. [CrossRef]
11. Varga, Z.; Flammer, A.J.; Steiger, P.; Haberecker, M.; Andermatt, R.; Zinkernagel, A.S.; Mehra, M.R.; Schuepbach, R.A.; Ruschitzka, F.; Moch, H. Endothelial cell infection and endotheliitis in COVID-19. *Lancet* **2020**, *395*, 1417–1418. [CrossRef]
12. Danzi, G.B.; Loffi, M.; Galeazzi, G.; Gherbesi, E. Acute pulmonary embolism and COVID-19 pneumonia: A random association? *Eur. Heart J.* **2020**, *41*, 1858. [CrossRef] [PubMed]
13. Tang, N.; Li, D.; Wang, X.; Sun, Z. Abnormal coagulation parameters are associated with poor prognosis in patients with novel coronavirus pneumonia. *J. Thromb. Haemost.* **2020**, *18*, 844–847. [CrossRef] [PubMed]
14. Han, H.; Yang, L.; Liu, R.; Liu, F.; Wu, K.-L.; Li, J.; Liu, X.-H.; Zhu, C.-L. Prominent changes in blood coagulation of patients with SARS-CoV-2 infection. *Clin. Chem. Lab. Med.* **2020**, *58*, 1116–1120. [CrossRef] [PubMed]
15. Tang, N.; Bai, H.; Chen, X.; Gong, J.; Li, D.; Sun, Z. Anticoagulant treatment is associated with decreased mortality in severe coronavirus disease 2019 patients with coagulopathy. *J. Thromb. Haemost.* **2020**, *18*, 1094–1099. [CrossRef]
16. Ren, B.; Yan, F.; Deng, Z.; Zhang, S.; Xiao, L.; Wu, M.; Cai, L. Extremely High Incidence of Lower Extremity Deep Venous Thrombosis in 48 Patients With Severe COVID-19 in Wuhan. *Circulation* **2020**, *142*, 181–183. [CrossRef] [PubMed]
17. Gralinski, L.E.; Bankhead, A.; Jeng, S.; Menachery, V.D.; Proll, S.; Belisle, S.E.; Matzke, M.; Webb-Robertson, B.-J.M.; Luna, M.L.; Shukla, A.K.; et al. Mechanisms of severe acute respiratory syndrome coronavirus-induced acute lung injury. *mBio* **2013**, *4*, e00271-13. [CrossRef]
18. Yao, X.H.; Li, T.Y.; He, Z.C.; Ping, Y.F.; Liu, H.W.; Yu, S.C.; Mou, H.M.; Wang, L.H.; Zhang, H.R.; Fu, W.J.; et al. A pathological report of three COVID-19 cases by minimal invasive autopsies. *Zhonghua Bing Li Xue Za Zhi* **2020**, *49*, 411–417. [CrossRef]

19. Wright, F.L.; Vogler, T.O.; Moore, E.E.; Moore, H.B.; Wohlauer, M.V.; Urban, S.; Nydam, T.L.; Moore, P.K.; McIntyre, R.C. Fibrinolysis Shutdown Correlation with Thromboembolic Events in Severe COVID-19 Infection. *J. Am. Coll. Surg.* **2020**, *231*, 193–203.e1. [CrossRef]
20. Tay, M.Z.; Poh, C.M.; Rénia, L.; MacAry, P.A.; Ng, L.F.P. The trinity of COVID-19: Immunity, inflammation and intervention. *Nat. Rev. Immunol.* **2020**, *20*, 363–374. [CrossRef]
21. Baldanzi, G.; Purghè, B.; Ragnoli, B.; Sainaghi, P.P.; Rolla, R.; Chiocchetti, A.; Manfredi, M.; Malerba, M. Circulating Peptidome Is Strongly Altered in COVID-19 Patients. *Int. J. Environ. Res. Public. Health* **2023**, *20*, 1564. [CrossRef]
22. Purghè, B.; Manfredi, M.; Ragnoli, B.; Baldanzi, G.; Malerba, M. Exosomes in chronic respiratory diseases. *Biomed. Pharmacother.* **2021**, *144*, 112270. [CrossRef]
23. Wool, G.D.; Miller, J.L. The Impact of COVID-19 Disease on Platelets and Coagulation. *Pathobiol. J. Immunopathol. Mol. Cell. Biol.* **2021**, *88*, 15–27. [CrossRef] [PubMed]
24. Malerba, M.; Clini, E.; Malagola, M.; Avanzi, G.C. Platelet activation as a novel mechanism of atherothrombotic risk in chronic obstructive pulmonary disease. *Expert Rev. Hematol.* **2013**, *6*, 475–483. [CrossRef] [PubMed]
25. Malerba, M.; Nardin, M.; Radaeli, A.; Montuschi, P.; Carpagnano, G.E.; Clini, E. The potential role of endothelial dysfunction and platelet activation in the development of thrombotic risk in COPD patients. *Expert Rev. Hematol.* **2017**, *10*, 821–832. [CrossRef] [PubMed]
26. Violi, F.; Cammisotto, V.; Pignatelli, P. Thrombosis in COVID-19 and non-COVID-19 pneumonia: Role of platelets. *Platelets* **2021**, *32*, 1009–1017. [CrossRef] [PubMed]
27. Polosa, R.; Malerba, M.; Cacciola, R.R.; Morjaria, J.B.; Maugeri, C.; Prosperini, G.; Gullo, R.; Spicuzza, L.; Radaeli, A.; Di Maria, G.U. Effect of acute exacerbations on circulating endothelial, clotting and fibrinolytic markers in COPD patients. *Intern. Emerg. Med.* **2013**, *8*, 567–574. [CrossRef]
28. Wiedmer, T.; Esmon, C.T.; Sims, P.J. Complement proteins C5b-9 stimulate procoagulant activity through platelet prothrombinase. *Blood* **1986**, *68*, 875–880. [CrossRef]
29. JCI Insight—The Complement System in COVID-19: Friend and Foe? Available online: https://insight.jci.org/articles/view/140711 (accessed on 20 April 2023).
30. Gupta, N.; Zhao, Y.-Y.; Evans, C.E. The stimulation of thrombosis by hypoxia. *Thromb. Res.* **2019**, *181*, 77–83. [CrossRef]
31. Leyfman, Y.; Erick, T.K.; Reddy, S.S.; Galwankar, S.; Nanayakkara, P.W.B.; Di Somma, S.; Sharma, P.; Stawicki, S.P.; Chaudry, I.H. Potential Immunotherapeutic Targets for Hypoxia Due to COVI-Flu. *Shock Augusta Ga* **2020**, *54*, 438–450. [CrossRef]
32. Kichloo, A.; Dettloff, K.; Aljadah, M.; Albosta, M.; Jamal, S.; Singh, J.; Wani, F.; Kumar, A.; Vallabhaneni, S.; Khan, M.Z. COVID-19 and Hypercoagulability: A Review. *Clin. Appl. Thromb. Hemost.* **2020**, *26*, 1076029620962853. [CrossRef]
33. Harzallah, I.; Debliquis, A.; Drénou, B. Lupus anticoagulant is frequent in patients with COVID-19. *J. Thromb. Haemost.* **2020**, *18*, 2064–2065. [CrossRef]
34. Iba, T.; Connors, J.M.; Levy, J.H. The coagulopathy, endotheliopathy, and vasculitis of COVID-19. *Inflamm. Res.* **2020**, *69*, 1181–1189. [CrossRef] [PubMed]
35. Levi, M.; van der Poll, T.; Schultz, M. Infection and inflammation as risk factors for thrombosis and atherosclerosis. *Semin. Thromb. Hemost.* **2012**, *38*, 506–514. [CrossRef] [PubMed]
36. Ekholm, M.; Kahan, T. The Impact of the Renin-Angiotensin-Aldosterone System on Inflammation, Coagulation, and Atherothrombotic Complications, and to Aggravated COVID-19. *Front. Pharmacol.* **2021**, *12*, 640185. [CrossRef] [PubMed]
37. Goeijenbier, M.; van Wissen, M.; van de Weg, C.; Jong, E.; Gerdes, V.E.A.; Meijers, J.C.M.; Brandjes, D.P.M.; van Gorp, E.C.M. Review: Viral infections and mechanisms of thrombosis and bleeding. *J. Med. Virol.* **2012**, *84*, 1680–1696. [CrossRef]
38. Branchford, B.R.; Carpenter, S.L. The Role of Inflammation in Venous Thromboembolism. *Front. Pediatr.* **2018**, *6*, 142. [CrossRef]
39. Iba, T.; Levy, J.H.; Levi, M.; Thachil, J. Coagulopathy in COVID-19. *J. Thromb. Haemost.* **2020**, *18*, 2103–2109. [CrossRef]
40. Fuchs, T.A.; Brill, A.; Wagner, D.D. Neutrophil extracellular trap (NET) impact on deep vein thrombosis. *Arterioscler. Thromb. Vasc. Biol.* **2012**, *32*, 1777–1783. [CrossRef]
41. Tsourouktsoglou, T.-D.; Warnatsch, A.; Ioannou, M.; Hoving, D.; Wang, Q.; Papayannopoulos, V. Histones, DNA, and Citrullination Promote Neutrophil Extracellular Trap Inflammation by Regulating the Localization and Activation of TLR4. *Cell Rep.* **2020**, *31*, 107602. [CrossRef]
42. Zuo, Y.; Yalavarthi, S.; Shi, H.; Gockman, K.; Zuo, M.; Madison, J.A.; Blair, C.; Weber, A.; Barnes, B.J.; Egeblad, M.; et al. Neutrophil extracellular traps in COVID-19. *JCI Insight* **2020**, *5*, 138999. [CrossRef]
43. Papageorgiou, C.; Jourdi, G.; Adjambri, E.; Walborn, A.; Patel, P.; Fareed, J.; Elalamy, I.; Hoppensteadt, D.; Gerotziafas, G.T. Disseminated Intravascular Coagulation: An Update on Pathogenesis, Diagnosis, and Therapeutic Strategies. *Clin. Appl. Thromb. Hemost.* **2018**, *24*, 8S–28S. [CrossRef]
44. van Gorp, E.C.; Suharti, C.; ten Cate, H.; Dolmans, W.M.; van der Meer, J.W.; ten Cate, J.W.; Brandjes, D.P. Review: Infectious diseases and coagulation disorders. *J. Infect. Dis.* **1999**, *180*, 176–186. [CrossRef] [PubMed]
45. Caci, G.; Albini, A.; Malerba, M.; Noonan, D.M.; Pochetti, P.; Polosa, R. COVID-19 and Obesity: Dangerous Liaisons. *J. Clin. Med.* **2020**, *9*, 2511. [CrossRef] [PubMed]
46. Sanchis-Gomar, F.; Lavie, C.J.; Mehra, M.R.; Henry, B.M.; Lippi, G. Obesity and Outcomes in COVID-19: When an Epidemic and Pandemic Collide. *Mayo Clin. Proc.* **2020**, *95*, 1445–1453. [CrossRef] [PubMed]

47. Lafontan, M. Fat cells: Afferent and efferent messages define new approaches to treat obesity. *Annu. Rev. Pharmacol. Toxicol.* **2005**, *45*, 119–146. [CrossRef]
48. Ragnoli, B.; Pochetti, P.; Raie, A.; Malerba, M. Comorbid Insomnia and Obstructive Sleep Apnea (COMISA): Current Concepts of Patient Management. *Int. J. Environ. Res. Public. Health* **2021**, *18*, 9248. [CrossRef]
49. Ragnoli, B.; Pochetti, P.; Pignatti, P.; Barbieri, M.; Mondini, L.; Ruggero, L.; Trotta, L.; Montuschi, P.; Malerba, M. Sleep Deprivation, Immune Suppression and SARS-CoV-2 Infection. *Int. J. Environ. Res. Public. Health* **2022**, *19*, 904. [CrossRef]
50. Spyropoulos, A.C.; Levy, J.H.; Ageno, W.; Connors, J.M.; Hunt, B.J.; Iba, T.; Levi, M.; Samama, C.M.; Thachil, J.; Giannis, D.; et al. Scientific and Standardization Committee communication: Clinical guidance on the diagnosis, prevention, and treatment of venous thromboembolism in hospitalized patients with COVID-19. *J. Thromb. Haemost.* **2020**, *18*, 1859–1865. [CrossRef]
51. Giannis, D.; Ziogas, I.A.; Gianni, P. Coagulation disorders in coronavirus infected patients: COVID-19, SARS-CoV-1, MERS-CoV and lessons from the past. *J. Clin. Virol. Off. Publ. Pan Am. Soc. Clin. Virol.* **2020**, *127*, 104362. [CrossRef]
52. Avnon, L.S.; Munteanu, D.; Smoliakov, A.; Jotkowitz, A.; Barski, L. Thromboembolic events in patients with severe pandemic influenza A/H1N1. *Eur. J. Intern. Med.* **2015**, *26*, 596–598. [CrossRef]
53. Fridlender, Z.G.; Khamaisi, M.; Leitersdorf, E. Association between cytomegalovirus infection and venous thromboembolism. *Am. J. Med. Sci.* **2007**, *334*, 111–114. [CrossRef] [PubMed]
54. Kahn, S.R.; Lim, W.; Dunn, A.S.; Cushman, M.; Dentali, F.; Akl, E.A.; Cook, D.J.; Balekian, A.A.; Klein, R.C.; Le, H.; et al. Prevention of VTE in nonsurgical patients: Antithrombotic Therapy and Prevention of Thrombosis, 9th ed: American College of Chest Physicians Evidence-Based Clinical Practice Guidelines. *Chest* **2012**, *141*, e195S–e226S. [CrossRef] [PubMed]
55. Connors, J.M.; Levy, J.H. COVID-19 and its implications for thrombosis and anticoagulation. *Blood* **2020**, *135*, 2033–2040. [CrossRef] [PubMed]
56. Lazzaroni, M.G.; Piantoni, S.; Masneri, S.; Garrafa, E.; Martini, G.; Tincani, A.; Andreoli, L.; Franceschini, F. Coagulation dysfunction in COVID-19: The interplay between inflammation, viral infection and the coagulation system. *Blood Rev.* **2021**, *46*, 100745. [CrossRef] [PubMed]
57. Mehta, P.; McAuley, D.F.; Brown, M.; Sanchez, E.; Tattersall, R.S.; Manson, J.J.; HLH Across Speciality Collaboration, UK. COVID-19: Consider cytokine storm syndromes and immunosuppression. *Lancet* **2020**, *395*, 1033–1034. [CrossRef]
58. Liu, B.; Li, M.; Zhou, Z.; Guan, X.; Xiang, Y. Can we use interleukin-6 (IL-6) blockade for coronavirus disease 2019 (COVID-19)-induced cytokine release syndrome (CRS)? *J. Autoimmun.* **2020**, *111*, 102452. [CrossRef]
59. Moore, J.B.; June, C.H. Cytokine release syndrome in severe COVID-19. *Science* **2020**, *368*, 473–474. [CrossRef]
60. Qin, C.; Zhou, L.; Hu, Z.; Zhang, S.; Yang, S.; Tao, Y.; Xie, C.; Ma, K.; Shang, K.; Wang, W.; et al. Dysregulation of Immune Response in Patients With Coronavirus 2019 (COVID-19) in Wuhan, China. *Clin. Infect. Dis. Off. Publ. Infect. Dis. Soc. Am.* **2020**, *71*, 762–768. [CrossRef]
61. Ye, Q.; Wang, B.; Mao, J. The pathogenesis and treatment of the 'Cytokine Storm' in COVID-19. *J. Infect.* **2020**, *80*, 607–613. [CrossRef]
62. Zhang, C.; Wu, Z.; Li, J.-W.; Zhao, H.; Wang, G.-Q. Cytokine release syndrome in severe COVID-19: Interleukin-6 receptor antagonist tocilizumab may be the key to reduce mortality. *Int. J. Antimicrob. Agents* **2020**, *55*, 105954. [CrossRef]
63. Levi, M.; van der Poll, T. Coagulation and sepsis. *Thromb. Res.* **2017**, *149*, 38–44. [CrossRef] [PubMed]
64. Folman, C.C.; Linthorst, G.E.; van Mourik, J.; van Willigen, G.; de Jonge, E.; Levi, M.; de Haas, M.; von dem Borne, A.E. Platelets release thrombopoietin (Tpo) upon activation: Another regulatory loop in thrombocytopoiesis? *Thromb. Haemost.* **2000**, *83*, 923–930. [CrossRef] [PubMed]
65. Levi, M.; van der Poll, T.; Schultz, M. Systemic versus localized coagulation activation contributing to organ failure in critically ill patients. *Semin. Immunopathol.* **2012**, *34*, 167–179. [CrossRef]
66. Fox, S.E.; Akmatbekov, A.; Harbert, J.L.; Li, G.; Quincy Brown, J.; Vander Heide, R.S. Pulmonary and cardiac pathology in African American patients with COVID-19: An autopsy series from New Orleans. *Lancet Respir. Med.* **2020**, *8*, 681–686. [CrossRef] [PubMed]
67. Yang, M.; Ng, M.H.; Li, C.K. Thrombocytopenia in patients with severe acute respiratory syndrome (review). *Hematology* **2005**, *10*, 101–105. [CrossRef]
68. Stouthard, J.M.; Levi, M.; Hack, C.E.; Veenhof, C.H.; Romijn, H.A.; Sauerwein, H.P.; van der Poll, T. Interleukin-6 stimulates coagulation, not fibrinolysis, in humans. *Thromb. Haemost.* **1996**, *76*, 738–742. [CrossRef]
69. Conti, P.; Caraffa, A.; Gallenga, C.E.; Ross, R.; Kritas, S.K.; Frydas, I.; Younes, A.; Ronconi, G. Coronavirus-19 (SARS-CoV-2) induces acute severe lung inflammation via IL-1 causing cytokine storm in COVID-19: A promising inhibitory strategy. *J. Biol. Regul. Homeost. Agents* **2020**, *34*, 1971–1975. [CrossRef]
70. Magro, G. SARS-CoV-2 and COVID-19: Is interleukin-6 (IL-6) the "culprit lesion" of ARDS onset? What is there besides Tocilizumab? SGP130Fc. *Cytokine X* **2020**, *2*, 100029. [CrossRef]
71. van de Veerdonk, F.L.; Netea, M.G. Blocking IL-1 to prevent respiratory failure in COVID-19. *Crit. Care* **2020**, *24*, 445. [CrossRef]
72. Zhao, Y.; Qin, L.; Zhang, P.; Li, K.; Liang, L.; Sun, J.; Xu, B.; Dai, Y.; Li, X.; Zhang, C.; et al. Longitudinal COVID-19 profiling associates IL-1RA and IL-10 with disease severity and RANTES with mild disease. *JCI Insight* **2020**, *5*, e139834. [CrossRef]
73. Satış, H.; Özger, H.S.; Aysert Yıldız, P.; Hızel, K.; Gulbahar, Ö.; Erbaş, G.; Aygencel, G.; Guzel Tunccan, O.; Öztürk, M.A.; Dizbay, M.; et al. Prognostic value of interleukin-18 and its association with other inflammatory markers and disease severity in COVID-19. *Cytokine* **2021**, *137*, 155302. [CrossRef] [PubMed]

74. Teuwen, L.-A.; Geldhof, V.; Pasut, A.; Carmeliet, P. COVID-19: The vasculature unleashed. *Nat. Rev. Immunol.* **2020**, *20*, 389–391. [CrossRef] [PubMed]
75. Martini, R. The compelling arguments for the need of microvascular investigation in COVID-19 critical patients. *Clin. Hemorheol. Microcirc.* **2020**, *75*, 27–34. [CrossRef] [PubMed]
76. Monteil, V.; Kwon, H.; Prado, P.; Hagelkrüys, A.; Wimmer, R.A.; Stahl, M.; Leopoldi, A.; Garreta, E.; Hurtado Del Pozo, C.; Prosper, F.; et al. Inhibition of SARS-CoV-2 Infections in Engineered Human Tissues Using Clinical-Grade Soluble Human ACE2. *Cell* **2020**, *181*, 905–913.e7. [CrossRef]
77. Stern, D.; Nawroth, P.; Handley, D.; Kisiel, W. An endothelial cell-dependent pathway of coagulation. *Proc. Natl. Acad. Sci. USA* **1985**, *82*, 2523–2527. [CrossRef] [PubMed]
78. Guang, C.; Phillips, R.D.; Jiang, B.; Milani, F. Three key proteases—Angiotensin-I-converting enzyme (ACE), ACE2 and renin—Within and beyond the renin-angiotensin system. *Arch. Cardiovasc. Dis.* **2012**, *105*, 373–385. [CrossRef]
79. Scialo, F.; Daniele, A.; Amato, F.; Pastore, L.; Matera, M.G.; Cazzola, M.; Castaldo, G.; Bianco, A. ACE2: The Major Cell Entry Receptor for SARS-CoV-2. *Lung* **2020**, *198*, 867–877. [CrossRef] [PubMed]
80. Marshall, R.P. The Pulmonary Renin-Angiotensin System. *Curr. Pharm. Des.* **2003**, *9*, 715–722. [CrossRef]
81. El-Arif, G.; Farhat, A.; Khazaal, S.; Annweiler, C.; Kovacic, H.; Wu, Y.; Cao, Z.; Fajloun, Z.; Khattar, Z.A.; Sabatier, J.M. The Renin-Angiotensin System: A Key Role in SARS-CoV-2-Induced COVID-19. *Molecules* **2021**, *26*, 6945. [CrossRef]
82. Yang, J.; Petitjean, S.J.L.; Koehler, M.; Zhang, Q.; Dumitru, A.C.; Chen, W.; Derclaye, S.; Vincent, S.P.; Soumillion, P.; Alsteens, D. Molecular interaction and inhibition of SARS-CoV-2 binding to the ACE2 receptor. *Nat. Commun.* **2020**, *11*, 4541. [CrossRef]
83. Reid, C.; Laird, B.; Travers, S.; McNiff, J.; Young, S.; Maddicks, J.; Bentley, A.; Fenning, S. Death from COVID-19: Management of breathlessness: A retrospective multicentre study. *BMJ Support. Palliat. Care* **2021**. [CrossRef]
84. Barkauskas, C.E.; Cronce, M.J.; Rackley, C.R.; Bowie, E.J.; Keene, D.R.; Stripp, B.R.; Randell, S.H.; Noble, P.W.; Hogan, B.L.M. Type 2 alveolar cells are stem cells in adult lung. *J. Clin. Investig.* **2013**, *123*, 3025–3036. [CrossRef]
85. Hoffmann, M.; Kleine-Weber, H.; Schroeder, S.; Krüger, N.; Herrler, T.; Erichsen, S.; Schiergens, T.S.; Herrler, G.; Wu, N.-H.; Nitsche, A.; et al. SARS-CoV-2 Cell Entry Depends on ACE2 and TMPRSS2 and Is Blocked by a Clinically Proven Protease Inhibitor. *Cell* **2020**, *181*, 271–280.e8. [CrossRef]
86. Rivellese, F.; Prediletto, E. ACE2 at the centre of COVID-19 from paucisymptomatic infections to severe pneumonia. *Autoimmun. Rev.* **2020**, *19*, 102536. [CrossRef]
87. Gemmati, D.; Bramanti, B.; Serino, M.L.; Secchiero, P.; Zauli, G.; Tisato, V. COVID-19 and Individual Genetic Susceptibility/Receptivity: Role of ACE1/ACE2 Genes, Immunity, Inflammation and Coagulation. Might the Double X-Chromosome in Females Be Protective against SARS-CoV-2 Compared to the Single X-Chromosome in Males? *Int. J. Mol. Sci.* **2020**, *21*, 3474. [CrossRef] [PubMed]
88. Patel, S.K.; Wai, B.; Ord, M.; MacIsaac, R.J.; Grant, S.; Velkoska, E.; Panagiotopoulos, S.; Jerums, G.; Srivastava, P.M.; Burrell, L.M. Association of ACE2 Genetic Variants With Blood Pressure, Left Ventricular Mass, and Cardiac Function in Caucasians With Type 2 Diabetes. *Am. J. Hypertens.* **2012**, *25*, 216–222. [CrossRef] [PubMed]
89. Luo, Y.; Liu, C.; Guan, T.; Li, Y.; Lai, Y.; Li, F.; Zhao, H.; Maimaiti, T.; Zeyaweiding, A. Association of ACE2 genetic polymorphisms with hypertension-related target organ damages in south Xinjiang. *Hypertens. Res.* **2019**, *42*, 681–689. [CrossRef]
90. Arnold, R.H. COVID-19—Does This Disease Kill Due to Imbalance of the Renin Angiotensin System (RAS) Caused by Genetic and Gender Differences in the Response to Viral ACE 2 Attack? *Heart Lung Circ.* **2020**, *29*, 964–972. [CrossRef] [PubMed]
91. Liu, M.-Y.; Zheng, B.; Zhang, Y.; Li, J.-P. Role and mechanism of angiotensin-converting enzyme 2 in acute lung injury in coronavirus disease 2019. *Chronic Dis. Transl. Med.* **2020**, *6*, 98–105. [CrossRef]
92. Shirbhate, E.; Pandey, J.; Patel, V.K.; Kamal, M.; Jawaid, T.; Gorain, B.; Kesharwani, P.; Rajak, H. Understanding the role of ACE-2 receptor in pathogenesis of COVID-19 disease: A potential approach for therapeutic intervention. *Pharmacol. Rep. PR* **2021**, *73*, 1539–1550. [CrossRef]
93. Wu, Y.P.; Wei, R.; Liu, Z.H.; Chen, B.; Lisman, T.; Ren, D.L.; Han, J.J.; Xia, Z.L.; Zhang, F.S.; Xu, W.B.; et al. Analysis of thrombotic factors in severe acute respiratory syndrome (SARS) patients. *Thromb. Haemost.* **2006**, *96*, 100–101. [CrossRef] [PubMed]
94. Reheman, A.; Gross, P.; Yang, H.; Chen, P.; Allen, D.; Leytin, V.; Freedman, J.; Ni, H. Vitronectin stabilizes thrombi and vessel occlusion but plays a dual role in platelet aggregation. *J. Thromb. Haemost.* **2005**, *3*, 875–883. [CrossRef] [PubMed]
95. Zhang, Y.; Xiao, M.; Zhang, S.; Xia, P.; Cao, W.; Jiang, W.; Chen, H.; Ding, X.; Zhao, H.; Zhang, H.; et al. Coagulopathy and Antiphospholipid Antibodies in Patients with COVID-19. *N. Engl. J. Med.* **2020**, *382*, e38. [CrossRef]
96. Borghi, M.O.; Beltagy, A.; Garrafa, E.; Curreli, D.; Cecchini, G.; Bodio, C.; Grossi, C.; Blengino, S.; Tincani, A.; Franceschini, F.; et al. Anti-Phospholipid Antibodies in COVID-19 Are Different From Those Detectable in the Anti-Phospholipid Syndrome. *Front. Immunol.* **2020**, *11*, 584241. [CrossRef]
97. Gómez-Mesa, J.E.; Galindo-Coral, S.; Montes, M.C.; Muñoz Martin, A.J. Thrombosis and Coagulopathy in COVID-19. *Curr. Probl. Cardiol.* **2021**, *46*, 100742. [CrossRef] [PubMed]
98. Li, Q.; Cao, Y.; Chen, L.; Wu, D.; Yu, J.; Wang, H.; He, W.; Chen, L.; Dong, F.; Chen, W.; et al. Hematological features of persons with COVID-19. *Leukemia* **2020**, *34*, 2163–2172. [CrossRef]
99. Liu, Y.; Sun, W.; Guo, Y.; Chen, L.; Zhang, L.; Zhao, S.; Long, D.; Yu, L. Association between platelet parameters and mortality in coronavirus disease 2019: Retrospective cohort study. *Platelets* **2020**, *31*, 490–496. [CrossRef] [PubMed]

100. Chabert, A.; Hamzeh-Cognasse, H.; Pozzetto, B.; Cognasse, F.; Schattner, M.; Gomez, R.M.; Garraud, O. Human platelets and their capacity of binding viruses: Meaning and challenges? *BMC Immunol.* **2015**, *16*, 26. [CrossRef]
101. Assinger, A. Platelets and infection—An emerging role of platelets in viral infection. *Front. Immunol.* **2014**, *5*, 649. [CrossRef]
102. Seyoum, M.; Enawgaw, B.; Melku, M. Human blood platelets and viruses: Defense mechanism and role in the removal of viral pathogens. *Thromb. J.* **2018**, *16*, 16. [CrossRef]
103. Aleem, A.; Nadeem, A.J. Coronavirus (COVID-19) Vaccine-Induced Immune Thrombotic Thrombocytopenia (VITT). In *StatPearls*; StatPearls Publishing: Treasure Island, FL, USA, 2023. Available online: http://www.ncbi.nlm.nih.gov/books/NBK570605/ (accessed on 20 April 2023).
104. Oldenburg, J.; Klamroth, R.; Langer, F.; Albisetti, M.; von Auer, C.; Ay, C.; Korte, W.; Scharf, R.E.; Pötzsch, B.; Greinacher, A. Diagnosis and Management of Vaccine-Related Thrombosis following AstraZeneca COVID-19 Vaccination: Guidance Statement from the GTH. *Hamostaseologie* **2021**, *41*, 184–189. [CrossRef]
105. Miller, E. Rapid evaluation of the safety of COVID-19 vaccines: How well have we done? *Clin. Microbiol. Infect.* **2022**, *28*, 477–478. [CrossRef] [PubMed]
106. Singer, M.; Deutschman, C.S.; Seymour, C.W.; Shankar-Hari, M.; Annane, D.; Bauer, M.; Bellomo, R.; Bernard, G.R.; Chiche, J.-D.; Coopersmith, C.M.; et al. The Third International Consensus Definitions for Sepsis and Septic Shock (Sepsis-3). *JAMA* **2016**, *315*, 801–810. [CrossRef] [PubMed]
107. McGonagle, D.; O'Donnell, J.S.; Sharif, K.; Emery, P.; Bridgewood, C. Immune mechanisms of pulmonary intravascular coagulopathy in COVID-19 pneumonia. *Lancet Rheumatol.* **2020**, *2*, e437–e445. [CrossRef] [PubMed]
108. Asakura, H.; Ogawa, H. COVID-19-associated coagulopathy and disseminated intravascular coagulation. *Int. J. Hematol.* **2021**, *113*, 45–57. [CrossRef]
109. Rahman, S.; Montero, M.T.V.; Rowe, K.; Kirton, R.; Kunik, F. Epidemiology, pathogenesis, clinical presentations, diagnosis and treatment of COVID-19: A review of current evidence. *Expert Rev. Clin. Pharmacol.* **2021**, *14*, 601–621. [CrossRef]
110. Zhang, X.; Yang, X.; Jiao, H.; Liu, X. Coagulopathy in patients with COVID-19: A systematic review and meta-analysis. *Aging* **2020**, *12*, 24535–24551. [CrossRef]
111. Fiorentino, G.; Benincasa, G.; Coppola, A.; Franzese, M.; Annunziata, A.; Affinito, O.; Viglietti, M.; Napoli, C. Targeted genetic analysis unveils novel associations between ACE I/D and APO T158C polymorphisms with D-dimer levels in severe COVID-19 patients with pulmonary embolism. *J. Thromb. Thrombolysis* **2023**, *55*, 51–59. [CrossRef]
112. Annunziata, A.; Coppola, A.; Di Spirito, V.; Cauteruccio, R.; Marotta, A.; Micco, P.D.; Fiorentino, G. The Angiotensin Converting Enzyme Deletion/Deletion Genotype Is a Risk Factor for Severe COVID-19: Implication and Utility for Patients Admitted to Emergency Department. *Medicina* **2021**, *57*, 844. [CrossRef]
113. Calabrese, C.; Annunziata, A.; Coppola, A.; Pafundi, P.C.; Guarino, S.; Di Spirito, V.; Maddaloni, V.; Pepe, N.; Fiorentino, G. ACE Gene I/D Polymorphism and Acute Pulmonary Embolism in COVID-19 Pneumonia: A Potential Predisposing Role. *Front. Med.* **2021**, *7*, 631148. Available online: https://www.frontiersin.org/articles/10.3389/fmed.2020.631148 (accessed on 14 May 2023). [CrossRef]
114. Gómez, J.; Albaiceta, G.M.; García-Clemente, M.; López-Larrea, C.; Amado-Rodríguez, L.; Lopez-Alonso, I.; Hermida, T.; Enriquez, A.I.; Herrero, P.; Melón, S.; et al. Angiotensin-converting enzymes (ACE, ACE2) gene variants and COVID-19 outcome. *Gene* **2020**, *762*, 145102. [CrossRef] [PubMed]
115. Sarangarajan, R.; Winn, R.; Kiebish, M.A.; Bountra, C.; Granger, E.; Narain, N.R. Ethnic Prevalence of Angiotensin-Converting Enzyme Deletion (D) Polymorphism and COVID-19 Risk: Rationale for Use of Angiotensin-Converting Enzyme Inhibitors/Angiotensin Receptor Blockers. *J. Racial Ethn. Health Disparities* **2021**, *8*, 973–980. [CrossRef] [PubMed]
116. Güngör, Y.; Kayataş, M.; Yıldız, G.; Özdemir, Ö.; Candan, F. The presence of PAI-1 4G/5G and ACE DD genotypes increases the risk of early-stage AVF thrombosis in hemodialysis patients. *Ren. Fail.* **2011**, *33*, 169–175. [CrossRef]
117. Di Tano, G.; Dede, M.; Pellicelli, I.; Martinelli, E.; Moschini, L.; Calvaruso, E.; Danzi, G.B. Pulmonary embolism in patients with COVID-19 pneumonia on adequate oral anticoagulation. *J. Thromb. Thrombolysis* **2022**, *53*, 576–580. [CrossRef]
118. Lubbe, L.; Cozier, G.E.; Oosthuizen, D.; Acharya, K.R.; Sturrock, E.D. ACE2 and ACE: Structure-based insights into mechanism, regulation and receptor recognition by SARS-CoV. *Clin. Sci. 1979* **2020**, *134*, 2851–2871. [CrossRef] [PubMed]
119. Makris, T.K.; Stavroulakis, G.A.; Dafni, U.G.; Gialeraki, A.E.; Krespi, P.G.; Hatzizacharias, A.N.; Tsoukala, C.G.; Vythoulkas, J.S.; Kyriakidis, M.K. ACE/DD genotype is associated with hemostasis balance disturbances reflecting hypercoagulability and endothelial dysfunction in patients with untreated hypertension. *Am. Heart J.* **2000**, *140*, 760–765. [CrossRef]
120. Kuo, C.-L.; Pilling, L.C.; Atkins, J.L.; Masoli, J.A.H.; Delgado, J.; Kuchel, G.A.; Melzer, D. APOE e4 Genotype Predicts Severe COVID-19 in the UK Biobank Community Cohort. *J. Gerontol. A Biol. Sci. Med. Sci.* **2020**, *75*, 2231–2232. [CrossRef]
121. Ghaffari, M.; Ansari, H.; Beladimoghadam, N.; Aghamiri, S.H.; Haghighi, M.; Nabavi, M.; Mansouri, B.; Mehrpour, M.; Assarzadegan, F.; Hesami, O.; et al. Neurological features and outcome in COVID-19: Dementia can predict severe disease. *J. Neurovirol.* **2021**, *27*, 86–93. [CrossRef]
122. Worldmeters.info. Available online: https://www.worldmeters.info/coronavirus/#countries (accessed on 14 May 2023).
123. Xiang, G.; Hao, S.; Fu, C.; Hu, W.; Xie, L.; Wu, Q.; Li, S.; Liu, X. The effect of coagulation factors in 2019 novel coronavirus patients. *Medicine* **2021**, *100*, e24537. [CrossRef]
124. Xiong, M.; Liang, X.; Wei, Y.-D. Changes in blood coagulation in patients with severe coronavirus disease 2019 (COVID-19): A meta-analysis. *Br. J. Haematol.* **2020**, *189*, 1050–1052. [CrossRef]

125. Wu, Z.; McGoogan, J.M. Characteristics of and Important Lessons from the Coronavirus Disease 2019 (COVID-19) Outbreak in China: Summary of a Report of 72 314 Cases from the Chinese Center for Disease Control and Prevention. *JAMA* **2020**, *323*, 1239–1242. [CrossRef]
126. Léonard-Lorant, I.; Delabranche, X.; Séverac, F.; Helms, J.; Pauzet, C.; Collange, O.; Schneider, F.; Labani, A.; Bilbault, P.; Molière, S.; et al. Acute Pulmonary Embolism in Patients with COVID-19 at CT Angiography and Relationship to d-Dimer Levels. *Radiology* **2020**, *296*, E189–E191. [CrossRef] [PubMed]
127. Wichmann, D.; Sperhake, J.-P.; Lütgehetmann, M.; Steurer, S.; Edler, C.; Heinemann, A.; Heinrich, F.; Mushumba, H.; Kniep, I.; Schröder, A.S.; et al. Autopsy Findings and Venous Thromboembolism in Patients With COVID-19: A Prospective Cohort Study. *Ann. Intern. Med.* **2020**, *173*, 268–277. [CrossRef] [PubMed]
128. Nahum, J.; Morichau-Beauchant, T.; Daviaud, F.; Echegut, P.; Fichet, J.; Maillet, J.-M.; Thierry, S. Venous Thrombosis Among Critically Ill Patients With Coronavirus Disease 2019 (COVID-19). *JAMA Netw. Open* **2020**, *3*, e2010478. [CrossRef]
129. Middeldorp, S.; Coppens, M.; van Haaps, T.F.; Foppen, M.; Vlaar, A.P.; Müller, M.C.A.; Bouman, C.C.S.; Beenen, L.F.M.; Kootte, R.S.; Heijmans, J.; et al. Incidence of venous thromboembolism in hospitalized patients with COVID-19. *J. Thromb. Haemost.* **2020**, *18*, 1995–2002. [CrossRef] [PubMed]
130. Shah, A.; Donovan, K.; McHugh, A.; Pandey, M.; Aaron, L.; Bradbury, C.A.; Stanworth, S.J.; Alikhan, R.; Von Kier, S.; Maher, K.; et al. Thrombotic and haemorrhagic complications in critically ill patients with COVID-19: A multicentre observational study. *Crit. Care* **2020**, *24*, 561. [CrossRef]
131. Cui, S.; Chen, S.; Li, X.; Liu, S.; Wang, F. Prevalence of venous thromboembolism in patients with severe novel coronavirus pneumonia. *J. Thromb. Haemost.* **2020**, *18*, 1421–1424. [CrossRef]
132. Carfora, V.; Spiniello, G.; Ricciolino, R.; Di Mauro, M.; Migliaccio, M.G.; Mottola, F.F.; Verde, N.; Coppola, N.; Coppola, N.; Sagnelli, C.; et al. Anticoagulant treatment in COVID-19: A narrative review. *J. Thromb. Thrombolysis* **2021**, *51*, 642–648. [CrossRef]
133. Shi, C.; Wang, C.; Wang, H.; Yang, C.; Cai, F.; Zeng, F.; Cheng, F.; Liu, Y.; Zhou, T.; Deng, B.; et al. The potential of low molecular weight heparin to mitigate cytokine storm in severe COVID-19 patients: A retrospective clinical study. *Clin. Transl. Sci.* **2020**, *13*, 1087–1095. [CrossRef]
134. Godino, C.; Scotti, A.; Maugeri, N.; Mancini, N.; Fominskiy, E.; Margonato, A.; Landoni, G. Antithrombotic therapy in patients with COVID-19? -Rationale and Evidence-. *Int. J. Cardiol.* **2021**, *324*, 261–266. [CrossRef]
135. Mangana, C.; Lorigo, M.; Cairrao, E. Implications of Endothelial Cell-Mediated Dysfunctions in Vasomotor Tone Regulation. *Biologics* **2021**, *1*, 231–251. [CrossRef]
136. Xu, J.; Zhang, X.; Pelayo, R.; Monestier, M.; Ammollo, C.T.; Semeraro, F.; Taylor, F.B.; Esmon, N.L.; Lupu, F.; Esmon, C.T. Extracellular histones are major mediators of death in sepsis. *Nat. Med.* **2009**, *15*, 1318–1321. [CrossRef] [PubMed]
137. Zhang, X.; Li, X. The Role of Histones and Heparin in Sepsis: A Review. *J. Intensive Care Med.* **2022**, *37*, 319–326. [CrossRef]
138. Mangiafico, M.; Caff, A.; Costanzo, L. The Role of Heparin in COVID-19: An Update after Two Years of Pandemics. *J. Clin. Med.* **2022**, *11*, 3099. [CrossRef] [PubMed]
139. Mousavi, S.; Moradi, M.; Khorshidahmad, T.; Motamedi, M. Anti-Inflammatory Effects of Heparin and Its Derivatives: A Systematic Review. *Adv. Pharmacol. Sci.* **2015**, *2015*, 507151. [CrossRef]
140. Thachil, J. The versatile heparin in COVID-19. *J. Thromb. Haemost.* **2020**, *18*, 1020–1022. [CrossRef] [PubMed]
141. Oduah, E.I.; Linhardt, R.J.; Sharfstein, S.T. Heparin: Past, Present, and Future. *Pharmaceuticals* **2016**, *9*, 38. [CrossRef]
142. Shukla, D.; Spear, P.G. Herpesviruses and heparan sulfate: An intimate relationship in aid of viral entry. *J. Clin. Investig.* **2001**, *108*, 503–510. [CrossRef] [PubMed]
143. Ghezzi, S.; Cooper, L.; Rubio, A.; Pagani, I.; Capobianchi, M.R.; Ippolito, G.; Pelletier, J.; Meneghetti, M.C.Z.; Lima, M.A.; Skidmore, M.A.; et al. Heparin prevents Zika virus induced-cytopathic effects in human neural progenitor cells. *Antivir. Res.* **2017**, *140*, 13–17. [CrossRef]
144. Mycroft-West, C.; Su, D.; Elli, S.; Guimond, S.; Miller, G.; Turnbull, J.; Yates, E.; Guerrini, M.; Fernig, D.; Lima, M.; et al. The 2019 coronavirus (SARS-CoV-2) surface protein (Spike) S1 Receptor Binding Domain undergoes conformational change upon heparin binding. *BioRxiv* **2020**. [CrossRef]
145. Di Castelnuovo, A.; Costanzo, S.; Antinori, A.; Berselli, N.; Blandi, L.; Bonaccio, M.; Cauda, R.; Guaraldi, G.; Menicanti, L.; Mennuni, M.; et al. Heparin in COVID-19 Patients Is Associated with Reduced In-Hospital Mortality: The Multicenter Italian CORIST Study. *Thromb. Haemost.* **2021**, *121*, 1054–1065. [CrossRef] [PubMed]
146. Gennaro, F.D. SARS-CoV-2 Transmission and Outcome in Neuro-rehabilitation patients hospitalized at Neuroscience Hospital in Italy: SARS-CoV-2 in severe neurological patients. *Mediterr. J. Hematol. Infect. Dis.* **2020**, *12*, e2020063. [CrossRef]
147. REMAP-CAP Investigators; ACTIV-4a Investigators; ATTACC Investigators; Goligher, E.C.; Bradbury, C.A.; McVerry, B.J.; Lawler, P.R.; Berger, J.S.; Gong, M.N.; Carrier, M.; et al. Therapeutic Anticoagulation with Heparin in Critically Ill Patients with COVID-19. *N. Engl. J. Med.* **2021**, *385*, 777–789. [CrossRef]
148. Stasi, C.; Fallani, S.; Voller, F.; Silvestri, C. Treatment for COVID-19: An overview. *Eur. J. Pharmacol.* **2020**, *889*, 173644. [CrossRef] [PubMed]
149. Mennuni, M.G.; Renda, G.; Grisafi, L.; Rognoni, A.; Colombo, C.; Lio, V.; Foglietta, M.; Petrilli, I.; Pirisi, M.; Spinoni, E.; et al. Clinical outcome with different doses of low-molecular-weight heparin in patients hospitalized for COVID-19. *J. Thromb. Thrombolysis* **2021**, *52*, 782–790. [CrossRef]

150. Rentsch, C.T.; Beckman, J.A.; Tomlinson, L.; Gellad, W.F.; Alcorn, C.; Kidwai-Khan, F.; Skanderson, M.; Brittain, E.; King, J.T.; Ho, Y.-L.; et al. Early initiation of prophylactic anticoagulation for prevention of coronavirus disease 2019 mortality in patients admitted to hospital in the United States: Cohort study. *BMJ* **2021**, *372*, n311. [CrossRef]
151. ISTH Interim Guidance on Recognition and Management of Coagulopathy in COVID-19—Journal of Thrombosis and Haemostasis. Available online: https://www.jthjournal.org/article/S1538-7836(22)00324-5/fulltext (accessed on 24 April 2023).
152. Hasan, S.S.; Radford, S.; Kow, C.S.; Zaidi, S.T.R. Venous thromboembolism in critically ill COVID-19 patients receiving prophylactic or therapeutic anticoagulation: A systematic review and meta-analysis. *J. Thromb. Thrombolysis* **2020**, *50*, 814–821. [CrossRef] [PubMed]
153. Thachil, J.; Tang, N.; Gando, S.; Falanga, A.; Cattaneo, M.; Levi, M.; Clark, C.; Iba, T. ISTH interim guidance on recognition and management of coagulopathy in COVID-19. *J. Thromb. Haemost.* **2020**, *18*, 1023–1026. [CrossRef] [PubMed]
154. Sayed Ahmed, H.A.; Merrell, E.; Ismail, M.; Joudeh, A.I.; Riley, J.B.; Shawkat, A.; Habeb, H.; Darling, E.; Goweda, R.A.; Shehata, M.H.; et al. Rationales and uncertainties for aspirin use in COVID-19: A narrative review. *Fam. Med. Community Health* **2021**, *9*, e000741. [CrossRef]
155. Bikdeli, B.; Madhavan, M.V.; Gupta, A.; Jimenez, D.; Burton, J.R.; Der Nigoghossian, C.; Chuich, T.; Nouri, S.N.; Dreyfus, I.; Driggin, E. Pharmacological Agents Targeting Thromboinflammation in COVID-19: Review and Implications for Future Research. *Thromb. Haemost.* **2020**, *120*, 1004–1024. [CrossRef] [PubMed]
156. Silasi, R.; Keshari, R.S.; Lupu, C.; Van Rensburg, W.J.; Chaaban, H.; Regmi, G.; Shamanaev, A.; Shatzel, J.J.; Puy, C.; Lorentz, C.U.; et al. Inhibition of contact-mediated activation of factor XI protects baboons against S aureus-induced organ damage and death. *Blood Adv.* **2019**, *3*, 658–669. [CrossRef] [PubMed]
157. Al-Horani, R.A. Potential Therapeutic Roles for Direct Factor Xa Inhibitors in Coronavirus Infections. *Am. J. Cardiovasc. Drugs Drugs Devices Interv.* **2020**, *20*, 525–533. [CrossRef] [PubMed]
158. Shatzel, J.J.; DeLoughery, E.P.; Lorentz, C.U.; Tucker, E.I.; Aslan, J.E.; Hinds, M.T.; Gailani, D.; Weitz, J.I.; McCarty, O.J.T.; Gruber, A. The contact activation system as a potential therapeutic target in patients with COVID-19. *Res. Pract. Thromb. Haemost.* **2020**, *4*, 500–505. [CrossRef]
159. Koulas, I.; Spyropoulos, A.C. A Review of FXIa Inhibition as a Novel Target for Anticoagulation. *Hamostaseologie* **2023**, *43*, 28–36. [CrossRef] [PubMed]
160. Di Gennaro, F.; Belati, A.; Tulone, O.; Diella, L.; Fiore Bavaro, D.; Bonica, R.; Genna, V.; Smith, L.; Trott, M.; Bruyere, O.; et al. Incidence of long COVID-19 in people with previous SARS-Cov2 infection: A systematic review and meta-analysis of 120,970 patients. *Intern. Emerg. Med.* **2022**, 1–9. [CrossRef]
161. Pasini, E.; Corsetti, G.; Romano, C.; Scarabelli, T.M.; Chen-Scarabelli, C.; Saravolatz, L.; Dioguardi, F.S. Serum Metabolic Profile in Patients With Long-Covid (PASC) Syndrome: Clinical Implications. *Front. Med.* **2021**, *8*, 714426. Available online: https://www.frontiersin.org/articles/10.3389/fmed.2021.714426 (accessed on 14 May 2023). [CrossRef]
162. Stefano, G.B.; Büttiker, P.; Weissenberger, S.; Martin, A.; Ptacek, R.; Kream, R.M. Editorial: The Pathogenesis of Long-Term Neuropsychiatric COVID-19 and the Role of Microglia, Mitochondria, and Persistent Neuroinflammation: A Hypothesis. *Med. Sci. Monit. Int. Med. J. Exp. Clin. Res.* **2021**, *27*, e933015. [CrossRef]
163. García-Abellán, J.; Fernández, M.; Padilla, S.; García, J.A.; Agulló, V.; Lozano, V.; Ena, N.; García-Sánchez, L.; Gutiérrez, F.; Masiá, M. Immunologic phenotype of patients with long-COVID syndrome of 1-year duration. *Front. Immunol.* **2022**, *13*, 920627. [CrossRef]
164. Chioh, F.W.; Fong, S.-W.; Young, B.E.; Wu, K.-X.; Siau, A.; Krishnan, S.; Chan, Y.-H.; Carissimo, G.; Teo, L.L.; Gao, F.; et al. Convalescent COVID-19 patients are susceptible to endothelial dysfunction due to persistent immune activation. *eLife* **2021**, *10*, e64909. [CrossRef]
165. Scurati, R.; Papini, N.; Giussani, P.; Alberti, G.; Tringali, C. The Challenge of Long COVID-19 Management: From Disease Molecular Hallmarks to the Proposal of Exercise as Therapy. *Int. J. Mol. Sci.* **2022**, *23*, 12311. [CrossRef]

International Journal of
Molecular Sciences

MDPI

Review

Determinants of COVID-19 Disease Severity–Lessons from Primary and Secondary Immune Disorders including Cancer

Antonio G. Solimando [1,*], Max Bittrich [2], Endrit Shahini [3], Federica Albanese [1], Georg Fritz [4] and Markus Krebs [5,6,*]

1 Guido Baccelli Unit of Internal Medicine, Department of Precision and Regenerative Medicine and Ionian Area—(DiMePRe-J), Aldo Moro Bari University, 70100 Bari, Italy
2 Department of Internal Medicine II, University Hospital Würzburg, 97080 Würzburg, Germany
3 Gastroenterology Unit, National Institute of Gastroenterology S. De Bellis, IRCCS Research Hospital, Via Turi 27, 70013 Castellana Grotte, Italy
4 Department of Anesthesiology, Intensive Care Medicine and Pain Therapy at the Immanuel Klinikum Bernau, Heart Center Brandenburg, 16321 Bernau, Germany
5 Comprehensive Cancer Center Mainfranken, University Hospital Würzburg, 97080 Würzburg, Germany
6 Department of Urology and Paediatric Urology, University Hospital Würzburg, 97080 Würzburg, Germany
* Correspondence: antonio.solimando@uniba.it (A.G.S.); krebs_m@ukw.de (M.K.)

Abstract: At the beginning of the COVID-19 pandemic, patients with primary and secondary immune disorders—including patients suffering from cancer—were generally regarded as a high-risk population in terms of COVID-19 disease severity and mortality. By now, scientific evidence indicates that there is substantial heterogeneity regarding the vulnerability towards COVID-19 in patients with immune disorders. In this review, we aimed to summarize the current knowledge about the effect of coexistent immune disorders on COVID-19 disease severity and vaccination response. In this context, we also regarded cancer as a secondary immune disorder. While patients with hematological malignancies displayed lower seroconversion rates after vaccination in some studies, a majority of cancer patients' risk factors for severe COVID-19 disease were either inherent (such as metastatic or progressive disease) or comparable to the general population (age, male gender and comorbidities such as kidney or liver disease). A deeper understanding is needed to better define patient subgroups at a higher risk for severe COVID-19 disease courses. At the same time, immune disorders as functional disease models offer further insights into the role of specific immune cells and cytokines when orchestrating the immune response towards SARS-CoV-2 infection. Longitudinal serological studies are urgently needed to determine the extent and the duration of SARS-CoV-2 immunity in the general population, as well as immune-compromised and oncological patients.

Keywords: COVID-19; SARS-CoV-2; disorder of immunity; cancer

Citation: Solimando, A.G.; Bittrich, M.; Shahini, E.; Albanese, F.; Fritz, G.; Krebs, M. Determinants of COVID-19 Disease Severity–Lessons from Primary and Secondary Immune Disorders including Cancer. *Int. J. Mol. Sci.* **2023**, *24*, 8746. https://doi.org/10.3390/ijms24108746

Academic Editors: Alexandru Schiopu, Emil Marian Arbănași and Eliza Russu

Received: 2 April 2023
Revised: 12 May 2023
Accepted: 12 May 2023
Published: 14 May 2023

1. Introduction

COVID-19 infection is a complex and heterogeneous disease, with the host response crucially determining its course: during the early phase of an infection, there is a substantial production of type 1 interferons, generated at the tissue level by infected as well as surrounding cells [1]. At the same time, SARS-CoV-2 infection can block type 1 interferon signaling in macrophages and dendritic cells [2,3]. Moreover, decreased interferon production—caused for instance by defects in Toll-like receptors (TLRs)—was linked to critically ill COVID-19 patients. Similar clinical courses were observed in patients with alterations in interferon receptors—leading to defective interferon sensing [4,5]. In line with this disease model, Bastard et al. discovered autoantibodies against type 1 interferon, which again hindered sufficient antiviral cellular signaling, in patients suffering from severe COVID-19 disease [4,6]. In general, these traits point towards a crucial role of interferon in preventing severe COVID-10 disease [7].

The cytokine production is usually maintained in the first week, when the virus replicates and the most overt clinical symptoms usually appear; next, the antibody production phase takes place together with the expansion of the T-cell compartment. During a viral infection, the peak in T-cell expansion usually occurs about a week from the infection. Consequently, inflammatory mediators are key drivers of COVID-19-related morbidity [1,8]. The knowledge that the cytokines' role is chiefly driving organ damage was what largely prompted the drug targeting. Commonly, the peripheral blood levels of cytokines are considered trustworthy in reflecting the immune response. Nonetheless, Daamen et al. provided evidence to warrant caution: chemokines and cytokines in peripheral blood differed significantly from those obtained from autoptic lung tissues and bronchoalveolar lavage [9]. This is unlikely to be limited to SARS-CoV-2 and will prompt additional research to map personalized and site-specific patients' immunomes in infections [10,11]. In this frame of mind, an unbiased immunophenotyping analysis revealed a selective clustering of individuals with severe COVID-19 courses [12].

It is possible to draw some distinctions based on the severity of the disease. T-cell activation, DR expression and monocytes are critical; significant differences were found in T-cell activation and MHC DR expression, as well as in the effector memory T-cell population (effector memory T cells re-expresses CD45RA, dubbed TEMRA) [12]. Many studies have investigated the role of immunity in COVID-19 [13–17]. Seminal findings revealed that monocytes correlate with symptoms, with CD169+-activated monocytes lacking in healthy controls [18]. The researchers also discovered a gamma interferon signature (high expression in patients with severe COVID-19 courses), that successfully distinguished patients based on their prognosis.

Furthermore, conditions associated with poor outcomes in COVID-19 appear to be associated with general risk factors, such as type 2 diabetes, obesity and COPD; it is worth noting that these are traditional markers of poor outcomes in almost any severe disease. Aside from organ transplantation, nothing has been discovered to identify the immune system's state as a major determinant [19]. Chronic inflammation is associated with kidney disease, diabetes and obesity, but these conditions do not result in immunosuppression [20]. Nonetheless, age is the single greatest risk factor for mortality and hospitalization, and immunosenescence represents an intriguing scenario for future research.

Because ACE2 and TMPRSS2 variants and expression can be candidates for gender and country differences in COVID-19 severity, host genetics is also important in COVID-19 [20,21]. There are two susceptibility loci for severe COVID-19 with respiratory failure [21]. Nonetheless, we review the current evidence pointing to novel aspects of immune-related conditions that may influence the outcome of SARS-CoV-2 infections (Figure 1).

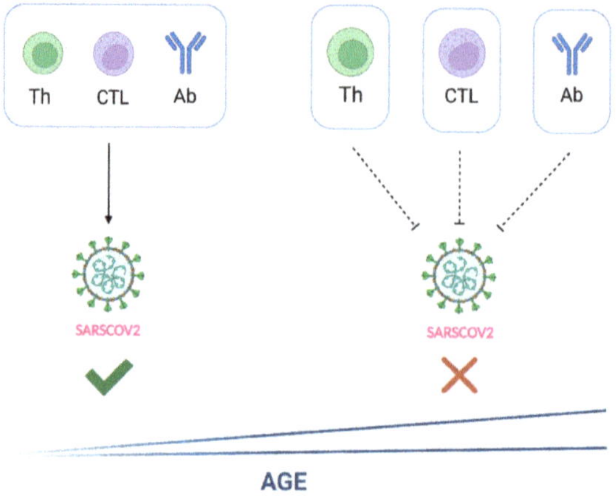

Figure 1. Higher age and a poor adaptive and humoral immune response as determinants of COVID-19 disease severity. Young patients and individuals with sufficient T-cell-based and humoral immune

response (left side) usually have self-limiting disease courses. In contrast, older patients and individuals with a limited immune response (right side) have a significantly worse prognosis in terms of COVID-19 outcome. Th: T helper cell; CTL: Cytotoxic T lymphocyte; Ab: Antibody.

2. Immunity, Immune Aging and COVID-19

2.1. Immune Response against SARS-CoV-2

Although infection with SARS-CoV-2 was expected to activate the host's immune response, data on this specific trait were initially scarce [22,23]. While SARS-CoV-2 infection results in both humoral and cellular immunity [24], the T-cell response does not differ significantly between mild and severe forms. Cross-reactions have been reported in unexposed subjects, most likely due to non-SARS-CoV-2 coronaviruses [24]. Compared to seronegative counterparts, seropositive individuals are significantly more protected against infection. Thus, the strong sequence homology and structural similarity with SARS-CoV-1 initially supported genetic and structural modelling, revealing an epitope-level similarity prediction. Despite being slightly less effective than mRNA vaccines (95%) [25–27], the humoral defense is protective against the virus in much the same way as the adenovirus-vectored vaccine (70%).

A test designed to determine which pieces of SARS-CoV-2 are recognized by the immune system was supported by CD4+ and CD8+ epitopes predicted to play significant roles in SARS-CoV-2 [22]. Specific analysis of SARS-CoV-2 human CD4 and CD8 T-cell epitope data proved 1400 additional SARS-CoV-2 epitopes and suggested different immunodominant regions of the virus as well as more commonly recognized epitopes.

T-cell and antibody responses in COVID-19 cases appear to be orchestrated by two main principles: in most humans, SARS-CoV-2 causes acute infections that resolve or cure. Both antibodies and T cells are important in modulating humoral responses, human vaccines and protecting against the virus [26]. A better understanding of SARS-CoV-2 T-cell and antibody adaptive responses prompted further investigation, leading to the measurement of SARS-CoV-2 immunity while identifying epitope pools detecting CD4+ in 100% and CD8+ T cells in 70% of convalescent COVID-19 patients. Furthermore, T-cell responses were discovered to be focused not only on the spike protein but also on M, N and other ORFs [28,29]. Additional details on the impact of different viral strains on the described groups would be informative in understanding disease severity and patient outcomes. For instance, recent studies have highlighted the importance of considering the viral strain in the context of COVID-19 prognosis. One study found that patients infected with the B.1.1.7 (Alpha) variant had a higher risk of hospitalization and death compared to patients infected with the original strain. Another study found that the B.1.351 (Beta) variant was associated with an increased risk of reinfection in patients who had previously recovered from COVID-19. Therefore, further research on the impact of different viral strains on disease severity and patient outcomes is needed to develop effective treatment strategies [30,31].

Of note, T-cell reactivity to SARS-CoV-2 epitopes has also been observed in non-exposed individuals [23]. In acute COVID-19 cases, disease severity correlates with adaptive immunity to SARS-CoV-2 underlining that a coordinated immune response is protective against the virus. T cells appear to be the major contributors to controlling SARS-CoV-2 infection. As the first line of defense against pathogens, the innate immune system plays a crucial role in combatting this novel virus. To better understand the interaction between SARS-CoV-2 and the human innate immune system, a conceptual framework is needed to link clinical observations with experimental findings from the first year of the pandemic. It has been observed that variations in innate immune system components among individuals contribute significantly to the diverse disease courses seen in COVID-19. Therefore, understanding the pathophysiological mechanisms of the cells and soluble mediators involved in innate immunity is essential to develop effective diagnostic markers and therapeutic strategies for COVID-19. However, more research is needed to establish the causality of events, which is currently lacking [32]. Several pathophysiological mechanisms of the innate immune system are involved in COVID-19. One of the most prominent mechanisms is the overactivation of the immune response, leading to a cytokine storm, which can cause severe damage to the lungs and other organs. This overactivation of the immune response can also result in the infiltration of immune cells, such as macrophages and neutrophils, into the lungs, leading to inflammation and tissue damage. Moreover, it has been observed that the innate immune system detects viral RNA through pattern recognition receptors, such as Toll-like receptors (TLRs) and retinoic acid-inducible gene 1 (RIG-I)-like receptors (RLRs), leading to the production of type I interferons (IFNs). However, SARS-CoV-2 can evade the innate immune system by inhibiting the production of type I IFNs, leading to uncontrolled viral replication and dissemination. In addition, there is evidence to suggest that the complement system, which is part of the innate immune system, is activated in COVID-19. Activation of the complement system can lead to the recruitment of immune cells, including neutrophils and macrophages, to the site of infection, contributing to inflammation and tissue damage. Furthermore, recent studies have suggested that the innate immune system may also play a role in the long-term effects of COVID-19, such as persistent fatigue and cognitive impairment. It has been proposed that the innate immune system may contribute to these long-term effects by inducing chronic inflammation and oxidative stress. Overall, a better understanding of the pathophysiological mechanisms involved in the innate immune system's response to SARS-CoV-2 is essential to develop effective diagnostic markers and therapeutic strategies for COVID-19 [33,33,34].

The adaptive immune system has three branches in its arsenal against the virus, but there is no strong evidence of a causal negative association between adaptive immunity and disease severity. Conversely, age is a major COVID-19 risk factor, and adaptive immunity shortcomings seem to be part of the dysfunctional response when poorly coordinated T-cell responses and limited naïve T cells are in place [35].

When considering the immune system ageing, we primarily consider T cells and thymic involution. The naive T-cell compartment contracts, thymus cells acquire senescent characteristics and some expanded oligoclonal T-cell populations are exhausted [36]. These phenomena also include herpes virus infections and susceptibility to bacteria [37]. The myeloid compartment also ages, as Lissner et al. demonstrated ex vivo and in vitro [38]. The authors used the Listeria monocytogenes infection as a model to assess the impact of a patient's age on the course of the disease.

Listeria infection is usually insignificant in most young adults. However, after the age of 80, the risk of stroke and poor outcome increases significantly [38,39]: in vitro, baseline differences in the monocyte response to listeria were significant between older and younger adults. Without any prior stimulation, older adults were already overproducing inflammatory cytokines. This specific trait has also been confirmed in bulk and single-cell analysis of PTX3 expression in COVID-19 patients' peripheral blood and lung tissue [40]. Regarding the six-hour time point, older adults had a longer persistence of inflammation in their monocytes. This finding sparked several investigations, including COVID-19 studies, into the myeloid compartment [37]. Corticosteroids are thus the foundation of therapeutic strategies to reduce mortality in clinical settings of COVID-19 respiratory failure. The discovery that age can influence immunological fitness prompted further research in a broader field typically associated with immunodeficiency and immune dysregulation.

T cells have been shown to contribute to a better outcome in SARS-CoV-2 infections with lower viral loads [41] and play an important role in the immune response [37]. In the monkey model, CD8+ T cells provide control. Individuals with agammaglobulinemia and B cell deficiency have a moderately increased risk of hospitalization. Moreover, COVID-19 is mostly mild in people with multiple sclerosis who take ocrelizumab (an antiCD20 antibody). In contrast, in the absence of detectable neutralizing antibodies, one single dose of Moderna or Pfizer vaccine provided substantial protection in most individuals [42]. Following that, researchers hope to determine how long SARS-CoV-2 immunological memory lasts. Dan et al. conducted an extensive analysis, highlighting significant immune memory in most individuals 8 months post-COVID-19 infection. Memory kinetics differ between T cells, memory B cells and antibodies. Immune memory is complex and heterogeneous, with an estimated half-life with a wide confidence interval due to COVID-19 heterogeneity and approximately 5% of individuals having low-level immune memory at 6 months [43].

2.2. Lessons from HIV Infection

The T-cell count has been discovered to be important in viral load control and infection eradication [44]. However, the first study on COVID-19-infected HIV patients from Spain found no significant difference between mild, moderate and severe courses due to HIV-related T-cell count. In large HIV cohorts, there were no differences in hospitalization rates, either. There was no dependence on T-cell count, specifically CD4+ T-cell count: Ho et al. reported a slightly higher rate of inflammatory cytokines but no differences in hospitalization in HIV-positive versus HIV-negative COVID-19 patients, and they were unable to identify a T-cell count that conferred an increased risk [45]. HIV infection, on the other hand, has been linked to a twofold increase in the risk of death in COVID-19-infected individuals in another study [46]. As a result, it is attractive to speculate that there is a disease spectrum associated with HIV viral load, immunosuppression, hospitalized cases and tuberculosis exposure that could explain clinical heterogeneity. Finally, HIV does not appear to be a major risk factor for highly aggressive COVID-19 courses, establishing a pathobiological stage in which T cells do not lead to disease aggressiveness. However, the frailty of this population subgroup prompted further research into vaccination and its prioritization for vulnerable patient subgroups.

Many studies have investigated the impact of HIV on COVID-19 outcomes and have suggested that the close monitoring of immune status and viral load, as well as adjustments to HIV treatment regimens, may be necessary for optimal management of COVID-19 in HIV-positive individuals. Additionally, early and aggressive treatment with antiviral therapy and corticosteroids has improved outcomes in COVID-19 patients, including those with HIV. COVID-19 vaccines are also recommended for HIV-positive individuals, although more research is needed to fully understand their safety and efficacy in this population. Finally, psychological and social support services are important considerations for HIV-positive individuals with COVID-19, as they may face unique challenges related to social isolation and stigma [47].

2.3. Vaccination and Immunity

The underlying trained innate immunity represents a significant breakthrough in COVID-19 prevention [48,49]. SARS-CoV-2 infection was tracked prospectively in 3720 healthcare workers who received two doses of the BNT162b2 vaccine between January 18 and March 31, 2021, with data collected until May 10, 2021. In subjects with symptoms suggestive of SARS-CoV-2 infection or contact with an infected subject, nasopharyngeal swabs were collected and tested for SARS-CoV-2 RNA positivity [25]. Surprisingly, subjects who had previously been infected and then vaccinated, thus receiving triple exposure to viral antigens, could benefit from a 50% risk reduction. All SARS-CoV-2-exposed subjects had a sustained level of SARS-CoV-2 neutralizing antibodies against all variants tested [25,50]. Significant responses to 25 mcg of Moderna mRNA-1273 vaccination spike were observed, as were RBD IgG antibody responses lasting up to 7 months [51]. A significant response has also been reported at various time points, higher at day 43 compared to day 15 and lasting up to day 209 [51].

CD4+ and CD8+ T cells exhibited similar behavior. The quality and duration of vaccination responses with various vaccine platforms have also been studied. Moderna, Pfizer, Johnson & Johnson, AstraZeneca and Novavax have all been tested for their ability to establish and maintain immune responses over time [52,53]. This will be useful in determining the magnitude and duration of vaccine-induced immunity, as well as in comparing different vaccine platforms in terms of responses induced by each other and in comparison to natural infection. Furthermore, this will help future vaccine designers determine when and if a booster is needed, as well as develop dose-sparing strategies [54]. Tarke et al. identified 280 different CD4+ restricted epitopes in this frame of mind (dominant epitopes are highly promiscuous, with implications for population coverage). They also discovered 523 distinct CD8+ epitopes, each recognizing multiple epitopes and antigens, yielding a conservative estimate of 15–20 epitopes recognized per donor, with important implications for viral immune escape [55].

3. Immune Dysregulation and Severity of COVID-19 Infection

3.1. COVID-19 in Patients with Cancer—Clinical Data, Risk Factors and Vaccination Response

When researchers examined factors contributing to COVID-19 mortality in European cancer patients, they discovered that onco-hematological pathologies, metastasis and additional comorbidities were risk factors for developing the severe disease [56]. Nonetheless, the retrospective nature of the available data significantly affected its quality. Furthermore, survival from symptom onset in hospitals was not influenced by a cancer diagnosis per se but rather by suboptimal ICU measures used on cancer subjects versus non-oncologists used on COVID-19 patients also suffering from cancer compared to COVID-19 patients without cancer [57]. Table 1 summarizes the available evidence on this topic.

Table 1. Available data obtained from SARS-CoV-2 infection and cancer.

Study	N, Neoplasms	Type	Risk Factors of Severe Outcome
China, Hubei [56]	205, mixed	Retrospective	Hematological tumors, chemo <4 weeks, metastatic disease progression
China, Wuhan [57]	232, mixed	Case-matched control	Advanced stage, ECOG, older patients
China, Wuhan [58]	28, mixed	Retrospective	Antineoplastic tx <2 weeks, CT patchy consolidation
France, Paris [59]	76, breast cancer	Prospective registry	Hypertension, older age
France, Lyon [60]	302, mixed	Retrospective	Male gender, ECOG, PD cancer
CCC19 (USA, Canada, Spain) [61]	928, mixed	Crowdsourcing	Age, male gender, NCDs, ECOG, PD cancer, smoking
TERAVOLT [62]	200, thoracic cancer	Crowdsourcing	Smoking
US, NYC [63]	20, childhood cancer	Retrospective	No increased risk of infection vs. non-cancer patients
US, NYC [64]	334, mixed	Case-matched control	Older age

Kuderer et al. defined factors associated with COVID-19 mortality in cancer patients, describing a not significant increase in risk for non-cytotoxic therapy (targeted agents, endocrine therapy, immunotherapy, radiation). At the same time, they confirmed increased mortality for subjects with hemato-oncological conditions, the elderly, and patients with comorbid conditions [61,65]. Large studies were initiated to examine iatrogenic immunosuppression, which surprisingly excluded an additional risk conferred by active chemotherapy for COVID-19 hospitalization severity or mortality. Indeed, a larger study by Kuderer et al. identified progressive disease as a risk factor for COVID-related mortality [61]. The authors' findings are consistent with the CDC's risk stratification for mortality [19]. Nonetheless, they discovered that, besides already known secondary effects [66], immune checkpoint inhibitor-based therapies are linked to an increased risk of mortality and disease severity. Remarkably, chemotherapy did not affect prognosis in this study [61].

Regarding humoral and cellular immunity, cancer patients are no exception to the general concept of vaccine responsiveness [67]. Passive immunization is also an option for subjects with ineffective vaccine responses [68]. In COVID-19 cancer patients, older age, the number of comorbidities, ECOG PS $\geq$2, active cancer and chemotherapy alone or in combination all increase the risk of death.

There is very little information available on the antibody responses against SARS-CoV-2 in cancer patients. The first prospective multicenter observational study evaluated the antibody response in cancer patients and oncology healthcare workers with confirmed or clinically suspected COVID-19 [69], demonstrating that cancer patients infected with SARS-CoV-2 have IgG antibody responses comparable to subjects not suffering from cancer. SARS-CoV-2 laboratory testing that is both timely and accurate is critical in managing COVID-19. Combining antibody testing and RT-PCR on swab specimens may improve COVID-19 detection [69]. This evidence was corroborated by Kamar et al., who discovered that three doses of an mRNA COVID-19 vaccine were effective in organ transplant recipients [70].

A prospective, multicenter cohort study conducted in 2022 aimed to compare the spike IgG seropositivity rate in blood samples from 776 cancer patients and 715 non-cancer volunteers following inactive SARS-CoV-2 vaccination. The cancer patient group had a seropositivity rate of 85.2%, while the control group had a rate of 97.5%. Cancer patients not only had a significantly lower seropositivity rate but also lower antibody levels ($p < 0.001$). Finally, lower seropositivity in cancer patients was associated with age and chemotherapy ($p < 0.001$) [71].

A study from 2021 aimed to assess the SARS-CoV2 IgG seroprevalence in 74 older patients (aged $\geq$ 80 years) with cancer one month after receiving the second dose of the BNT162b2 vaccine. While median serum IgG levels in older cancer patients were lower compared to control (2396.10 AU/mL vs. 8737.49 AU/mL; $p < 0.0001$), this study still was the first to describe a positive immune response in this vulnerable patient subgroup [72]. A 2022 meta-analysis, on the other hand, looked at factors predicting poor seroconversion in 5499 cancer patients. The authors discovered that age, male gender and metastatic disease were associated with a lower seropositivity after COVID-19 vaccination. Additionally associated with seropositivity were immunoglobulin heavy chain variable mutation status and high concentrations of IgG, IgM and IgA. Regarding cancer treatment strategies, anti-CD20 therapy within the last 12 months and chemotherapy were found to be negatively associated with seroconversion. These findings suggested that improved vaccination strategies would be beneficial for the elderly, males or patients receiving active chemotherapy and that prevention should be prioritized even after a full course of vaccination [73]. Another recent study examined COVID-19 vaccine uptake trends in 579 sequential cancer patients previously infected with SARS-CoV-2. Specifically, older age and female sex were significantly associated with higher vaccine uptake in univariate and multivariate models (age (OR = 1.18, $p < 0.001$), and female sex (OR = 1.80, $p = 0.003$), respectively) [74].

Notably, the aim of Mai et al.'s systematic review and meta-analysis was to determine the proportion of non-responders to COVID-19 primary vaccination in 849 patients with hematological cancer and 82 patients with solid cancer who seroconverted after a booster dose. Seroconversion occurred in 44% of patients with hematological malignancies, while a significantly higher seroconversion (80%) was observed among solid tumor patients. Higher antibody titers were found to be significantly associated with an increased duration between the second and third dose (OR = 1.02, $p \leq 0.05$), patient age (OR = 0.960, $p \leq 0.05$) and cancer type. Therefore, administering a COVID-19 vaccine booster dose improved seroconversion and antibody levels. Patients with solid cancer consistently responded better to booster vaccines than patients with hematological cancer [75].

Another recent systematic review and meta-analysis of 28 articles assessed the efficacy and safety of COVID-19 vaccines in patients with active malignancies. In contrast to the previous meta-analysis, they discovered higher overall seroconversion rates of 70% and 88% in patients with solid tumors and hematologic malignancies, respectively, after receiving a second dose of the COVID-19 vaccine [76].

In particular, a recent study compared the development of neutralizing antibodies against SARS-CoV-2 in non-vaccinated patients with multiple myeloma (MM) and COVID-19 to patients who received two doses of the BNT162b2 vaccine, most likely due to immunoparesis [77,78]. Patients with MM and COVID-19 had a better humoral response than vaccinated patients with MM. COVID-19-positive patients had a higher median neutralizing antibodies titer than vaccinated patients (87.6% vs. 58.7%; $p = 0.01$). However, there was no difference in neutralizing antibody production between COVID-19-positive and vaccinated patients who did not receive treatment ($p = 0.14$). As a result, it was suggested by the authors that vaccinated patients with MM on treatment who have not previously received a COVID-19 infection should be considered for booster vaccination [79].

There is little information in the literature about the levels of autoantibodies in patients with paraneoplastic syndromes and whether these autoantibodies could interfere with the vaccine response in any fashion.

Immunologic self-tolerance defects increase the risk of paraneoplastic autoimmune diseases and immune-mediated toxicity, which have been examined in patients with thymic epithelial tumors. Common COVID-19 vaccine adverse events among 54 participants in a 2021 US study included injection site pain, fatigue and headaches [80]. Among the 19 patients previously been diagnosed with paraneoplastic autoimmune disease, 3 experienced autoimmune flares after the first dose, and 3 experienced autoimmune flares after the second dose. The majority of paraneoplastic autoimmune disease flares were mild and self-limiting. Following vaccination, one patient (2%) was diagnosed with a new paraneoplastic autoimmune disease. As a result, the overall tolerability of COVID-19 mRNA vaccines in patients with thymic tumors was comparable to that of the general population [78,79].

Prioritizing these populations who will benefit the most from SARS-CoV-2 vaccination and thus have a positive impact on the pandemic's trajectory is critical. Patients with cancer, immunological disorders and close contacts should be prioritized. Customizing vaccination schedules could be one approach to developing more effective health policies based on evidence-based data. Alternative vaccine schedules are not insignificant, and they frequently affect vaccine efficacy. Similarly, adjusting the schedules to account for the risk of severe COVID-19 outcomes, as well as individuals' ability to mount and sustain an immune response, is critical [81,82].

3.2. Immune Dysregulation and Severity of COVID-19 Infection

Researchers also investigated the potential contribution of systemic autoimmune disease (SAD) to COVID-19 disease severity. For this, they investigated the prognostic impact of SAD on COVID-19 mortality in a nationwide Spanish registry study performed before the introduction of SARS-CoV-2 vaccination. The presence of SAD in COVID-19 patients was generally associated with higher mortality. However, after adjusting for patient characteristics and comorbidities, SAD did not have a statistically significant effect on mortality [83]. While case-control studies did not confirm an isolated effect of autoimmune disease on COVID-19 severity, further population-based studies implied higher mortality in SAD patients—with advanced age, male gender and comorbidities again being the relevant predictive factors [84].

The use of biologics and other immunosuppressive therapies has been a concern during the COVID-19 pandemic, as it was initially believed that these treatments could increase the risk of severe disease. However, studies have shown that the risk factors for COVID-19 hospitalization are similar in patients receiving biologics compared to the general population [85]. Treatment with biologics has not been found to affect the severity of COVID-19 [6,86]. In some cases, patients with COVID-19 were found to have autoantibodies to type I interferons, which can contribute to uncontrolled inflammation and worsen disease severity [1,5,6,16]. In patients with autoimmune diseases, the use of biologics and other immunosuppressive therapies is common. However, it is important to balance the need for disease control with the potential risk of infection. A study by Haberman et al. found that treatment with TNF inhibitors, IL-17 inhibitors, IL-23 inhibitors, IL-12 inhibitors and JAK inhibitors did not increase the risk of COVID-19 severity [87]. These cytokine inhibitors may even be beneficial in preventing endothelial toxicities and systemic complications associated with COVID-19 [87,88]. While iatrogenic immunosuppression can increase the risk of infection, it is also important to consider the potential role of autoimmunity and uncontrolled inflammation in COVID-19 severity. Inflammation and immunity play important roles in medicine, including the systemic inflammatory chronic state [89]. Therefore, interception of autoimmunity and uncontrolled inflammation may be a potential therapeutic strategy for severe COVID-19 cases [5,90,91].

Recent studies have also shown that the IL-31/IL-33 axis plays an essential role in the immune response against SARS-CoV-2. In particular, the axis is involved in the regulation of cytokine production and immune cell activation [92]. Therefore, further research is needed to investigate the potential therapeutic targets for COVID-19 using IL-31/IL-33 axis modulation. Understanding the immune response to SARS-CoV-2 in different patient populations, including cancer patients and those with immune deficiencies, is critical in developing effective treatment strategies. The impact of different viral strains on disease severity and patient outcomes should also be considered. The IL-31/IL-33 axis has emerged as a key player in the immune response against SARS-CoV-2, and further research is needed to fully understand its potential as a therapeutic target for COVID-19 [93]. In summary, while the use of biologics and other immunosuppressive therapies was a concern during the COVID-19 pandemic, studies have shown that these treatments do not increase the risk of COVID-19 severity. Additionally, in patients with autoimmune diseases, cytokine inhibitors may even be beneficial in preventing complications associated with COVID-19. The potential role of autoimmunity and uncontrolled inflammation in COVID-19 severity highlights the importance of considering these factors in therapeutic strategies. More research is needed to better understand the complex interaction between SAD and COVID-19—this is also reflected by the recent discovery of SAD—and cancer-specific antinuclear antibodies in COVID-19 patients [94]. Moreover, Böröcz et al. recently reported compound-dependent expression levels of natural autoantibodies after COVID-19 vaccination [95].

The discovery of inborn errors in type I IFN immunity in patients with life-threatening COVID-19 paved the way for further research in this area [5]. Inborn errors of immunity are an archetypical field that should be further investigated in terms of patient care and a better understanding of the host defense against SARS-CoV-2. Despite emphasizing the lack of high-quality evidence, the CDC lists primary immune deficiencies as a risk factor [19]. Immune deficiencies are listed as comorbid conditions in three large studies, but they are not further defined, and there is a lack of pre-specified iatrogenic immune-compromising conditions [96]. Focusing on B cells, Quinti et al. began with a small cohort of seven patients with antibody deficiency—two patients had agammaglobulinemia with no B cells, and five patients suffered from common variable immunodeficiency (CVID): one of seven patients died [97,98]. The two patients with agammaglobulinemia, in the authors' opinion, had a better outcome, including a shorter hospital stay, than the patients with CVID [97]. In line with this, Soresina et al. described two individuals with X-linked agammaglobulinemia, another condition characterized by the absence of B cells; both subjects developed pneumonia which was presumed to be bacterial but recovered uneventfully and did not seem to have any evidence of ARDS or any evidence of complications leading to ICU admission [98].

Based on this evidence, it is tempting to conclude that B cells can be harmful, especially considering additional evidence regarding acalabrutinib intake. Even though the study was small and uncontrolled, the authors assumed that acalabrutinib was extremely beneficial in their COVID-19 cohort [99]. Moreover, the authors proposed that the underlying mechanism could be IL-6 monocytic production, with IL-6 levels decreasing in treated patients [99], as confirmed by in silico analyses [1,100]. Nevertheless, achieving the statistical power required to corroborate conclusions about inborn errors of immunity is difficult.

Meyts et al. were the first to describe 94 patients with primary immunodeficiency (PID, IEI) and coinfection with COVID-19. Specifically, COVID-19 was found in 20–25% of IEI patients, with 75–80% developing mild SARS-CoV-2 disease [101]. IEIs, in particular, could predispose patients to more severe forms of COVID-19, with a variable, unpredictable disease course in cases of antibody deficiency. Overall, 60 patients were hospitalized with a mortality rate of 11%, comparable to the general population (between 10% and 13%). When comparing the CDC and the Meyts' cohort mortality rates, it is important to compare the age of the patients who died, as well as the per cent mortality: age is the prognostically most relevant risk factor. The key points highlight a link between age and clinical phenotype, with young kids being relatively resilient. A two-year-old with a chronic granulomatous disease that was not diagnosed had hemophagocytic lymphohistiocytosis and Burkholderia cepacia infection at the time of death; however, we do not know the precise impact of COVID-19 in this specific case [101]. The second, young combined-immune deficiency patient died from sepsis and hemophagocytic lymphohistiocytosis [101]. The underlying pathobiology was unclear. Ancillary to these examples, two patients with antibody deficiency had cardiomyopathy or lymphoma, and two subjects experienced sepsis, renal failure and heart failure as the ultimate cause of death [101], as published recently [102–104]. Moreover, two patients with antibody deficiency, lung disease and heart disease as comorbid conditions died because of sepsis and renal failure, respectively. Despite this heterogeneous cohort, a proportion of 7% HLH, 6% renal insufficiency and 4% autoimmune cytopenias are unquestionably higher than in the general population. This raises the possibility of an increased risk of autoimmune diseases, such as autoimmune cytopenias and Guillain–Barré neuropathy.

Collectively, we may pave the way for representing two major causes of death, namely HLH in younger subjects and sepsis or renal failure in older subjects [101]. Buccioli et al. confirmed these fundings. Indeed, 57% of SCID pre-HSCT and 75% of Good syndrome subjects were admitted to ICU. Subjects with the autoimmune polyendocrine syndrome type 1 (APS) behaved similarly, with 15% mortality [101]. At baseline, APS (APECED) with autoimmune polyendocrine syndrome type 1, mucocutaneous candidiasis, hypoparathyroidism and hypoadrenocorticism appear to neutralize anti-IFN antibodies (alpha or omega). FACT, rare genetic variants with compromised IFN type I immunity, reduced the production of TLR3-, MDA5- and APECED activity and reduced the cellular response to STAT1- and STAT2-signaling [105]. In these circumstances, it appears that a compromised immune response is the driving force behind more severe forms of COVID-19.

Hypersecretion of IFN-I, on the other hand, causes severe forms of Multisystem Inflammatory Syndrome in Children (MIS-C), a SOCS1-driven condition [106]. Additionally, type I IFN appears to be related to pernio (chilblains) severity in COVID-19 [107].

Other IEIs, such as X-linked agammaglobulinemia or states with reduced or absent B lymphocytes, have a lower ability to eliminate the virus with a longer duration of infection [108]. In these cases, combining monoclonal antibodies and antiviral drugs can ensure a good outcome. They are not more severe in other forms of the disease, such as phagocyte disorders, autoinflammatory diseases and hereditary angioedema.

Furthermore, data from the IPINet network's 2021 and 2022 studies on a large population of Italian subjects with IEI revealed 74 cases of SARS-CoV-2 infection in 1161 patients with CVID, with an incidence comparable to that of the general adult population. The cumulative incidence is even lower in the pediatric population [109,110]. In terms of the severity of the infection in patients with IEI (IPINet, 2021), according to age, subjects <18 years have a lower incidence of severe symptoms than older subjects, with no deaths following the infection in patients <30 years.

The mortality rate was higher in Good syndrome and Del 22q11, both associated with a T-cell defect [109,110]. Four deaths were reported in the adult age group in the IPINet, with an overall death rate from COVID-19 of 3.5% in IEI vs. 2.5% in the Italian population. The median age at death in subjects >18 years with IEI was 48 years vs. 80 years in the Italian population, with a range from 5.7% in CVID to 33% in Good syndrome. Mortality was also higher in the 50–60-year age group (14.3 vs. 0.6%). Greater comorbidities at a younger age appear to best distinguish these patients from the general population [109,110]. STAT1 alterations are no exception, potentially posing a life-threatening situation, resulting in bone marrow failure and poor outcomes [91,111]. This bone marrow failure phenotype [90,112–114] seems particularly relevant due to the possibility of targeting the JAK/STAT pathway in COVID-19 [115].

The risk factors for increased severity of COVID-19 suggest that a more severe outcome correlates with the same risk factors seen in the general population, namely the male sex and associated comorbidities, such as chronic lung disease and chronic liver disease. On the contrary, rheumatological manifestations would not affect mortality. The same factors determine the duration of the infection (2 weeks vs. 2–3 months) [116]. This may be a risk factor for viral spread.

4. Conclusions

The immunocompromised patient is an excellent candidate for an intense clinical investigation into the relationship between SARS-CoV-2 infection and host defenses. Three emerging paradigms in cancer treatment prioritization and frailty have a greater impact on the clinical outcome than cancer-related immune dysfunction. Of note, cancer-related immune dysfunction did not play a crucial role in COVID-19 disease severity in contrast to cancer-related frailty. SARS-CoV-2 infection was contracted by 20–25% of subjects with inborn errors of immunity, with 75–80% having a mild or asymptomatic clinical course. COVID-19 severity and mortality appear to be associated with comorbidities that manifest younger than the general population.

Ultimately, the COVID-19 vaccines are safe for cancer patients, but they may be less effective than in healthy people, especially those with compromised immune systems.

Author Contributions: Writing—original draft preparation, A.G.S., E.S. and M.K.; methodology, A.G.S., G.F. and M.B.; software, M.B., F.A. and M.B.; validation, M.K.; formal analysis, A.G.S., M.B., G.F. and M.K.; investigation, A.G.S., F.A. and M.K.; resources, A.G.S., F.A. and M.K.; data curation, A.G.S. and F.A.; writing—review and editing, A.G.S., G.F. and M.K.; visualization, A.G.S., F.A. and M.K.; supervision, E.S., G.F. and M.K. All authors have read and agreed to the published version of the manuscript.

Funding: This research received no external funding.

Institutional Review Board Statement: Not applicable.

Informed Consent Statement: Not applicable.

Data Availability Statement: Not applicable.

Acknowledgments: We thank Mary Victoria Pragnell, BA, at the School of Medicine and Surgery at the University of Bari. The authors acknowledge Biorender for providing comprehensive medical and biological figures and fruitful datasets for the international scientific community. Publication license n. MN24UVSCXY.

Conflicts of Interest: The authors declare no conflict of interest.

References

1. Karami, H.; Derakhshani, A.; Ghasemigol, M.; Fereidouni, M.; Miri-Moghaddam, E.; Baradaran, B.; Tabrizi, N.J.; Najafi, S.; Solimando, A.G.; Marsh, L.M.; et al. Weighted Gene Co-Expression Network Analysis Combined with Machine Learning Validation to Identify Key Modules and Hub Genes Associated with SARS-CoV-2 Infection. *J. Clin. Med.* **2021**, *10*, 3567. [CrossRef] [PubMed]
2. Abdelmoaty, M.M.; Yeapuri, P.; Machhi, J.; Olson, K.E.; Shahjin, F.; Kumar, V.; Zhou, Y.; Liang, J.; Pandey, K.; Acharya, A.; et al. Defining the Innate Immune Responses for SARS-CoV-2-Human Macrophage Interactions. *Front. Immunol.* **2021**, *12*, 741502. [CrossRef] [PubMed]
3. Yang, D.; Chu, H.; Hou, Y.; Chai, Y.; Shuai, H.; Lee, A.C.-Y.; Zhang, X.; Wang, Y.; Hu, B.; Huang, X.; et al. Attenuated Interferon and Proinflammatory Response in SARS-CoV-2-Infected Human Dendritic Cells Is Associated with Viral Antagonism of STAT1 Phosphorylation. *J. Infect. Dis.* **2020**, *222*, 734–745. [CrossRef] [PubMed]
4. Meffre, E.; Iwasaki, A. Interferon Deficiency Can Lead to Severe COVID. *Nature* **2020**, *587*, 374–376. [CrossRef]
5. Zhang, Q.; Bastard, P.; Liu, Z.; Le Pen, J.; Moncada-Velez, M.; Chen, J.; Ogishi, M.; Sabli, I.K.D.; Hodeib, S.; Korol, C.; et al. Inborn Errors of Type I IFN Immunity in Patients with Life-Threatening COVID-19. *Science* **2020**, *370*, eabd4570. [CrossRef] [PubMed]
6. Bastard, P.; Rosen, L.B.; Zhang, Q.; Michailidis, E.; Hoffmann, H.-H.; Zhang, Y.; Dorgham, K.; Philippot, Q.; Rosain, J.; Béziat, V.; et al. Autoantibodies against Type I IFNs in Patients with Life-Threatening COVID-19. *Science* **2020**, *370*, eabd4585. [CrossRef]
7. Su, H.C.; Jing, H.; Zhang, Y.; Casanova, J.-L. Interfering with Interferons: A Critical Mechanism for Critical COVID-19 Pneumonia. *Annu. Rev. Immunol.* **2023**, *41*, 561–585. [CrossRef]

8. Garcia-Beltran, W.F.; Lam, E.C.; Astudillo, M.G.; Yang, D.; Miller, T.E.; Feldman, J.; Hauser, B.M.; Caradonna, T.M.; Clayton, K.L.; Nitido, A.D.; et al. COVID-19-Neutralizing Antibodies Predict Disease Severity and Survival. *Cell* **2021**, *184*, 476–488.e11. [CrossRef]
9. Daamen, A.R.; Bachali, P.; Owen, K.A.; Kingsmore, K.M.; Hubbard, E.L.; Labonte, A.C.; Robl, R.; Shrotri, S.; Grammer, A.C.; Lipsky, P.E. Comprehensive Transcriptomic Analysis of COVID-19 Blood, Lung, and Airway. *Sci. Rep.* **2021**, *11*, 7052. [CrossRef]
10. Gardinassi, L.G.; Souza, C.O.S.; Sales-Campos, H.; Fonseca, S.G. Immune and Metabolic Signatures of COVID-19 Revealed by Transcriptomics Data Reuse. *Front. Immunol.* **2020**, *11*, 1636. [CrossRef]
11. Dwivedi, P.; Alam, S.I.; Tomar, R.S. Secretome, Surfome and Immunome: Emerging Approaches for the Discovery of New Vaccine Candidates against Bacterial Infections. *World J. Microbiol. Biotechnol.* **2016**, *32*, 155. [CrossRef] [PubMed]
12. Kuri-Cervantes, L.; Pampena, M.B.; Meng, W.; Rosenfeld, A.M.; Ittner, C.A.G.; Weisman, A.R.; Agyekum, R.S.; Mathew, D.; Baxter, A.E.; Vella, L.A.; et al. Comprehensive Mapping of Immune Perturbations Associated with Severe COVID-19. *Sci. Immunol.* **2020**, *5*, eabd7114. [CrossRef] [PubMed]
13. Tay, M.Z.; Poh, C.M.; Rénia, L.; MacAry, P.A.; Ng, L.F.P. The Trinity of COVID-19: Immunity, Inflammation and Intervention. *Nat. Rev. Immunol.* **2020**, *20*, 363–374. [CrossRef] [PubMed]
14. Randolph, H.E.; Barreiro, L.B. Herd Immunity: Understanding COVID-19. *Immunity* **2020**, *52*, 737–741. [CrossRef] [PubMed]
15. Calder, P.C. Nutrition, Immunity and COVID-19. *BMJ Nutr. Prev. Health* **2020**, *3*, 74–92. [CrossRef] [PubMed]
16. Solimando, A.G.; Susca, N.; Borrelli, P.; Prete, M.; Lauletta, G.; Pappagallo, F.; Buono, R.; Inglese, G.; Forina, B.M.; Bochicchio, D.; et al. Short-Term Variations in Neutrophil-to-Lymphocyte and Urea-to-Creatinine Ratios Anticipate Intensive Care Unit Admission of COVID-19 Patients in the Emergency Department. *Front. Med.* **2020**, *7*, 625176. [CrossRef] [PubMed]
17. Bavaro, D.F.; Diella, L.; Solimando, A.G.; Cicco, S.; Buonamico, E.; Stasi, C.; Ciannarella, M.; Marrone, M.; Carpagnano, F.; Resta, O.; et al. Bamlanivimab and Etesevimab Administered in an Outpatient Setting for SARS-CoV-2 Infection. *Pathog. Glob. Health* **2022**, 1–8. [CrossRef]
18. Chevrier, S.; Zurbuchen, Y.; Cervia, C.; Adamo, S.; Raeber, M.E.; de Souza, N.; Sivapatham, S.; Jacobs, A.; Bachli, E.; Rudiger, A.; et al. A Distinct Innate Immune Signature Marks Progression from Mild to Severe COVID-19. *Cell Rep. Med.* **2021**, *2*, 100166. [CrossRef]
19. Centers for Disease Control and Prevention Factors That Affect Your Risk of Getting Very Sick from COVID-19 2022. Available online: https://www.cdc.gov/coronavirus/2019-ncov/your-health/risks-getting-very-sick.html (accessed on 11 May 2023).
20. Caramelo, F.; Ferreira, N.; Oliveiros, B. Estimation of Risk Factors for COVID-19 Mortality—Preliminary Results. *medRxiv Epidemiology* **2020**. [CrossRef]
21. The Severe COVID-19 GWAS Group Genomewide Association Study of Severe COVID-19 with Respiratory Failure. *N. Engl. J. Med.* **2020**, *383*, 1522–1534. [CrossRef]
22. Grifoni, A.; Sidney, J.; Vita, R.; Peters, B.; Crotty, S.; Weiskopf, D.; Sette, A. SARS-CoV-2 Human T Cell Epitopes: Adaptive Immune Response against COVID-19. *Cell Host Microbe* **2021**, *29*, 1076–1092. [CrossRef] [PubMed]
23. Grifoni, A.; Weiskopf, D.; Ramirez, S.I.; Mateus, J.; Dan, J.M.; Moderbacher, C.R.; Rawlings, S.A.; Sutherland, A.; Premkumar, L.; Jadi, R.S.; et al. Targets of T Cell Responses to SARS-CoV-2 Coronavirus in Humans with COVID-19 Disease and Unexposed Individuals. *Cell* **2020**, *181*, 1489–1501.e15. [CrossRef] [PubMed]
24. Cassaniti, I.; Percivalle, E.; Bergami, F.; Piralla, A.; Comolli, G.; Bruno, R.; Vecchia, M.; Sambo, M.; Colaneri, M.; Zuccaro, V.; et al. SARS-CoV-2 Specific T-Cell Immunity in COVID-19 Convalescent Patients and Unexposed Controls Measured by Ex Vivo ELISpot Assay. *Clin. Microbiol. Infect.* **2021**, *27*, 1029–1034. [CrossRef] [PubMed]
25. Rovida, F.; Cassaniti, I.; Percivalle, E.; Sarasini, A.; Paolucci, S.; Klersy, C.; Cutti, S.; Novelli, V.; Marena, C.; Luzzaro, F.; et al. Incidence of SARS-CoV-2 Infection in Health Care Workers from Northern Italy Based on Antibody Status: Immune Protection from Secondary Infection- A Retrospective Observational Case-Controlled Study. *Int. J. Infect. Dis.* **2021**, *109*, 199–202. [CrossRef]
26. Baden, L.R.; El Sahly, H.M.; Essink, B.; Kotloff, K.; Frey, S.; Novak, R.; Diemert, D.; Spector, S.A.; Rouphael, N.; Creech, C.B.; et al. Efficacy and Safety of the MRNA-1273 SARS-CoV-2 Vaccine. *N. Engl. J. Med.* **2021**, *384*, 403–416. [CrossRef]
27. Voysey, M.; Clemens, S.A.C.; Madhi, S.A.; Weckx, L.Y.; Folegatti, P.M.; Aley, P.K.; Angus, B.; Baillie, V.L.; Barnabas, S.L.; Bhorat, Q.E.; et al. Safety and Efficacy of the ChAdOx1 NCoV-19 Vaccine (AZD1222) against SARS-CoV-2: An Interim Analysis of Four Randomised Controlled Trials in Brazil, South Africa, and the UK. *Lancet* **2021**, *397*, 99–111. [CrossRef]
28. Peng, Y.; Mentzer, A.J.; Liu, G.; Yao, X.; Yin, Z.; Dong, D.; Dejnirattisai, W.; Rostron, T.; Supasa, P.; Liu, C.; et al. Broad and Strong Memory CD4+ and CD8+ T Cells Induced by SARS-CoV-2 in UK Convalescent Individuals Following COVID-19. *Nat. Immunol.* **2020**, *21*, 1336–1345. [CrossRef]
29. Moss, P. The T Cell Immune Response against SARS-CoV-2. *Nat. Immunol.* **2022**, *23*, 186–193. [CrossRef]
30. Telenti, A.; Arvin, A.; Corey, L.; Corti, D.; Diamond, M.S.; García-Sastre, A.; Garry, R.F.; Holmes, E.C.; Pang, P.S.; Virgin, H.W. After the Pandemic: Perspectives on the Future Trajectory of COVID-19. *Nature* **2021**, *596*, 495–504. [CrossRef]
31. Callaway, E. Beyond Omicron: What's next for COVID's Viral Evolution. *Nature* **2021**, *600*, 204–207. [CrossRef]
32. Schultze, J.L.; Aschenbrenner, A.C. COVID-19 and the Human Innate Immune System. *Cell* **2021**, *184*, 1671–1692. [CrossRef] [PubMed]
33. Diamond, M.S.; Kanneganti, T.-D. Innate Immunity: The First Line of Defense against SARS-CoV-2. *Nat. Immunol.* **2022**, *23*, 165–176. [CrossRef] [PubMed]
34. Hu, B.; Huang, S.; Yin, L. The Cytokine Storm and COVID-19. *J. Med. Virol.* **2021**, *93*, 250–256. [CrossRef] [PubMed]

35. Rydyznski Moderbacher, C.; Ramirez, S.I.; Dan, J.M.; Grifoni, A.; Hastie, K.M.; Weiskopf, D.; Belanger, S.; Abbott, R.K.; Kim, C.; Choi, J.; et al. Antigen-Specific Adaptive Immunity to SARS-CoV-2 in Acute COVID-19 and Associations with Age and Disease Severity. *Cell* **2020**, *183*, 996–1012.e19. [CrossRef] [PubMed]
36. Weyand, C.M.; Goronzy, J.J. Aging of the Immune System. Mechanisms and Therapeutic Targets. *Ann. Am. Thorac. Soc.* **2016**, *13* (Suppl. 5), S422–S428. [CrossRef]
37. Nikolich-Zugich, J.; Goodrum, F.; Knox, K.; Smithey, M.J. Known Unknowns: How Might the Persistent Herpesvirome Shape Immunity and Aging? *Curr. Opin. Immunol.* **2017**, *48*, 23–30. [CrossRef]
38. Lissner, M.M.; Thomas, B.J.; Wee, K.; Tong, A.-J.; Kollmann, T.R.; Smale, S.T. Age-Related Gene Expression Differences in Monocytes from Human Neonates, Young Adults, and Older Adults. *PLoS ONE* **2015**, *10*, e0132061. [CrossRef]
39. Fasano, R.; Malerba, E.; Prete, M.; Solimando, A.G.; Buonavoglia, A.; Silvestris, N.; Leone, P.; Racanelli, V. Impact of Antigen Presentation Mechanisms on Immune Response in Autoimmune Hepatitis. *Front. Immunol.* **2021**, *12*, 814155. [CrossRef]
40. Brunetta, E.; Folci, M.; Bottazzi, B.; De Santis, M.; Gritti, G.; Protti, A.; Mapelli, S.N.; Bonovas, S.; Piovani, D.; Leone, R.; et al. Macrophage Expression and Prognostic Significance of the Long Pentraxin PTX3 in COVID-19. *Nat. Immunol.* **2021**, *22*, 19–24. [CrossRef]
41. WHO Rapid Evidence Appraisal for COVID-19 Therapies (REACT) Working Group; Sterne, J.A.C.; Murthy, S.; Diaz, J.V.; Slutsky, A.S.; Villar, J.; Angus, D.C.; Annane, D.; Azevedo, L.C.P.; Berwanger, O.; et al. Association between Administration of Systemic Corticosteroids and Mortality among Critically Ill Patients with COVID-19: A Meta-Analysis. *JAMA* **2020**, *324*, 1330–1341. [CrossRef]
42. Kalimuddin, S.; Tham, C.Y.L.; Qui, M.; de Alwis, R.; Sim, J.X.Y.; Lim, J.M.E.; Tan, H.-C.; Syenina, A.; Zhang, S.L.; Le Bert, N.; et al. Early T Cell and Binding Antibody Responses Are Associated with COVID-19 RNA Vaccine Efficacy Onset. *Med* **2021**, *2*, 682–688.e4. [CrossRef] [PubMed]
43. Dan, J.M.; Mateus, J.; Kato, Y.; Hastie, K.M.; Yu, E.D.; Faliti, C.E.; Grifoni, A.; Ramirez, S.I.; Haupt, S.; Frazier, A.; et al. Immunological Memory to SARS-CoV-2 Assessed for up to 8 Months after Infection. *Science* **2021**, *371*, eabf4063. [CrossRef]
44. Vizcarra, P.; Pérez-Elías, M.J.; Quereda, C.; Moreno, A.; Vivancos, M.J.; Dronda, F.; Casado, J.L.; COVID-19 ID Team. Description of COVID-19 in HIV-Infected Individuals: A Single-Centre, Prospective Cohort. *Lancet HIV* **2020**, *7*, e554–e564. [CrossRef] [PubMed]
45. Ho, H.-E.; Peluso, M.J.; Margus, C.; Matias Lopes, J.P.; He, C.; Gaisa, M.M.; Osorio, G.; Aberg, J.A.; Mullen, M.P. Clinical Outcomes and Immunologic Characteristics of Coronavirus Disease 2019 in People With Human Immunodeficiency Virus. *J. Infect. Dis.* **2021**, *223*, 403–408. [CrossRef] [PubMed]
46. Davies, M.-A. HIV and Risk of COVID-19 Death: A Population Cohort Study from the Western Cape Province, South Africa. *MedRxiv Prepr. Serv. Health Sci.* **2020**. [CrossRef]
47. Chenneville, T.; Gabbidon, K.; Hanson, P.; Holyfield, C. The Impact of COVID-19 on HIV Treatment and Research: A Call to Action. *Int. J. Environ. Res. Public. Health* **2020**, *17*, 4548. [CrossRef]
48. Mantovani, A.; Netea, M.G. Trained Innate Immunity, Epigenetics, and COVID-19. *N. Engl. J. Med.* **2020**, *383*, 1078–1080. [CrossRef]
49. Tregoning, J.S.; Brown, E.S.; Cheeseman, H.M.; Flight, K.E.; Higham, S.L.; Lemm, N.-M.; Pierce, B.F.; Stirling, D.C.; Wang, Z.; Pollock, K.M. Vaccines for COVID-19. *Clin. Exp. Immunol.* **2020**, *202*, 162–192. [CrossRef]
50. Cassaniti, I.; Bergami, F.; Percivalle, E.; Gabanti, E.; Sammartino, J.C.; Ferrari, A.; Adzasehoun, K.M.G.; Zavaglio, F.; Zelini, P.; Comolli, G.; et al. Humoral and Cell-Mediated Response against SARS-CoV-2 Variants Elicited by MRNA Vaccine BNT162b2 in Healthcare Workers: A Longitudinal Observational Study. *Clin. Microbiol. Infect. Off. Publ. Eur. Soc. Clin. Microbiol. Infect. Dis.* **2022**, *28*, 301.e1–301.e8. [CrossRef]
51. Mateus, J.; Dan, J.M.; Zhang, Z.; Rydyznski Moderbacher, C.; Lammers, M.; Goodwin, B.; Sette, A.; Crotty, S.; Weiskopf, D. Low-Dose MRNA-1273 COVID-19 Vaccine Generates Durable Memory Enhanced by Cross-Reactive T Cells. *Science* **2021**, *374*, eabj9853. [CrossRef]
52. Self, W.H.; Tenforde, M.W.; Rhoads, J.P.; Gaglani, M.; Ginde, A.A.; Douin, D.J.; Olson, S.M.; Talbot, H.K.; Casey, J.D.; Mohr, N.M.; et al. Comparative Effectiveness of Moderna, Pfizer-BioNTech, and Janssen (Johnson & Johnson) Vaccines in Preventing COVID-19 Hospitalizations among Adults without Immunocompromising Conditions - United States, March-August 2021. *MMWR Morb. Mortal. Wkly. Rep.* **2021**, *70*, 1337–1343. [CrossRef] [PubMed]
53. Zheng, C.; Shao, W.; Chen, X.; Zhang, B.; Wang, G.; Zhang, W. Real-World Effectiveness of COVID-19 Vaccines: A Literature Review and Meta-Analysis. *Int. J. Infect. Dis.* **2022**, *114*, 252–260. [CrossRef] [PubMed]
54. Zhang, Z.; Mateus, J.; Coelho, C.H.; Dan, J.M.; Moderbacher, C.R.; Gálvez, R.I.; Cortes, F.H.; Grifoni, A.; Tarke, A.; Chang, J.; et al. Humoral and Cellular Immune Memory to Four COVID-19 Vaccines. *Cell* **2022**, *185*, 2434–2451.e17. [CrossRef] [PubMed]
55. Tarke, A.; Sidney, J.; Methot, N.; Yu, E.D.; Zhang, Y.; Dan, J.M.; Goodwin, B.; Rubiro, P.; Sutherland, A.; Wang, E.; et al. Impact of SARS-CoV-2 Variants on the Total CD4+ and CD8+ T Cell Reactivity in Infected or Vaccinated Individuals. *Cell Rep. Med.* **2021**, *2*, 100355. [CrossRef] [PubMed]
56. Yang, K.; Sheng, Y.; Huang, C.; Jin, Y.; Xiong, N.; Jiang, K.; Lu, H.; Liu, J.; Yang, J.; Dong, Y.; et al. Clinical Characteristics, Outcomes, and Risk Factors for Mortality in Patients with Cancer and COVID-19 in Hubei, China: A Multicentre, Retrospective, Cohort Study. *Lancet Oncol.* **2020**, *21*, 904–913. [CrossRef]

57. Tian, J.; Yuan, X.; Xiao, J.; Zhong, Q.; Yang, C.; Liu, B.; Cai, Y.; Lu, Z.; Wang, J.; Wang, Y.; et al. Clinical Characteristics and Risk Factors Associated with COVID-19 Disease Severity in Patients with Cancer in Wuhan, China: A Multicentre, Retrospective, Cohort Study. *Lancet Oncol.* **2020**, *21*, 893–903. [CrossRef]
58. Zhang, L.; Zhu, F.; Xie, L.; Wang, C.; Wang, J.; Chen, R.; Jia, P.; Guan, H.Q.; Peng, L.; Chen, Y.; et al. Clinical Characteristics of COVID-19-Infected Cancer Patients: A Retrospective Case Study in Three Hospitals within Wuhan, China. *Ann. Oncol. Off. J. Eur. Soc. Med. Oncol.* **2020**, *31*, 894–901. [CrossRef]
59. Vuagnat, P.; Frelaut, M.; Ramtohul, T.; Basse, C.; Diakite, S.; Noret, A.; Bellesoeur, A.; Servois, V.; Hequet, D.; Laas, E.; et al. COVID-19 in Breast Cancer Patients: A Cohort at the Institut Curie Hospitals in the Paris Area. *Breast Cancer Res. BCR* **2020**, *22*, 55. [CrossRef]
60. Assaad, S.; Avrillon, V.; Fournier, M.-L.; Mastroianni, B.; Russias, B.; Swalduz, A.; Cassier, P.; Eberst, L.; Steineur, M.-P.; Kazes, M.; et al. High Mortality Rate in Cancer Patients with Symptoms of COVID-19 with or without Detectable SARS-CoV-2 on RT-PCR. *Eur. J. Cancer Oxf. Engl. 1990* **2020**, *135*, 251–259. [CrossRef]
61. Kuderer, N.M.; Choueiri, T.K.; Shah, D.P.; Shyr, Y.; Rubinstein, S.M.; Rivera, D.R.; Shete, S.; Hsu, C.-Y.; Desai, A.; de Lima Lopes, G.; et al. Clinical Impact of COVID-19 on Patients with Cancer (CCC19): A Cohort Study. *Lancet* **2020**, *395*, 1907–1918. [CrossRef]
62. Garassino, M.C.; Whisenant, J.G.; Huang, L.-C.; Trama, A.; Torri, V.; Agustoni, F.; Baena, J.; Banna, G.; Berardi, R.; Bettini, A.C.; et al. COVID-19 in Patients with Thoracic Malignancies (TERAVOLT): First Results of an International, Registry-Based, Cohort Study. *Lancet Oncol.* **2020**, *21*, 914–922. [CrossRef]
63. Boulad, F.; Kamboj, M.; Bouvier, N.; Mauguen, A.; Kung, A.L. COVID-19 in Children with Cancer in New York City. *JAMA Oncol.* **2020**, *6*, 1459–1460. [CrossRef]
64. Miyashita, H.; Mikami, T.; Chopra, N.; Yamada, T.; Chernyavsky, S.; Rizk, D.; Cruz, C. Do Patients with Cancer Have a Poorer Prognosis of COVID-19? An Experience in New York City. *Ann. Oncol.* **2020**, *31*, 1088–1089. [CrossRef] [PubMed]
65. Lisco, G.; De Tullio, A.; Stragapede, A.; Solimando, A.G.; Albanese, F.; Capobianco, M.; Giagulli, V.A.; Guastamacchia, E.; De Pergola, G.; Vacca, A.; et al. COVID-19 and the Endocrine System: A Comprehensive Review on the Theme. *J. Clin. Med.* **2021**, *10*, 2920. [CrossRef]
66. Solimando, A.G.; Crudele, L.; Leone, P.; Argentiero, A.; Guarascio, M.; Silvestris, N.; Vacca, A.; Racanelli, V. Immune Checkpoint Inhibitor-Related Myositis: From Biology to Bedside. *Int. J. Mol. Sci.* **2020**, *21*, 3054. [CrossRef] [PubMed]
67. Lasagna, A.; Agustoni, F.; Percivalle, E.; Borgetto, S.; Paulet, A.; Comolli, G.; Sarasini, A.; Bergami, F.; Sammartino, J.C.; Ferrari, A.; et al. A Snapshot of the Immunogenicity, Efficacy and Safety of a Full Course of BNT162b2 Anti-SARS-CoV-2 Vaccine in Cancer Patients Treated with PD-1/PD-L1 Inhibitors: A Longitudinal Cohort Study. *ESMO Open* **2021**, *6*, 100272. [CrossRef] [PubMed]
68. De Gasparo, R.; Pedotti, M.; Simonelli, L.; Nickl, P.; Muecksch, F.; Cassaniti, I.; Percivalle, E.; Lorenzi, J.C.C.; Mazzola, F.; Magrì, D.; et al. Bispecific IgG Neutralizes SARS-CoV-2 Variants and Prevents Escape in Mice. *Nature* **2021**, *593*, 424–428. [CrossRef]
69. Marra, A.; Generali, D.; Zagami, P.; Cervoni, V.; Gandini, S.; Venturini, S.; Morganti, S.; Passerini, R.; Orecchia, R.; Curigliano, G. Seroconversion in Patients with Cancer and Oncology Health Care Workers Infected by SARS-CoV-2. *Ann. Oncol.* **2021**, *32*, 113–119. [CrossRef]
70. Kamar, N.; Abravanel, F.; Marion, O.; Couat, C.; Izopet, J.; Del Bello, A. Three Doses of an MRNA COVID-19 Vaccine in Solid-Organ Transplant Recipients. *N. Engl. J. Med.* **2021**, *385*, 661–662. [CrossRef]
71. Yasin, A.I.; Aydin, S.G.; Sümbül, B.; Koral, L.; Şimşek, M.; Geredeli, Ç.; Öztürk, A.; Perkin, P.; Demirtaş, D.; Erdemoglu, E.; et al. Efficacy and Safety Profile of COVID-19 Vaccine in Cancer Patients: A Prospective, Multicenter Cohort Study. *Future Oncol. Lond. Engl.* **2022**, *18*, 1235–1244. [CrossRef]
72. Iacono, D.; Cerbone, L.; Palombi, L.; Cavalieri, E.; Sperduti, I.; Cocchiara, R.A.; Mariani, B.; Parisi, G.; Garufi, C. Serological Response to COVID-19 Vaccination in Patients with Cancer Older than 80 Years. *J. Geriatr. Oncol.* **2021**, *12*, 1253–1255. [CrossRef] [PubMed]
73. Yang, W.; Zhang, D.; Li, Z.; Zhang, K. Predictors of Poor Serologic Response to COVID-19 Vaccine in Patients with Cancer: A Systematic Review and Meta-Analysis. *Eur. J. Cancer Oxf. Engl. 1990* **2022**, *172*, 41–50. [CrossRef] [PubMed]
74. Shahid, Z.; Patrick, A.L.; Wallander, M.L.; Donahue, E.E.; Trufan, S.J.; Tan, A.R.; Hwang, J.J.; Burgess, E.F.; Ragon, B.; Ghosh, N.; et al. COVID-19 Vaccine Uptake Trends in SARS-CoV-2 Previously Infected Cancer Patients. *Vaccine X* **2023**, *14*, 100289. [CrossRef] [PubMed]
75. Mai, A.S.; Lee, A.R.Y.B.; Tay, R.Y.K.; Shapiro, L.; Thakkar, A.; Halmos, B.; Grinshpun, A.; Herishanu, Y.; Benjamini, O.; Tadmor, T.; et al. Booster Doses of COVID-19 Vaccines for Patients with Haematological and Solid Cancer: A Systematic Review and Individual Patient Data Meta-Analysis. *Eur. J. Cancer Oxf. Engl. 1990* **2022**, *172*, 65–75. [CrossRef] [PubMed]
76. Javadinia, S.A.; Alizadeh, K.; Mojadadi, M.-S.; Nikbakht, F.; Dashti, F.; Joudi, M.; Harati, H.; Welsh, J.S.; Farahmand, S.A.; Attarian, F. COVID-19 Vaccination in Patients With Malignancy; A Systematic Review and Meta-Analysis of the Efficacy and Safety. *Front. Endocrinol.* **2022**, *13*, 860238. [CrossRef]
77. Desantis, V.; Saltarella, I.; Lamanuzzi, A.; Melaccio, A.; Solimando, A.G.; Mariggiò, M.A.; Racanelli, V.; Paradiso, A.; Vacca, A.; Frassanito, M.A. MicroRNAs-Based Nano-Strategies as New Therapeutic Approach in Multiple Myeloma to Overcome Disease Progression and Drug Resistance. *Int. J. Mol. Sci.* **2020**, *21*, 3084. [CrossRef]

78. Vacca, A.; Melaccio, A.; Sportelli, A.; Solimando, A.G.; Dammacco, F.; Ria, R. Subcutaneous Immunoglobulins in Patients with Multiple Myeloma and Secondary Hypogammaglobulinemia: A Randomized Trial. *Clin. Immunol. Orlando Fla* **2018**, *191*, 110–115. [CrossRef]
79. Gavriatopoulou, M.; Terpos, E.; Malandrakis, P.; Ntanasis-Stathopoulos, I.; Briasoulis, A.; Gumeni, S.; Fotiou, D.; Papanagnou, E.-D.; Migkou, M.; Theodorakakou, F.; et al. Myeloma Patients with COVID-19 Have Superior Antibody Responses Compared to Patients Fully Vaccinated with the BNT162b2 Vaccine. *Br. J. Haematol.* **2022**, *196*, 356–359. [CrossRef]
80. Ballman, M.; Swift, S.; Mullenix, C.; Mallory, Y.; Zhao, C.; Szabo, E.; Shelat, M.; Sansone, S.; Steinberg, S.M.; McAdams, M.J.; et al. Tolerability of Coronavirus Disease 2019 Vaccines, BNT162b2 and MRNA-1273, in Patients with Thymic Epithelial Tumors. *JTO Clin. Res. Rep.* **2021**, *2*, 100229. [CrossRef]
81. Trapani, D.; Curigliano, G. COVID-19 Vaccines in Patients with Cancer. *Lancet Oncol.* **2021**, *22*, 738–739. [CrossRef]
82. Shahini, E.; Pesce, F.; Argentiero, A.; Solimando, A.G. Can Vitamin D Status Influence Seroconversion to SARS-CoV2 Vaccines? *Front. Immunol.* **2022**, *13*, 1038316. [CrossRef] [PubMed]
83. Moreno-Torres, V.; De Mendoza, C.; Mellor-Pita, S.; Martínez-Urbistondo, M.; Durán-del Campo, P.; Tutor-Ureta, P.; Vázquez-Comendador, J.-M.; Calderón-Parra, J.; Múñez-Rubio, E.; Ramos-Martínez, A.; et al. Systemic Autoimmune Diseases in Patients Hospitalized with COVID-19 in Spain: A Nation-Wide Registry Study. *Viruses* **2022**, *14*, 1631. [CrossRef] [PubMed]
84. Brito-Zerón, P.; Sisó-Almirall, A.; Flores-Chavez, A.; Retamozo, S.; Ramos-Casals, M. SARS-CoV-2 Infection in Patients with Systemic Autoimmune Diseases. *Clin. Exp. Rheumatol.* **2021**, *39*, 676–687. [CrossRef] [PubMed]
85. Gianfrancesco, M.; Yazdany, J.; Robinson, P.C. Epidemiology and Outcomes of Novel Coronavirus 2019 in Patients with Immune-Mediated Inflammatory Diseases. *Curr. Opin. Rheumatol.* **2020**, *32*, 434–440. [CrossRef] [PubMed]
86. Gianfrancesco, M.; Hyrich, K.L.; Al-Adely, S.; Carmona, L.; Danila, M.I.; Gossec, L.; Izadi, Z.; Jacobsohn, L.; Katz, P.; Lawson-Tovey, S.; et al. Characteristics Associated with Hospitalisation for COVID-19 in People with Rheumatic Disease: Data from the COVID-19 Global Rheumatology Alliance Physician-Reported Registry. *Ann. Rheum. Dis.* **2020**, *79*, 859–866. [CrossRef]
87. Haberman, R.H.; Um, S.; Axelrad, J.E.; Blank, R.B.; Uddin, Z.; Catron, S.; Neimann, A.L.; Mulligan, M.J.; Herat, R.S.; Hong, S.J.; et al. Methotrexate and TNF Inhibitors Affect Long-Term Immunogenicity to COVID-19 Vaccination in Patients with Immune-Mediated Inflammatory Disease. *Lancet Rheumatol.* **2022**, *4*, e384–e387. [CrossRef]
88. Quartuccio, L.; Valent, F.; Pasut, E.; Tascini, C.; De Vita, S. Prevalence of COVID-19 among Patients with Chronic Inflammatory Rheumatic Diseases Treated with Biologic Agents or Small Molecules: A Population-Based Study in the First Two Months of COVID-19 Outbreak in Italy. *Joint Bone Spine* **2020**, *87*, 439–443. [CrossRef]
89. Kotas, M.E.; Medzhitov, R. Homeostasis, Inflammation, and Disease Susceptibility. *Cell* **2015**, *160*, 816–827. [CrossRef]
90. Solimando, A.G.; Vacca, A.; Ribatti, D. Inborn Error of Immunity: A Journey Through Novel Genes and Clinical Presentation. In *Encyclopedia of Infection and Immunity*; Elsevier: Amsterdam, The Netherlands, 2022; pp. 798–818. ISBN 978-0-323-90303-5.
91. Solimando, A.G.; Desantis, V.; Palumbo, C.; Marasco, C.; Pappagallo, F.; Montagnani, M.; Ingravallo, G.; Cicco, S.; Di Paola, R.; Tabares, P.; et al. STAT1 Overexpression Triggers Aplastic Anemia: A Pilot Study Unravelling Novel Pathogenetic Insights in Bone Marrow Failure. *Clin. Exp. Med.* **2023**. [CrossRef]
92. Murdaca, G.; Paladin, F.; Tonacci, A.; Borro, M.; Greco, M.; Gerosa, A.; Isola, S.; Allegra, A.; Gangemi, S. Involvement of Il-33 in the Pathogenesis and Prognosis of Major Respiratory Viral Infections: Future Perspectives for Personalized Therapy. *Biomedicines* **2022**, *10*, 715. [CrossRef]
93. Murdaca, G.; Greco, M.; Tonacci, A.; Negrini, S.; Borro, M.; Puppo, F.; Gangemi, S. IL-33/IL-31 Axis in Immune-Mediated and Allergic Diseases. *Int. J. Mol. Sci.* **2019**, *20*, 5856. [CrossRef] [PubMed]
94. Bossuyt, X.; Vulsteke, J.-B.; Van Elslande, J.; Boon, L.; Wuyts, G.; Willebrords, S.; Frans, G.; Geukens, N.; Carpentier, S.; Tejpar, S.; et al. Antinuclear Antibodies in Individuals with COVID-19 Reflect Underlying Disease: Identification of New Autoantibodies in Systemic Sclerosis (CDK9) and Malignancy (RNF20, RCC1, TRIP13). *Autoimmun. Rev.* **2023**, *22*, 103288. [CrossRef]
95. Böröcz, K.; Kinyó, Á.; Simon, D.; Erdő-Bonyár, S.; Németh, P.; Berki, T. Complexity of the Immune Response Elicited by Different COVID-19 Vaccines, in the Light of Natural Autoantibodies and Immunomodulatory Therapies. *Int. J. Mol. Sci.* **2023**, *24*, 6439. [CrossRef] [PubMed]
96. Gao, Y.; Chen, Y.; Liu, M.; Shi, S.; Tian, J. Impacts of Immunosuppression and Immunodeficiency on COVID-19: A Systematic Review and Meta-Analysis. *J. Infect.* **2020**, *81*, e93–e95. [CrossRef] [PubMed]
97. Quinti, I.; Lougaris, V.; Milito, C.; Cinetto, F.; Pecoraro, A.; Mezzaroma, I.; Mastroianni, C.M.; Turriziani, O.; Bondioni, M.P.; Filippini, M.; et al. A Possible Role for B Cells in COVID-19? Lesson from Patients with Agammaglobulinemia. *J. Allergy Clin. Immunol.* **2020**, *146*, 211–213.e4. [CrossRef]
98. Soresina, A.; Moratto, D.; Chiarini, M.; Paolillo, C.; Baresi, G.; Focà, E.; Bezzi, M.; Baronio, B.; Giacomelli, M.; Badolato, R. Two X-Linked Agammaglobulinemia Patients Develop Pneumonia as COVID-19 Manifestation but Recover. *Pediatr. Allergy Immunol. Off. Publ. Eur. Soc. Pediatr. Allergy Immunol.* **2020**, *31*, 565–569. [CrossRef] [PubMed]
99. Roschewski, M.; Lionakis, M.S.; Sharman, J.P.; Roswarski, J.; Goy, A.; Monticelli, M.A.; Roshon, M.; Wrzesinski, S.H.; Desai, J.V.; Zarakas, M.A.; et al. Inhibition of Bruton Tyrosine Kinase in Patients with Severe COVID-19. *Sci. Immunol.* **2020**, *5*, eabd0110. [CrossRef]
100. Jenner, A.L.; Aogo, R.A.; Alfonso, S.; Crowe, V.; Deng, X.; Smith, A.P.; Morel, P.A.; Davis, C.L.; Smith, A.M.; Craig, M. COVID-19 Virtual Patient Cohort Suggests Immune Mechanisms Driving Disease Outcomes. *PLoS Pathog.* **2021**, *17*, e1009753. [CrossRef]

101. Meyts, I.; Bucciol, G.; Quinti, I.; Neven, B.; Fischer, A.; Seoane, E.; Lopez-Granados, E.; Gianelli, C.; Robles-Marhuenda, A.; Jeandel, P.-Y.; et al. Coronavirus Disease 2019 in Patients with Inborn Errors of Immunity: An International Study. *J. Allergy Clin. Immunol.* **2021**, *147*, 520–531. [CrossRef]
102. Solimando, A.G.; Annese, T.; Tamma, R.; Ingravallo, G.; Maiorano, E.; Vacca, A.; Specchia, G.; Ribatti, D. New Insights into Diffuse Large B-Cell Lymphoma Pathobiology. *Cancers* **2020**, *12*, 1869. [CrossRef]
103. Shadbad, M.A.; Safaei, S.; Brunetti, O.; Derakhshani, A.; Lotfinejad, P.; Mokhtarzadeh, A.; Hemmat, N.; Racanelli, V.; Solimando, A.G.; Argentiero, A.; et al. A Systematic Review on the Therapeutic Potentiality of PD-L1-Inhibiting MicroRNAs for Triple-Negative Breast Cancer: Toward Single-Cell Sequencing-Guided Biomimetic Delivery. *Genes* **2021**, *12*, 1206. [CrossRef] [PubMed]
104. Susca, N.; Solimando, A.G.; Borrelli, P.; Marziliano, D.; Monitillo, F.; Raimondo, P.; Vestito, D.; Lopizzo, A.; Brindicci, G.; Abumayyaleh, M.; et al. Electrocardiographic Pathological Findings Caused by the SARS-CoV-2 Virus Infection: Evidence from a Retrospective Multicenter International Cohort Longitudinal Pilot Study of 548 Subjects. *J. Cardiovasc. Dev. Dis.* **2023**, *10*, 58. [CrossRef] [PubMed]
105. Gray, P.E.; Bartlett, A.W.; Tangye, S.G. Severe COVID-19 Represents an Undiagnosed Primary Immunodeficiency in a High Proportion of Infected Individuals. *Clin. Transl. Immunol.* **2022**, *11*, e1365. [CrossRef]
106. Cazzato, G.; Cascardi, E.; Colagrande, A.; Foti, C.; Stellacci, A.; Marrone, M.; Ingravallo, G.; Arezzo, F.; Loizzi, V.; Solimando, A.G.; et al. SARS-CoV-2 and Skin: New Insights and Perspectives. *Biomolecules* **2022**, *12*, 1212. [CrossRef]
107. Solimando, A.G.; Marziliano, D.; Ribatti, D. SARS-CoV-2 and Endothelial Cells: Vascular Changes, Intussusceptive Microvascular Growth and Novel Therapeutic Windows. *Biomedicines* **2022**, *10*, 2242. [CrossRef] [PubMed]
108. Brown, L.-A.K.; Moran, E.; Goodman, A.; Baxendale, H.; Bermingham, W.; Buckland, M.; AbdulKhaliq, I.; Jarvis, H.; Hunter, M.; Karanam, S.; et al. Treatment of Chronic or Relapsing COVID-19 in Immunodeficiency. *J. Allergy Clin. Immunol.* **2022**, *149*, 557–561.e1. [CrossRef]
109. Milito, C.; Lougaris, V.; Giardino, G.; Punziano, A.; Vultaggio, A.; Carrabba, M.; Cinetto, F.; Scarpa, R.; Delle Piane, R.M.; Baselli, L.; et al. Clinical Outcome, Incidence, and SARS-CoV-2 Infection-Fatality Rates in Italian Patients with Inborn Errors of Immunity. *J. Allergy Clin. Immunol. Pract.* **2021**, *9*, 2904–2906.e2. [CrossRef]
110. Giardino, G.; Milito, C.; Lougaris, V.; Punziano, A.; Carrabba, M.; Cinetto, F.; Scarpa, R.; Dellepiane, R.M.; Ricci, S.; Rivalta, B.; et al. The Impact of SARS-CoV-2 Infection in Patients with Inborn Errors of Immunity: The Experience of the Italian Primary Immunodeficiencies Network (IPINet). *J. Clin. Immunol.* **2022**, *42*, 935–946. [CrossRef]
111. Rosenberg, J.M.; Peters, J.M.; Hughes, T.; Lareau, C.A.; Ludwig, L.S.; Massoth, L.R.; Austin-Tse, C.; Rehm, H.L.; Bryson, B.; Chen, Y.-B.; et al. JAK Inhibition in a Patient with a STAT1 Gain-of-Function Variant Reveals STAT1 Dysregulation as a Common Feature of Aplastic Anemia. *Med* **2022**, *3*, 42–57.e5. [CrossRef]
112. Fattizzo, B.; Kulasekararaj, A.G.; Hill, A.; Benson-Quarm, N.; Griffin, M.; Munir, T.; Arnold, L.; Riley, K.; Ireland, R.; De Lavallade, H.; et al. Clinical and Morphological Predictors of Outcome in Older Aplastic Anemia Patients Treated with Eltrombopag. *Haematologica* **2019**, *104*, e494–e496. [CrossRef]
113. Argentiero, A.; Solimando, A.G.; Brunetti, O.; Calabrese, A.; Pantano, F.; Iuliani, M.; Santini, D.; Silvestris, N.; Vacca, A. Skeletal Metastases of Unknown Primary: Biological Landscape and Clinical Overview. *Cancers* **2019**, *11*, 1270. [CrossRef] [PubMed]
114. Notarangelo, L.D. Primary Immunodeficiencies (PIDs) Presenting with Cytopenias. *Hematol. Am. Soc. Hematol. Educ. Program* **2009**, 139–143. [CrossRef] [PubMed]
115. Ferrarini, A.; Vacca, A.; Solimando, A.G.; Tavio, M.; Acquaviva, R.; Rocchi, M.; Nitti, C.; Salvi, A.; Menditto, V.; Luchetti Gentiloni, M.M.; et al. Early Administration of Tofacitinib in COVID-19 Pneumonitis: An Open Randomised Controlled Trial. *Eur. J. Clin. Invest.* **2022**, *53*, e13898. [CrossRef] [PubMed]
116. Shields, A.M.; Burns, S.O.; Savic, S.; Richter, A.G.; Anantharachagan, A.; Arumugakani, G.; Baker, K.; Bahal, S.; Bermingham, W.; Bhole, M.; et al. COVID-19 in Patients with Primary and Secondary Immunodeficiency: The United Kingdom Experience. *J. Allergy Clin. Immunol.* **2021**, *147*, 870–875.e1. [CrossRef] [PubMed]

International Journal of
Molecular Sciences

MDPI

Review

Thrombotic Mechanism Involving Platelet Activation, Hypercoagulability and Hypofibrinolysis in Coronavirus Disease 2019

Hideo Wada [1,*], Katsuya Shiraki [1], Hideto Shimpo [2], Motomu Shimaoka [3], Toshiaki Iba [4] and Katsue Suzuki-Inoue [5]

1 Department of General and Laboratory Medicine, Mie Prefectural General Medical Center, Yokkaichi 5450-132, Japan; katsuya-shiraki@mie-gmc.jp
2 Mie Prefectural General Medical Center, Yokkaichi 5450-132, Japan; hideto-shimpo@mie-gmc.jp
3 Department of Molecular Pathobiology and Cell Adhesion Biology, Mie University Graduate School of Medicine, Tsu 514-0001, Japan; motomushimaoka@gmail.com
4 Department of Emergency and Disaster Medicine, Juntendo University Graduate School of Medicine, Tokyo 113-8431, Japan; toshiiba@juntendo.ac.jp
5 Department of Clinical and Laboratory Medicine, Yamanashi Medical University, Yamanashi 409-3821, Japan; katsuei@yamanashi.ac.jp
* Correspondence: wadahide@clin.medic.mie-u.ac.jp; Tel.: +81-59-345-2321

Abstract: Coronavirus disease 2019 (COVID-19) has spread, with thrombotic complications being increasingly frequently reported. Although thrombosis is frequently complicated in septic patients, there are some differences in the thrombosis noted with COVID-19 and that noted with bacterial infections. The incidence (6–26%) of thrombosis varied among reports in patients with COVID-19; the incidences of venous thromboembolism and acute arterial thrombosis were 4.8–21.0% and 0.7–3.7%, respectively. Although disseminated intravascular coagulation (DIC) is frequently associated with bacterial infections, a few cases of DIC have been reported in association with COVID-19. Fibrin-related markers, such as D-dimer levels, are extremely high in bacterial infections, whereas soluble C-type lectin-like receptor 2 (sCLEC-2) levels are high in COVID-19, suggesting that hypercoagulable and hyperfibrinolytic states are predominant in bacterial infections, whereas hypercoagulable and hypofibrinolytic states with platelet activation are predominant in COVID-19. Marked platelet activation, hypercoagulability and hypofibrinolytic states may cause thrombosis in patients with COVID-19.

Keywords: COVID-19; bacterial infection; thrombosis; platelet activation; sCLEC-2; hypofibrinolytic state

Citation: Wada, H.; Shiraki, K.; Shimpo, H.; Shimaoka, M.; Iba, T.; Suzuki-Inoue, K. Thrombotic Mechanism Involving Platelet Activation, Hypercoagulability and Hypofibrinolysis in Coronavirus Disease 2019. *Int. J. Mol. Sci.* **2023**, *24*, 7975. https://doi.org/10.3390/ijms24097975

Academic Editors: Eliza Russu, Alexandru Schiopu and Emil Marian Arbănași

Received: 7 April 2023
Revised: 26 April 2023
Accepted: 26 April 2023
Published: 28 April 2023

1. Introduction

Coronavirus disease 2019 (COVID-19) has spread worldwide from China [1,2], resulting in a pandemic [3]. It was previously reported that approximately 2% of patients with COVID-19 died, and 5–10% developed severe and life-threatening acute respiratory distress syndrome (ARDS) [4–6], with many more patients developing COVID-19 developing mild or moderate illness [7,8]. Following the appearance of the omicron variants of COVID-19 [9], the mortality rate was reduced, but the incidence of infections markedly increased, resulting in a relative increase in deaths. Therefore the management of complications of COVID-19 has become increasingly important.

2. Macrothrombotic Complications

The relationship between COVID-19 and thrombosis including venous thromboembolism (VTE) [10], such as pulmonary embolism (PE), and deep vein thrombosis (DVT) and arterial thrombosis, such as acute cerebral infarction (ACI) [11] and acute coronary syndrome (ACS) [12], has attracted attention [13]. On the other hand, many reports on thrombotic complications, such as disseminated intravascular coagulation (DIC) [14] and thrombotic microangiopathy (TMA) [15] have been previously reported in severe sepsis due to bacterial infection. A soluble C-type lectin-like receptor 2 (sCLEC-2) assay has been recently developed as a biomarker for platelet activation [16–18].

We herein review, based on a large number of reports, the mechanism underlying the development of thrombosis in COVID-19, which differs from that in bacterial infection.

3. Incidence of Macrothrombotic Complications in COVID-19

There have been many reports on macrothrombosis, such as VTE, ACS and ACI, in general, and the incidence of all thrombosis has varied substantially (6–26%) among patients with COVID-19 [19] (Table 1).

3.1. VTE

There have been many systematic reviews and meta-analyses concerning VTE [10,19–21], and the incidence of VTE, including DVT with PE and DVT, has been reported to vary in COVID-19. VTE was reportedly found more frequently in patients who were admitted to the intensive-care unit (ICU) than in those not admitted to the ICU. More than half of COVID-19 patients with PE (57.6%) lacked DVT [20], suggesting that some cases of PE might be caused by vascular injury instead of embolism. The incidence of VTE was higher when assessed according to screening or prospective studies [10] and postmortem studies [21] than in retrospective studies. These findings suggest that the incidence of VTE is high but varies depending on the incidence and severity of COVID-19, the age and race of patients, and the details of hospitalization and prophylaxis.

3.2. Arterial Thrombosis

The incidence of arterial thrombosis was low (0.7–3.7%) in overall patients [20,21] and 5% among ICU admissions [21]. The frequency of ACS in patients with COVID-19 was 1.0% in overall patients and 6.0–33.0% in cases of severe disease [12,22]. A review of cardiac autopsy cases of COVID-19 found that the most common comorbidities were coronary artery disease (33%) and acute ischemia (8%) [23]. A higher mortality rate among patients with COVID-19 and ST-segment elevation myocardial infarction (STEMI) was noted in comparison to previous studies, with reported concerns being late presentation due to fear of infection, delayed care time, and poor resource allocation [24].

On the neuroimaging of COVID-19 patients, especially critically ill patients, 3.4% of patients showed COVID-19-related neuroimaging findings [25,26], such as white matter abnormalities, followed by acute/subacute ischemic infarction and encephalopathy. The incidence of ACI in patients with COVID-19 is low (0.4–1.3%) [11,26–28]. The risk factors for ACS and ACI in patients with COVID-19 include old age, hypertension, diabetes mellitus, coronary artery disease, and severe infection [11,28]. Accurately diagnosing arterial thrombosis is difficult in COVID-19 patients with critical illnesses and there are no routine markers for ACI (such as D-dimer for VTE), which suggests that the true incidence of arterial thrombosis may be increased in COVID-19.

Table 1. Pooled incidence and thromboembolism in patients with COVID-19 infections.

	ICU+Non-ICU	ICU	Non-ICU	Japan
		Pooled incidence (%)		
TH	6–26 [19]	—	—	1.86 [22]
PE	7.1–16.5 [10,20,21]	19.0–24.7 [20,21]	10.5–19.0 [20,21]	0.5 [22]
DVT	12.1–20.0 [10,20,21]	28.0 [21]	—	0.7 [22]
VTE	17.0–21.0 [10,21]	4.8–31.0 [10,19,21]	1.5–46.1 [10,19]	1.2 [22]
ACI	0.4–1.3 [11,22,29,30]	—	—	0.4 [22]
ACS	1.0 [12]	6–33 [23]	—	0.1 [22]

TH, thrombosis; PE, pulmonary embolism; DVT, deep vein thrombosis; TE, thromboembolism; ACI, acute cerebral infarction; ACS. Acute coronary thrombosis, DIC, disseminated intravascular coagulation; COVID-19; coronavirus disease 2019; ICU, intensive-care unit; Reference [10] Jiménez D et al.: 48 studies with 18,093 patients; [11] Nannoni S et al.: 61 studies with 108,571 patients; [12] Zhao YH et al.: 2277 articles with 108,571 patients; [19] Cheng NM et al.: 68 studies; [20] Suh YJ et al.; 27 studies with 3342 patients; [21] Malas MB et al.: 42 studies with 8271 patients; [22] Peiris S et al.: 63 studies; [23] Roshdy A et al.: 316 cases; [26] Kim PH et al.: 17 studies with 1394; [27] Horiuchi H et al.: one questionnaire with 5807 patients; [28] Qureshi AI et al.: 8163 patients; [29] Xiao, D. et al.: systemic review. [30] Pepera, G. et al.; systemic review.

3.3. *Mortality*

The pooled mortality rate among patients with all types of thrombosis was 23%, while that among patients without any types of thrombosis was 13%. The pooled odds of mortality were 74% higher among patients who developed thrombosis than among those who did not [21]. A systematic review of reports on COVID-19 demonstrated that thrombosis increased the risk of mortality by 161% and the risk of a critical status by 190% [29]. In addition, preexisting cerebrovascular diseases (CVDs) were linked to poor outcomes and an increased risk of death in patients with COVID-19 [30].

3.4. *After Discharge*

The incidence of events in patients with COVID-19 after discharge was 1.55% for VTE, 0.45% for acute CVD, 0.49% for ACS, 0.77% for other arterial thromboses and 1.73% for major bleeding [31]. In an analysis of patients with and without COVID-19, the incidence of ACI was 1.3% in those with COVID-19 and 1.0% in those without COVID-19, suggesting that the risk of thrombosis continues after discharge and that the management of comorbidities is important for patients with COVID-19. ACI usually occurs in the presence of other cardiovascular risk factors and is associated with a twofold increase in the risk of long hospitalization or death in patients with COVID-19 [28].

3.5. *Asia including Japan*

The incidence of acute CVD in patients with COVID-19 was shown to be higher in Asia (3.1%) than in Europe (1.1%) and North America (1.1%) [11]. A questionnaire on COVID-19-related thrombosis in 6202 patients hospitalized in Japan showed that thrombotic events occurred in 1.86% of the 5807 patients with available data including symptomatic ACI (0.4%), AMI (0.1%), DVT (0.7%), PE (0.5%), and other thrombotic events (0.4%) [27], suggesting that the frequency of VTE is low in Japan due to the low incidence and severity of COVID-19 and sufficient prophylaxis with heparin.

3.6. *Variety of Severity and Complications of Thrombosis in COVID-19*

There are large differences in severity or mortality among the COVID-19 variants. Furthermore, an increased number of patients causes an increase in severe patients with COVID-19. The level of the medical system, such as bed numbers for COVID-19, quality of ICU, medical insurance and medication, can decrease mortality or thrombotic complications. Although high mortality was observed in 2019, low mortality due to COVID-19 was observed in 2023. As many factors affect mortality or complications of thrombosis in patients with COVID-19, the evaluation of thrombosis in COVID-19 should be carefully performed (Figure 1).

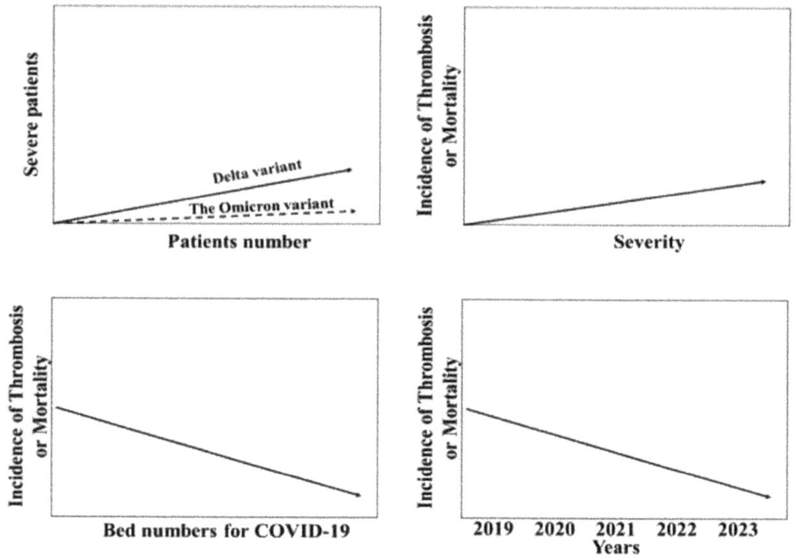

Figure 1. Variety of severity and complications of thrombosis in COVID-19.

4. Microangiopathy as DIC and TMA in COVID-19 and Other Infections

4.1. DIC

Although the relationship between DIC and COVID-19 has sometimes been reviewed [32], few systematic reviews have been conducted and the incidence of typical DIC in patients with COVID-19 was shown to be very low [33]. However, it has been generally reported that DIC is frequently associated with patients with other infectious diseases, and the incidence of DIC in other infectious diseases suspected to be bacterial infections is 20–70% [34,35], considering that the incidence of complications with DIC is higher in patients with bacterial infections than in those with COVID-19. The outcome of DIC in septic patients is extremely low [14]. There have been many systematic reviews and studies based on big data of the effects of DIC or sepsis treatments [36,37]. In a recent report that compared COVID-19 to bacterial infection, the mortality rate was 17.0% in patients with other pneumonia, 16.7% in patients with sepsis, and 4.3% in patients with COVID-19, suggesting that the mortality rate due to sepsis is higher than that due to COVID-19 [36]. In addition, thrombosis such as VTE, ACI or ACS is not frequently detected in patients with bacterial infection [38]. There are many differences between septic DIC and COVID-19 coagulopathy. In particular, a clot waveform analysis (CWA) [39] of activated partial thromboplastin time (APTT) showed a large difference between the two diseases. Significant prolongation of the peak time and a marked reduction in the peak height of CWA-APTT were observed in patients with overt DIC [40], whereas moderate prolongation of the peak time and a significant increase in the peak height of CWA-APTT were observed in patients with COVID-19 coagulopathy [41]. Based on these findings, a markedly increased peak height suggests hypercoagulability, while a markedly decreased peak height suggests hypocoagulability (Figure 2). These differences may be caused by hypofibrinogenemia and hyperfibrinolysis in overt DIC and hypercoagulability induced by thrombin burst and hypofibrinolysis in COVID-19 coagulopathy.

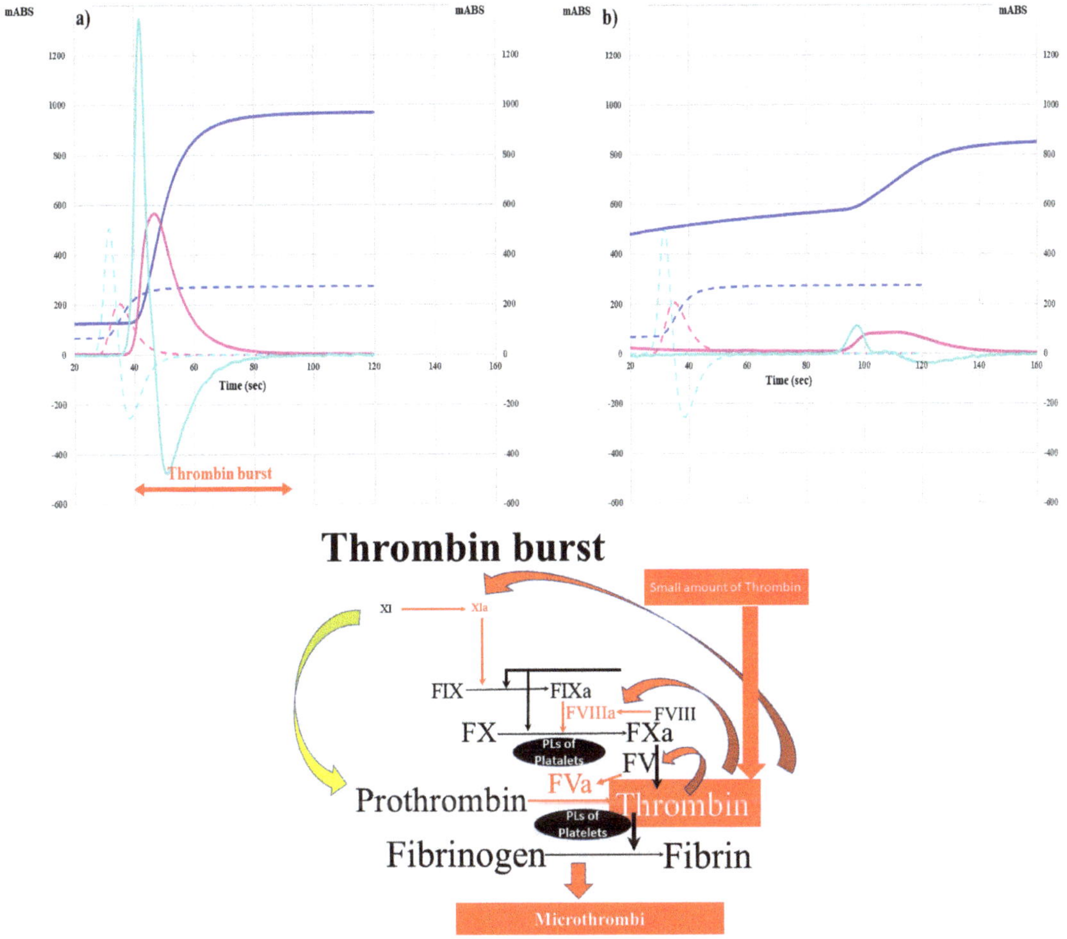

Figure 2. Difference in the CWA-APTT between COVID-19 coagulopathy with thrombin burst (**a**) and overt-DIC (**b**). CWA, clot waveform analysis; APTT, activated partial thromboplastin time; HV, healthy volunteer; COVID-19, coronavirus disease 2019; DIC, disseminated intravascular coagulation; navy line, fibrin formation curve; pink line, 1st derivative curve (velocity); light blue, 2nd derivative curve (acceleration); solid line, patient; dotted line, HV. A significant reduction in the peak height suggests bleeding, and a significant increase in the peak height suggest hypercoagulability and thrombotic risk. FX, activated FX; PLs, phospholipids; FVIIIa, activated FVIII, FVa, activated FV; FIXa, activated FIX; FXIa, activated FXI. A schematic illustration of thrombin burst in hypercoagulability with COVID-19.

4.2. TMA

The association with TMA in patients with COVID-19 has been reviewed [42] and several reports described TMA in patients with COVID-19 [43], with the frequency of TMA being reported to be 1.0–20% and the outcome of TMA varying but quite poor [15]. TMA involves Shiga toxin-producing Escherichia coli (STEC)-hemolytic uremic syndrome (HUS), thrombotic thrombocytopenic purpura (TTP), atypical HUS and secondary HUS [15]. Acquired TTP is caused by the inhibitor for a disintegrin-like and metalloproteinase with thrombospondin type 1 motifs 13 (ADAMTS13) and aHUS is mainly caused by an hereditary abnormality of compliment regulation.

As ADAMTS-13 activity and the complement system are not usually examined, TTP and aHUS may not usually be diagnosed in general hospitals. However, decreased ADAMTS-13 activity and elevated C5b-9 levels have been reported in patients with COVID-19 [41,44,45]. The low incidence of TMA may be due to the lack of diagnostic biomarkers for TMA in clinical use. Elevated sCLEC-2 levels suggest that critically ill patients with COVID-19 have some degree of microangiopathy [46]. A marked elevation of sCLEC-2 levels was also reported in patients with TMA [17], suggesting the marked activation of platelets in patients with COVID-19 as well as in patients with TMA. Many critically ill patients with COVID-19 are also associated with thrombocytopenia, anemia and organ failure, suggesting that these patients met the diagnostic criteria of TMA [47] and necessitating further investigation for TMA in patients with COVID-19. COVID-19 complicated with TMA is expected to increase in frequency going forward.

5. Biomarkers for Thrombosis in COVID-19

5.1. Routine Biomarkers

Although conventional PT and APTT are hemostatic markers and cannot show hypercoagulability and thrombotic risk, CWA-APTT and a small amount of TF-induced FIX activation assay (sTF/FIXa) can show hypercoagulability [39]. D-dimer values have been reported to be useful biomarkers with a high sensitivity for thrombosis in patients with COVID-19 and are correlated with the severity of COVID-19 [19,20] (Table 2). Although elevated D-dimer levels are a well-known risk factor for thrombosis, the D-dimer cutoff level is low in COVID-19 [48]. Although D-dimer is useful for the exclusion of VTE in patients with COVID-19, it may not be useful for the diagnosis of VTE in patients with COVID-19 [15,19,20]. D-dimer levels were reported to be significantly higher in patients with other pneumonia and sepsis due to bacterial infections than in patients with COVID-19, whereas there was no significant difference in D-dimer levels between patients with unidentified clinical syndrome and those with COVID-19 [14,15,46].

Platelet counts were extremely low in patients with sepsis and other pneumonia due to bacterial infection, especially DIC or pre-DIC, but only moderately low in COVID-19 patients with critical illness [14,15,46]. As multiple viruses interfere with hematopoiesis, thrombocytopenia is a common phenomenon in various viral infections including COVID-19 [49]. However, thrombocytopenia is suggested to be associated with increased platelet consumption and destruction in COVID-19. The prothrombin time (PT) and APTT were significantly prolonged in septic patients with DIC but not in patients with COVID-19 [14,15,46]. Therefore, DIC and sepsis-induced coagulopathy are generally diagnosed using a scoring system based on PT, platelet counts and fibrin-related products, such as D-dimer levels [50–52]. Fibrinogen levels were significantly increased in patients with COVID-19 compared with patients with sepsis. No significant differences have been noted in platelet counts, PT or APTT among the four stages of COVID-19, although platelet counts tend to be reduced in severe or critical illness [46]. Therefore, the above scoring system may not be useful for diagnosing thrombosis in patients with COVID-19, suggesting that coagulation factor abnormalities may not be significant in COVID-19.

5.2. Platelet Activation

Platelet activation can be evaluated to detect substances such as P selectin [53] or phosphatidylserine [54] on the platelet surface via flow cytometry. However, this method is not routine laboratory work. Platelet–leukocyte aggregates are often detected to show platelet activation [55], but this method is not quantitative (Table 3). Microparticles with tissue factor (TF) from platelets or vessels have been reported to be increased in patients with thrombosis [56], but this method is still being researched. Although, the β-thromboglobulin (β-TG), platelet factor 4 (PF4), and P-selectin are considered biomarkers of platelet activation, their diagnostic specificity for thrombosis due to platelet activation is not high, and their clinical laboratory use is inconvenient [57].

Soluble platelet membrane glycoprotein VI (sGPVI) and soluble C-type lectin-like receptor 2 (sCLEC-2) have been reported as new biomarkers for platelet activation [16,17,57]. Both sGPVI and sCLEC-2 were significantly elevated in patients with TMA and DIC [17,51]. Elevated sCLEC-2 levels were also reported in patients with ACS [18], ACI [58] and COVID-19 [46]. Specifically, the sCLEC-2/platelet ratio is useful for evaluating the severity of COVID-19. Furthermore, the plasma sCLEC-2 levels in patients with the mild stage of COVID-19 were similar to those in patients with other pneumonias, suggesting that the activation of platelets may occur in the early stage of COVID-19 without symptoms of microangiopathy [36]. Activated platelets in patients with COVID-19 may release large amounts of sCLEC-2 into the blood before causing severe microangiopathy. Although many reports have demonstrated decreased ADAMTS13 activity and increased von Willebrand factor (VWF) in patients with COVID-19 [59,60], ADAMTS-13 activity was not less than 10% in COVID-19 and the clinical usefulness of a mild decrease in ADAMTS-13 is not clear. Anti-PF 4 antibodies have often been reported in COVID-19 patients associated with thrombosis [61,62], suggesting that one of the thrombotic mechanisms in patients with COVID-19 is heparin-induced thrombocytopenia (HIT).

Table 2. Routine biomarkers for coagulopathy in COVID-19 infections and sepsis.

	COVID-19 Infection [14,15,52,54,55]			Sepsis Due to Bacterial Infection [37,38,57,59]		
	Cutoff Value	Sensitivity	Specificity	Cutoff Value	Sensitivity	Specificity
D-dimer	1.0–3.0 μg/mL	high	low	5–10 μg/mL	moderately high	moderately high
Platelet counts	16.0×10^{10}/L	low	low	12.0×10^{10}/L	moderately high	moderately high
PT-INR	1.20	low	low	1.20	moderately high	moderately high
Fibrinogen	increased	-	-	1.5 g/L	slightly high	high
Antithrombin	-	-	-	70%	moderately high	moderately high
WBC	decreased (at first)			markedly increased		
Hemoglobin	decreased (at severe or critical illness)			no change		

PT-INR, prothrombin time-internationalized ratio; WBC, white blood cells; COVID-19, coronavirus disease 2019.

Table 3. Examinations for platelet activation.

	Methods	Quantitative	Multiple Assay	Easy Assay	Specificity
Activated substance on platelet	flow cytometry	NA	NA	adequate	specific
Microparticles from platelet	flow cytometry, immunoassay	NA	NA	adequate	semispecific
Platelet–leukocyte aggregates	flow cytometry, microscopy	NA	NA	adequate	specific
β-TG, platelet factor 4 (PF4)	ELISA	PA	PA	NA	specific
P-secretin	ELISA	adequate	adequate	adequate	semispecific
GP-VI,	ELISA	adequate	adequate	adequate	specific
sCLEC-2	CLEIA	adequate	adequate	SA	specific

β-TG, β-thromboglobulin; PF4, platelet factor 4; NA, not adequate; PA, partially adequate; SA, strongly adequate; sGPVI, soluble platelet membrane glycoprotein VI; sCLEC-2, soluble C-type lectin-like receptor 2; ELISA, enzyme-linked immunosorbent assay, CLEIA, chemiluminescent enzyme immunoassay.

5.3. *Hypofibrinolysis and Vascular Endothelial Cell Injury Markers*

Increased fibrinogen [63] and plasminogen activator inhibitor-1 (PAI-I) levels [64], slightly increased D-dimer levels [65], and viscoelastic whole blood coagulation testing with and without tissue plasminogen activator [66,67] suggested a hypercoagulable and hypofibrinolytic state in patients with COVID-19. Most studies that reported hypofibrinolysis in patients with COVID-19 [66–68] used thromboelastography (TEG), and conducting statistical analyses for hypofibrinolysis proved difficult. Therefore, the hypofibrinolytic state in COVID-19 has not yet been sufficiently evaluated. Although it has been emphasized that D-dimer levels are increased in COVID-19 patients with severe or critical illness [36], the increase in D-dimer values in patients with COVID-19 has been shown to be significantly lower than that in other pneumonia patients [69]. Organ failure is worse in advanced COVID-19 patients, so vascular endothelial cell injury markers such as soluble thrombomodulin (sTM), VWF and PAI-I are high, while AT levels are low, suggesting that hypofibrinolysis may be related to organ failure and vascular endothelial cell injury.

5.4. *Inflammatory Marker*

Increased values for the white blood cell count, C-reactive protein (CRP) level [8], procalcitonin level [70], presepsin level [71], C5b-9 and C5a levels [44], and levels of inflammatory cytokines, such as tumor necrosis factor α, interleukin-1, interleukin-2, interleukin-6, interleukin-10 and interferon γ, were reported in patients with severe COVID-19; elevation in these inflammatory factors can lead to cytokine storm [72]. As procalcitonin is a biomarker for bacterial infection, presepsin may be more useful for diagnosing COVID-19 than procalcitonin [73]. These inflammatory mediators can further cause hypercoagulability, platelet activation, hypofibrinolysis, and vascular endothelial cell injuries by activating leukocytes, vascular endothelial cells and platelets.

6. Mechanisms for Thrombosis in COVID-19 and Sepsis

Several mechanisms for thrombosis underlying the worsening of the condition of COVID-19 patients, such as old age, long time-bed rest and comorbidities [23,28], inflammation and cytokine storms [12], vascular endothelial injuries [74], primary pulmonary thrombosis [75], hypoventilation, a hypercoagulable state (including activation of the TF pathway) [74], neutrophil extracellular traps (NETs) [76], hypofibrinolysis [66] and platelet activation [60], have been proposed. The mechanism underlying thrombosis in COVID-19 (Figure 3) and in bacterial infection (Figure 4) is shown.

6.1. *Platelet Activation*

Severe acute respiratory syndrome coronavirus-2 (SARS-CoV-2) binds to the CD-147 receptor of platelets [77]. Early and intense platelet activation, which was reproduced in vitro by stimulating platelets with SARS-CoV-2 depending on the CD147 receptor, has been reported [53]. Platelet activation and platelet–monocyte aggregate formation trigger TF expression in patients with severe COVID-19 [78]. SARS-CoV-2-induced platelet activation may participate in thrombus formation and inflammatory responses in COVID-19 patients. The early accumulation of extracellular vesicles with the soluble P-selectin and high mobility group box 1 (HMGB-1) protein which platelets release, was shown to predict worse clinical outcomes [53]. The plasma sCLEC-2 levels in patients with COVID-19 were significantly higher than those in patients with other infections and reflected the progression of the severity of COVID-19 although these levels were significantly higher in patients with sepsis due to bacterial infection [46] (Figure 4).

Thrombocytopenia is often observed in COVID-19 patients with severe disease as well as in septic patients with DIC [79]. The sCLEC-2/platelet ratio was significantly higher in COVID-19 patients with severe and critical illness than in those with mild illness, suggesting that one of the causes of thrombocytopenia might be consumption due to microthrombi formation, suggesting that COVID-19 has microangiopathy as well as DIC or TMA. Low-dose aspirin was reported to be useful for managing COVID-19 [80].

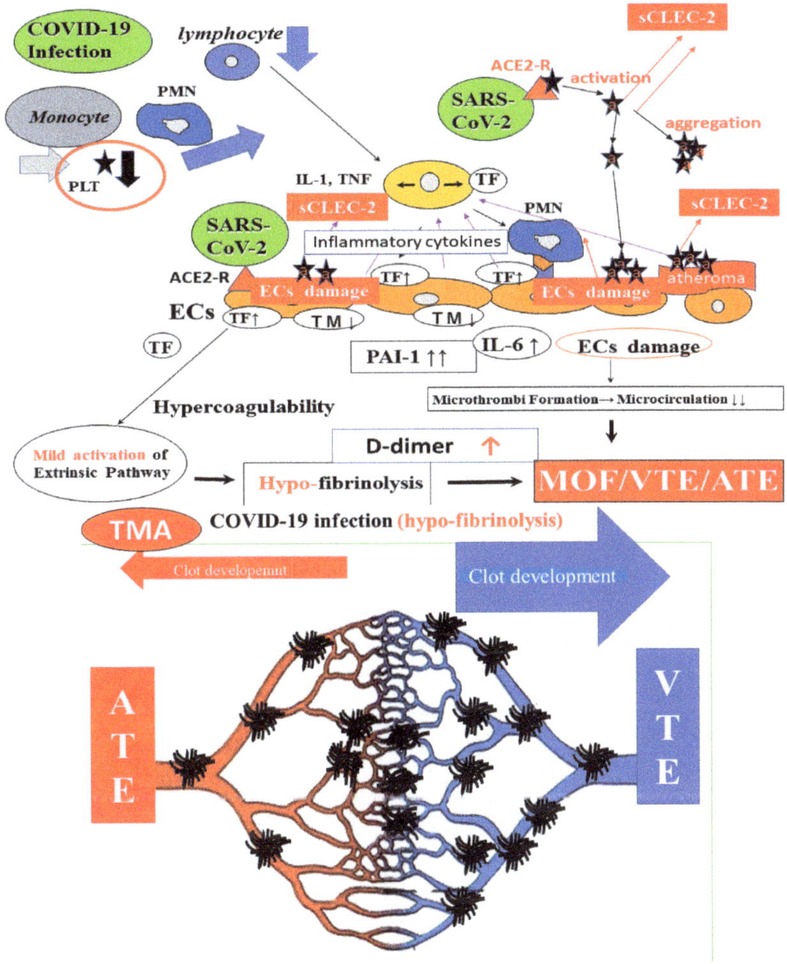

Figure 3. The mechanism underlying thrombosis in COVID-19. MΦ, macrophage; PMN, polymorphonuclear cell; NETS, neutrophil extracellular traps; ECs, endothelial cells; IFN, interferon; LPS, lipopolysaccharide; TF, tissue factor; IL, interleukin; TNF, tumor necrosis factor; TM, thrombomodulin; PAI-I, plasminogen activator inhibitor-1; AT-III, antithrombin; MOF, multiple organ failure; VTE, venous thromboembolism; DIC, disseminated intravascular coagulation; a★, activated platelet; PLT, platelet; COVID-19, coronavirus disease 2019; SARS-CoV-2, severe acute respiratory syndrome related coronavirus-2; sCLEC-2, soluble C-type lectin-like receptor 2; TMA, thrombotic microangiopathy; VTE, venous thromboembolism; ATE, arterial thromboembolism.

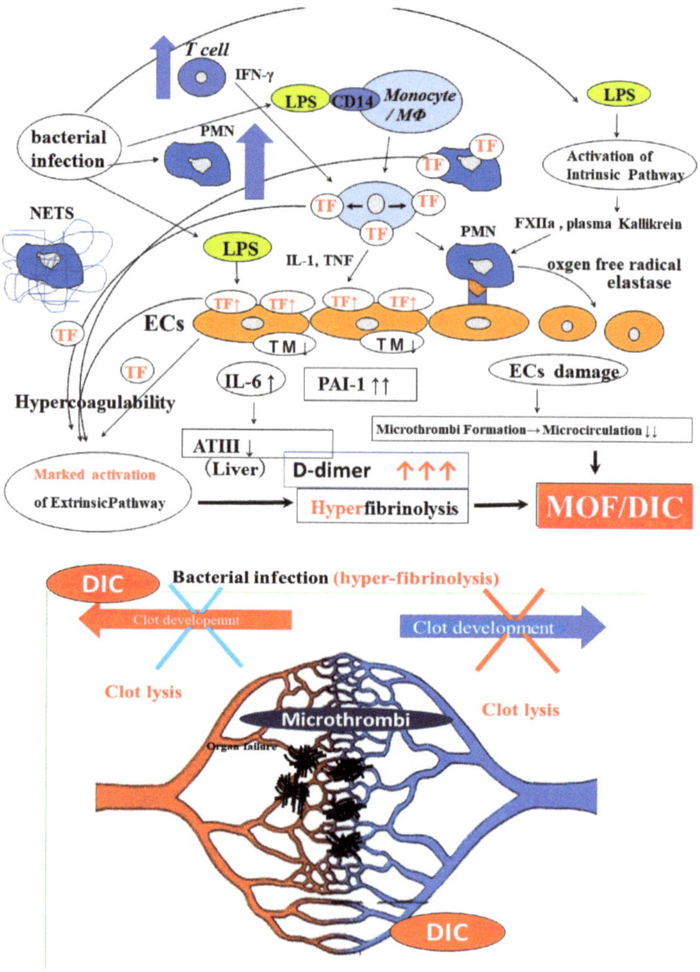

Figure 4. The mechanism underlying thrombosis in bacterial infection. MΦ, macrophage; PMN, polymorphonuclear cell; NETS, neutrophil extracellular traps; ECs, endothelial cells; IFN, interferon; LPS, lipopolysaccharide; TF, tissue factor; IL, interleukin; TNF, tumor necrosis factor; TM, thrombomodulin; PAI-I, plasminogen activator inhibitor-1; AT-III, antithrombin; MOF, multiple organ failure; VTE, venous thromboembolism; DIC, disseminated intravascular coagulation.

6.2. Hypercoagulable State

Marked activation of leukocytes and the overexpression of TF are considered some of the most important causes of thrombosis or DIC due to bacterial infection [14,79]. Markedly increased values of white blood cell count, plasma TF, and TF messenger RNA levels in white blood cells have been reported in patients with sepsis [81]. Increased levels of inflammatory cytokines, fibrin-related products (e.g., D-dimer), vascular endothelial cell injury markers (e.g., thrombomodulin [TM]), and PAI-I and decreased antithrombin, thrombocytopenia, and a prolonged PT were also reported in septic patients [14,38,82]. Such cases of sepsis are frequently associated with DIC [38]. Severe septic patients with elevated sCLEC-2 levels may also have microangiopathy [46]. There are some differences in the mechanism underlying thrombocytopenia between DIC and TMA [79], although thrombocytopenia in both diseases is caused by platelet consumption. Regarding COVID -19 (Figure 3), leukocyte counts are generally decreased early in COVID-19 [8], suggesting that activated platelets and injured vascular endothelial cells may play an important role in the onset of thrombosis through CD-147 [53]. However, CWA-APTT and CWA-sTF/FIXa showed hypercoagulability in patients with COVID-19 [41] suggesting that thrombin burst (Figure 2) [83] which is enhanced by activated platelets, causes hypercoagulability in this state.

6.3. *Hypofibrinolysis*

Although both severe COVID-19 and bacterial infections may have similar microangiopathy, complications with VTE are frequent in patients with COVID-19 but are not frequent in septic patients. DIC is caused by hypercoagulation and hyperfibrinolysis [38], most microthrombi in the microvasculature may dissolve promptly in DIC, whereas microthrombi in COVID-19 may develop into venous thrombosis. Vascular injuries are observed in COVID-19 [74], suggesting that elevated PAI-I may inhibit fibrinolysis [84] (Tables 4 and 5). In addition, the sCLEC-2/D-dimer ratio in patients with COVID-19 was significantly higher than that in patients with other infections [69], suggesting that hypercoagulable and hypofibrinolysis states are more predominant in patients with COVID-19 than in other pneumonia patients. Markedly increased TF and D-dimer levels are observed in cases of bacterial infection [38,81], suggesting that hypercoagulable and hyperfibrinolytic states exist in severe bacterial infections. Regarding COVID-19 infection, the sCLEC-2/D-dimer ratio in cases with critical illness was significantly lower than that in cases with mild illness, suggesting that most patients with early-stage COVID-19 infection show only platelet activation with hypofibrinolysis, and that severe COVID-19 causes even further hypercoagulability [69] through a thrombin burst induced by platelet activation (Figure 4).

Table 4. Differences and similarities between COVID-19 and severe sepsis bacterial infections.

	COVID-19 Infection	**Severe Sepsis Due to Bacterial Infections**
Activation of platelets	+++++	+++
Activation of leukocytes	+	+++++
Tissue factor generation	++++	+++++
Cytokine generation	+++++	++++
Lung injury	+++++	+++
Organ failure excluding lung	+	+++
Development of atheroma	+++	+
Development of venous thrombosis	+++++	++
Fibrinolysis	+	+++++

Table 5. Differences and similarities between COVID-19 and severe sepsis bacterial infections.

	COVID-19 Infection	**Severe Sepsis Due to Bacterial Infections**
Venous thromboembolism	frequent	not frequent
Arterial thrombosis	relatively frequent	not frequent
Mortality rate	approximately 2%	20–45% in severe sepsis
Incidence of infection	markedly high	relatively high
Death number	markedly high	relatively high
Microangiopathy	positive	positive
Coagulation	mild or hypercoagulable states	hypercoagulable state
Fibrinolysis	hypofibrinolytic state	hyperfibrinolytic state
DIC	not frequent	frequent

DIC, disseminated intravascular coagulation; COVID-19, coronavirus disease 2019.

7. Treatment and Prophylaxis for Thrombosis

Although antithrombotic agents such as heparin reduce the risk of thromboembolism in severely ill patients, there are a few recommendations for patients with COVID-19 in the ISTH guidelines on antithrombotic treatment [85]. Among non-critically ill patients hospitalized for COVID-19, there is a strong recommendation for the use of prophylactic doses of low molecular weight heparin (LMWH) or unfractionated heparin (UFH) and for select patients in this group; the use of therapeutic doses LMWH/UFH is preferred over prophylactic doses, but without the addition of an antiplatelet agent. There are weak recommendations for adding an antiplatelet agent to prophylactic LMWH/UFH in select critically ill patients and prophylactic rivaroxaban for select patients after discharge. A recent review of RCTs [86] in critically ill patients demonstrated that a therapeutic dose of anticoagulation does not improve outcomes and results in more bleeding than a prophylactic dose of anticoagulant in these patients. Trials in noncritically ill hospitalized patients showed that anticoagulation at a therapeutic dose with a heparin formulation might improve clinical outcomes. Anticoagulation with a direct oral anticoagulant may improve outcomes of posthospital discharge; the results of a large RCT that is currently in progress are awaited [87]. There is not sufficient evidence that therapeutic anticoagulant can be recommended in critically ill patients at the present time.

8. Conclusions

A hypercoagulable state, platelet activation (observed as the marked elevation of sCLEC-2), and hypofibrinolysis due to vascular injuries are observed in patients with COVID-19, suggesting that SARS-CoV-2 may cause thrombogenicity via a mechanism different from that involved in bacterial infection.

Author Contributions: Conceptualization, H.W.; methodology, K.S.-I.; validation, K.S.; formal analysis, M.S.; investigation, T.I.; writing—original draft preparation, H.W.; writing—review and editing, M.S.; visualization, T.I.; supervision, H.S.; project administration, K.S.; funding acquisition, H.W. All authors have read and agreed to the published version of the manuscript.

Funding: This research was funded by the Japanese Ministry of Health, Labor and Welfare (grant number 21FC1008). The APC was funded by Mie University.

Institutional Review Board Statement: The study protocol (2020-S25) was approved by the Human Ethics Review committees of Mie Prefectural General Medical Center. This study was faithfully carried out in accordance with the principles of the Declaration of Helsinki.

Informed Consent Statement: We did not directly use patient data that required informed consent.

Data Availability Statement: Yes, available in References.

Conflicts of Interest: The measurements of sCLEC-2 and D-dimer levels were partially supported by LSI Medience. The authors declare no other conflict of interest in association with the present study.

References

1. Zhou, F.; Yu, T.; Du, R.; Fan, G.; Liu, Y.; Liu, Z.; Xiang, J.; Wang, Y.; Song, B.; Gu, X.; et al. Clinical course and risk factors for mortality of adult inpatients with COVID-19 in Wuhan, China: A retrospective cohort study. *Lancet* **2020**, *395*, 1054–1062. [CrossRef] [PubMed]
2. Jiang, F.; Deng, L.; Zhang, L.; Cai, Y.; Cheung, C.W.; Xia, Z.J. Review of the Clinical Characteristics of Coronavirus Disease 2019 (COVID-19). *Gen. Intern. Med.* **2020**, *35*, 1545–1549. [CrossRef] [PubMed]
3. Gavriatopoulou, M.; Ntanasis-Stathopoulos, I.; Korompoki, E.; Fotiou, D.; Migkou, M.; Tzanninis, I.-G.; Psaltopoulou, T.; Kastritis, E.; Terpos, E.; Dimopoulos, M.A. Emerging treatment strategies for COVID-19 infection. *Clin. Exp. Med.* **2020**, *21*, 167–179. [CrossRef] [PubMed]
4. Machhi, J.; Herskovitz, J.; Senan, A.M.; Dutta, D.; Nath, B.; Oleynikov, M.D.; Blomberg, W.R.; Meigs, D.D.; Hasan, M.; Patel, M.; et al. The Natural History, Pathobiology, and Clinical Manifestations of SARS-CoV-2 Infections. *J. Neuroimmune Pharmacol.* **2020**, *15*, 359–386. [CrossRef]
5. Hertanto, D.M.; Wiratama, B.S.; Sutanto, H.; Wungu, C.D.K. Immunomodulation as a Potent COVID-19 Pharmacotherapy: Past, Present and Future. *J. Inflamm. Res.* **2021**, *14*, 3419–3428. [CrossRef]
6. Berlin, D.A.; Gulick, R.M.; Martinez, F.J. Severe COVID-19. *N. Engl. J. Med.* **2020**, *383*, 2451–2460. [CrossRef]

7. Gandhi, R.T.; Lynch, J.B.; Del Rio, C. Mild or Moderate COVID-19. *N. Engl. J. Med.* **2020**, *383*, 1757–1766. [CrossRef]
8. Yamamoto, A.; Wada, H.; Ichikawa, Y.; Mizuno, H.; Tomida, M.; Masuda, J.; Makino, K.; Kodama, S.; Yoshida, M.; Fukui, S.; et al. Evaluation of Biomarkers of Severity in Patients with COVID-19 Infection. *J. Clin. Med.* **2021**, *10*, 3775. [CrossRef]
9. Karim, S.S.A.; Karim, Q.A. Omicron SARS-CoV-2 variant: A new chapter in the COVID-19 pandemic. *Lancet* **2021**, *398*, 2126–2128. [CrossRef]
10. Jiménez, D.; García-Sanchez, A.; Rali, P.; Muriel, A.; Bikdeli, B.; Ruiz-Artacho, P.; Le Mao, R.; Rodríguez, C.; Hunt, B.J.; Monreal, M. Incidence of VTE and Bleeding Among Hospitalized Patients With Coronavirus Disease 2019: A Systematic Review and Meta-analysis. *Chest* **2021**, *159*, 1182–1196. [CrossRef]
11. Nannoni, S.; de Groot, R.; Bell, S.; Markus, H.S. Stroke in COVID-19: A systematic review and meta-analysis. *Int. J. Stroke* **2021**, *16*, 137–149. [CrossRef] [PubMed]
12. Zhao, Y.H.; Zhao, L.; Yang, X.C.; Wang, P. Cardiovascular complications of SARS-CoV-2 infection (COVID-19): A systematic review and meta-analysis. *Rev. Cardiovasc. Med.* **2021**, *22*, 159–165. [CrossRef] [PubMed]
13. Chan, N.C.; Weitz, J.I. COVID-19 coagulopathy, thrombosis, and bleeding. *Blood* **2020**, *136*, 381–383. [CrossRef] [PubMed]
14. Wada, H.; Thachil, J.; Di Nisio, M.; Mathew, P.; Kurosawa, S.; Gando, S.; Kim, H.K.; Nielsen, J.D.; Dempfle, C.E.; Levi, M.; et al. The Scientific Standardization Committee on DIC of the International Society on Thrombosis Haemostasis: Guidance for diagnosis and treatment of DIC from harmonization of the recommendations from three guidelines. *J. Thromb. Haemost.* **2013**, *11*, 761–767. [CrossRef]
15. Wada, H.; Matsumoto, T.; Yamashita, Y. Natural History of Thrombotic Thrombocytopenic Purpura and Hemolytic Uremic Syndrome. *Semin. Thromb. Hemost.* **2014**, *40*, 866–873.
16. Suzuki-Inoue, K.; Fuller, G.L.; Garcia, A.; Eble, J.A.; Pohlmann, S.; Inoue, O.; Gartner, T.K.; Hughan, S.C.; Pearce, A.C.; Laing, G.D.; et al. A novel Syk-dependent mechanism of platelet activation by the C-type lectin receptor sCLEC-2. *Blood* **2006**, *107*, 542–549. [CrossRef]
17. Yamashita, Y.; Suzuki, K.; Mastumoto, T.; Ikejiri, M.; Ohishi, K.; Katayama, N.; Suzuki-Inoue, K.; Wada, H. Elevated plasma levels of soluble C-type lectin-like receptor 2 (sCLEC-2) in patients with thrombotic microangiopathy. *Thromb. Res.* **2019**, *178*, 54–58. [CrossRef]
18. Inoue, O.; Osada, M.; Nakamura, J.; Kazama, F.; Shirai, T.; Tsukiji, N.; Sasaki, T.; Yokomichi, H.; Dohi, T.; Kaneko, M.; et al. Soluble CLEC-2 is generated independently of ADAM10 and is increased in plasma in acute coronary syndrome: Comparison with soluble GPVI. *Int. J. Hematol.* **2019**, *110*, 285–294. [CrossRef]
19. Cheng, N.M.; Chan, Y.C.; Cheng, S.W. COVID-19 related thrombosis: A mini-review. *Phlebology* **2022**, *10*, 2683555211052170. [CrossRef]
20. Suh, Y.J.; Hong, H.; Ohana, M.; Bompard, F.; Revel, M.P.; Valle, C.; Gervaise, A.; Poissy, J.; Susen, S.; Hékimian, G.; et al. Pulmonary Embolism and Deep Vein Thrombosis in COVID-19: A Systematic Review and Meta-Analysis. *Radiology* **2021**, *298*, E70–E80. [CrossRef]
21. Malas, M.B.; Naazie, I.N.; Elsayed, N.; Mathlouthi, A.; Marmor, R.; Clary, B. Thromboembolism risk of COVID-19 is high and associated with a higher risk of mortality: A systematic review and meta-analysis. *eClin. Med.* **2020**, *29*, 100639. [CrossRef] [PubMed]
22. Peiris, S.; Ordunez, P.; DiPette, D.; Padwal, R.; Ambrosi, P.; Toledo, J.; Stanford, V.; Lisboa, T.; Aldighieri, S.; Reveiz, L. Cardiac Manifestations in Patients with COVID-19: A Scoping Review. *Glob. Heart* **2022**, *17*, 2. [CrossRef] [PubMed]
23. Roshdy, A.; Zaher, S.; Fayed, H.; Coghlan, J.G. COVID-19 and the Heart: A Systematic Review of Cardiac Autopsies. *Front. Cardiovasc. Med.* **2021**, *7*, 626975. [CrossRef] [PubMed]
24. Thakker, R.A.; Elbadawi, A.; Chatila, K.F.; Goel, S.S.; Reynoso, D.; Berbarie, R.F.; Gilani, S.; Rangasetty, U.; Khalife, W. Comparison of Coronary Artery Involvement and Mortality in STEMI Patients with and without SARS-CoV-2 during the COVID-19 Pandemic: A Systematic Review and Meta-Analysis. *Curr. Probl. Cardiol.* **2022**, *47*, 101032. [CrossRef] [PubMed]
25. Choi, Y.; Lee, M.K. Neuroimaging findings of brain MRI and CT in patients with COVID-19: A systematic review and meta-analysis. *Eur. J. Radiol.* **2020**, *133*, 109393. [CrossRef] [PubMed]
26. Kim, P.H.; Kim, M.; Suh, C.H.; Chung, S.R.; Park, J.E.; Kim, S.C.; Choi, Y.J.; Lee, J.H.; Kim, H.S.; Baek, J.H.; et al. Neuroimaging Findings in Patients with COVID-19: A Systematic Review and Meta-Analysis. *Korean J. Radiol.* **2021**, *22*, 1875–1885. [CrossRef]
27. Horiuchi, H.; Morishita, E.; Urano, T.; Yokoyama, K. Questionnaire-survey Joint Team on The COVID-19-related thrombosis: COVID-19-Related Thrombosis in Japan: Final Report of a Questionnaire-Based Survey in 2020. *J. Atheroscler. Thromb.* **2021**, *28*, 400–406. [CrossRef]
28. Qureshi, A.I.; Baskett, W.I.; Huang, W.; Shyu, D.; Myers, D.; Raju, M.; Lobanova, I.; Suri, M.F.K.; Naqvi, S.H.; French, B.R.; et al. Acute ischemic stroke and COVID-19: An analysis of 27 676 patients. *Stroke* **2021**, *52*, 905–912. [CrossRef]
29. Xiao, D.; Tang, F.; Chen, L.; Gao, H.; Li, X. Cumulative Evidence for the Association of Thrombosis and the Prognosis of COVID-19: Systematic Review and Meta-Analysis. *Front. Cardiovasc. Med.* **2022**, *8*, 819318. [CrossRef]
30. Pepera, G.; Tribali, M.S.; Batalik, L.; Petrov, I.; Papathanasiou, J. Epidemiology, risk factors and prognosis of cardiovascular disease in the Coronavirus Disease 2019 (COVID-19) pandemicera: A systematic review. *Rev. Cardiovasc. Med.* **2022**, *23*, 28. [CrossRef]

31. Giannis, D.; Allen, S.L.; Tsang, J.; Flint, S.; Pinhasov, T.; Williams, S.; Tan, G.; Thakur, R.; Leung, C.; Snyder, M.; et al. Postdischarge thromboembolic outcomes and mortality of hospitalized patients with COVID-19: The CORE-19 registry. *Blood* **2021**, *137*, 2838–2847. [CrossRef] [PubMed]
32. Iba, T.; Levy, J.H.; Levi, M.; Thachil, J. Coagulopathy in COVID-19. *J. Thromb. Haemost.* **2020**, *18*, 2103–2109. [CrossRef] [PubMed]
33. Zhou, X.; Cheng, Z.; Luo, L.; Zhu, Y.; Lin, W.; Ming, Z.; Chen, W.; Hu, Y. Incidence and impact of disseminated intravascular coagulation in COVID-19 a systematic review and meta-analysis. *Thromb. Res.* **2021**, *201*, 23–29. [CrossRef] [PubMed]
34. Larsen, J.B.; Aggerbeck, M.A.; Granfeldt, A.; Schmidt, M.; Hvas, A.M.; Adelborg, K. Res Pract: Disseminated intravascular coagulation diagnosis: Positive predictive value of the ISTH score in a Danish population. *Thromb. Haemost.* **2021**, *5*, e12636.
35. Gando, S.; Shiraishi, A.; Yamakawa, K.; Ogura, H.; Saitoh, D.; Fujishima, S.; Mayumi, T.; Kushimoto, S.; Abe, T.; Shiino, Y.; et al. Role of disseminated intravascular coagulation in severe sepsis. Japanese Association for Acute Medicine (JAAM) Focused Outcomes Research in Emergency Care in Acute Respiratory Distress Syndrome, Sepsis and Trauma (FORECAST) Study Group. *Thromb. Res.* **2019**, *178*, 182–188. [CrossRef] [PubMed]
36. Yamakawa, K.; Aihara, M.; Ogura, H.; Yuhara, H.; Hamasaki, T.; Shimazu, T. Recombinant human soluble thrombomodulin in severe sepsis: Systematic review and meta-analysis. *J. Thromb. Haemost.* **2015**, *13*, 508–519. [CrossRef]
37. Tagami, T. Antithrombin concentrate use in sepsis-associated disseminated intravascular coagulation: Re-evaluation of a 'pendulum effect' drug using a nationwide database. *J. Thromb. Haemost.* **2018**, *16*, 458–461. [CrossRef]
38. Wada, H.; Matsumoto, T.; Yamashita, Y. Diagnosis and treatment of disseminated intravascular coagulation (DIC) according to four DIC guidelines. *J. Intensive Care* **2014**, *2*, 15. [CrossRef]
39. Wada, H.; Matsumoto, T.; Ohishi, K.; Shiraki, K.; Shimaoka, M. Update on the Clot Waveform Analysis. *Clin. Appl. Thromb. Hemost.* **2020**, *26*, 1076029620912027. [CrossRef]
40. Suzuki, K.; Wada, H.; Imai, H.; Iba, T.; Thachil, J.; Toh, C.H. Subcommittee on Disseminated Intravascular Coagulation. A re-evaluation of the D-dimer cut-off value for making a diagnosis according to the ISTH overt-DIC diagnostic criteria: Communication from the SSC of the ISTH. *J. Thromb. Haemost.* **2018**, *16*, 1442–1444. [CrossRef]
41. Suzuki1, K.; Wada, H.; Ikejiri, K.; Ito, A.; Matsumoto, T.; Tone, S.; Hasegawa, M.; Shimaoka, M.; Iba, T.; Imai, H. Prolongation of Peak Time but an Elevated Peak Height of a Clot Wave Form Analysis in Severe Coronavirus Disease 2019. *Med. Res. Arch.* **2023**, *11*. Available online: https://esmed.org/MRA/index.php/mra/article/view/3549 (accessed on 25 April 2023).
42. Tiwari, N.R.; Phatak, S.; Sharma, V.R.; Agarwal, S.K. COVID-19 and thrombotic microangiopathies. *Thromb. Res.* **2021**, *202*, 191–198. [CrossRef]
43. Diorio, C.; McNerney, K.O.; Lambert, M.; Paessler, M.; Anderson, E.M.; Henrickson, S.E.; Chase, J.; Liebling, E.J.; Burudpakdee, C.; Lee, J.H.; et al. Evidence of thrombotic microangiopathy in children with SARS-CoV-2 across the spectrum of clinical presentations. *Blood Adv.* **2020**, *4*, 6051–6063. [CrossRef] [PubMed]
44. Detsika, M.G.; Diamanti, E.; Ampelakiotou, K.; Jahaj, E.; Tsipilis, S.; Athanasiou, N.; Dimopoulou, I.; Orfanos, S.E.; Tsirogianni, A.; Kotanidou, A. C3a and C5b-9 Differentially Predict COVID-19 Progression and Outcome. *Life* **2022**, *12*, 1335. [CrossRef] [PubMed]
45. Mancini, I.; Baronciani, L.; Artoni, A.; Colpani, P.; Biganzoli, M.; Cozzi, G.; Novembrino, C.; Anzoletti, M.B.; De Zan, V.; Pagliari, M.T.; et al. The ADAMTS13-von Willebrand factor axis in COVID-19 patients. *J. Thromb. Haemost.* **2021**, *19*, 513–521. [CrossRef] [PubMed]
46. Wada, H.; Ichikawa, Y.; Ezaki, M.; Yamamoto, A.; Tomida, M.; Yoshida, M.; Fukui, S.; Moritani, I.; Shiraki, K.; Shimaoka, M.; et al. Elevated Plasma Soluble C-Type Lectin-like Receptor 2 Is Associated with the Worsening of Coronavirus Disease 2019. *J. Clin. Med.* **2022**, *11*, 985. [CrossRef]
47. Wada, H.; Shiraki, K.; Matsumoto, T.; Shimpo, H.; Yamashita, Y.; Shimaoka, M. The evaluation of a scoring system for diagnosing atypical hemolytic uremic syndrome—A review analysis for Japanese aHUS. *Thrmbosis Update* **2020**, *1*, 100012. [CrossRef]
48. Matsunaga, N.; Hayakawa, K.; Terada, M.; Ohtsu, H.; Asai, Y.; Tsuzuki, S.; Suzuki, S.; Toyoda, A.; Suzuki, K.; Endo, M.; et al. Clinical epidemiology of hospitalized patients with COVID-19 in Japan: Report of the COVID-19 Registry Japan. *Clin. Infect. Dis.* **2021**, *73*, e3677–e3689. [CrossRef]
49. Yang, X.; Yang, Q.; Wang, Y.; Wu, Y.; Xu, J.; Yu, Y.; Shang, Y. Thrombocytopenia and its association with mortality in patients with COVID-19. *J. Thromb. Haemost.* **2020**, *18*, 1469–1472. [CrossRef]
50. Wada, H.; Takahashi, H.; Uchiyama, T.; Eguchi, Y.; Okamoto, K.; Kawasugi, K.; Madoiwa, S.; Asakura, H. DIC subcommittee of the Japanese Society on Thrombosis and Hemostasis: The approval of revised diagnostic criteria for DIC from the Japanese Society on Thrombosis and Hemostasis. *Thromb. J.* **2017**, *15*, 17. [CrossRef]
51. Iba, T.; Levy, J.H.; Raj, A.; Warkentin, T.E. Advance in the Management of Sepsis-Induced Coagulopathy and Disseminated Intravascular Coagulation. *J. Clin. Med.* **2019**, *8*, 728. [CrossRef] [PubMed]
52. Wada, H.; Yamamoto, A.; Tomida, M.; Ichikawa, Y.; Ezaki, M.; Masuda, J.; Yoshida, M.; Fukui, S.; Moritani, I.; Inoue, H.; et al. Proposal of Quick Diagnostic Criteria for Disseminated Intravascular Coagulation. *J. Clin. Med.* **2022**, *11*, 1028. [CrossRef] [PubMed]
53. Maugeri, N.; De Lorenzo, R.; Clementi, N.; Antonia; Diotti, R.; Criscuolo, E.; Godino, C.; Tresoldi, C.; Bonini, C.; Clementi, M.; et al. Unconventional CD147-dependent platelet activation elicited by SARS-CoV-2 in COVID-19. *J. Thromb. Haemost.* **2022**, *20*, 434–448. [CrossRef] [PubMed]

54. Lee, C.S.M.; Selvadurai, M.V.; Pasalic, L.; Yeung, J.; Konda, M.; Kershaw, G.W.; Favaloro, E.J.; Chen, V.M. Measurement of procoagulant platelets provides mechanistic insight and diagnostic potential in heparin-induced thrombocytopenia. *J. Thromb. Haemost.* **2022**, *20*, 975–988. [CrossRef]
55. Jennings, L.K. Mechanisms of platelet activation: Need for new strategies to protect against platelet-mediated atherothrombosis. *Thromb. Haemost.* **2009**, *102*, 248–257. [CrossRef]
56. Sánchez-López, V.; Gao, L.; Ferrer-Galván, M.; Arellano-Orden, E.; Elías-Hernández, T.; Jara-Palomares, L.; Asensio-Cruz, M.I.; Castro-Pérez, M.J.; Rodríguez-Martorell, F.J.; Lobo-Beristain, J.L.; et al. Differential biomarker profiles between unprovoked venous thromboembolism and cancer. *Ann. Med.* **2020**, *52*, 310–320. [CrossRef]
57. Yamashita, Y.; Naitoh, K.; Wada, H.; Ikejiri, M.; Mastumoto, T.; Ohishi, K.; Hosaka, Y.; Nishikawa, M.; Katayama, N. Elevated plasma levels of soluble platelet glycoprotein VI (GPVI) in patients with thrombotic microangiopathy. *Thromb. Res* **2014**, *133*, 440–444. [CrossRef]
58. Nishigaki, A.; Ichikawa, Y.; Ezaki, E.; Yamamoto, A.; Suzuki, K.; Tachibana, K.; Kamon, T.; Horie, S.; Masuda, J.; Makino, K.; et al. Soluble C-type lectin-like receptor 2 elevation in patients with acute cerebral infarction. *J. Clin. Med.* **2021**, *10*, 3408. [CrossRef]
59. Favaloro, E.J.; Henry, B.M.; Lippi, G. Increased VWF and Decreased ADAMTS-13 in COVID-19: Creating a Milieu for (Micro)Thrombosis. *Semin. Thromb. Hemost.* **2021**, *47*, 400–418. [CrossRef]
60. Sweeney, J.M.; Barouqa, M.; Krause, G.J.; Gonzalez-Lugo, J.D.; Rahman, S.; Gil, M.R. Low ADAMTS13 Activity Correlates with Increased Mortality in COVID-19 Patients. *TH Open* **2021**, *5*, e89–e103.
61. Nazy, I.; Jevtic, S.D.; Moore, J.C.; Huynh, A.; Smith, J.W.; Kelton, J.G.; Arnold, D.M. Platelet-activating immune complexes identified in critically ill COVID-19 patients suspected of heparin-induced thrombocytopenia. *J. Thromb. Haemost.* **2021**, *19*, 1342–1347. [CrossRef] [PubMed]
62. Favaloro, E.J.; Henry, B.M.; Lippi, G. The complicated relationships of heparin-induced thrombocytopenia and platelet factor 4 antibodies with COVID-19. *Int. J. Lab. Hematol.* **2021**, *43*, 547–558. [CrossRef] [PubMed]
63. Schrick, D.; Tőkés-Füzesi, M.; Réger, B.; Molnár, T. Metabolites: Plasma Fibrinogen Independently Predicts Hypofibrinolysis in Severe COVID-19. *Metabolities* **2021**, *11*, 826. [CrossRef]
64. Nougier, C.; Benoit, R.; Simon, M.; Desmurs-Clavel, H.; Marcotte, G.; Argaud, L.; David, J.S.; Bonnet, A.; Negrier, C.; Dargaud, Y.J. Hypofibrinolytic state and high thrombin generation may play a major role in SARS-COV2 associated thrombosis. *J. Thromb. Haemost.* **2020**, *18*, 2215–2219. [CrossRef] [PubMed]
65. Kruse, J.M.; Magomedov, A.; Kurreck, A.; Münch, F.H.; Koerner, R.; Kamhieh-Milz, J.; Kahl, A.; Gotthardt, I.; Piper, S.K.; Eckardt, K.U.; et al. Thromboembolic complications in critically ill COVID-19 patients are associated with impaired fibrinolysis. *Crit. Care* **2020**, *24*, 676. [CrossRef]
66. Bachler, M.; Bösch, J.; Stürzel, D.P.; Hell, T.; Giebl, A.; Ströhle, M.; Klein, S.J.; Schäfer, V.; Lehner, G.F.; Joannidis, M.; et al. Impaired fibrinolysis in critically ill COVID-19 patients. *Br. J. Anaesth.* **2021**, *126*, 590–598. [CrossRef]
67. Bareille, M.; Hardy, M.; Douxfils, J.; Roullet, S.; Lasne, D.; Levy, J.H.; Stépanian, A.; Susen, S.; Frère, C.; Lecompte, T.; et al. Viscoelastometric Testing to Assess Hemostasis of COVID-19: A Systematic Review. *J. Clin. Med.* **2021**, *10*, 1740. [CrossRef]
68. Pavoni., V.; Gianesello, L.; Pazzi, M.; Dattolo, P.; Prisco, D. Questions about COVID-19 associated coagulopathy: Possible answers from the viscoelastic tests. *J. Clin. Monit. Comput.* **2022**, *36*, 55–69. [CrossRef]
69. Wada, H.; Shiraki, K.; Suzuki-Inoue, K. Comments to: Unconventional CD147-platelet activation elicited by SARS-CoV-2 in COVID-19: sCLEC-2 is new marker for platelet activation by COVID-19. *J. Thromb. Haemost.* **2022**, *20*, 2159–2160. [CrossRef]
70. Zhao, Y.; Yin, L.; Patel, J.; Tang, L.; Huang, Y. The inflammatory markers of multisystem inflammatory syndrome in children (MIS-C) and adolescents associated with COVID-19: A meta-analysis. *J. Med. Virol.* **2021**, *93*, 4358–4369. [CrossRef]
71. Guarino, M.; Perna, B.; Maritati, M.; Remelli, F.; Trevisan, C.; Spampinato, M.D.; Costanzini, A.; Volpato, S.; Contini, C.; De Giorgio, R. Presepsin levels and COVID-19 severity: A systematic review and meta-analysis. *Clin. Exp. Med.* **2022**, 1–10. [CrossRef] [PubMed]
72. Montazersaheb, S.; Hosseiniyan Khatibi, S.M.; Hejazi, M.S.; Tarhriz, V.; Farjami, A.; Ghasemian Sorbeni, F.; Farahzadi, R.; Ghasemnejad, T. COVID-19 infection: An overview on cytokine storm and related interventions. *Virol. J.* **2022**, *19*, 92. [CrossRef] [PubMed]
73. Fukui, S.; Ikeda, K.; Kobayashi, M.; Nishida, K.; Yamada, K.; Horie, S.; Shimada, Y.; Miki, H.; Goto, H.; Hayashi, K.; et al. Predictive prognostic biomarkers in patients with COVID-19 infection. *Mol. Med. Rep.* **2023**, *27*, 15. [CrossRef] [PubMed]
74. Connors, J.M.; Levy, J.H. COVID-19 and its implications for thrombosis and anticoagulation. *Blood* **2020**, *135*, 2033–2040. [CrossRef]
75. Gabrielli, M.; Lamendola, P.; Esperide, A.; Valletta, F.; Franceschi, F. COVID-19 and thrombotic complications: Pulmonary thrombosis rather than embolism? *Thromb. Res.* **2020**, *193*, 98. [CrossRef]
76. Zuo, Y.; Yalavarthi, S.; Shi, H.; Gockman, K.; Zuo, M.; Madison, J.A.; Blair, C.; Weber, A.; Barnes, B.J.; Egeblad, M.; et al. Neutrophil extracellular traps (NETs) in COVID-19. *JCI Insight* **2020**, *5*, e138999.
77. Zhang, S.; Liu, Y.; Wang, X.; Yang, L.; Li, H.; Wang, Y.; Liu, M.; Zhao, X.; Xie, Y.; Yang, Y.; et al. SARS-CoV-2 binds platelet ACE2 to enhance thrombosis in COVID-19. *J. Hematol. Oncol.* **2020**, *13*, 120. [CrossRef]
78. Hottz, E.D.; Azevedo-Quintanilha, I.G.; Palhinha, L.; Teixeira, L.; Barreto, E.A.; Pão, C.R.R.; Righy, C.; Franco, S.; Souza, T.M.L.; Kurtz, P.; et al. Platelet activation and platelet-monocyte aggregate formation trigger tissue factor expression in patients with severe COVID-19. *Blood* **2020**, *136*, 1330–1341. [CrossRef]

79. Wada, H.; Matsumoto, T.; Suzuki, K.; Imai, H.; Katayama, N.; Iba, T.; Matsumoto, M. Differences and similarities between disseminated intravascular coagulation and thrombotic microangiopathy. *Thromb. J.* **2018**, *16*, 14. [CrossRef]
80. Salah, H.M.; Mehta, J.L. Meta-Analysis of the Effect of Aspirin on Mortality in COVID-19. *Am. J. Cardiol.* **2021**, *142*, 158–159. [CrossRef]
81. Sase, T.; Wada, H.; Kamikura, Y.; Kaneko, T.; Abe, Y.; Nishioka, J.; Nobori, T.; Shiku, H. Tissue factor messenger RNA levels in leukocytes compared with tissue factor antigens in plasma from patients in hypercoagulable state caused by various diseases. *Thromb. Haemost.* **2004**, *92*, 132–139. [CrossRef] [PubMed]
82. Wada, H.; Minamikawa, K.; Wakita, Y.; Nakase, T.; Kaneko, T.; Ohiwa, M.; Tamaki, S.; Deguchi, K.; Shirakawa, S.; Hayashi, T.; et al. Increased vascular endothelial cell markers in patients with disseminated intravascular coagulation. *Am. J. Hematol.* **1993**, *44*, 85–88. [CrossRef] [PubMed]
83. Wada, H.; Ichikawa, Y.; Ezaki, E.; Matsumoto, T.; Yamashita, Y.; Shiraki, K.; Shimaoka, M.; Shimpo, H. The reevaluation of thrombin time using a clot waveform analysis. *J. Clin. Med.* **2021**, *10*, 4840. [CrossRef] [PubMed]
84. Han, M.; Pandey, D. ZMPSTE24 Regulates SARS-CoV-2 Spike Protein-enhanced Expression of Endothelial PAI-1. *Am. J. Respir. Cell Mol. Biol.* **2021**, *65*, 300–308. [CrossRef] [PubMed]
85. Connors, J.M.; Falanga, A.; Iba, T.; Kaatz, S.; Levy, J.H.; Middeldorp, S.; Minichiello, T.; Ramacciotti, E.; Samama, C.M.; Thachil, J. International Society on Thrombosis and Haemostasis. ISTH guidelines for antithrombotic treatment in COVID-19. *J. Thromb. Haemost.* **2022**, *20*, 2214–2225.
86. Rizk, J.G.; Gupta, A.; Lazo JGJr Sardar, P.; Henry, B.M.; Lavie, C.J.; Effron, M.B. To Anticoagulate or Not to Anticoagulate in COVID-19: Lessons after 2 Years. *Semin. Thromb. Hemost.* **2023**, *49*, 62–72. [CrossRef]
87. Berger, J.S.; Van Tassell, B.W.; Middeldorp, S.; Piazza, G.; Weitz, J.I.; Cushman, M.; Lip, G.Y.H.; Goldhaber, S.Z.; Bikdeli, B. Use of novel antithrombotic agents for COVID-19: Systematic summary of ongoing randomized controlled trials. *J. Thromb. Haemost.* **2021**, *19*, 3080–3089.

International Journal of *Molecular Sciences*

MDPI

Case Report

Prenatal and Neonatal Pulmonary Thrombosis as a Potential Complication of SARS-CoV-2 Infection in Late Pregnancy

Gazala Abdulaziz-Opiela [1,†], Anna Sobieraj [1,†], Greta Sibrecht [2], Julia Bajdor [3], Bartłomiej Moroziński [4], Zuzanna Kozłowska [2], Rafał Iciek [5], Katarzyna Wróblewska-Seniuk [2,*], Ewa Wender-Ożegowska [5] and Tomasz Szczapa [2]

1 Faculty of Medicine, Poznan University of Medical Sciences, 61-701 Poznan, Poland
2 II Department of Neonatology, Poznan University of Medical Sciences, 61-701 Poznan, Poland
3 Department of Radiology, Nicolaus Copernicus Hospital, 80-803 Gdansk, Poland
4 Department of Pediatric Cardiology, Poznan University of Medical Sciences, 61-701 Poznan, Poland
5 Department of Reproduction, Poznan University of Medical Sciences, 61-701 Poznan, Poland
* Correspondence: kwroblewska@ump.edu.pl
† These authors contributed equally to this work.

Abstract: Neonatal venous thrombosis is a rare condition that can be iatrogenic or occur due to viral infections or genetic mutations. Thromboembolic complications are also commonly observed as a result of SARS-CoV-2 infections. They can affect pediatric patients, especially the ones suffering from multisystem inflammatory syndrome in children (MIS-C) or multisystem inflammatory syndrome in neonates (MIS-N). The question remains whether the maternal SARS-CoV-2 infection during pregnancy can lead to thromboembolic complications in fetuses and neonates. We report on a patient born with an embolism in the arterial duct, left pulmonary artery, and pulmonary trunk, who presented several characteristic features of MIS-N, suspecting that the cause might have been the maternal SARS-CoV2 infection in late pregnancy. Multiple genetic and laboratory tests were performed. The neonate presented only with a positive result of IgG antibodies against SARS-CoV-2. He was treated with low molecular weight heparin. Subsequent echocardiographic tests showed that the embolism dissolved. More research is necessary to evaluate the possible neonatal complications of maternal SARS-CoV-2 infection.

Keywords: pulmonary thrombosis; SARS-CoV-2; neonatal thrombosis; COVID-19 complications

Citation: Abdulaziz-Opiela, G.; Sobieraj, A.; Sibrecht, G.; Bajdor, J.; Mroziński, B.; Kozłowska, Z.; Iciek, R.; Wróblewska-Seniuk, K.; Wender-Ożegowska, E.; Szczapa, T. Prenatal and Neonatal Pulmonary Thrombosis as a Potential Complication of SARS-CoV-2 Infection in Late Pregnancy. *Int. J. Mol. Sci.* **2023**, *24*, 7629. https://doi.org/10.3390/ijms24087629

Academic Editors: Eliza Russu, Alexandru Schiopu and Emil Marian Arbănași

Received: 9 March 2023
Revised: 18 April 2023
Accepted: 19 April 2023
Published: 21 April 2023

1. Introduction

Neonatal venous thrombosis is a rare condition that occurs most often in infants born between the 22nd and 27th week of pregnancy [1]. Up to 90% of venous thromboembolisms are iatrogenic and are associated with central venous catheters [2,3]. Other predisposing factors are mechanical ventilation, infections with cardiotropic viruses (e.g., parvovirus B19, influenza virus, human immunodeficiency virus, cytomegalovirus, herpes simplex virus) [4], hospital stays equal or longer than five days [5], and genetic mutations (e.g., Factor V, Factor II, methylenetetrahydrofolate reductase (MTHFR) genes, protein S or C deficiencies) [6].

While SARS-CoV-2 infection most often leads to respiratory disease, it must be acknowledged that the virus might affect other systems and organs as well. The non-respiratory complications of SARS-CoV-2 infection such as preeclampsia [7] or neurological diseases [8] have been described in the literature. Thromboembolic complications are commonly observed due to SARS-CoV-2 infections, especially among adults [9]. They can also affect pediatric patients, particularly those suffering from the multisystem inflammatory syndrome in children (MIS-C) [10]. The hypothesis of maternal infection playing the pathophysiological role in neonatal thrombosis development has already been described in the literature [11]. As SARS-CoV-2 can be transmitted through the placenta [12], the neonate can develop multisystem inflammatory syndrome in neonates (MIS-N) after birth due to maternal infection [13]. We present a case of a neonate born with a pulmonary embolism in the arterial duct, left pulmonary artery, and pulmonary trunk and several characteristic features of MIS-N potentially associated with the maternal SARS-CoV-2 infection.

2. Case Presentation

The mother, in the 40th week of pregnancy, was admitted to the hospital with no uterine contractions for observation before labor. She reported having had an infection of probable viral etiology in the 38th week of pregnancy with fever, headache, fatigue, and intense cough. The disease happened during the COVID-19 pandemic, while the number of daily new cases was reaching peak values. Despite the symptoms of SARS-CoV-2 infection, the mother did not perform a test. She has not been vaccinated against SARS-CoV-2 either. A fetal ultrasound on admission showed an enlarged heart, asymmetrical atria, and fluid in the pericardium and abdomen cavity. Previous ultrasound scans did not show such abnormalities. Due to the suspicion of circulatory failure, the patient was transferred to a third-level referral hospital, and a cesarean section was performed.

The neonate was hypotrophic (<3rd percentile), with a birth weight of 2580 g. However, there was no evidence of fetal growth restriction in ultrasound scans performed in the 3rd trimester. The Apgar score was 8 in the 1st and 10 in the 5th minute of life. For the first five minutes of life, he required Continuous Positive Airway Pressure (CPAP) respiratory support with a maximal FiO_2 of 25%. Blood samples from the umbilical cord were collected, and pH values from umbilical vessels were within the normal range (pH 7.31 and 7.36, BE: -0.65 and -1.81, respectively). During the first and second days of life, he had recurrent desaturations and required constant passive oxygen therapy with FiO_2 between 25 and 30%.

Echocardiography was performed twice during the initial hospital stay—in the 1st and 12th hour of life. It revealed enlarged heart atria and a spherical structure with a diameter of 4.5 mm at the connection point between the arterial duct and the left pulmonary artery. Moreover, the right ventricle's systolic dysfunction was observed. To confirm the presence of the suspected pulmonary embolism, on the 3rd day of life, chest computed tomography angiography (chest angio-CT) was performed (Figure 1), which demonstrated the presence of an embolism located in the arterial duct, left pulmonary artery, and pulmonary trunk (size 15 mm $\times$ 4.5 mm $\times$ 4.5 mm). In the cross-section image, the thrombus occupied more than half of the lumen of the pulmonary trunk and narrowed the blood inflow to the left pulmonary artery.

The abdominal ultrasonography performed on the first day of life showed an enlarged liver and free peritoneal fluid with no other abnormalities. The additional laboratory tests in the neonate suggested an abnormal liver function (ALT: 172 IU/L, AST: 178 IU/L) and normalized with time. The albumin level was initially low (2.51 g/dL) and increased later (3.31 g/dL). The initial C-reactive protein level was 11.53 mg/L and decreased to 2.5 mg/L on the 9th day of life. Cranial ultrasound was performed twice (on the 6th and 12th day of life) and showed higher echogenicity of white matter along lateral ventricles. A follow-up ultrasound was recommended on an outpatient basis.

Multiple genetic tests were performed to find the cause of embolism formation, such as factor II, factor V, the MTHFR gene, and PAI-1 gene. The patient only tested heterozygous in the MTHFR C677T and A1298C polymorphisms and positive in the PAI-1 5G/4G polymorphism. The results of the remaining tests were normal. The biological mother had not had any medical history of thrombotic diseases, nor other members of the neonate's family.

Moreover, laboratory tests were performed for infections with cardiotropic viruses, ruling out cytomegalovirus, adenovirus, parvovirus-B19, enteroviruses, Coxsackie B viruses, human herpes virus 6, and influenza A and B virus infections. Furthermore, a reverse transcription polymerase chain reaction (RT-PCR) test and an antibodies test for SARS-CoV-2 were performed. The neonate presented with a positive result of IgG antibodies against SARS-CoV-2.

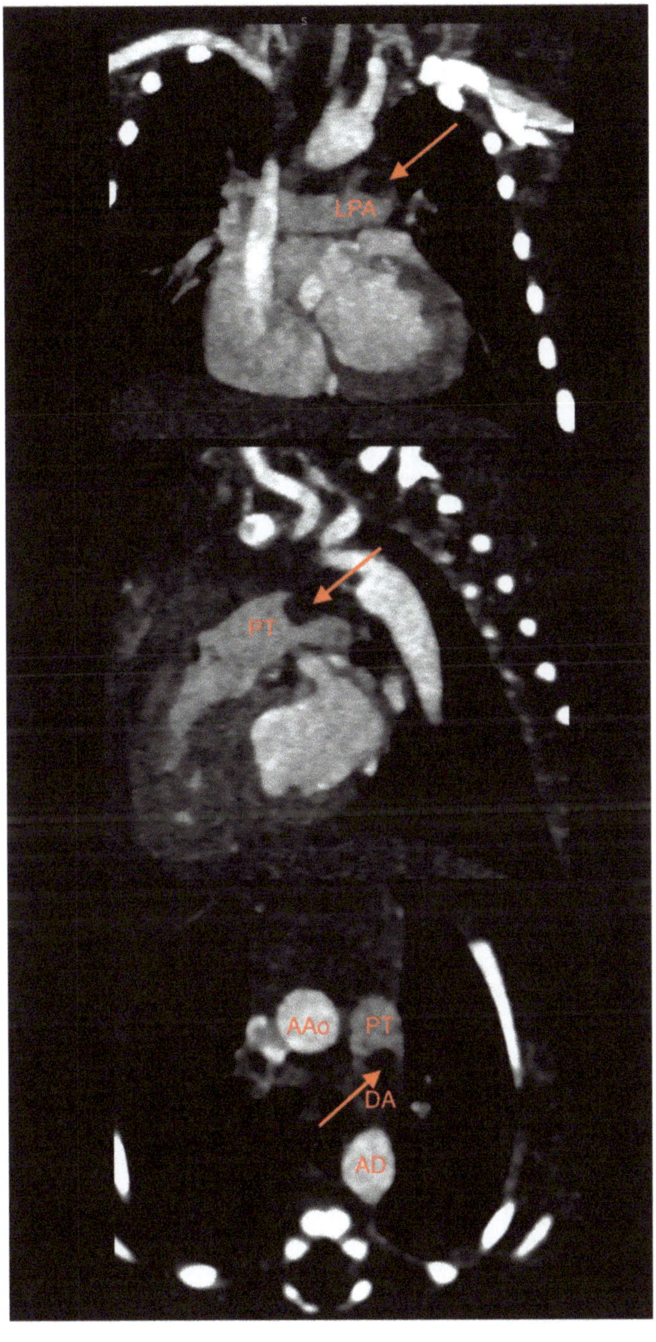

Figure 1. Angio-CT scan of 4-day-old neonate presenting thrombus extending into the left pulmonary artery, pulmonary trunk, and arterial duct. LPA: Left pulmonary artery; PT: Pulmonary trunk; DA: Arterial duct; AAo: Ascending aorta; AD: Descending aorta.

In coagulation tests, we observed increased D-Dimers levels (7.42 mg/L), standard prothrombin times (15.8 s), and a reduced number of platelets (100 G/L). Protein C and Protein S activity was normal (28% and 48%, respectively). Troponin I was 202.8 ng/L, and the N-terminal prohormone of brain natriuretic peptide (NT-proBNP) was >35.000 pg/mL, suggesting myocardial damage and heart failure.

The neonate received two treatment doses of 4.5 milligrams of a low molecular weight heparin (LMWH) on the second day of life. Prolonged bleeding time from injection sites was observed. Coagulation tests showed activated partial thromboplastin time (APTT) above 400 s, decreased fibrinogen (1.61 G/L), and elevated anty-Xa activity (1.92 U/mL). Fresh frozen plasma was transfused, and normalization of the coagulation parameters was observed.

The neonate was transferred to the Cardiology Department on the 3rd day of life, where he received a continuous infusion of unfractionated heparin. However, due to the difficulties in maintaining appropriate APTT values and observed thrombocytopenia, the treatment was changed to LMWH. The activity of anti-Xa was monitored regularly. Moreover, antithrombin III was supplemented as its activity was reduced to 35%. Subsequent echocardiographic tests were performed to monitor the effects of the applied treatment. The echocardiography performed on the 9th and 12th day of life did not show the embolism, suggesting it had resorbed completely. The results of the follow-up abdominal ultrasound did not show any abnormalities. On the 12th day of life, the patient was discharged home in good condition.

3. Discussion

SARS-CoV-2 is a single-stranded ribonucleic acid (RNA) β-coronavirus. Using a specific host protease, transmembrane serine protease 2 (TMPRSS2) [14], it binds to the host cell receptor-angiotensin-converting enzyme 2 receptor (ACE2-R) with the major spike glycoprotein (S1) [15]. ACE2-R is expressed in various tissues and organs, e.g., the lungs, heart, intestine, muscles, liver, pancreas, or kidneys and on the epithelial cells of oral mucosa and the tongue [16,17]. Both arterial and vascular endothelium is characterized by high levels of ACE2-R expression as well [18]. The binding of the virus causes a decrease in the receptor activity, resulting in the accumulation of angiotensin II, which triggers intracellular signaling pathways (caspase 3, p83 MAPK, ROS, cytochrome C) and, subsequently, leads to vasoconstriction, increased oxidative stress, cellular damage, proinflammatory effect, and fibrosis [19]. Moreover, the replication of the virus inside the host cells may promote the immune response, releasing interferon-γ and interleukins: IL-1β and IL-6, which facilitates endothelial activation and inflammation [19,20].

Healthy endothelium is antithrombotic but might become prothrombotic when activated. COVID-19 infection determines endothelial activation by angiopoietin-2, a mediator stored in the Weibel–Palade body, which shows elevated circulating levels in COVID-19 and an association with the induction of procoagulant and proinflammatory reactions [21]. Endothelial activation promotes platelet recruitment through the secretion of the von Willebrand factor and expression of fibrinogen and P-selectin on the surface. Platelet aggregation might generate a deposition of platelet-rich clots in the lung microcirculation. This event is the key mechanism leading to respiratory failure. Furthermore, endothelial cells upregulate the expression of adhesion molecules: VCAM-1, ICAM-1, and E-selectin, which promote leukocyte adhesion and activation. The interaction of platelets and leukocytes facilitates the coagulation pathway and proinflammatory molecules secretion [20]. After the systemic activation of the coagulation and the development of disseminated microthrombosis, multiple organs will be affected.

Ackermann et al., in their study, presented results from autopsies performed on patients who died because of COVID-19. They examined their lungs and described that endothelial cells in the specimens were swollen, the intercellular junctions were disrupted, and there was a lack of contact with the basal membrane. The findings proved that infection with SARS-CoV-2 caused injury to the endothelium and can promote thromboembolism formation [22]. It was predicted that the injury of pulmonary endothelial cells contributed significantly to diffuse alveolar damage and the development of acute respiratory distress syndrome (ARDS) [23]. In another study, a post-mortem autopsy of severe COVID-19 patients confirmed diffuse alveolar damage and inflammatory infiltrations with hyaline membrane formation in the lung and, also, inflammation of the myocardium, focal pancreatitis, axon injury, glomerular microthrombosis, macrophage accumulation in the brain, and lymphocyte infiltrations of the liver [24].

The possible complications of SARS-CoV-2 infections are currently the subject of many studies. However, knowledge regarding the neonatal population is relatively scarce. During the COVID-19 pandemic, the prevalence of prothrombotic and cardiovascular complications increased. They occurred in about 9% of all adult patients [25], with up to 50% of those with severe manifestations [26]. These patients were more susceptible to developing deep vein thrombosis, arterial thrombosis, pulmonary embolisms, or intracatheter thrombosis [20], which were usually related to poorer prognosis and higher mortality rates [27]. However, among pediatric patients suffering from COVID-19, these complications were rather rare [28]. The incidence of thromboembolisms was lower in this group than in adults [29].

Schulze-Schiappacasse et al. published a case report of a 27-day-old neonate with a severe SARS-CoV-2 infection. At first, he presented with watery diarrhea and food refusal for 48 h, and, later, he developed pulmonary thrombosis. Despite the therapy with LMWH, the thrombus continued to grow. Therefore, the neonate required two courses of alteplase, which improved his clinical condition. Many factors could have contributed to the development of the disease, but SARS-CoV-2 infection might be treated as a condition promoting the thrombotic event [30]. However, to the best of our knowledge, no case report has been published where pulmonary thrombosis occurred in utero and caused circulatory failure in the fetus.

Multisystem inflammatory syndrome in neonates (MIS-N) is a syndrome similar to MIS-C, which has been well-described in pediatric patients. The reasons for neonates developing the syndrome are maternal infection and transplacental transfer of SARS-CoV2 antibodies or disease after birth [31]. Possible symptoms include increased CRP and cardiac enzymes, abnormal coagulation tests, cardiomegaly, hepatomegaly and splenomegaly, abnormal liver and kidney function tests, free peritoneal fluid, abnormalities in the brain, and low albumin levels. Compared to MIS-C, fever is not always observed. The outcome is favorable in most cases. However, the observed mortality rate can be up to 9.2% in neonates with MIS-N. The neonate presented in this case report had several MIS-N features such as elevated CRP, increased cardiac enzymes, cardiomegaly, free peritoneal fluid, hepatomegaly, abnormal liver tests, and low albumin level. However, he did not present with abnormalities in the brain, leukocytosis with lymphopenia, or hyponatremia, which are also common.

The molecular mechanisms of MIS-C and MIS-N have been the subject of many studies. SARS-CoV-2 infection preceding MIS-C is usually asymptomatic, but it appears to activate several immunological pathways. SARS-CoV-2 infection is believed to stimulate T-cells, which results in the stimulation of macrophages, monocytes, B-cells, and plasma cells. All of the immune mechanisms, along with the cytokine release (cytokine storm), lead to hyperinflammation and the development of MIS-C [32]. A reduced number of NK cells and lower NK cell degranulation was also identified as a possible factor in the immunopathogenesis of MIS-C [33].

Distinguishing MIS-C from other similar inflammatory syndromes remains challenging, given the lack of information about possible SARS-CoV-2 exposure in many cases. In order to facilitate the differential diagnosis, signatures of MIS-C were compared with severe COVID-19, Kawasaki disease, toxic shock syndrome, or hemophagocytic lymphohistiocytosis (HLH) [32,34]. The comparison studies aimed to identify a profile of inflammatory biomarkers that would be unique for MIS-C. The results indicated that MIS-C and Kawasaki have partially overlapping cytokine profiles, with elevated inflammatory markers such as

IL-6, IL-18, IL-17a, or IFN-γ [35,36]. However, higher levels of IL-17a in Kawasaki disease might suggest different immunopathology. It has been proven that cytokine and chemokine profiles differed in severe COVID-19 and MIS-C. However, there is no consensus on MIS-C distinctive biomarkers [35,37,38]. MIS-C patients were characterized by higher expression of IL-6, higher levels of IFN-γ-induced chemokines (CXCL9 and CXCL10), and higher expression of IFN-γ in T-cells [33,39].

Comparing patients with MIS-C and with HLH, T-cell activation and TH1 cytokines were found in both groups but they differed in amplitude [34]. Hyperinflammation and cytokine storms were described in severe COVID-19 patients as well. According to the studies on COVID-19 complications, the cytokine storm might contribute to thromboembolism formation and multiorgan damage [20].

Thromboembolic complications have been described among the pediatric population both in COVID-19 patients and MIS-C [10,40,41]. Thromboembolisms occur more often among children suffering from MIS-C, with an incidence rate ranging from 1.4% to 6.5% [41]. There are several molecular mechanisms involved in thromboembolism formation. Hyperinflammation and cytokine storms contribute to endothelial dysfunction and hyperactivation of platelets. Moreover, activation of the complement described in MIS-C patients is suspected to increase the risk of thrombosis development.

Although MIS-C and COVID-19 are both unique risk factors, the pathogenesis of thromboembolism formation remains very complex and many factors play a role, including genetic mutations. There has been much research on various types of thrombophilia. It is known that factor V Leiden or prothrombin mutations increase the risk of venous thromboembolisms during SARS-CoV-2 infections [42,43]. PAI-1 gene mutation is a risk factor for myocardial infarctions and venous thromboembolism formation [44]. It may contribute to the severity of COVID-19 infection and lead to coagulopathy characterized by thrombi formation [45]. However, the impact of PAI-1 5G/4G polymorphism on COVID-19 severity has not been confirmed yet [27]. Moreover, the most frequent MTHFR gene polymorphisms C677T and A1298C had also been alleged to contribute to the more severe course of COVID-19. The possible impact of these polymorphisms is still being evaluated in the research studies [27]. However, according to the guidelines established by the American College of Medical Genetics in 2013 [46], the compound 677/1298 heterozygote polymorphism is unlikely to be an independent risk factor for thrombosis occurrence [47]. Given all of these examples, the genetic mutations of the presented neonate do not seem to be a leading factor contributing to pulmonary embolism formation. The possible causes of pulmonary thrombosis appear to be maternal SARS-CoV-2 infection and MIS-N.

The treatment of neonates with pulmonary thrombosis remains a challenge, as there is no consensus on the most favorable method. They include low molecular weight heparin, unfractionated heparin, thrombolytic therapy with alteplase, and catheter-based embolectomy [48]. Coagulation tests must be performed frequently to monitor the treatment. Decisions should be made carefully based on the extent of the thrombosis and modified as the patient is observed day by day to minimize the side effects of the treatment. More research regarding thrombosis treatment strategies is necessary. The usage of novel technologies such as artificial intelligence and machine learning has been described in the literature and might contribute to further search for possible therapies [49,50].

4. Conclusions

Given the positive result of IgG antibodies against SARS-CoV-2 and the mother's infection in late pregnancy with symptoms suggesting COVID-19, we suspected that SARS-CoV-2 was a major factor associated with the formation of the pulmonary embolism in the presented newborn.

More research is necessary to evaluate the possible neonatal complications of maternal SARS-CoV-2 infection. In the described case, the neonate's heart failure was diagnosed prenatally, which resulted in the admission to a 3rd reference-level hospital. A correct diagnosis was made, allowing for effective treatment. It is essential that pregnant women suffering from COVID-19 are monitored to detect possible abnormalities.

Author Contributions: G.A.-O., A.S. and J.B. described the case and drafted the manuscript. B.M., Z.K., T.S., R.I. and E.W.-O. participated in the diagnostics and treatment of the neonate and provided the medical records. G.S., K.W.-S. and T.S. coordinated, edited, and revised the manuscript. All authors contributed to the article. All authors have read and agreed to the published version of the manuscript.

Funding: This research received no external funding.

Institutional Review Board Statement: Ethical review and approval were waived for this study as it is a case report and not an experimental study.

Informed Consent Statement: Written informed consent has been obtained from the patient's mother to publish this paper.

Conflicts of Interest: The authors declare that the research was conducted in the absence of any commercial or financial relationships that could be construed as potential conflict of interest.

References

1. Makatsariya, A.; Bitsadze, V.; Khizroeva, J.; Vorobev, A.; Makatsariya, N.; Egorova, E.; Mischenko, A.; Mashkova, T.; Antonova, A. Neonatal thrombosis. *J. Matern.-Fetal Neonatal Med.* **2020**, *35*, 1169–1177. [CrossRef] [PubMed]
2. Amankwah, E.K.; Atchison, C.M.; Arlikar, S.; Ayala, I.; Barrett, L.; Branchford, B.R.; Streiff, M.; Takemoto, C.; Goldenberg, N.A. Risk factors for hospital-sssociated venous thromboembolism in the neonatal intensive care unit. *Thromb. Res.* **2014**, *134*, 305–309. [CrossRef] [PubMed]
3. Easterlin, M.C.; Li, Y.; Yieh, L.; Gong, C.L.; Jaffray, J.; Hall, M.; Friedlich, P.S.; Lakshmanan, A. Predictors of venous thromboembolism among infants in children's hospitals in the United States: A retrospective Pediatric Health Information Study. *J. Perinatol.* **2022**, *42*, 103–109. [CrossRef] [PubMed]
4. Boulet, S.L.; Grosse, S.D.; Thornburg, C.D.; Yusuf, H.; Tsai, J.; Hooper, W.C. Trends in Venous Thromboembolism-Related Hospitalizations, 1994–2009. *Pediatrics* **2012**, *130*, e812–e820. [CrossRef] [PubMed]
5. Branchford, B.R.; Mourani, P.; Bajaj, L.; Manco-Johnson, M.; Wang, M.; Goldenberg, N.A. Risk factors for in-hospital venous thromboembolism in children: A case-control study employing diagnostic validation. *Haematologica* **2012**, *97*, 509–515. [CrossRef]
6. Nowak-Göttl, U.; Dübbers, A.; Kececioglu, D.; Koch, H.G.; Kotthoff, S.; Runde, J.; Vielhaber, H. Factor V Leiden, protein C, and lipoprotein (a) in catheter-related thrombosis in childhood: A prospective study. *J. Pediatr.* **1997**, *131*, 608–612. [CrossRef]
7. Tossetta, G.; Fantone, S.; Delli Muti, N.; Balercia, G.; Ciavattini, A.; Giannubilo, S.R.; Marzioni, D. Preeclampsia and severe acute respiratory syndrome coronavirus 2 infection: A systematic review. *J. Hypertens.* **2022**, *40*, 1629–1638. [CrossRef]
8. Dale, L. Neurological Complications of COVID-19: A Review of the Literature. *Cureus* **2022**, *14*, e27633. [CrossRef]
9. Helms, J.; Tacquard, C.; Severac, F.; Leonard-Lorant, I.; Ohana, M.; Delabranche, X.; Merdji, H.; Clere-Jehl, R.; Schenck, M.; Fagot Gandet, F.; et al. High risk of thrombosis in patients with severe SARS-CoV-2 infection: A multicenter prospective cohort study. *Intensive Care Med.* **2020**, *46*, 1089–1098. [CrossRef]
10. Whitworth, H.; Sartain, S.E.; Kumar, R.; Armstrong, K.; Ballester, L.; Betensky, M.; Cohen, C.T.; Diaz, R.; Diorio, C.; Goldenberg, N.A.; et al. Rate of thrombosis in children and adolescents hospitalized with COVID-19 or MIS-C. *Blood* **2021**, *138*, 190–198. [CrossRef]
11. Campi, F.; Longo, D.; Bersani, I.; Savarese, I.; Lucignani, G.; Haass, C.; Paolino, M.C.; Vadalà, S.; De Liso, P.; Di Capua, M.; et al. Neonatal Cerebral Venous Thrombosis following Maternal SARS-CoV-2 Infection in Pregnancy. *Neonatology* **2022**, *119*, 268–272. [CrossRef] [PubMed]
12. Vivanti, A.J.; Vauloup-Fellous, C.; Prevot, S.; Zupan, V.; Suffee, C.; Do Cao, J.; Benachi, A.; De Luca, D. Transplacental transmission of SARS-CoV-2 infection. *Nat. Commun.* **2020**, *11*, 3572. [CrossRef]
13. Lima, A.R.O.; Cardoso, C.C.; Bentim, P.R.B.; Voloch, C.M.; Rossi, Á.D.; da Costa, R.M.M.S.C.; da Paz, J.A.S.; Agostinho, R.F.; Figueiredo, V.R.F.S.; Júnior, J.S.S.; et al. Maternal SARS-CoV-2 Infection Associated to Systemic Inflammatory Response and Pericardial Effusion in the Newborn: A Case Report. *J. Pediatr. Infect. Dis. Soc.* **2020**, *10*, 536–539. [CrossRef]
14. Jin, Y.; Ji, W.; Yang, H.; Chen, S.; Zhang, W.; Duan, G. Endothelial activation and dysfunction in COVID-19: From basic mechanisms to potential therapeutic approaches. *Signal Transduct. Target. Ther.* **2020**, *5*, 293. [CrossRef]
15. Batah, S.S.; Fabro, A.T. Pulmonary pathology of ARDS in COVID-19: A pathological review for clinicians. *Respir. Med.* **2021**, *176*, 106239. [CrossRef]
16. Gheblawi, M.; Wang, K.; Viveiros, A.; Nguyen, Q.; Zhong, J.C.; Turner, A.J.; Raizada, M.K.; Grant, M.B.; Oudit, G.Y. Angiotensin-Converting Enzyme 2: SARS-CoV-2 Receptor and Regulator of the Renin-Angiotensin System: Celebrating the 20th Anniversary of the Discovery of ACE2. *Circ. Res.* **2020**, *126*, 1456–1474. [CrossRef]
17. Xu, H.; Zhong, L.; Deng, J.; Peng, J.; Dan, H.; Zeng, X.; Li, T.; Chen, Q. High expression of ACE2 receptor of 2019-nCoV on the epithelial cells of oral mucosa. *Int. J. Oral Sci.* **2020**, *12*, 8. [CrossRef] [PubMed]

18. Hamming, I.; Timens, W.; Bulthuis, M.L.; Lely, A.T.; Navis, G.; van Goor, H. Tissue distribution of ACE2 protein, the functional receptor for SARS coronavirus. A first step in understanding SARS pathogenesis. *J. Pathol.* **2004**, *203*, 631–637. [CrossRef] [PubMed]
19. Silva Andrade, B.; Siqueira, S.; de Assis Soares, W.R.; de Souza Rangel, F.; Santos, N.O.; Dos Santos Freitas, A.; Ribeiro da Silveira, P.; Tiwari, S.; Alzahrani, K.J.; Góes-Neto, A.; et al. Long-COVID and Post-COVID Health Complications: An Up-to-Date Review on Clinical Conditions and Their Possible Molecular Mechanisms. *Viruses* **2021**, *13*, 700. [CrossRef]
20. Ribes, A.; Vardon-Bounes, F.; Mémier, V.; Poette, M.; Au-Duong, J.; Garcia, C.; Minville, V.; Sié, P.; Bura-Rivière, A.; Voisin, S.; et al. Thromboembolic events and COVID-19. *Adv. Biol. Regul.* **2020**, *77*, 100735. [CrossRef]
21. Smadja, D.M.; Guerin, C.L.; Chocron, R.; Yatim, N.; Boussier, J.; Gendron, N.; Khider, L.; Hadjadj, J.; Goudot, G.; DeBuc, B.; et al. Angiopoietin-2 as a marker of endothelial activation is a good predictor factor for intensive care unit admission of COVID-19 patients. *Angiogenesis* **2020**, *23*, 611–620.
22. Ackermann, M.; Verleden, S.E.; Kuehnel, M.; Haverich, A.; Welte, T.; Laenger, F.; Vanstapel, A.; Werlein, C.; Stark, H.; Tzankov, A.; et al. Pulmonary Vascular Endothelialitis, Thrombosis, and Angiogenesis in Covid-19. *N. Engl. J. Med.* **2020**, *383*, 120–128. [CrossRef]
23. Teuwen, L.A.; Geldhof, V.; Pasut, A.; Carmeliet, P. COVID-19: The vasculature unleashed. Nature reviews. *Immunology* **2020**, *20*, 389–391. [CrossRef]
24. Eketunde, A.O.; Mellacheruvu, S.P.; Oreoluwa, P. A review of postmortem findings in patients with COVID-19. *Cureus* **2020**, *12*, e9438.
25. Blondon, M.; Cereghetti, S.; Pugin, J.; Marti, C.; Darbellay Farhoumand, P.; Reny, J.; Calmy, A.; Combescure, C.; Mazzolai, L.; Pantet, O.; et al. Therapeutic anticoagulation to prevent thrombosis, coagulopathy, and mortality in severe COVID-19: The Swiss COVID-HEP randomized clinical trial. *Res. Pract. Thromb. Haemost.* **2022**, *6*, e12712. [CrossRef]
26. Zhou, F.; Yu, T.; Du, R.; Fan, G.; Liu, Y.; Liu, Z.; Xiang, J.; Wang, Y.; Song, B.; Gu, X.; et al. Clinical course and risk factors for mortality of adult inpatients with COVID-19 in Wuhan, China: A retrospective cohort study. *Lancet* **2020**, *395*, 1054–1062. [CrossRef] [PubMed]
27. Lapić, I.; Radić Antolic, M.; Horvat, I.; Premužić, V.; Palić, J.; Rogić, D.; Zadro, R. Association of polymorphisms in genes encoding prothrombotic and cardiovascular risk factors with disease severity in COVID-19 patients: A pilot study. *J. Med. Virol.* **2022**, *94*, 3669–3675. [CrossRef] [PubMed]
28. Aguilera-Alonso, D.; Murias, S.; Martínez-de-Azagra Garde, A.; Soriano-Arandes, A.; Pareja, M.; Otheo, E.; Moraleda, C.; Tagarro, A.; Calvo, C. Prevalence of thrombotic complications in children with SARS-CoV-2. *Arch. Dis. Child.* **2021**, *106*, 1129–1132. [CrossRef] [PubMed]
29. Chalmers, E.A. Epidemiology of venous thromboembolism in neonates and children. *Thromb. Res.* **2006**, *118*, 3–12. [CrossRef] [PubMed]
30. Schulze-Schiappacasse, C.; Alarcón-Andrade, G.; Valenzuela, G.; Ferreiro, M.; Cavagnaro, A.; García-Salum, T.; Gutiérrez, M.; Medina, R.A. Pulmonary Artery Thrombosis in a Newborn With Severe Coronavirus Disease 2019. *Pediatr. Infect. Dis. J.* **2021**, *40*, e252–e254. [CrossRef]
31. More, K.; Aiyer, S.; Goti, A.; Parikh, M.; Sheikh, S.; Patel, G.; Kallem, V.; Soni, R.; Kumar, P. Multisystem inflammatory syndrome in neonates (MIS-N) associated with SARS-CoV2 infection: A case series. *Eur. J. Pediatr.* **2022**, *181*, 1883–1898. [CrossRef]
32. Nakra, N.A.; Blumberg, D.A.; Herrera-Guerra, A.; Lakshminrusimha, S. Multi-System Inflammatory Syndrome in Children (MIS-C) Following SARS-CoV-2 Infection: Review of Clinical Presentation, Hypothetical Pathogenesis, and Proposed Management. *Children* **2020**, *7*, 69. [CrossRef]
33. Rey-Jurado, E.; Espinosa, Y.; Astudillo, C.; Jimena Cortés, L.; Hormazabal, J.; Noguera, L.P.; Cofré, F.; Piñera, C.; González, R.; Bataszew, A.; et al. Deep immunophenotyping reveals biomarkers of multisystemic inflammatory syndrome in children in a Latin American cohort. *J. Allergy Clin. Immunol.* **2022**, *150*, 1074–1085.e11. [CrossRef] [PubMed]
34. Kumar, D.; Rostad, C.A.; Jaggi, P.; Villacis Nunez, D.S.; Prince, C.; Lu, A.; Hussaini, L.; Nguyen, T.H.; Malik, S.; Ponder, L.A.; et al. Distinguishing immune activation and inflammatory signatures of multisystem inflammatory syndrome in children (MIS-C) versus hemophagocytic lymphohistiocytosis (HLH). *J. Allergy Clin. Immunol.* **2022**, *149*, 1592–1606.e16. [CrossRef]
35. Consiglio, C.R.; Cotugno, N.; Sardh, F.; Pou, C.; Amodio, D.; Rodriguez, L.; Tan, Z.; Zicari, S.; Ruggiero, A.; Pascucci, G.R.; et al. The Immunology of Multisystem Inflammatory Syndrome in Children with COVID-19. *Cell* **2020**, *183*, 968–981.e7. [CrossRef]
36. Esteve-Sole, A.; Anton, J.; Pino-Ramirez, R.M.; Sanchez-Manubens, J.; Fumadó, V.; Fortuny, C.; Rios-Barnes, M.; Sanchez-de-Toledo, J.; Girona-Alarcón, M.; Mosquera, J.M.; et al. Similarities and differences between the immunopathogenesis of COVID-19-related pediatric multisystem inflammatory syndrome and Kawasaki disease. *J. Clin. Investig.* **2021**, *131*, e144554. [CrossRef]
37. Gurlevik, S.L.; Ozsurekci, Y.; Sağ, E.; Derin Oygar, P.; Kesici, S.; Akca, Ü.K.; Cuceoglu, M.K.; Basaran, O.; Göncü, S.; Karakaya, J.; et al. The difference of the inflammatory milieu in MIS-C and severe COVID-19. *Pediatr. Res.* **2022**, *92*, 1805–1814. [CrossRef] [PubMed]
38. Sacco, K.; Castagnoli, R.; Vakkilainen, S.; Liu, C.; Delmonte, O.M.; Oguz, C.; Kaplan, I.M.; Alehashemi, S.; Burbelo, P.D.; Bhuyan, F.; et al. Immunopathological signatures in multisystem inflammatory syndrome in children and pediatric COVID-19. *Nat. Med.* **2022**, *28*, 1050–1062. [CrossRef]

39. Caldarale, F.; Giacomelli, M.; Garrafa, E.; Tamassia, N.; Morreale, A.; Poli, P.; Timpano, S.; Baresi, G.; Zunica, F.; Cattalini, M.; et al. Plasmacytoid Dendritic Cells Depletion and Elevation of IFN-γ Dependent Chemokines CXCL9 and CXCL10 in Children with Multisystem Inflammatory Syndrome. *Front. Immunol.* **2021**, *12*, 654587. [CrossRef]
40. Trapani, S.; Rubino, C.; Lasagni, D.; Pegoraro, F.; Resti, M.; Simonini, G.; Indolfi, G. Thromboembolic complications in children with COVID-19 and MIS-C: A narrative review. *Front. Pediatr.* **2022**, *10*, 944743. [CrossRef] [PubMed]
41. Amonkar, P.S.; Gavhane, J.B.; Kharche, S.N.; Kadam, S.S.; Bhusare, D.B. Aortic thrombosis in a neonate with COVID-19-related fetal inflammatory response syndrome requiring amputation of the leg: A case report. *Paediatr. Int. Child Health* **2021**, *41*, 211–216. [CrossRef] [PubMed]
42. Matsuyama, T.; Kubli, S.P.; Yoshinaga, S.K.; Pfeffer, K.; Mak, T.W. An aberrant STAT pathway is central to COVID-19. *Cell Death Differ.* **2020**, *27*, 3209–3225. [CrossRef]
43. Stevens, H.; Canovas, R.; Tran, H.; Peter, K.; McFadyen, J.D. Inherited Thrombophilias Are Associated With a Higher Risk of COVID-19–Associated Venous Thromboembolism: A Prospective Population-Based Cohort Study. *Circulation* **2022**, *145*, 940–942. [CrossRef] [PubMed]
44. Sillen, M.; Declerck, P.J. Targeting PAI-1 in Cardiovascular Disease: Structural Insights into PAI-1 Functionality and Inhibition. *Front. Cardiovasc. Med.* **2020**, *7*, 622473. [CrossRef] [PubMed]
45. Hickey, S.E.; Curry, C.J.; Toriello, H.V. ACMG Practice Guideline: Lack of evidence for MTHFR polymorphism testing. *Genet. Med.* **2013**, *15*, 153–156. [CrossRef] [PubMed]
46. Graydon, J.S.; Claudio, K.; Baker, S.; Kocherla, M.; Ferreira, M.; Roche-Lima, A.; Rodríguez-Maldonado, J.; Duconge, J.; Ruaño, G. Ethnogeographic prevalence and implications of the 677C>T and 1298A>C MTHFR polymorphisms in US primary care populations. *Biomark. Med.* **2019**, *13*, 649–661. [CrossRef] [PubMed]
47. ElHassan, N.O.; Sproles, C.; Sachdeva, R.; Bhutta, S.T.; Szabo, J.S. A neonate with left pulmonary artery thrombosis and left lung hypoplasia: A case report. *J. Med. Case Rep.* **2010**, *4*, 284. [CrossRef] [PubMed]
48. Sawyer, T.; Antle, A.; Studer, M.; Thompson, M.; Perry, S.; Mahnke, C.B. Neonatal Pulmonary Artery Thrombosis Presenting as Persistent Pulmonary Hypertension of the Newborn. *Pediatr. Cardiol.* **2008**, *30*, 520–522. [CrossRef] [PubMed]
49. Datta, A.; Flynn, N.R.; Barnette, D.A.; Woeltje, K.F.; Miller, G.P.; Swamidass, S.J. Machine learning liver-injuring drug interactions with non-steroidal anti-inflammatory drugs (NSAIDs) from a retrospective electronic health record (EHR) cohort. *PLoS Comput. Biol.* **2021**, *17*, e1009053. [CrossRef]
50. Datta, A.; Matlock, M.K.; Le Dang, N.; Moulin, T.; Woeltje, K.F.; Yanik, E.L.; Joshua Swamidass, S. 'Black Box' to 'Conversational' Machine Learning: Ondansetron Reduces Risk of Hospital-Acquired Venous Thromboembolism. *IEEE J. Biomed. Health Inform.* **2021**, *25*, 2204–2214. [CrossRef]

International Journal of
Molecular Sciences

MDPI

Article

Elevated FAI Index of Pericoronary Inflammation on Coronary CT Identifies Increased Risk of Coronary Plaque Vulnerability after COVID-19 Infection

Botond Barna Mátyás [1,2,3], Imre Benedek [1,2,4], Emanuel Blîndu [1,2,3], Renáta Gerculy [1,2,3], Aurelian Roșca [1,2,3], Nóra Rat [1,2,4,*], István Kovács [1,2,4], Diana Opincariu [2,4], Zsolt Parajkó [1,2,3], Evelin Szabó [1,2,3], Bianka Benedek [5] and Theodora Benedek [1,2,4]

1 Clinic of Cardiology, Mureș County Emergency Clinical Hospital, 540142 Târgu Mureș, Romania; matyas_botond@yahoo.com (B.B.M.); imre.benedek@umfst.ro (I.B.); emi.blindu@yahoo.com (E.B.); gerculy_renata@yahoo.com (R.G.); rosca_aurelian@yahoo.com (A.R.); istvan.kovacs@umfst.ro (I.K.); p_zsolt92@yahoo.com (Z.P.); szaboevelin22@yahoo.com (E.S.); theodora.benedek@umfst.ro (T.B.)
2 Center of Advanced Research in Multimodality Cardiac Imaging, CardioMed Medical Center, 540124 Târgu Mureș, Romania; diana.opincariu@yahoo.ro
3 Doctoral School of Medicine and Pharmacy, University of Medicine, Pharmacy, Science and Technology "George Emil Palade" of Târgu-Mures, 540139 Târgu-Mures, Romania
4 Department of Cardiology, University of Medicine, Pharmacy, Science and Technology "George Emil Palade" of Târgu-Mures, 540139 Târgu Mureș, Romania
5 Faculty of Medicine and Pharmacy, University of Medicine, Pharmacy, Science and Technology "George Emil Palade" of Târgu-Mures, 540139 Târgu Mureș, Romania; benedekb.krisztina@gmail.com
* Correspondence: nora.rat@umfst.ro; Tel.: +40-265-215-551

Abstract: Inflammation is a key factor in the development of atherosclerosis, a disease characterized by the buildup of plaque in the arteries. COVID-19 infection is known to cause systemic inflammation, but its impact on local plaque vulnerability is unclear. Our study aimed to investigate the impact of COVID-19 infection on coronary artery disease (CAD) in patients who underwent computed tomography angiography (CCTA) for chest pain in the early stages after infection, using an AI-powered solution called CaRi-Heart®. The study included 158 patients (mean age was 61.63 ± 10.14 years) with angina and low to intermediate clinical likelihood of CAD, with 75 having a previous COVID-19 infection and 83 without infection. The results showed that patients who had a previous COVID-19 infection had higher levels of pericoronary inflammation than those who did not have a COVID-19 infection, suggesting that COVID-19 may increase the risk of coronary plaque destabilization. This study highlights the potential long-term impact of COVID-19 on cardiovascular health, and the importance of monitoring and managing cardiovascular risk factors in patients recovering from COVID-19 infection. The AI-powered CaRi-Heart® technology may offer a non-invasive way to detect coronary artery inflammation and plaque instability in patients with COVID-19.

Keywords: COVID-19; vascular inflammation; fat attenuation index; plaque vulnerability; thrombosis; chronic coronary syndrome; pericoronary adipose tissue

Citation: Mátyás, B.B.; Benedek, I.; Blîndu, E.; Gerculy, R.; Roșca, A.; Rat, N.; Kovács, I.; Opincariu, D.; Parajkó, Z.; Szabó, E.; et al. Elevated FAI Index of Pericoronary Inflammation on Coronary CT Identifies Increased Risk of Coronary Plaque Vulnerability after COVID-19 Infection. *Int. J. Mol. Sci.* **2023**, *24*, 7398. https://doi.org/10.3390/ijms24087398

Academic Editors: Alexandru Schiopu, Emil Marian Arbănași and Eliza Russu

Received: 11 March 2023
Revised: 14 April 2023
Accepted: 15 April 2023
Published: 17 April 2023

1. Introduction

1.1. The Impact of Vascular Inflammation in Atherosclerosis

It is well-established that vascular inflammation is a key factor in the development and progression of atherosclerosis. Plaques that are stable have a chronic inflammatory response, while those that are vulnerable or have ruptured have an "active" inflammation that can compromise the protective fibrous cap and raises the risk of rupture, which is the main cause of acute vascular events (AVE) [1].

Atherosclerosis is a prevalent condition that affects the blood vessels and increases the risk of serious AVE, such as acute coronary syndrome (ACS) and cerebrovascular events.

These events occur when the plaques rupture and form clots, which can lead to severe complications and even death. The concept of "vulnerable plaque" (VP) was introduced to describe the unpredictable nature of the progression of atherosclerosis [2], a VP is one that is more likely to rupture and cause an AVE [3]. In recent years, research has focused on understanding the mechanisms that lead to plaque instability and rupture. However, there are also factors outside of the plaque that can increase a person's risk for an event, leading to the concept of "vulnerable patient" [3,4]. A vulnerable patient is someone who is at a higher risk of developing an AVE or sudden cardiac death based on factors such as the characteristics of the plaque, perivascular inflammation, blood flow, and myocardial vulnerability [3–5].

In recent years, epicardial adipose tissue (EAT) and perivascular adipose tissue (PVAT) have been extensively researched for their roles as markers and promoters of local coronary inflammation [6,7]. PVAT is a layer of fat that surrounds the coronary arteries and other blood vessels, and is composed of lipid-filled cells (adipocytes), connective tissue cells (such as preadipocytes), and interstitial tissue. PVAT is considered part of the vessel and has a close anatomical and physiological relationship with the arterial wall [8]. EAT and PVAT also contribute to systemic inflammation by releasing cytokines into the circulation through paracrine signaling pathways [9]. Non-invasive imaging methods have been used to effectively quantify EAT and PVAT, which has been shown to predict the risk of AVE across a variety of cardiovascular disorders, and also correlates with markers for systemic inflammation, increased oxidative stress, severity of atherosclerosis, and patient prognosis [10,11].

1.2. COVID-19 Inflammatory Response: Pathophysiology

The COVID-19 pandemic has had a considerable impact on cardiovascular health, due to its effects on inflammation and destabilization of the immune system, both during the acute phase of the infection and over the course of the disease, as well as in long-COVID syndrome [12,13]. SARS-CoV-2 infection can exacerbate underlying cardiovascular diseases (CVD) or promote vulnerability of coronary atherosclerotic plaques due to high levels of pro-inflammatory cytokines and chemokines in the bloodstream. These substances can lead to microvascular and vascular thrombosis, coronary vasospasm, modulation of shear stress, and platelet activation, which can further contribute to plaque vulnerability [14]. The intensity of the cytokine storm, or excessive release of cytokines, has been identified as a significant component in predicting the clinical progression of extrapulmonary organ failure and mortality in COVID-19 patients [15].

1.3. PVAT-FAI Mapping for Inflammation Detection

The optimal method to detect inflammation in the PVAT using coronary computed tomography angiography (CCTA) is through the use of the fat attenuation index (FAI). The FAI is a measure of the CT attenuation gradients in the perivascular space and is calculated by comparing the attenuation values of the PVAT and the adjacent vessel. In cases of coronary inflammation, the composition of the PVAT undergoes a change towards higher aqueous and lower lipophilic content, which can be observed in the FAI due to a decrease in the CT attenuation of the PVAT. Chronic inflammation can also lead to unfavorable fibrotic and other remodeling of the PVAT, which can be identified using progressed radiomic texture analysis of the perivascular adipose tissue [16,17]. The FAI has several advantages as a measure of vascular inflammation; it is not affected by the degree of coronary calcification, is not influenced by individual systemic inflammation as measured by hs-CRP, and is not associated with the severity of coronary stenosis [18,19].

CCTA is commonly used in COVID-19 patients with diagnosed or suspected CVD, especially when the results are likely to significantly affect the patient's treatment plan or save their life [8,20]. As previously discussed, local vascular inflammation can be quantified non-invasively using CT imaging with the computation of the FAI, using artificial intelligence algorithms [21,22].

2. Results

2.1. Baseline Characteristics of the Study Population

This study recruited 158 patients who reported chest pain and had a low to intermediate clinical likelihood of CAD. In total, 47.46% of the participants (n = 75) had a history of COVID-19 infection a few months prior to the CCTA examination, while the remaining 52.53% did not have any prior infection. The participants had an average age of 61.63 ± 10.14 years, and 67.08% (n = 106) of them were male. There were no statistically significant differences between the two groups in terms of gender, age, and comorbidities such as hypertension, diabetes, and obesity. In contrast, it was observed that group 1 exhibited a lower incidence of hypercholesterolemia in comparison to group 2 (40.00% vs. 59.04%, p = 0.02), alongside having a higher body mass index (28.51 ± 4.21 vs. 26.93 ± 4.25, p = 0.03) and significantly reduced levels of triglycerides (134.1 ± 75.04 vs. 154.0 ± 64.58, p = 0.03). The groups did not show any significant differences in terms of PCI after CCTA, multi-vessel PCI, heart failure, left ventricular ejection fraction (LVEF), serum creatinine, and total cholesterol. The average time from COVID-19 infection to CCTA examination for group 2 was 138.1 ± 103.2 days and there were no significant differences between the groups in terms of vaccination against COVID-19. The baseline characteristics, comorbidities, and risk factors of the two study groups are presented in Table 1.

Table 1. Baseline characteristics, comorbidities, and risk factors in the study population.

Parameters	Whole Study Sample (n = 158)	Group 1 (COVID-19) (n = 75)	Group 2 (non COVID-19) (n = 83)	p Value *
Male gender, n (%)	106 (67.08%)	46 (61.33%)	60 (72.29%)	NS
Age at time of scan, mean ± SD	61.63 ± 10.14	60.29 ± 10.30	62.84 ± 9.90	NS
Smoking, n (%)	29 (18.35%)	10 (13.33%)	19 (22.89%)	NS
Hypertension, n (%)	135 (85.44%)	61 (81.33%)	74 (89.16%)	NS
Hypercholesterolemia, n (%)	79 (50.00%)	30 (40.00%)	49 (59.04%)	0.02
Diabetes, n (%)	44 (27.84%)	18 (24.00%)	26 (31.33%)	NS
Obesity, n (%)	41 (25.94%)	25 (33.33%)	16 (20.25%)	0.07
BMI, mean ± SD	27.57 ± 4.29	28.51 ± 4.21	26.93 ± 4.25	0.03
PCI after CCTA, n (%)	69 (43.67%)	27 (36.99%)	42 (50.60%)	NS
Multi-vessel PCI, n (%)	23 (14.55%)	7 (25.93%)	16 (38.10%)	NS
Heart failure, n (%)	117 (74.05%)	57 (76.00%)	60 (75.95%)	NS
LVEF (%), mean ± SD	47.69 ± 5.07	48.34 ± 4.18	47.12 ± 5.71	NS
Creatinine (mg/dL), mean ± SD	0.97 ± 0.26	0.93 ± 0.23	1.00 ± 0.27	NS
Total cholesterol (mg/dL), mean ± SD	167.3 ± 47.13	161.4 ± 43.55	171.0 ± 49.24	0.07
Triglycerides (mg/dL), mean ± SD	145.7 ± 69.49	134.1 ± 75.04	154.0 ± 64.58	0.03
COVID-19 vaccine, n (%)	99 (62.65%)	43 (57.33%)	56 (60.22%)	NS
Time from COVID-19 to CCTA (days), mean ± SD		138.1 ± 103.2		

* BMI—body mass index > 30 kg/m^2; PCI—percutaneous coronary intervention; LVEF—left ventricular ejection fraction; NS—non-significance.

Figure 1 demonstrates the case of a single patient who underwent CCTA among the 158 patients referred to the partner center for further assessment utilizing AI algorithms.

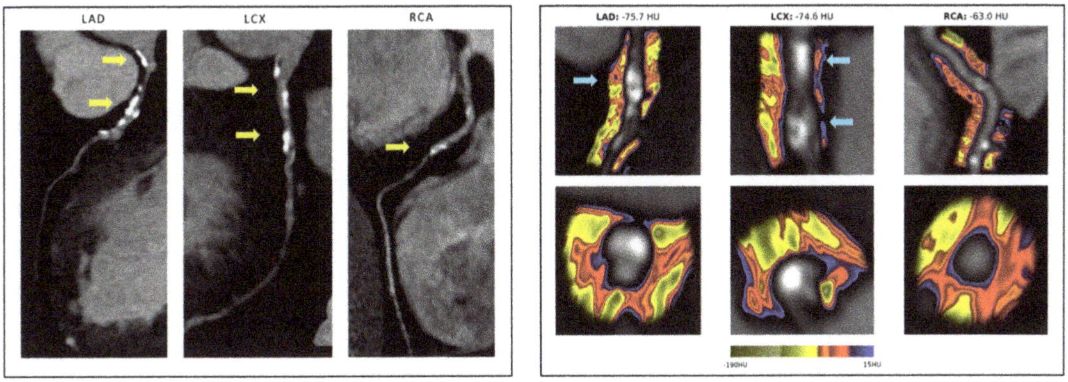

(a) (b)

Figure 1. Conventional CCTA image of the three major coronary arteries (**a**) and a colored mapping representation of an abnormal FAI for the same patient (**b**). Figure shows CCTA images of the three major coronary arteries with a stable atherosclerotic lesion (yellow arrows) in a patient who had a COVID-19 infection a few months prior to CCTA examination (**a**) and delineated pericoronary fat with the FAI colored mapping around the non-culprit lesions (blue arrows) demonstrating abnormal FAI in the same patient (**b**). Using the CaRi-Heart® v2.4.2 platform (panel **b**), FAI-Score was evaluated for each individual at baseline in the proximal LAD, LCX, and RCA.

2.2. PVAT-FAI Values and Scores

According to the standard adipose tissue Hounsfield unit range (−190 to −30 HU), there were no significant differences in the coronary FAI index values between the two groups as revealed by the conventional CT scan. The FAI-score was consistently higher in the non COVID-19 group; more precisely: LAD (group 1—9.32 ± 6.00 vs. group 2—11.61 ± 7.60, $p = 0.05$), LCX (group 1—10.48 ± 6.24 vs. group 2—12.43 ± 6.65, $p = 0.05$), FAI-score TOTAL (group 1—10.47 ± 7.19 vs. group 2—12.81 ± 8.28, $p = 0.001$) (Table 2).

Table 2. PVAT-FAI Score Centile of Coronary Inflammation for Age and Gender.

Parameters	Whole Study Sample (n = 158)	Group 1 (COVID-19) (n = 75)	Group 2 (non COVID-19) (n = 83)	*p* Value *
FAI HU LAD, mean ± SD	−76.08 ± 7.66	−75.07 ± 7.59	−76.46 ± 7.74	NS
FAI HU LCX, mean ± SD	−71.32 ± 7.50	−71.44 ± 7.88	−71.21 ± 7.16	NS
FAI HU RCA, mean ± SD	−73.11 ± 8.94	−72.97 ± 9.38	−73.23 ± 9.61	NS
FAI-Score LAD, mean ± SD	10.54 ± 6.97	9.32 ± 6.00	11.61 ± 7.60	0.05
FAI-Score LCX, mean ± SD	11.48 ± 6.50	10.48 ± 6.24	12.43 ± 6.65	0.05
FAI-Score RCA, mean ± SD	15.00 ± 11.71	14.54 ± 12.17	15.40 ± 11.36	NS
FAI-Score TOTAL, mean ± SD	11.72 ± 7.87	10.47 ± 7.19	12.81 ± 8.28	0.001
FAI-Score Centile LAD, mean ± SD	0.61 ± 0.28	0.66 ± 0.29	0.58 ± 0.28	0.05
FAI-Score Centile LCX, mean ± SD	0.73 ± 0.22	0.79 ± 0.16	0.68 ± 0.26	0.03
FAI-Score Centile RCA, mean ± SD	0.73 ± 0.26	0.83 ± 0.20	0.68 ± 0.29	0.05

* By Mann–Whitney test or chi-square test or Fisher-exact test, when appropriate; Passed D'Agostino and Pearson normality test; NS — non-significance.

2.3. PVAT-FAI Score Centile of Coronary Inflammation

The FAI-score of the LAD, LCX, and RCA was used to create percentile curves across various age and sex groups. These curves were evaluated for their prognostic significance in Cox models that were adjusted for hypertension, diabetes mellitus, smoking, hyperlipidemia, high-risk plaque characteristics, and the modified Duke prognostic CAD index (Figure 2).

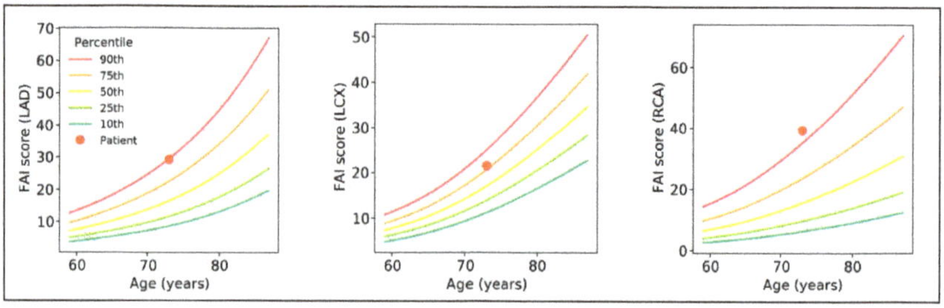

Figure 2. Nomograms with percentile curves for FAI-Score, adjusted for age, gender, and risk factors for each major coronary territory.

For the FAI-score Centile, the overall pattern shifts significantly, as the values for all three coronary arteries are higher for the subjects in the COVID-19 positive group, as follows: FAI-Score Centile LAD (group 1—0.66 ± 0.29 vs. group 2—0.58 ± 0.28, $p = 0.05$), FAI-Score Centile LCX (group 1—0.79 ± 0.16 vs. group 2—0.68 ± 0.26, $p = 0.03$), FAI-Score Centile RCA (group 1—0.83 ± 0.20 vs. group 2—0.68 ± 0.29, $p = 0.05$). FAI-Score Centile values of the two study groups are presented in Figure 3.

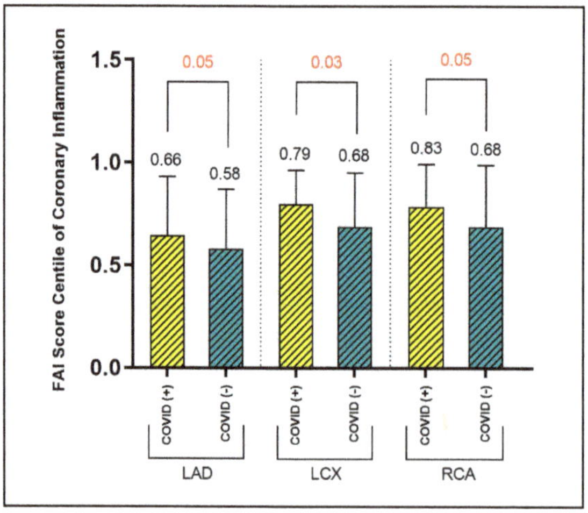

Figure 3. PVAT-FAI Score Centile of Coronary Inflammation for each coronary artery.

3. Discussion

A major challenge in the field of coronary atherosclerosis research is to find markers that can detect coronary inflammation, which is closely connected to the vulnerability of plaques. By doing so, it would be possible to identify patients who are at an elevated risk of AVE even before they show any clinical symptoms. Additionally, addressing inflammation may be a viable approach for preventing and managing this disease [23].

The ongoing coronavirus pandemic has had a significant impact on our society, including a significant effect on cardiovascular health [24], which was initially thought to be primarily a respiratory illness. The increased incidence of COVID-19 has presented healthcare professionals with various challenges, including assessing inflammation in PVAT as a marker of cardiovascular involvement. The respiratory issues caused by COVID-19 can lead to severe hypoxemia, which can result in multi-organ failure and cardiac damage [25].

The virus induces inflammation by triggering the release of cytokines and chemokines from respiratory epithelial cells, dendritic cells, and macrophages, as well as promoting the accumulation of EAT and PVAT. This can lead to local vascular inflammation and endothelial dysfunction, resulting in plaque formation and progression [26,27]. Certain biomarkers, such as inflammatory markers, chest CT findings, and nutritional status scores, have been shown in studies to predict adverse outcomes in COVID-19 patients. These results suggest that early identification and management of high-risk patients could lead to better outcomes [28–30].

Several studies have reported that COVID-19 infected patients have a higher incidence of cardiovascular events, including acute myocardial infarction, stroke, and heart failure, within one year of infection [31]. Additionally, Katsoularis et al. conducted a self-controlled case series and matched cohort study in Sweden, which showed an increased risk of acute myocardial infarction and ischemic stroke following COVID-19 [32]. Moreover, the Liuzzo and Volpe article highlighted the substantially elevated long-term cardiovascular risk linked to SARS-CoV-2 infection [33]. Collectively, these studies suggest that COVID-19 may have a significant impact on cardiovascular health and can potentially lead to long-term consequences. The importance of closely monitoring and managing cardiovascular health in COVID-19 patients is emphasized, and further research is necessary to fully comprehend the cardiovascular effects of COVID-19.

CCTA has become the first-line test for investigating suspected CAD. However, as its use expands in different clinical settings, it is essential to enhance its accuracy while also improving its diagnostic and prognostic importance in the early stages of coronary atherosclerosis [34–36]. The main findings of our study are as follows.

Firstly, our study revealed that the study population had a high FAI Score, and in all cases, the FAI Score was consistently higher in the non COVID-19 group. The new FAI Score for each coronary artery is a more dependable way of measuring coronary inflammation and a more accurate predictor of the risk of cardiac mortality than previous FAI methods [16,24].

Secondly, we discovered that the existence of lesions with greater pericoronary FAI-Score Centile value in the studied population were more commonly associated with patients who had previously been infected with COVID-19. It is established that the FAI-Score tends to increase with age. The percentile curves associated with the FAI Score are estimates of how the score is distributed among a group of patients who have undergone a clinically indicated CCTA. These curves provide a way to compare an individual's FAI Score to the others in the same age and gender group. It is important to note that the FAI Score is just one factor among many that can affect an individual's overall cardiovascular risk. In our opinion, this may be the reason why the COVID-19 group shows higher values of FAI-Score Centile.

Our study suggests that the PVAT-FAI Score is a trustworthy marker of coronary immune-inflammatory activation and its correlation with plaque vulnerability. This has important implications for assessing vascular involvement beyond typical conditions encountered by cardiologists, particularly in the context of the COVID-19 pandemic [37]. Further research is needed to understand the impact of plaque location on hemodynamic characteristics and the relationship between the specific vulnerable plaque phenotype and the degree of PVAT inflammation.

In the last decade, CCTA has been established as an excellent comprehensive tool for investigating suspected coronary artery disease. Mapping the PVAT-FAI on routine CCTA can detect coronary artery inflammation non-invasively by measuring changes in the composition of pericoronary fat. At the same time, systemic inflammation can be enhanced due to various infectious diseases, including SARS-CoV-2 infection. Thus, it is postulated that COVID-19 can modulate pericoronary FAI via systemic inflammatory pathways and plaque composition towards a higher vulnerability degree, which, in turn, can alter patient prognosis. There are scarce data regarding the evolution of FAI, and, therefore, of local coronary inflammation following SARS-CoV-2 infection, which could interfere with the development and progression of coronary atherosclerosis.

4. Materials and Methods

4.1. Study Design and Population

Our cross-sectional observational study, conducted at the Center of Advanced Research in Multimodality Cardiac Imaging, Cardio-Med Medical Center (Târgu Mureș, Romania) included 158 patients presenting with pain in the chest area and a low to intermediate likelihood of CAD. The patients underwent 128-slice CCTA to assess coronary anatomy and atherosclerosis, determine FAI score, and perform plaque analysis. The study participants were categorized into two main groups based on their COVID-19 status: group 1 (n = 75) included patients who had a previous COVID-19 infection and group 2 (n = 83) included patients matched for age and gender who did not have a COVID-19 infection prior to the CCTA examination. We ensured the accuracy of patient selection in the first group by only including individuals who had laboratory-confirmed COVID-19, exhibited mild to moderate symptoms, and had not received any treatment in healthcare facilities. Demographic and laboratory characteristics, cardiovascular risk factors, and symptom development were all monitored and assessed for each patient before the CCTA examination.

Patients with high coronary calcification, irregular heart rate, inability to achieve heart rate below 65 beats per minute, morbid obesity, inability to follow breath-hold instructions, or any other condition that could affect image quality were excluded from the study. In addition, those with chest pain caused by factors other than CAD, a history of myocardial infarction, high clinical probability of CAD, severe symptoms, or ACS requiring percutaneous coronary intervention (PCI) were also excluded.

4.2. CCTA Acquisition Procedure and Image Post-Processing

All participants underwent a CCTA scan using a 128-slice Siemens Somatom Definition AS (Siemens Healthcare, Erlangen, Germany) from the Centre of Cardio-Med (Târgu Mureș, Romania). The scan was retrospectively gated with a heart rate below 65 beats per minute and the parameters included a tube voltage of 120 kV, gantry rotation time of 0.33 s, and a collimation of 128 × 0.6. Beta-blockers were given to patients with a resting heart rate above 65 beats per minute, and blood pressure was monitored during the administration of intravenous or oral beta blockers. The acquisition process began with a native scan for coronary calcium assessment, followed by the administration of 80–100 mL of iodine-based contrast material based on body weight with a 50-mL saline chase at a flow rate of 5.5–6 mL/s during inspiratory breath-hold. All obtained scans were saved in a devoted electronic imaging database for offline image post-processing and for cloud delivery.

All the acquired images were converted to DICOM format, then anonymized and transferred to the partner center (Centre of CARISTO Diagnostics, Oxford, UK) via the cloud for post-processing. The inclusion criteria for the analysis included the presence of plaques with a stenosis effect of at least 50% and with at least one vulnerability marker present (low attenuation noncalcified plaque—LAP, positive remodeling—PR, spotty calcifications—SC and the napkin ring sign—NRS). The FAI and AI-based FAI scores were determined for each of the major coronary arteries in all patients.

The calculation of the PVAT-FAI employs AI-enhanced algorithms (CaRi-Heart®, CARISTO Diagnostics, Oxford, UK) that deliver precise and consistent attenuation measurements in concentric 1-mm 3D layers of perivascular adipose tissue surrounding the human arterial wall [16,38]. The PVAT-FAI calculation process involves multiple complex steps, including segmenting the heart and analyzing the perivascular space and adipose tissue using AI algorithms. The algorithms correct for various factors and technical aspects of the scan to differentiate PVAT-FAI from conventional CT attenuation and accurately interpret coronary inflammation [39]. In order to enhance comprehensibility, Table 3 illustrates the distinction between FAI (HU) and FAI-Score.

Table 3. The interpretation of FAI (HU) and FAI-Score.

Fat Attenuation Index (HU)	A non-adjusted, graphic illustration of the level of inflammation in the three primary epicardial coronary arteries.
Fat Attenuation Index-Score	A personalized measurement of the quantification of coronary inflammation in the three primary epicardial coronary arteries, adjusted for age and gender, expressed as a relative risk.

4.3. Statistical Analysis

After quantifying the PVAT-FAI for each coronary artery, all collected data were sent back to our center and stored in an electronic Microsoft Excel database (Microsoft Corporation, Redmond, WA, USA). Statistical analysis was performed using GraphPad Prism 9.5 software (GraphPad Software, Inc., San Diego, CA, USA). The study included a PCAT-FAI analysis of 474 coronary arteries: 158 on the left anterior descending artery (LAD), 158 on the circumflex artery (LCX), and 158 on the right coronary artery (RCA). In addition, the CaRi-Heart® risk and the Duke score were also determined for each individual [37].

The data were analyzed comparatively between patients with and without previous SARS-CoV-2 infection. Nominal (categorical) variables were reported as integer values (percentages) and compared between groups using the Chi-square test (χ^2) and its variables. Numeric data were expressed as mean ± standard deviation, and a Mann–Whitney or unpaired Student's *t*-test was used. Pearson correlation analysis was conducted to determine correlations between the PVAT-FAI and other variables as appropriate. Results were considered statistically significant if the two-sided *p*-value was 0.05.

5. Study Limitations and Future Directions

The purpose of this study was to assess the impact of COVID-19 infection on CAD in patients who underwent CCTA examinations for chest pain in the early stages after the infection, using the new AI—powered CaRi-Heart® medical device which combines standardized FAI mapping with plaque metrics and clinical risk factors to provide personalized cardiovascular risk assessment.

Our study has a few limitations that should be acknowledged. Firstly, the patients were only recruited from a single center, which may not accurately represent the entire population. Additionally, the study did not include a follow-up period, nor the measurement of serum inflammatory biomarkers, which could provide more insight into the correlation between coronary inflammation and risk of acute events. Secondly, the study only included lesions with at least 50% stenosis, so it is unclear if FAI-Score can identify cases with a high risk of events before significant stenosis. In addition, non-ST elevation ACS patients, who may have an increased inflammatory burden, were not included in the study (according to the 2020 ESC guidelines that recommend CCTA as a substitute for invasive angiography in cases with low to intermediate CAD likelihood). Although these limitations exist, additional research is required to validate the clinical significance of the FAI-Score in managing coronary inflammation.

In order to expand on the results of this proof-of-concept study, future research plans include conducting a follow-up period to evaluate the outcome prediction capability of the FAI mapping technique and its correlation with systemic inflammation as measured by biomarker analysis. Additionally, to address the limitations of this study, our research team intends to explore the correlation between local vascular inflammation and hemodynamic differences in vessels by computing shear stress using CCTA imaging. In an effort to gain a comprehensive understanding of overall coronary vulnerability, future studies will incorporate computerized plaque analysis, which provides insight into intrinsic vulnerability, in conjunction with FAI.

6. Conclusions

Lesions with higher pericoronary FAI-Score Centile values were more commonly found in patients who had previously been infected with COVID-19. The pericoronary FAI-Score percentile curves illustrate the level of coronary inflammation and provide a uniform interpretation of perivascular FAI mapping on CCTA. Patients in the upper percentile curves have an increased risk of cardiovascular disease, regardless of the presence of traditional risk factors or established atherosclerotic changes.

An association has been observed between COVID-19 infection and an elevated risk of destabilizing coronary plaque, as indicated by higher levels of inflammation in the pericoronary adipose tissue. The use of pericoronary FAI as a marker for identifying vulnerable patients at high risk for cardiovascular events could have significant implications in the deployment of targeted prevention strategies. However, further validation of these findings through larger studies with more consistent data is necessary to establish the utility of FAI in clinical practice.

Author Contributions: Conceptualization, B.B.M., I.B. and T.B.; methodology, T.B. and I.B.; validation, B.B.M., I.B., E.B., R.G., A.R., N.R., E.S. and T.B.; formal analysis, I.B., I.K., D.O. and Z.P.; investigation, B.B.M., E.B., I.K. and T.B.; resources, I.B.; data curation, N.R., D.O. and B.B.; writing—original draft preparation, B.B.M. and T.B.; writing—review and editing, B.B.M. and T.B.; visualization, B.B.M., R.G., N.R., D.O. and T.B.; supervision, I.B.; project administration, I.B. and T.B.; funding acquisition, I.B. and T.B. All authors have read and agreed to the published version of the manuscript.

Funding: This work was supported by the University of Medicine, Pharmacy, Science and Technology "George Emil Palade" of Târgu Mureș Research Grant number 164/20/10 January 2023, project title: "The Role of Epicardial Pericoronary Adipose Tissue Inflammation in the Progression and Vulnerability of Atherosclerotic Plaques".

Institutional Review Board Statement: All study procedures were conducted in accordance with good clinical practice guidelines and the Declaration of Helsinki and were reviewed and approved by the institution's ethics committee (protocol code 26884/10 on November 2021) and the Scientific Research Ethics Committee of the University of Medicine, Pharmacy, Science and Technology "George Emil Palade" from Târgu Mureș (protocol code 1513/9 on December 2021).

Informed Consent Statement: Informed consent was obtained from all subjects involved in the study.

Data Availability Statement: The data presented in this study are available on request from the corresponding author. The data are not publicly available due to privacy reasons.

Acknowledgments: This manuscript is a part of a Ph.D. thesis from the Doctoral School of Medicine and Pharmacy at the University of Medicine, Pharmacy, Science and Technology "George Emil Palade" of Târgu-Mures entitled "The Role of Epicardial Pericoronary Adipose Tissue Inflammation in the Progression and Vulnerability of Atherosclerotic Plaques", which will be presented by Botond Barna Mátyás, having the approval of all authors.

Conflicts of Interest: The authors declare no conflict of interest. The funders had no role in the design of the study; in the collection, analyses, or interpretation of data; in the writing of the manuscript; or in the decision to publish the results.

References

1. Spagnoli, L.G.; Bonanno, E.; Sangiorgi, G.; Mauriello, A. Role of inflammation in atherosclerosis. *J. Nucl. Med.* **2007**, *48*, 1800–1815. [CrossRef] [PubMed]
2. Arbab-Zadeh, A.; Fuster, V. From Detecting the Vulnerable Plaque to Managing the Vulnerable Patient: JACC State-of-the-Art Review. *J. Am. Coll. Cardiol.* **2019**, *74*, 1582–1593. [CrossRef] [PubMed]
3. Naghavi, M.; Libby, P.; Falk, E. From vulnerable plaque to vulnerable patient: A call for new definitions and risk assessment strategies: Part I. *Circulation* **2003**, *108*, 1664–1672. [CrossRef] [PubMed]
4. O'Connel, J.L.; Pehna de Aleida, R.; Roever, L. The challenge to detect and to treat vulnerable plaques and vulnerable patients. *Interv. Cardiol.* **2016**, *8*, 721–723.
5. Benedek, T.; Maurovich Horvath, P.; Ferdinandy, P.; Merkely, B. The Use of Biomarkers for the Early Detection of Vulnerable Atherosclerotic Plaques and Vulnerable Patients. A Review. *J. Cardiovasc. Emerg.* **2016**, *2*, 106–113. [CrossRef]

6. Raț, N.; Opincariu, D.; Márton, E.; Zavate, R.; Pintican, M.; Benedek, T. The Effect of Periplaque Fat on Coronary Plaque Vulnerability in Patients with Stable Coronary Artery Disease—A 128-multislice CT-based Study. *J. Interdiscip. Med.* **2018**, *3*, 69–76. [CrossRef]
7. Nyulas, T.; Marton, E.; Rus, V.; Rat, N.; Ratiu, M.; Benedek, T.; Benedek, I. Morphological Features and Plaque Composition in Culprit Atheromatous Plaques of Patients with Acute Coronary Syndromes. *J. Cardiovasc. Emerg.* **2018**, *4*, 84–94. [CrossRef]
8. Villines, T.C.; Al'Aref, S.J.; Andreini, D.; Chen, M.Y.; Choi, A.D.; De Cecco, C.N.; Dey, D.; Earls, J.P.; Ferencik, M.; Gransar, H.; et al. The Journal of Cardiovascular Computed Tomography: 2020 Year in review. *J. Cardiovasc. Comput. Tomogr.* **2021**, *15*, 180–189. [CrossRef]
9. Madonna, R.; Massaro, M.; Scoditti, E.; Pescetelli, I.; De Caterina, R. The epicardial adipose tissue and the coronary arteries: Dangerous liaisons. *Cardiovasc. Res.* **2019**, *115*, 1013–10255. [CrossRef]
10. Yang, X.; Li, Y.; Li, Y.; Ren, X.; Zhang, X.; Hu, D.; Gao, Y.; Xing, Y.; Shang, H. Oxidative Stress-Mediated Atherosclerosis: Mechanisms and Therapies. *Front. Physiol.* **2017**, *8*, 60. [CrossRef]
11. Monti, C.B.; Codari, M.; De Cecco, C.N.; Secchi, F.; Sardanelli, F.; Stillman, A.E. Novel imaging biomarkers: Epicardial adipose tissue evaluation. *Br. J. Radiol.* **2020**, *93*, 20190770. [CrossRef] [PubMed]
12. DePace, N.L.; Colombo, J. Long-COVID Syndrome and the Cardiovascular System: A Review of Neurocardiologic Effects on Multiple Systems. *Curr. Cardiol. Rep.* **2022**, *24*, 1711–1726. [CrossRef] [PubMed]
13. Raman, B.; Bluemke, D.A.; Lüscher, T.F.; Neubauer, S. Long COVID: Post-acute sequelae of COVID-19 with a cardiovascular focus. *Eur. Heart J.* **2022**, *43*, 1157–1172. [CrossRef] [PubMed]
14. Sheth, A.R.; Grewal, U.S.; Patel, H.P.; Thakkar, S.; Garikipati, S.; Gaddam, J.; Bawa, D. Possible mechanisms responsible for acute coronary events in COVID-19. *Med. Hypotheses.* **2020**, *143*, 110125. [CrossRef]
15. Wang, H.; Ma, S. The cytokine storm and factors determining the sequence and severity of organ dysfunction in multiple organ dysfunction syndrome. *Am. J. Emerg. Med.* **2008**, *26*, 711–715. [CrossRef]
16. Antonopoulos, A.S.; Sanna, F.; Sabharwal, N.; Thomas, S.; Oikonomou, E.K.; Herdman, L.; Margaritis, M.; Shirodaria, C.; Kampoli, A.M.; Akoumianakis, I.; et al. Detecting human coronary inflammation by imaging perivascular fat. *Sci. Transl. Med.* **2017**, *9*, eaal2658. [CrossRef]
17. Elnabawi, Y.A.; Oikonomou, E.K.; Dey, A.K.; Mancio, J.; Rodante, J.A.; Aksentijevich, M.; Choi, H.; Keel, A.; Erb-Alvarez, J.; Teague, H.L.; et al. Association of Biologic Therapy With Coronary Inflammation in Patients With Psoriasis as Assessed by Perivascular Fat Attenuation Index. *JAMA Cardiol.* **2019**, *4*, 885–891. [CrossRef] [PubMed]
18. Oikonomou, E.K.; West, H.W.; Antoniades, C. Cardiac Computed Tomography: Assessment of Coronary Inflammation and Other Plaque Features. *Arterioscler. Thromb. Vasc. Biol.* **2019**, *39*, 2207–2219. [CrossRef]
19. Oikonomou, E.K.; Marwan, M.; Desai, M.Y.; Mancio, J.; Alashi, A.; Hutt Centeno, E.; Thomas, S.; Herdman, L.; Kotanidis, C.P.; Thomas, K.E.; et al. Non-invasive detection of coronary inflammation using computed tomography and prediction of residual cardiovascular risk (the CRISP CT study): A post-hoc analysis of prospective outcome data. *Lancet* **2018**, *392*, 929–939. [CrossRef]
20. Skulstad, H.; Cosyns, B.; Popescu, B.A.; Galderisi, M.; Salvo, G.D.; Donal, E.; Petersen, S.; Gimelli, A.; Haugaa, K.H.; Muraru, D.; et al. COVID-19 pandemic and cardiac imaging: EACVI recommendations on precautions, indications, prioritization, and protection for patients and healthcare personnel. *Eur. Heart J. Cardiovasc. Imaging* **2020**, *21*, 592–598. [CrossRef]
21. Lin, A.; Kolossváry, M.; Motwani, M.; Išgum, I.; Maurovich-Horvat, P.; Slomka, P.J.; Dey, D. Artificial Intelligence in Cardiovascular Imaging for Risk Stratification in Coronary Artery Disease. *Radiol. Cardiothorac. Imaging* **2021**, *3*, e2005. [CrossRef] [PubMed]
22. Oikonomou, E.K.; Antonopoulos, A.S.; Schottlander, D.; Marwan, M.; Mathers, C.; Tomlins, P. Standardized measurement of coronary inflammation using cardiovascular computed tomography: Integration in clinical care as a prognostic medical device. *Cardiovasc. Res.* **2021**, *117*, 2677–2690. [CrossRef] [PubMed]
23. Wong, B.W.; Meredith, A.; Lin, D.; McManus, B.M. The biological role of inflammation in atherosclerosis. *Can. J. Cardiol.* **2012**, *28*, 631–641. [CrossRef] [PubMed]
24. Shi, S.; Qin, M.; Shen, B.; Cai, Y.; Liu, T.; Yang, F.; Gong, W.; Liu, X.; Liang, J.; Zhao, Q.; et al. Association of Cardiac Injury With Mortality in Hospitalized Patients With COVID-19 in Wuhan, China. *JAMA Cardiol.* **2020**, *5*, 802–810. [CrossRef] [PubMed]
25. Huang, C.; Wang, Y.; Li, X.; Ren, L.; Zhao, J.; Hu, Y.; Zhang, L.; Fan, G.; Xu, J.; Gu, X.; et al. Clinical features of patients infected with 2019 novel coronavirus in Wuhan, China. *Lancet* **2020**, *395*, 497–506. [CrossRef] [PubMed]
26. Law, H.K.; Cheung, C.Y.; Ng, H.Y.; Sia, S.F.; Chan, Y.O.; Luk, W.; Nicholls, J.M.; Peiris, J.S.; Lau, Y.L. Chemokine up-regulation in SARS-coronavirus-infected, monocyte-derived human dendritic cells. *Blood* **2005**, *106*, 2366–2374. [CrossRef]
27. Mester, A.; Benedek, I.; Rat, N.; Tolescu, C.; Polexa, S.A.; Benedek, T. Imaging Cardiovascular Inflammation in the COVID-19 Era. *Diagnostics* **2021**, *11*, 1114. [CrossRef]
28. Matyas, B.; Polexa, S.; Benedek, I.; Buicu, A.; Benedek, T. Biomarkers of Systemic Versus Local Inflammation During the Acute Phase of Myocardial Infarction, as Predictors of Post-infarction Heart Failure. *J. Cardiovasc. Emerg.* **2021**, *7*, 70–76. [CrossRef]
29. Arbănași, E.M.; Halmaciu, I.; Kaller, R.; Mureșan, A.V.; Arbănași, E.M.; Suciu, B.A.; Coșarcă, C.M.; Cojocaru, I.I.; Melinte, R.M.; Russu, E. Systemic Inflammatory Biomarkers and Chest CT Findings as Predictors of Acute Limb Ischemia Risk, Intensive Care Unit Admission, and Mortality in COVID-19 Patients. *Diagnostics* **2022**, *12*, 2379. [CrossRef]

30. Mureșan, A.V.; Hălmaciu, I.; Arbănași, E.M.; Kaller, R.; Arbănași, E.M.; Budișcă, O.A.; Melinte, R.M.; Vunvulea, V.; Filep, R.C.; Mărginean, L.; et al. Prognostic Nutritional Index, Controlling Nutritional Status (CONUT) Score, and Inflammatory Biomarkers as Predictors of Deep Vein Thrombosis, Acute Pulmonary Embolism, and Mortality in COVID-19 Patients. *Diagnostics* **2022**, *12*, 2757. [CrossRef]
31. Ortega-Paz, L.; Arévalos, V.; Fernández-Rodríguez, D.; Jiménez-Díaz, V.; Bañeras, J.; Campo, G. One-year cardiovascular outcomes after coronavirus disease 2019: The cardiovascular COVID-19 registry. *PLoS ONE* **2022**, *17*, e0279333. [CrossRef] [PubMed]
32. Katsoularis, I.; Fonseca-Rodríguez, O.; Farrington, P.; Lindmark, K.; Fors Connolly, A.M. Risk of acute myocardial infarction and ischaemic stroke following COVID-19 in Sweden: A self-controlled case series and matched cohort study. *Lancet* **2021**, *398*, 599–607. [CrossRef] [PubMed]
33. Liuzzo, G.; Volpe, M. SARS-CoV-2 infection markedly increases long-term cardiovascular risk. *Eur Heart J.* **2022**, *43*, 1899–1900. [CrossRef] [PubMed]
34. Budoff, M.J.; Dowe, D.; Jollis, J.G.; Gitter, M.; Sutherland, J.; Halamert, E.; Scherer, M.; Bellinger, R.; Martin, A.; Benton, R.; et al. Diagnostic performance of 64-multidetector row coronary computed tomographic angiography for evaluation of coronary artery stenosis in individuals without known coronary artery disease: Results from the prospective multicenter ACCURACY (Assessment by Coronary Computed Tomographic Angiography of Individuals Undergoing Invasive Coronary Angiography) trial. *J. Am. Coll. Cardiol.* **2008**, *52*, 1724–1732. [PubMed]
35. Min, J.K.; Dunning, A.; Lin, F.Y.; Achenbach, S.; Al-Mallah, M.; Budoff, M.J.; Cademartiri, F.; Callister, T.Q.; Chang, H.J.; Cheng, V.; et al. Age- and sex-related differences in all-cause mortality risk based on coronary computed tomography angiography findings results from the International Multicenter CONFIRM (Coronary CT Angiography Evaluation for Clinical Outcomes: An International Multicenter Registry) of 23,854 patients without known coronary artery disease. *J. Am. Coll. Cardiol.* **2011**, *58*, 849–860. [PubMed]
36. Oikonomou, E.K.; Antoniades, C. The role of adipose tissue in cardiovascular health and disease. *Nat. Rev. Cardiol.* **2019**, *16*, 83–99. [CrossRef]
37. Guzik, T.J.; Mohiddin, S.A.; Dimarco, A.; Patel, V.; Savvatis, K.; Marelli-Berg, F.M.; Madhur, M.S.; Tomaszewski, M.; Maffia, P.; D'Acquisto, F.; et al. COVID-19 and the cardiovascular system: Implications for risk assessment, diagnosis, and treatment options. *Cardiovasc. Res.* **2020**, *116*, 1666–1687. [CrossRef]
38. Antoniades, C.; Kotanidis, C.P.; Berman, D.S. State-of-the-art review article. Atherosclerosis affecting fat: What can we learn by imaging perivascular adipose tissue? *J. Cardiovasc. Comput. Tomogr.* **2019**, *13*, 288–296. [CrossRef]
39. Kotanidis, C.P.; Antoniades, C. Perivascular fat imaging by computed tomography (CT): A virtual guide. *Br. J. Pharmacol.* **2021**, *178*, 4270–4290. [CrossRef]

International Journal of
Molecular Sciences

MDPI

Article

The Long Term Residual Effects of COVID-Associated Coagulopathy

Marco Ranucci [1,*,†], Ekaterina Baryshnikova [1,†], Martina Anguissola [1], Sara Pugliese [1], Mara Falco [2] and Lorenzo Menicanti [3]

1 Department of Cardiovascular Anesthesia and Intensive Care, IRCCS Policlinico San Donato, 20097 Milan, Italy
2 Department of Radiology, Koelliker Hospital, 10134 Turin, Italy
3 Scientific Directorate, IRCCS Policlinico San Donato, 20097 Milan, Italy
* Correspondence: marco.ranucci@grupposandonato.it
† These authors contributed equally to the work.

Abstract: During the acute phase of COVID-19, many patients experience a complex coagulopathy characterized by a procoagulant pattern. The present study investigates the persistence of hemostatic changes in post-COVID patients at a long-term follow up, and the link with the persistence of physical and neuropsychological symptoms. We completed a prospective cohort study on 102 post-COVID patients. Standard coagulation and viscoelastic tests were performed, along with an assessment of persistent symptoms and recording of acute phase details. A procoagulant state was adjudicated in the presence of fibrinogen > 400 mg/dL, or D-dimer > 500 ng/mL, or platelet count > 450,000 cells/μL, or a maxim clot lysis at viscoelastic test < 2%. A procoagulant state was identified in 75% of the patients at 3 months follow up, 50% at 6 months, and 30% at 12–18 months. Factors associated with the persistence of a procoagulant state were age, severity of the acute phase, and persistence of symptoms. Patients with major physical symptoms carry a procoagulant state relative risk of 2.8 (95% confidence interval 1.17–6.7, $p = 0.019$). The association between persistent symptoms and a procoagulant state raises the hypothesis that an ongoing process of thrombi formation and/or persistent microthrombosis may be responsible for the main physical symptoms in long-COVID patients.

Keywords: COVID-19; post-acute COVID-19 syndrome; coagulopathy; fibrinolysis; thrombosis

Citation: Ranucci, M.; Baryshnikova, E.; Anguissola, M.; Pugliese, S.; Falco, M.; Menicanti, L. The Long Term Residual Effects of COVID-Associated Coagulopathy. *Int. J. Mol. Sci.* **2023**, *24*, 5514. https://doi.org/10.3390/ijms24065514

Academic Editors: Alexandru Schiopu, Emil Arbanasi and Eliza Russu

Received: 14 February 2023
Revised: 9 March 2023
Accepted: 10 March 2023
Published: 14 March 2023

1. Introduction

The COVID-19 associated coagulopathy (CoAC) is a complex syndrome complicating the acute phase of COVID-19 infection, first recognized at the beginning of the pandemic in Italy through the use of standard coagulation tests, point-of-care viscoelastic tests (VET), and a biochemical measure of markers of thrombin generation, fibrin generation, platelet activation, and fibrinolysis [1–3].

Recognized patterns of CoAC are increased thrombin generation [4–6], thrombocytosis in the early phases and thrombocytopenia in late severe conditions [7,8], blunted fibrinolysis [6,9], and high levels of D-dimer [10–12].

This complex pattern clearly shows a dynamic behavior, where phases of activation are followed by phases of coagulation factor consumption, exhaustion of the hemostatic system, and, in more severe cases, disseminated intravascular coagulopathy. The main clinical consequences of CoAC are thromboembolic complications, most frequently represented by pulmonary embolism [13,14]. However, thrombi formation may be observed practically everywhere, even in minor, subclinical manifestations of CoAC [15,16]. Extensive imaging analyses clearly confirm the presence of micro and macro thrombotic formation in different organs [17].

Whether this pattern and/or the consequences of CoAC resist and leave a long-term signature in the hemostatic system after the closure of the acute phase of the disease is still not well defined. There is an Indian study with a 3-month and a 6-month follow up where elevated D-dimer values were associated with persistence of symptoms [18]; however, prolonged elevation of D-dimer levels seems not to be associated with the severity of acute phase response [19]. The only study assessing the hemostatic profile after 1 year from the acute phase shows the persistence of high D-dimer and factor VIII levels in 18% and 49% of the patients, respectively, with an increased thrombin generation [20].

Since the first reports of hypercoagulability during the acute phase of COVID-19 were based on point-of-care viscoelastic testing (VET), it is reasonable to use this approach to investigate the long-term residual effects of the disease on the hemostatic system. The present study aims to investigate the hemostatic pattern of COVID-19 patients at a long-term follow up, and to assess the association between patterns of the acute phase, persistence of clinical symptoms, and hemostatic system profile.

2. Results

The general characteristics of the patient population during the acute phase and at follow-up are shown in Table 1. The hemostatic profile at follow-up is shown in Table 2, separately for patients with or without persistent major physical symptoms (MPS) and/or major neuropsychological symptoms (MNS). During the acute phase, a procoagulant pattern was identified in 99 (97.1%) of the patients, with one or more of the following conditions: peak fibrinogen levels > 400 mg/dL in 99 (97.1%) patients; peak D-Dimer > 500 ng/mL in 87 (84.8%) patients; peak platelet count > 450,000 cells/μL in 17 (15.8%) patients and nadir antithrombin (AT) activity < 70% in 6 (5.9%) patients. After discharge from the hospital, a procoagulant state was still present at follow-up in 38 (37.3%), presenting one or more of the following conditions: fibrinogen levels > 400 mg/dL in 7 (6.9%) patients; D-Dimer > 500 ng/mL in 28 (27.4%) patients; platelet count > 450,000 cells/μL in 17 (15.8%) patients, AT activity < 70% in 4 (3.9%) patients, and ClotPro EXtest maximum lysis (ML) < 2% in 7 (6.9%) patients.

Table 1. Patient population (N = 102) details during the acute phase of the disease and at follow-up.

ACUTE PHASE	
Item	**Value**
Age at hospital admission (years)	63.8 (13.1)
Gender male	67 (65.7%)
Weight (kgs)	80.4 (17.8)
Body mass index (kg/m^2)	27.6 (5.4)
Hospital stay (days)	14 (10–23)
Unit of admission	
Ward	97 (95.1%)
Intensive Care Unit	5 (4.9%)
Vaccination (at least 2 doses)	15 (14.7%)
Obesity	24 (23.5%)
Arterial hypertension	44 (43.1%)
Diabetes	15 (14.7%)
Coronaropathy	12 (11.8%)
Heart failure	6 (5.9%)
Smoking habit	
No	50 (49%)
Previous	48 (47.1%)
Ongoing	4 (3.9%)
Atrial fibrillation	7 (6.9%)
Active cancer previous 5 years	9 (8.8%)
Chronic obstructive pulmonary disease	5 (4.9%)
Chronic kidney failure	6 (5.9%)
Previous cerebrovascular accident	3 (2.9%)
Anxiety	16 (15.7%)

Table 1. *Cont.*

ACUTE PHASE	
Item	**Value**
Depression	12 (11.8%)
Chronic liver failure	3 (2.9%)
Therapy	
Beta-blockers	17 (16.7%)
Angiotensin converting enzyme inhibitors	13 (12.7%)
Sartans	8 (7.8%)
Warfarin	2 (2%)
Direct oral anticoagulants	3 (2.9%)
Antiplatelet agents	18 (17.6%)
Calcium antagonists	14 (13.7%)
Statins	15 (14.7%)
Laboratory exams (acute phase)	
Peak fibrinogen (mg/dL)	611 (152)
Peak D-dimer (ng/mL)	3118 (7620)
Peak platelet count (×1000 cells/μL)	329 (110)
Nadir platelet count (×1000 cells/μL)	180 (68)
Nadir antithrombin (%)	100 (15)
Procoagulant state at any time	99 (97.1%)
FOLLOW-UP	
Item	**Value**
Follow-up time (months)	17 (13–18.5)
Persistent major physical symptoms	60 (58.8%)
Fatigue	50 (49%)
Dyspnea	44 (43.1%)
Cough	13 (12.7%)
Fever	2 (2%)
Persistent major neuropsychological symptoms	44 (43.1%)
Anxiety	23 (22.5%)
Depression	21 (20.6%)
Memory dysfunction	34 (33.3%)
Brain fog	10 (9.8%)
Anticoagulant/antiplatelet therapy	
Dual antiplatelet therapy	4 (3.9%)
Warfarin	1 (1%)
Direct oral anticoagulants	7 (6.9%)
Procoagulant state after hospital discharge	38 (37.3%)

Data are mean (standard deviation), median (interquartile range) or number (%).

Table 2. Hemostatic profile at follow up according to the presence of persistent major physical or neuropsychological symptoms. N = 102.

Item	MPS	No MPS	Mean Difference	p	MNS	No MNS	Mean Difference	p
	N = 60	N = 42	(95% C.I.)		N = 44	N = 58	(95% C.I.)	
INR	1.09 (0.09)	1.1 (0.24)	0.03 (−0.05 to 0.09)	0.578	1.09 (0.09)	1.1 (0.2)	0.01 (−0.06 to 0.07)	0.867
aPTT (s)	28.8 (5.0)	28.4 (4.4)	0.96 (−2.4 to 1.4)	0.607	28.4 (3.8)	28.9 (5.4)	0.45 (−1.4 to 2.3)	0.641
Fibrinogen (mg/dL)	313 (68)	283 (58)	−31 (−56 to −4.7)	0.021	299 (70)	302 (64)	2.7 (−24 to 29)	0.836
D-dimer (ng/mL)	564 (577)	476 (645)	−88 (−331–154)	0.473	544 (479)	514 (690)	−30 (−272–211)	0.806
Platelet count (×1000 cells/μL)	216 (65)	222 (62)	6.2 (−19 to 32)	0.628	218 (76)	219 (52)	0.9 (−24 to 26)	0.943
Antithrombin (%)	90 (13.4)	94 (10.5)	4.8 (−0.5 to 10)	0.073	92 (12)	91 (13)	−1.4 (−6.7 to 3.9)	0.603
EXtest CT (s)	69 (14)	69 (14)	−0.19 (−5.8 to 5.4)	0.947	68 (13)	69 (14)	1.6 (−3.9 to 7.1)	0.567
EXtest MCF (mm)	61 (49)	60 (3.4)	−1.4 (−2.8 to 0.2)	0.090	62 (4.2)	60 (3.4)	0.8 (−2.7 to 0.3)	0.127
EXtest maximum lysis (%)	4.5 (2.3)	5.9 (2.6)	1.42 (0.44 to 2.39)	0.005	5.0 (2.4)	5.2 (2.6)	0.16 (−0.85 to 1.18)	0.753
INtest CT	157 (30)	158 (18)	1.16 (−9.1 to 11.4)	0.823	152 (27)	162 (24)	5.1 (−0.2 to 20)	0.056
INtest MCF	60 (3.9)	59 (3.3)	−1.7 (−3.1 to −0.2)	0.026	60 (4)	59 (3.4)	0.74 (−2.5 to 0.4)	0.171
INtest maximum lysis (%)	4.1 (2.3)	5.5 (2.5)	1.37 (0.40 to 2.33)	0.006	4.6 (2.5)	4.8 (2.5)	0.50 (−0.81 to 1.18)	0.713
FIBtest MCF	20 (4.9)	18 (3.9)	−1.5 (−3.3 to 0.4)	0.117	20 (4.7)	19 (4.3)	−1.0 (−2.8 to 0.79)	0.265
TPAtest lysis time (s)	227 (47)	209 (36)	−18 (−35 to −0.7)	0.033	232 (47)	210 (39)	−22 (−38 to −5)	0.012
TPAtest maximum lysis (%)	95 (1.3)	95 (1.0)	−0.22 (−0.7 to 0.26)	0.346	95 (1.1)	94.5 (1.2)	−0.7 (−1.1 to −0.22)	0.005

Data are mean (standard deviation). aPTT: activated partial thromboplastin time; C.I.: confidence interval; CT: clotting time; EXtest: extrinsic pathway test; INR: international normalized ratio; INtest: intrinsic pathway test; FIBtest: fibrinogen test; MCF: maximum clot firmness; MNS: major neuropsychological symptoms; MPS: major physical symptoms; TPA: tissue plasminogen activator.

The probability of a persistent procoagulant state during follow up is shown in Figure 1 (cubic regression analysis, R^2 0.415, $p = 0.001$). Overall, a persistent procoagulant state was still present in 75% of the patient population at 3 months, 50% at 6 months, and 25% at 12 months of follow-up, with a slight increase to 35% at 18 months. The R^2 value justifies 41% of the follow-up time based relationship, and there are certainly other factors affecting the persistence of a procoagulant state. Among these, persistence of MPS carries a higher rate of a procoagulant state (46.7% vs. 23.8%, relative risk 2.8, 95% confidence interval 1.17–6.7, $p = 0.019$), whereas persistence of MNS did not (40.9% vs. 34.5%). Among the acute phase factors, only age class and the severity of the disease were significantly associated with a procoagulant state at follow up (Figure 2). For increasing age higher than 50 years, there is a significant ($p = 0.001$) incremental increase of the procoagulant state rate, up to 90% in elderly people (> 80 years), and the severity of the disease carries a significant ($p = 0.05$) impact on the procoagulant state rate, especially for patients with a severe pattern that show a risk of procoagulant state at follow up that is almost double the risk for mild to moderate patterns of the disease in the acute phase.

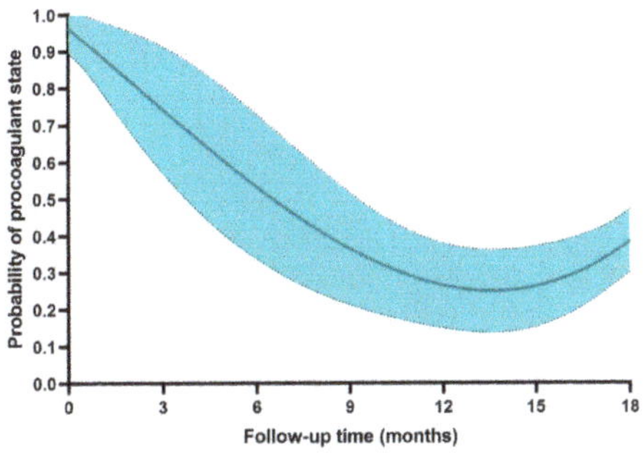

Figure 1. Probability of the persistence of a procoagulant state. Cubic regression function with 95% confidence interval bands.

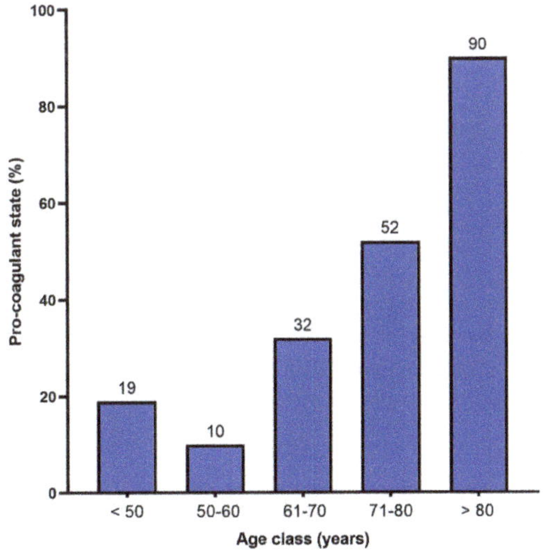

(A)

Figure 2. *Cont.*

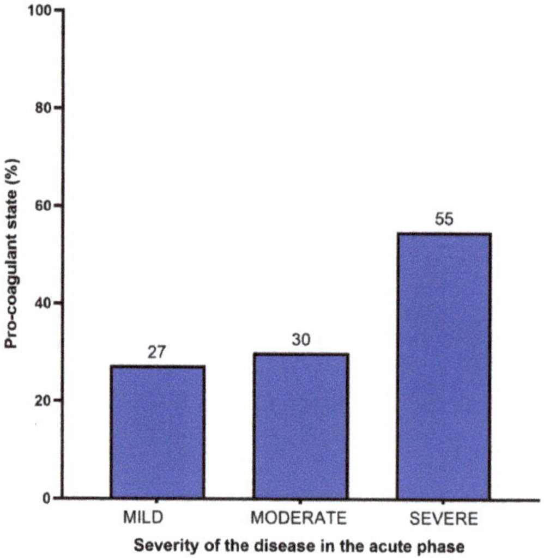

(B)

Figure 2. Rate of procoagulant state persistence based on the age at acute phase stage (Panel (**A**)) and severity of the acute phase disease (Panel (**B**)).

Table 2 reports the hemostatic profile of the patients at follow up, according to the presence of persistent MPS or MNS. Patients with MPS had significantly ($p = 0.021$) higher levels of fibrinogen and of MCF (maximum clot firmness) at the INtest ($p = 0.026$), with a reduced ML (maximum lysis) at both the EXtest ($p = 0.005$) and the INtest ($p = 0.006$), and a longer lysis time at the TPAtest ($p = 0.033$). Patients with MNS had a significantly longer lysis time at the TPAtest ($p = 0.012$). Overall, the general pattern of patients with persistent symptoms is representative of an increased clot firmness, mainly due to fibrinogen contribution, with an impaired fibrinolysis. D-Dimer levels were not different between patients with or without persistent symptoms. Overall, individual and mean standard coagulation data of the patient population are reported in Figure 3. The most evident finding is the presence of high levels of D-dimer in about 30% of the patients. Figure 4 reports the main differences between patients with or without persistent symptoms with respect to VET. For both persistent MPS and MNS, there is evidence of a decreased fibrinolysis with respect to asymptomatic patients.

A sensitivity analysis was conducted on patients with ($n = 44$) or without ($n = 58$) persistent dyspnea. Patients with persistent dyspnea had significantly lower values of EXtest ML (4.4% ± 2.3 vs. 5.6% ± 2.6, mean difference 1.2, 95% confidence interval 0.22 to 2.2, $p = 0.017$) and of INtest ML (3.9% ± 2.1 vs. 5.3% ± 2.6, mean difference 1.42, 95% confidence interval 0.47 to 2.38, $p = 0.004$). The severity of the disease in the acute phase did not affect the fibrinolysis at the EXtest ML (5.3 % ± 2.3 for non-severe cases vs. 4.5% ± 2.9% for severe cases, $p = 0.172$) but affected the fibrinolysis at the INtest ML ((5 % ± 2.4 for non-severe cases vs. 3.9% ± 2.6% for severe cases, $p = 0.033$). When corrected for the severity of the disease, persistent dyspnea remained independently associated with a reduced fibrinolysis both at the EXtest ML ($p = 0.028$) and at the INtest ML ($p = 0.002$).

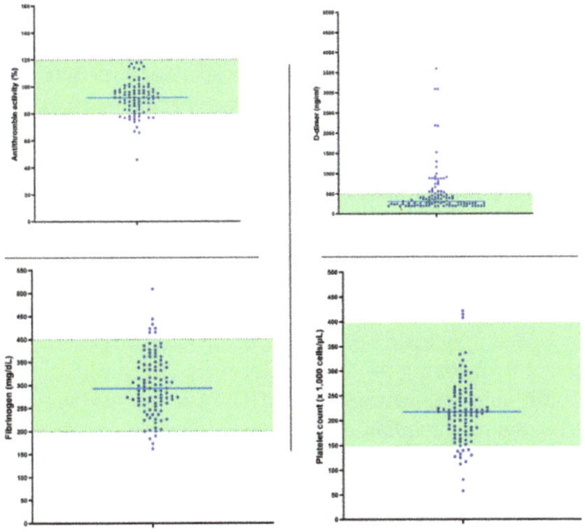

Figure 3. Individual and mean standard coagulation data at follow up. Green area is the normality range.

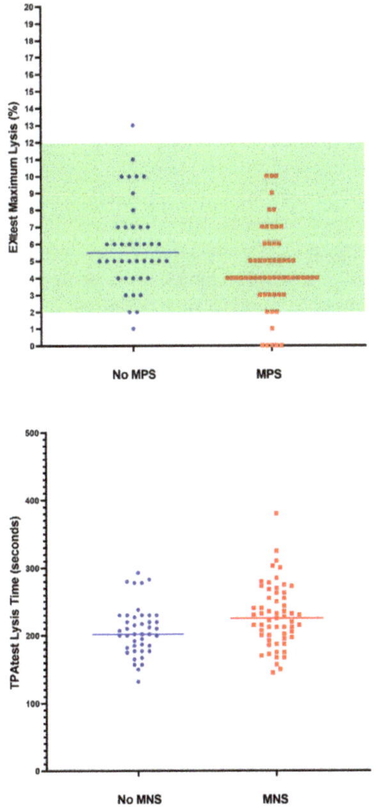

Figure 4. Individual and mean values of fibrinolysis according to the presence of major physical symptoms (MPS) and major neurological symptoms (MNS). Green area is the normality range. No defined normal range exists for TPAtest.

3. Discussion

The main results of our study are (i) persistent hemostatic changes are detectable in 37% of patients hospitalized for COVID-19 at a median follow-up of 17 months; (ii) the main pattern is suggestive of an ongoing fibrinolytic process; and (iii) patients with residual MPS (especially persistent dyspnea) and MNS have significantly lower levels of fibrinolysis. The severity of the disease partially affects the fibrinolysis shutdown.

Much is known about the procoagulant profile of COVID-19 patients during the acute phase of the disease. Much less is known about the short- and long-term sequelae of this pattern. Persistent organ dysfunction, even after several months from the acute phase, has already been observed, and this is a reasonable finding, considering that organs directly (lung) or indirectly (heart, brain, kidney) and severely damaged by the disease take time to recover, and may even not recover at all. Conversely, the hemostatic system is a dynamic structure comprising proteases, glycoproteins, proteins, and cells. All these components are continuously re-synthesized by the liver and the bone marrow, so once the acute insult represented by the inflammatory reaction to virus or bacterial sepsis is overcome, it could be logical to assume that the system comes back to normal, unless in the presence of an ongoing or unresolved process elsewhere in the human body.

Actually, the information on the coagulation profile in long-COVID patients is scarce and mainly limited to short-term follow up. Townsend and associates [19] studied 150 COVID-19 patients at a median of 80 days from the diagnosis, both hospitalized and outpatients. The mean D-Dimer was 327 ng/mL (lower than in our series), with 25% of the patients showing abnormally elevated values (27% in our series). Elevation of D-Dimer was more frequent in older patients and in those with severe acute disease. Our results are basically in agreement with these findings, and the difference in mean D-Dimer values is probably to be ascribed to the different patient population (100% hospitalized in our series vs. 55% in Townsend's series). Of notice, our follow-up time was 6-fold longer, thus demonstrating that elevated D-Dimers persist over time. Kalaivani et al. [18] checked the D-Dimer levels after 3 and 6 months from the acute phase. After 3 months, 42% of the patients had elevated (>500 ng/mL) D-Dimer levels, with a decrease to 32% at 6 months. These results, again, confirm our finding both in terms of the incidence and the persistence of elevated D-Dimer levels. These rates were found in a population of patients with long-COVID symptoms, and are in-line with our rates of the procoagulant pattern in patients with persistent MPS. A more sound analysis of the coagulation profile at a mean follow up of 12 months after the acute phase was offered by Fan et al. [20], but, unfortunately, in a small series of 39 patients, of whom only 9 suffered a severe pattern of the disease. When compared to a control group, these patients showed significantly higher D-Dimer levels and Factor VIII activity, and a significantly lower AT activity. Thrombin generation and markers of endotheliopathy were significantly higher in long-COVID patients. An increased thrombin generation and endothelial cell activation is confirmed at a 2-month follow up by the study of Gerotfiazas et al. [21], and by von Meijenfeldt et al. [22] at a 4-month follow up in a series of 29 patients, which found an increased thrombin generation and an inhibition of fibrinolysis induced by high levels of plasmin activator inhibitor. Finally, increased levels of antiplasmin were identified in long-COVID patients by Pretorius et al. [23].

Overall, the combined information coming from both our and previous studies is suggestive of persistent or even ongoing micro-thrombi formation and fibrinolysis. This pattern may derive from (i) a continuous process of fibrinolysis of thrombi formed during the acute phase and (ii) an ongoing thrombi formation triggered by endothelial dysfunction and thrombin generation. Of notice, in both our and previous studies, this pattern is more frequent in elderly patients, in those with severe patterns of the disease during the acute phase, and in those with a persistence of major physical symptoms. These results stress the role of the patient-related procoagulant state (a common feature in elderly patients) as well as disease-related procoagulant conditions (more pronounced in severe states during the acute phase). This complex pattern includes an apparent paradox: high levels of fibrin degradation products (D-Dimer) and a concomitant blunting of fibrinolysis. This condition, which was observed even during the acute phase of the disease, has been interpreted in terms of a fibrinolytic process that is present but inadequate to completely counteract the overwhelming amount of fibrin generated by the thrombin burst [2]. Nielsen et al. [24] proposed a very sound and interesting theory to explain the fibrinolysis paradox in COVID-19 patients. They hypothesized that, since the lungs are the primary location of fibrin breakdown and the main source of the D-dimer found in the systemic circulation, hyperfibrinolysis can occur in the pulmonary extra- and intravascular compartments while a systemic hypofibrinolytic state co-exists.

There are many studies addressing thrombotic complications during the acute phase of COVID-19. Tamayo-Velasco et al. retrospectively investigated 2894 patients in the Spanish territory, detecting a rate of major thromboembolic events reaching 3.5%, with a higher associated morbidity and mortality [25]. In an interesting propensity-matched study, De Vita and associates compared thromboembolic events in COVID-19 versus other kinds of infectious respiratory diseases [26]. Before adjustment for the confounders, the thromboembolic event rate was significantly (p = 0.001) higher in non-COVID-19 patients (6.9%) than in COVID-19 patients (4.7%); however, after propensity matching, this difference lost significance.

How this long-lasting condition may evolve into clinically relevant effects (namely thrombotic or thromboembolic events) remains an unsolved issue.

Follow-up studies of COVID-19 patients have addressed the incidence of deep vein thrombosis and pulmonary embolism. In a large nationwide study conducted in Sweden [27], patients who tested positive for SARS-CoV-2 were matched to tested negative and were followed for 180 days after the acute phase. The authors found that there was a significant increased incidence rate of deep venous thrombosis and pulmonary embolism, and that the risk of thromboembolic events was higher in patients who experienced a severe pattern of COVID-19. In a series of 83 patients with persistent respiratory symptoms after 2 months from the acute phase, Iqbal et al. [28] found a pulmonary embolism rate of 12.5%. Indirect signs of pulmonary vessel microthrombosis were investigated in a wide series of 767 patients studied 3 months after the acute phase [29]. Impaired lung diffusion was found in 17% of the patient population, and many case reports of pulmonary embolism were reported in long-COVID patients [30]. Pulmonary angiogram in long-COVID patients has been suggested following a specific algorithm based on persistence of respiratory symptoms, lung diffusion tests, and perfusion imaging [31]. The hypothesis that lung vasculature could be the main site of thrombus formation or deposition is supported, in our series, by the finding of significantly higher levels of D-Dimer in patients with persistent dyspnea.

In conclusion, the hemostatic system continues to react to the residual effects of the COVID-19 in a considerable amount of patients, even several months after the acute phase. Unfortunately, there are no studies linking the finding of a long-term procoagulant pattern to overt clinical manifestations. This kind of study would require patient populations larger than the one in our and previously published series, but could provide important information to trigger pre-emptive pharmacological strategies in patients with a long-lasting procoagulant profile.

4. Materials and Methods

This is a single-center, prospective cohort study conducted at the IRCCS San Donato, a Clinical Research Hospital partially funded by the Italian Ministry of Health. The Local Ethics Committee (San Raffaele Hospital) approved the experimental design on March 9, 2022, registry number 28/INT/2022. All the patients gave written informed consent. The study has been financed by a grant from the Italian Ministry of Health, within the research projects of the Cardiac Network of the Italian IRCCS (Clinical Research Hospitals). The primary endpoint of this study was the identification of the hemostatic system profile and its link with the acute phase pattern and the persistence of major physical and neuropsychological symptoms from 3 all the way up to 12–18 months from hospital discharge.

4.1. Patient Population and Study Procedures

The patients were recruited through a first telephone contact, and those who were reachable and agreed to participate received a date for the study procedure at our hospital. The eligible patient population was represented by subjects hospitalized at our Institution with a diagnosis of COVID-19 infection between 1 January 2021 and 31 July 2022. The planned patient population was 100 patients. The final patient population comprised 102 subjects.

4.2. Data Collection and Definitions

Data collection was based on (i) retrieval of the relevant data from the original patient's files, (ii) a personal interview conducted in a hospital office by dedicated biologists and medical doctors, and (iii) the coagulation parameters measured through standard laboratory tests and viscoelastic tests.

The following items regarding the acute phase hospitalization were collected: demographics (with age classes $\leq$ 50 years, 51–60 years, 61–70 years, 71–80 years, and > 80 years); disease severity (mild: no oxygen therapy; moderate: nasal oxygen or oxygen mask; severe: non-invasive or invasive ventilation), hospital stay, unit of admission, vaccination (2 doses) at the time of hospital admission; co-morbidities (obesity, hypertension, diabetes, history of coronary disease, heart failure, atrial fibrillation, chronic obstructive pulmonary disease, asthma, active cancer, chronic kidney failure, chronic liver failure, previous cerebrovascular accident, anxiety, depression); and therapy at the time of hospitalization; laboratory exams (peak fibrinogen levels, peak D-Dimer, peak platelet count, nadir platelet count, nadir antithrombin).

Follow-up items included: follow-up duration; any symptom after discharge; work capacity reduced; fatigue, fever, cough, or dyspnea (these last four items combined as "Major physical symptoms"—MPS); and chest pain, arrythmias, headache, sleep disturbances, anxiety, depression (not pre-existing or worsened), memory dysfunction, brain fog, (these last four items combined as "Major Neuropsychological Symptoms"—MNS), paresthesias, muscle pain, joint pain, and sensorial deficit. For each symptom or combination of symptoms, there was a distinction between resolved and ongoing status. Details on ongoing therapies acting on the hemostatic system at the date of follow up were collected.

A blood sample was collected during the same follow-up visit. The coagulation profile was assessed both through standard laboratory analysis and a point-of-care analysis by ClotPro (Haemonetics, Boston, MA, USA).

Standard laboratory assessment included coagulation tests (activated Partial Thrombin Time, aPTT, seconds; international normalized ratio, INR; fibrinogen, mg/dL; D-dimer, ng/mL; antithrombin activity, %) and platelet count (cells/µL).

ClotPro is a CE-marked semi-automatic viscoelastic in vitro point-of-care device featuring the Active Tip™ technology with ready-to-use tips pre-filled with reagents and working with 340 µL citrated blood. The system is composed by a stationary pin and a rotating cup and a typical viscoelastic curve is produced as the clot develops. Samples were analyzed within 30 min of blood draw. Four kind of tests were performed: EXtest (tissue factor activated), INtest (ellagic acid activated), FIBtest (functional fibrinogen), and TPAtest (r-tPA induced fibrinolysis with extrinsic pathway activation). For the EXtest, INtest, and FIBtest, the following parameters were considered: CT (coagulation time, seconds), MCF (maximum clot firmness, mm) and ML (maximum lysis, %). For the TPA test, the LT (lysis time, time required to dissolve 50% of the MCF of the clot once MCF is reached, seconds) and ML (%) were included in the analysis. Data were collected in an electronic platform (Research Electronic Data Capture–RedCAP).

4.3. Statistical Analysis

Data are shown as number (percentage), mean (standard deviation), or median (interquartile range), as appropriate. The differences between categorical variables were assessed using a Pearson's chi square, while differences in continuous variables were explored with a student's t test (normally distributed variables) or a non-parametric test (non-normally distributed variables). The association between the duration of the follow-up (months) and the persistence of a procoagulant profile was assessed using polynomial function regressions (best fit based on R^2 value) with a 95% confidence interval. For the statistical calculations and graphical support, data were exported from RedCAP into statistical packages (SPSS 20.0, IBM, Chicago, IL, USA and GraphPad 9.2.0, GraphPad Software, Inc., San Diego, CA, USA). For all tests, a p value < 0.05 was considered significant.

Author Contributions: Conceptualization, M.R., M.F. and L.M.; methodology, E.B.; formal analysis, M.R.; investigation, E.B., M.A. and S.P.; data curation, E.B., M.A. and S.P.; writing—original draft preparation, M.R. and M.F.; writing—review and editing, M.R. and E.B.; supervision, M.R. and L.M.; project administration, E.B., M.A. and S.P.; funding acquisition, M.R. and L.M. All authors have read and agreed to the published version of the manuscript.

Funding: The study has been financed by a grant from the Italian Ministry of Health, within the research projects of the Cardiac Network of the Italian IRCCS (Clinical Research Hospitals).

Institutional Review Board Statement: The study was conducted in accordance with the Declaration of Helsinki, and approved by the Local Ethics Committee (San Raffaele Hospital) on 9 March 2022, registry number 28/INT/2022. All the patients gave a written informed consent.

Informed Consent Statement: Informed consent was obtained from all subjects involved in the study.

Data Availability Statement: The original dataset supporting the findings of this study will be deposited in the public repository, Zenodo, after the publication of the paper, and accessible upon a reasonable request to the corresponding author.

Conflicts of Interest: M.R. received research grants and a speaker's fee from CSL Behring and a speaker's fee from Werfen and LFB. E.B. has received speakers' fees from Stago and a travel grant from HemoSonics. Other authors declare no conflict of interest.

References

1. Ranucci, M.; Ballotta, A.; Di Dedda, U.; Baryshnikova, E.; Poli, M.D.; Resta, M.; Falco, M.; Albano, G.; Menicanti, L. The procoagulant pattern of patients with COVID 19 acute respiratory distress syndrome. *J. Thromb. Haemost.* **2020**, *18*, 1747–1751 [CrossRef] [PubMed]
2. Ranucci, M.; Sitzia, C.; Baryshnikova, E.; Di Dedda, U.; Cardani, R.; Martelli, F.; Corsi Romanelli, M. COVID-19-Associated Coagulopathy: Biomarkers of Thrombin Generation and Fibrinolysis Leading the Outcome. *J. Clin. Med.* **2020**, *9*, 3487. [CrossRef] [PubMed]
3. Panigada, M.; Bottino, N.; Tagliabue, P.; Grasselli, G.; Novembrino, C.; Chantarangkul, V.; Pesenti, A.; Peyvandi, F.; Tripodi, A. Hypercoagulability of COVID-19 patients in intensive care unit: A report of thromboelastography findings and other parameters of hemostasis. *J. Thromb. Haemost.* **2020**, *18*, 1738–1742. [CrossRef] [PubMed]
4. Blasi, A.; von Meijenfeldt, F.A.; Adelmeijer, J.; Calvo, A.; Ibañez, C.; Perdomo, J.; Reverter, J.C.; Lisman, T. In vitro hypercoagulability and ongoing in vivo activation of coagulation and fibrinolysis in COVID-19 patients on anticoagulation. *J. Thromb. Haemost.* **2020**, *18*, 2646–2653. [CrossRef] [PubMed]
5. Al-Samkari, H.; Song, F.; Van Cott, E.M.; Kuter, D.J.; Rosovsky, R. Evaluation of the prothrombin fragment 1.2 in patients with coronavirus disease 2019 (COVID-19). *Am. J. Hematol.* **2020**, *95*, 1479–1485. [CrossRef]
6. Nougier, C.; Benoit, R.; Simon, M.; Desmurs-Clavel, H.; Marcotte, G.; Argaud, L.; David, J.S.; Bonnet, A.; Negrier, C.; Dargaud, Y. Hypofibrinolytic state and high thrombin generation may play a major role in SARS-CoV-2 associated thrombosis. *J. Thromb. Haemost.* **2020**, *18*, 2215–2219. [CrossRef]
7. Barrett, T.J.; Lee, A.H.; Xia, Y.; Lin, L.H.; Black, M.; Cotzia, P.; Hochman, J.; Berger, J.S. Platelet and Vascular Biomarkers Associate With Thrombosis and Death in Coronavirus Disease. *Circ. Res.* **2020**, *127*, 945–947. [CrossRef]
8. Zaid, Y.; Puhm, F.; Allaeys, I.; Naya, A.; Oudghiri, M.; Khalki, L.; Limami, Y.; Zaid, N.; Sadki, K.; Ben El Haj, R.; et al. Platelets can associate with SARS-CoV-2 RNA and are hyperactivated in COVID-19. *Circ. Res.* **2020**, *127*, 1404–1418. [CrossRef]
9. Prabhakaran, P.; Ware, L.B.; White, K.E.; Cross, M.T.; Matthay, M.A.; Olman, M.A. Elevated levels of plasminogen activator inhibitor-1 in pulmonary edema fluid are associated with mortality in acute lung injury. *Am. J. Physiol. Lung Cell Mol. Physiol.* **2003**, *285*, L20–L28. [CrossRef]
10. Choi, J.J.; Wehmeyer, G.T.; Li, H.A.; Alshak, M.N.; Nahid, M.; Rajan, M.; Liu, B.; Schatoff, E.M.; Elahjji, R.; Abdelghany, Y.; et al. D-dimer cut-off points and risk of venous thromboembolism in adult hospitalized patients with COVID-19. *Thromb. Res.* **2020**, *196*, 318–321. [CrossRef]
11. Naymagon, L.; Zubizarreta, N.; Feld, J.; van Gerwen, M.; Alsen, M.; Thibaud, S.; Kessler, A.; Venugopal, S.; Makki, I.; Qin, Q.; et al. Admission D-dimer levels, D-dimer trends, and outcomes in COVID-19. *Thromb. Res.* **2020**, *196*, 99–105. [CrossRef]

12. Chocron, R.; Duceau, B.; Gendron, N.; Ezzouhairi, N.; Khider, L.; Trimaille, A.; Goudot, G.; Weizman, O.; Alsac, J.M.; Pommier, T.; et al. D-dimer at hospital admission for COVID-19 are associated with in-hospital mortality, independent of venous thromboembolism: Insights from a French multicenter cohort study. *Arch. Cardiovasc. Dis.* **2021**, *114*, 381–393. [CrossRef]
13. Gervaise, A.; Bouzad, C.; Peroux, E.; Helissey, C. Acute pulmonary embolism in non-hospitalized COVID-19 patients referred to CTPA by emergency department. *Eur. Radiol.* **2020**, *30*, 6170–6177. [CrossRef]
14. Fang, C.; Garzillo, G.; Batohi, B.; Teo, J.T.H.; Berovic, M.; Sidhu, P.S.; Robbie, H. Extent of pulmonary thromboembolic disease in patients with COVID-19 on CT: Relationship with pulmonary parenchymal disease. *Clin. Radiol.* **2020**, *75*, 780–788. [CrossRef]
15. Cui, S.; Chen, S.; Li, X.; Siu, S.; Wang, F. Prevalence of venous thromboembolism in patients with severe novel coronavirus pneumonia. *J. Thromb. Haemost.* **2020**, *18*, 1421–1424. [CrossRef]
16. Klok, F.A.; Kruip, M.J.H.A.; Van der Meer, N.J.M.; Arbous, M.S.; Gommers, D.A.M.P.J.; Kant, K.M.; Kaptein, F.H.J.; van Paassen, J.; Stals, M.A.M.; Huisman, M.V.; et al. Incidence of thrombotic complications in critically ill ICU patiens with COVID-19. *Thromb. Res.* **2020**, *191*, 145–147. [CrossRef]
17. Abhinaya, S.; Baskaran, V.; Dillibabu, E.; Hemanth, S.; Abdul Rahman, H.; Srinvasan, K. Systemic arterio-venous thrombosis in COVID-19: A pictorial review. *World J. Radiol.* **2021**, *13*, 19–28.
18. Kalaivani, M.K.; Dinakar, S. Association between D-dimer levels and post-acute sequelae of SARS-CoV-2 in patients from a tertiary care center. *Biomark Med.* **2022**, *16*, 833–838. [CrossRef]
19. Townsend, L.; Fogarty, H.; Dyer, A.; Martin-Loeches, I.; Bannan, C.; Nadarajan, P.; Bergin, C.; Farrelly, C.O.; Conlon, N.; Bourke, N.M.; et al. Prolonged elevation of D-dimer levels in convalescent COVID-19 patients is independent of the acute phase response. *J. Thromb. Haemost.* **2021**, *19*, 1064–1070. [CrossRef]
20. Fan, B.E.; Wong, S.W.; Sum, C.L.L.; Lim, G.H.; Leung, B.P.; Tan, C.W.; Ramanathan, K.; Dalan, R.; Cheung, C.; Lim, X.R.; et al. Hypercoagulability, endotheliopathy, and inflammation approximating 1 year after recovery: Assessing the long-term outcomes in COVID-19 patients. *Am. J. Hematol.* **2022**, *97*, 915–923. [CrossRef]
21. Gerotziafas, G.T.; Van Dreden, P.; Sergentanis, T.N.; Politou, M.; Rousseau, A.; Grusse, M.; Sabbah, M.; Elalamy, I.; Pappa, V.; Skourti, T.; et al. Persisting endothelial cell activation and hypercoagulability after COVID-19 recovery—The Prospective Observational ROADMAP-PostCOVID-19 study. *Hemato* **2022**, *3*, 111–121. [CrossRef]
22. Von Meijenfeldt, F.A.; Thålin, C.; Lisman, T. Sustained prothrombotic changes in convalescent patients with COVID-19. *Lancet Haematol.* **2021**, *8*, e475. [CrossRef] [PubMed]
23. Pretorius, E.; Vlok, M.; Venter, C.; Bezuidenhout, J.A.; Laubscher, G.J.; Steenkamp, J.; Kell, D.B. Persistent clotting protein pathology in Long COVID/Post-Acute Sequelae of COVID-19 (PASC) is accompanied by increased levels of antiplasmin. *Cardiovasc. Diabetol.* **2021**, *20*, 172. [CrossRef] [PubMed]
24. Nielsen, N.D.; Rollins-Raval, M.A.; Raval, J.S.; Thachil, J. Is it hyperfibrinolysis or fibrinolytic shutdown in severe COVID-19? *Thromb. Res.* **2022**, *210*, 1–3. [CrossRef]
25. Tamayo-Velasco, A.; Bombín-Canal, C.; Cebeira, M.J.; Prada, L.S.-D.; Miramontes-González, J.P.; Martín-Fernández, M.; Peñarrubia-Ponce, M.J. Full Characterization of Thrombotic Events in All Hospitalized COVID-19 Patients in a Spanish Tertiary Hospital during the First 18 Months of the Pandemic. *J. Clin. Med.* **2022**, *11*, 3443. [CrossRef]
26. De Vita, A.; De Matteis, G.; d'Aiello, A.; Ravenna, S.E.; Liuzzo, G.; Lanza, G.A.; Massetti, M.; Crea, F.; Gasbarrini, A.; Franceschi, F.; et al. Incidence and Predictors of Thrombotic Complications in 4272 Patients with COVID-19 or Other Acute Infectious Respiratory Diseases: A Propensity Score-Matched Study. *J. Clin. Med.* **2021**, *10*, 4973. [CrossRef]
27. Katsoularis, I.; Fonseca-Rodríguez, O.; Farrington, P.; Jerndal, H.; Lundevaller, E.H.; Sund, M.; Lindmark, K.; Connolly, A.-M.F. Risks of deep vein thrombosis, pulmonary embolism, and bleeding after COVID-19: Nationwide self-controlled cases series and matched cohort study. *BMJ* **2022**, *377*, e069590. [CrossRef]
28. Venturelli, S.; Benatti, S.V.; Casati, M.; Binda, F.; Zuglian, G.; Imeri, G.; Conti, C.; Biffi, A.M.; Spada, M.S.; Bondi, E.; et al. Post COVID-19 sequelae of the respiratory system. A single center experience reporting the compromise of the airway, alveolar and vascular components. *Monaldi Arch. Chest. Dis.* **2022**. [CrossRef]
29. Venturelli, S.; Benatti, S.V.; Casati, M.; Binda, F.; Zuglian, G.; Imeri, G.; Conti, C.; Biffi, A.M.; Spada, M.S.; Bondi, E.; et al. Surviving COVID-19 in Bergamo province: A post-acute outpatient re-evaluation. *Epidemiol. Infect.* **2021**, *149*, e32. [CrossRef]
30. Mouzarou, A.; Ioannou, M.; Leonidou, E.; Chaziri, I. Pulmonary Embolism in Post-COVID-19 Patients, a Literature Review: Red Flag for Increased Awareness? *SN Compr. Clin. Med.* **2022**, *4*, 190. [CrossRef]
31. Dhawan, R.T.; Gopalan, D.; Howard, L.; Vicente, A.; Park, M.; Manalan, K.; Wallner, I.; Marsden, P.; Dave, S.; Branley, H.; et al. Beyond the clot: Perfusion imaging of the pulmonary vasculature after COVID-19. *Lancet Respir. Med.* **2021**, *9*, 107–116. [CrossRef]

International Journal of
Molecular Sciences

MDPI

Review

Pathways of Coagulopathy and Inflammatory Response in SARS-CoV-2 Infection among Type 2 Diabetic Patients

Orsolya-Zsuzsa Akácsos-Szász [1], Sándor Pál [2,*], Kinga-Ilona Nyulas [1], Enikő Nemes-Nagy [3], Ana-Maria Fárr [4], Lóránd Dénes [5], Mónika Szilveszter [6], Erika-Gyöngyi Bán [7], Mariana Cornelia Tilinca [8] and Zsuzsánna Simon-Szabó [4,*]

1 Doctoral School, Faculty of Medicine, George Emil Palade University of Medicine Pharmacy, Science, and Technology of Târgu Mureş, 540142 Târgu-Mureș, Romania
2 Department of Transfusion Medicine, Medical School, University of Pécs, 7624 Pécs, Hungary
3 Department of Chemistry and Medical Biochemistry, Faculty of Medicine in English, George Emil Palade University of Medicine, Pharmacy, Science, and Technology of Târgu Mureş, 540142 Târgu-Mureș, Romania
4 Department of Pathophysiology, Faculty of Medicine, George Emil Palade University of Medicine, Pharmacy, Science, and Technology of Târgu Mureş, 540142 Târgu-Mureș, Romania
5 Department of Anatomy, Faculty of Medicine, George Emil Palade University of Medicine, Pharmacy, Science, and Technology of Târgu Mureş, 540142 Târgu-Mureș, Romania
6 Clinic of Plastic Surgery, Mureș County Emergency Hospital, 540136 Târgu Mureș, Romania
7 Department of Pharmacology, Faculty of Medicine in English, George Emil Palade University of Medicine, Pharmacy, Science, and Technology of Târgu Mureş, 540142 Târgu-Mureș, Romania
8 Department of Internal Medicine I, Faculty of Medicine in English, George Emil Palade University of Medicine, Pharmacy, Science, and Technology of Târgu Mureş, 540142 Târgu-Mureș, Romania
* Correspondence: pal.sandor@pte.hu (S.P.); zsuzsanna.simon-szabo@umfst.ro (Z.S.-S.); Tel.: +36-30-693-2933 (S.P.)

Citation: Akácsos-Szász, O.-Z.; Pál, S.; Nyulas, K.-I.; Nemes-Nagy, E.; Fárr, A.-M.; Dénes, L.; Szilveszter, M.; Bán, E.-G.; Tilinca, M.C.; Simon-Szabó, Z. Pathways of Coagulopathy and Inflammatory Response in SARS-CoV-2 Infection among Type 2 Diabetic Patients. *Int. J. Mol. Sci.* **2023**, *24*, 4319. https://doi.org/10.3390/ijms24054319

Academic Editors: Eliza Russu, Alexandru Schiopu and Emil Arbanasi

Received: 7 January 2023
Revised: 14 February 2023
Accepted: 18 February 2023
Published: 21 February 2023

Abstract: Chronic inflammation and endothelium dysfunction are present in diabetic patients. COVID-19 has a high mortality rate in association with diabetes, partially due to the development of thromboembolic events in the context of coronavirus infection. The purpose of this review is to present the most important underlying pathomechanisms in the development of COVID-19-related coagulopathy in diabetic patients. The methodology consisted of data collection and synthesis from the recent scientific literature by accessing different databases (Cochrane, PubMed, Embase). The main results are the comprehensive and detailed presentation of the very complex interrelations between different factors and pathways involved in the development of arteriopathy and thrombosis in COVID-19-infected diabetic patients. Several genetic and metabolic factors influence the course of COVID-19 within the background of diabetes mellitus. Extensive knowledge of the underlying pathomechanisms of SARS-CoV-2-related vasculopathy and coagulopathy in diabetic subjects contributes to a better understanding of the manifestations in this highly vulnerable group of patients; thus, they can benefit from a modern, more efficient approach regarding diagnostic and therapeutic management.

Keywords: COVID-19; thrombosis; coagulopathy; vasculopathy; inflammation; diabetes mellitus

1. Introduction

Diabetes mellitus (DM) is a major and common public health issue in both developed and developing countries, due to its high mortality rate and induced disabilities.

COVID-19 is caused by the SARS-CoV-2 virus, and since its appearance it became a public health problem due to its rapid spread, the severity of the symptoms, and increased mortality, causing a pandemic, with serious medical, social, and economic consequences globally [1–3].

Chronic inflammation, present in DM, enhances the synthesis of several cytokines. This chronic inflammatory state is preceded by a subclinical inflammatory response, represented by elevated IL-1β and IL-6 before the onset of T2DM [4]. Multiple studies reported during the pandemic that severe forms of COVID-19 are associated with elevated inflammatory markers, and comorbidities [5–8].

Endothelial dysfunction is also a consequence of DM and leads to micro- and macroangiopathy, and concomitantly to hypercoagulability [9].

Scientists had reported from the beginning of the pandemic the association of thrombosis and hypercoagulability with COVID-19, and the urgent need to understand the underlying mechanism for adequate management [10–12]. COVID-19-associated coagulopathy (CAC) is potentially lethal and can lead to disabilities [13–16]. To prevent severe complications and reduce the mortality of COVID-19 patients, targeted therapies for the associated pathologies are required.

The authors have undertaken to write a review that integrates the mechanisms of COVID-19 coagulopathy in patients with type 2 diabetes mellitus (T2DM). To synthesize the paper, a comprehensive literature search on PubMed, Embase, and Cochrane Library was performed, using the following keywords: "SARS-CoV-2", "T2DM", "COVID-19 and diabetes mellitus", "coagulopathy and T2DM", "mechanism", "inflammation" "cytokine storm", "gene polymorphism", "COVID-19 and coagulopathy", "hypercoagulability and endothelial dysfunction", "role of MASP-2 and COVID-19 hypercoagulability", "complement activation and COVID-19". Open-access, full-text English language articles published between the 1st of January 2020 and the 2nd of December 2022 were accessed. The first search included clinical trials, meta-analyses, and randomized controlled clinical trials, and returned 1126 results. In the second step, we narrowed our search area by screening the articles using titles and abstracts, reducing the number of articles to 200. After eliminating duplicates, full-text analysis and further reduction occurred, and finally, 101 manuscripts were selected and integrated into this review, without taking into consideration the scientific impact or citation numbers of each article.

The authors aimed to assess the links between the altered molecular pathways of coagulation on the background of chronic low-grade inflammation of diabetes mellitus and the pathomechanisms of COVID-19-associated coagulopathy and extreme inflammatory response. The secondary goal was to identify possible mechanisms that may be responsible for the higher risk of severe COVID-19 progression in diabetic patients.

The originality of the article is derived from the multiple interactions presented, which are involved in the pathomechanism of COVID-19-related vasculopathy and coagulopathy in type 2 diabetic patients. Novel research results are included, based on the latest articles in scientific literature, and the connections between different pathways are presented in the text and on a complex, original diagram.

A limitation of the study is the lack of long-term experience in basic research related to COVID-19 mechanisms, taking into consideration the relatively recent occurrence of this special epidemiological situation of the coronavirus pandemic. Another limitation is that exclusively open-access articles were used and the authors used only articles written in English, so data that were published in other languages or not in open access were not included in this review.

2. The Pathophysiology of COVID-19 and T2DM Coagulopathy

2.1. The Pathways of Diabetic Endothelial Dysfunction

The most common form of diabetes is T2DM, a heterogeneous disorder, characterized by relative insulin deficiency, and insulin resistance in target tissues. Insulin resistance could be the key mechanism in the development of T2DM and other pathologies, such as hypertension, obesity, coronary artery disease, and metabolic syndrome [17]. The lack of insulin response is the result of the decrease of insulin receptors on the target cell's surface. Some authors have reported that altered endothelial cell signaling and activation of redox regulated transcription factors are contributors as well [18,19]. Normally, insulin binding to its receptors activates two major signaling pathways: the phosphatidylinositol 3-kinase (PI3K)-dependent insulin signaling pathway and the mitogen-activated protein kinase

(MAPK)-dependent insulin signaling pathway. PI3K is responsible for metabolic changes and is regulating glucose transporter type 4 (GLUT4) translocation in adipose cells, while MAPK regulates mitogenesis, growth, and differentiation [17]. Endothelial production of nitric oxide (NO) is regulated by a PI3K-dependent insulin signaling pathway, with a vasodilator effect, also enhancing glucose uptake of skeletal muscles [17]. It was also described that insulin stimulates endothelin-1 (ET-1) secretion via the MAPK signaling pathway, leading to vasoconstriction. In T2DM, the overproduction of advanced glycation end products (AGEs) and inflammatory cytokines contribute to the development of macroangiopathy, and its main form, atherosclerosis. It was also described that oxidative stress and excess production of reactive oxygen species (ROS) are the consequences of the activated major pathways involved in the development of diabetes- related complications: polyol pathway, protein kinase C (PKC) isoforms, excess formation of AGEs, increased expression of AGEs receptor and its activating ligands, and overactivity of the hexosamine pathway [20–22]. Hyperglycemia in T2DM is also responsible for endothelial dysfunction as the consequence of insulin resistance and excessive production of ROS [17]. Oxidative stress will lead to decreased antioxidant effect and excess synthesis of hydrogen peroxide anion, which directly deactivates NO, resulting in decreased NO activity [20]. ROS in excess can induce epigenetic changes. All these mechanisms can be the common links between the development of diabetes, chronic inflammatory response, and cardiovascular diseases (CVD). Cardiovascular complications are present in approximately 80% of T2DM patients [18].

Vascular complications of T2DM include macrovascular, microvascular, cerebrovascular lesions, and peripheral artery disease [18,23].

Macrovascular arteriopathy can affect the central and peripheral arteries, while microvascular diseases affect the small blood vessels in multiple organs, leading to chronic kidney disease (CKD), retinopathy, and the most common type, peripheral neuropathy [24].

The vascular endothelium secretes vasoactive substances to maintain vascular homeostasis by regulating vasoconstriction and vasodilation. Angiotensin II (AT-II), thromboxane A2, and ET-1 have vasoconstrictor effects, while prostaglandin I2 and NO are vasodilators under physiological conditions [20].

The homeostasis of vascular function, especially blood pressure and volume control, is under the regulation of the renin–angiotensin–aldosterone system (RAAS), but RAAS is also known to be involved in local tissue homeostasis, with anti-inflammatory, anticoagulant, antiproliferative, antifibrotic, and antiapoptotic effects on epithelial cells via the ACE2 activated Mas-receptor axis [25].

In T2DM, vascular homeostasis is disturbed by endothelial dysfunction, oxidative stress, platelet hyperreactivity, and inflammation [26], causing alteration in the physicochemical properties of the vascular wall, and enhance the development of atherosclerosis. All these events will aggravate thrombosis and hypercoagulability [27].

2.2. The Pathomechanism of Endothelial Dysfunction in COVID-19

SARS-CoV-2 infects human cells using the ACE2 receptor and a specific transmembrane serine protease 2 (TMPRSS2), for the priming of the spike protein [28].

ACE2 is expressed in various tissues and organs, including endothelium, lung, heart, intestine, kidney, pancreas, and on the epithelial cells of oral mucosa and the tongue [29]. Reportedly, in T2DM patients the ACE2 receptors are upregulated. It has been hypothesized by many that overexpression of ACE2 receptors in T2DM potentially increases the susceptibility to COVID-19 [30,31].

Once SARS-CoV-2 binds to ACE2 receptors and blocks their activity, the RAAS will be affected. Consequently, accumulation of angiotensin 2 (AngII) will occur, which triggers intracellular signaling pathways (caspase 3, p83 MAPK, ROS, cytochrome C) [32], and leads to vasoconstriction, increased oxidative stress, inflammation, cellular damage, and fibrosis. The regulation of RAAS is influenced by the interaction between ACE2 and bradykinin (BK). Normally, BK acts as a negative regulator of RAAS by dilating blood vessels via local NO release. BK is known for its anti-inflammatory and antioxidant properties and has a role in regulating cytokine production and blood vessel permeability. It also has a stimulating effect on plasminogen secretion and thrombus formation. In COVID-19, the internalization of ACE2 will enhance the activation of different types of BK receptors, leading to increased inflammation and local vascular hyperpermeability. Indirectly, it may activate the coagulation cascade through the resulting endothelial damage [33]. The activation of p83 MAPK can contribute to inflammation and oxidative stress, and the activation of caspase 3 can lead to cellular death [33]. ROS formation will induce oxidative damage to cells and tissues and will release cytochrome C from mitochondria, which can trigger the activation of apoptotic signaling pathways and contribute to cell death as well [34].

Nuclear factor kappa B (NF-κB) is a key molecule involved in the nuclear translocation and activation of controlled genes. Overactivation of NF-κB will lead to the extensive synthesis of proinflammatory mediators, uncontrolled inflammatory response, and eventually to cytochrome storm, as observed in COVID-19 patients [35].

After the endothelial infection by the SARS-CoV-2, von Willebrand factor (vWF) is released into the circulation. The vWF is stored in the Weibel–Palade bodies of the endothelial cells. Platelet aggregation initiated by the increased release of vWF [14] will generate a deposition of platelet-rich clots in the lung microcirculation. This event is the key mechanism leading to respiratory failure [36]. Hypercoagulability will be sustained because of the associated release of factor VIII [14], but it is also the consequence of the virus replication within the endothelial cells. The infection causes endothelial cell death and consequently, the endothelial damage will launch the procoagulant reaction [37].

CAC is characterized by clot formation in the lungs, and elevated D-dimer levels at an early stage of COVID-19, but after the systemic activation of the coagulation and the development of disseminated microthrombosis, multiple organs will be affected [38]. Post-mortem autopsy of severe COVID-19 patients found diffuse alveolar damage, and inflammatory infiltrations with hyaline membrane formation in the lung, but also inflammation of the myocardium, focal pancreatitis, axon injury, glomerular microthrombosis, macrophage accumulation in the brain, and lymphocyte infiltrations of the liver [39].

COVID-19 infection determines endothelial activation by angiopoietin-2, a mediator stored also in the Weibel–Palade body, which is released as well, showing elevated circulating levels in COVID-19 and an association with the induction of procoagulant and proinflammatory reactions [40].

2.3. *Inflammatory Response in COVID-19*

The development of inflammatory processes is a key pathological feature of SARS-CoV-2 infection. From the early beginning of the pandemic, several studies have suggested that massive inflammatory cytokines and chemokines are released in COVID-19 [41].

The innate immune system plays an important role, so proinflammatory cytokine production is a desired phase of the immune response against a pathogen. However, in some cases of COVID-19 infection, proinflammatory cytokine release and synthesis are rapidly overactivated, leading to multisystemic damage to the infected host. Interleukin (IL) 2 and 6 (IL-2, IL-6), tumor necrosis factor-alpha (TNF-α), interferon-gamma (IFN-γ), macrophage inflammatory protein (MIP), and monocyte chemoattractant protein 1 (MCP-1) are among many other cytokines that are present in seriously ill COVID-19 patients [42,43].

2.3.1. From Cytokine Formation to Cytokine Storm

During inflammation, IL-6-induced tissue factor is released by macrophages [44].

IL-6 is a proinflammatory cytokine that can stimulate the release of other cytokines and activate immune cells, contributing to the overall systemic inflammation observed in severe COVID-19 cases [45].

AngII triggers NF-κB activation, leading to hyperinflammation, mostly through increased synthesis of IL-6 and IL-1b, and subsequently enhancing the transcription of proinflammatory cytokines. These interleukins presented extremely elevated levels in case of severe COVID-19 [46,47].

The exaggerated expression of IL-6 and IL-6 receptor in COVID-19 leads to endothelial cell hyperactivation and a large amount of tissue factor is released, both processes leading to infection-induced coagulopathy. This event plays an important role in thrombocytopenia, although the cytokine storm is the trigger of thrombocytosis. IL-6 is also participating in the production of some coagulation factors (fibrinogen, factor VIII). Acting on the endothelium, IL-6 enhances the synthesis of vascular endothelial growth factor (VEGF), leading to vascular hyperpermeability and hypotension [48]. Additionally, other cytokines, such as TNF-α, IFN-γ, and IL-1β, have also been implicated in the cytokine storm observed in COVID-19 patients and can contribute to increased inflammation and hypercoagulability.

IL-6 and IL-1α have the crucial role of linking inflammation with the coagulation system. During the proinflammatory phase, these cytokines are present on activated platelets, monocytes, and endothelial cells. IL-1α has the role of activating the inflammatory cascade in thrombo-inflammatory conditions, but is also a key element of thrombogenesis, through its granulocyte recruitment effect, prolongation of clot-lysis time, and increasing thrombocyte activity [43]. Combined with TNF, IL-1 is the most important mediator of endogenous coagulation cascade suppression [44].

The exact mechanisms and interplay between cytokines in diabetes with SARS-CoV-2 infection remains an area of active research.

2.3.2. Complement Cascade Activation

The activation of the complement system following infection with SARS-CoV-2, as the main participant of innate immunity plays an important role in thrombotic events, combined with endothelium disturbances, thrombocytopenia, and bleeding, all representing risk factors of poor clinical outcome [34].

The literature describes three pathways of complement activation (host–antigen contact, antigen–antibody complex trigger, lectin pathway), all in the defense of the host, leading to the synthesis of C3 and derivatives and activation of plasma proteins [49]. The host–antigen contact will activate the first pathway, the activation of the second pathway is caused by antigen–antibody complexes, and the third one is activated by the lectin pathway, which will bind polysaccharides on antigen surfaces to host cells [50]. At this point, the virus will invade host cells that express the ACE2 receptor and damage them, causing a thrombotic–inflammatory response, which further activates the complement system [51]. The particularity of COVID-19 is related to the lectin pathway component, the mannose-associated serine protease 2 (MASP-2), with a key function of thrombin activation and fibrin mesh formation. Complement cascade participants dysregulate the endothelial cells, affecting the action of clotting cascade proteins [50].

In diabetic patients, the complement system, as an innate humoral defense, will become dysregulated, with the consequences of chronic low-grade inflammation and increased risk of infections [52].

Factor XII (FXIIa) activation has a trigger effect on complement complex C1. A further procoagulant effect of complement activation is the initiation of thrombocyte aggregation [53]. These pathomechanisms reveal a close relationship between complement and coagulation cascade, leading to the reciprocal up-regulation of both processes.

In COVID-19 the complement (C3 and C5) is the mediator for developing inflammation [54]. The terminal C5b-C9 complement activation leads to a release of C3b and C5b fragments, with a proinflammatory role [50]. C3b is involved in the opsonization process, marking the SARS-CoV-2, to be destroyed by immune cells. It is important as well for recruiting macrophages and neutrophils, which can release cytokines, signaling molecules that coordinate the immune response. This will induce prostaglandin and leukotriene synthesis, boosting further proinflammatory cytokine production. In some cases, the release of cytokines can become excessive, leading to an overactive immune response [54].

Normally, these processes occur with the purpose of self-defense of the host. However, uncontrolled complement activation results in exaggerated inflammation and systemic procoagulation status with the installation of disseminated intravascular coagulopathy and cellular damage [50].

In the later stages of the complement cascade activation, C5b is involved in the formation of the membrane attack complex (MAC). MAC formation has a role in direct cell lysis. In COVID-19 patients, activation of C5b and formation of the MAC can contribute to inflammation and tissue damage in the lungs and can induce the development of severe symptoms and complications [55–57].

2.4. *The Cytotoxicity of Neutrophil Extracellular Trap*

Neutrophil extracellular trap (NET) release is a mechanism of the innate immune response, as a result of the interaction with activated platelets. It occurs through the explosive intravascular destruction of neutrophils and the release of nucleic substances in the extracellular space, providing a source of extracellular histones with significant cytotoxicity [58]. With the ability to trigger inflammation and thrombosis, NETs release into the extracellular space oxidizes enzymes (NADPH oxidase, nitric oxide synthase) [44,59].

It has also been reported that NETs are among the main drivers of immune-thrombosis in severe COVID-19 cases [60]. Some authors hypothesize that SARS-CoV-2 can directly activate platelets through interaction with its surface spike protein [61], which triggers the release of platelet granules containing proinflammatory and procoagulant factors. Additionally, cytokine release as the result of the immune response to infected cells can also contribute to platelet activation. In COVID-19, platelets are activated and play a role in microvascular thrombosis, leading to serious complications such as acute respiratory distress syndrome (ARDS) and multi-organ failure (MOF) [62].

From the outbreak of the SARS-CoV-2 pandemic, Nicolai et al., among others, hypothesized that activated platelets might induce severe forms of NETosis in some COVID-19 patients with severe symptoms, leading to immune-thrombosis and higher mortality. The team superfused neutrophils isolated from healthy patients with platelet-rich plasma from severe COVID-19 patients and healthy subjects, revealing that the thrombocytes of severe COVID-19 patients adhered at a significantly increased rate to neutrophils compared to the controls [63].

The release of prothrombotic FXII, vWF, TF, and fibrinogen by NETosis will also lead to a procoagulant microenvironment. Circulating histones will also activate further platelets through their Toll-like receptors, resulting in clot formation [34].

NETosis is considered by a few authors to be a prothrombotic risk factor in COVID-19. Thus, a possible therapeutic option for thrombosis risk mitigation is proposedly NET inhibition using neutrophil elastase inhibitors and adenosine receptor agonists [64].

2.5. *Hypercoagulability*

The hypercoagulability present in T2DM will be enhanced by SARS-CoV-2's binding to the ACE2 receptor and the receptor's internalization will alter ACE2 functionality. Normally the enzyme binds to AngII, transforming it into angiotensin 1-7 (Ang1-7) peptide with anti-inflammatory effects. Ang1-7 binds and activates a MAS-related transmembrane G-protein coupled receptor (MRGPCR) [34], this reaction will assure anti-inflammatory, antioxidant, and antithrombotic effects. The downregulation of ACE2 receptors will alter RAAS leading to the above-mentioned hypercoagulability, but also hyper-inflammation, hypertension, hypertrophy, and apoptosis [33].

Moreover, platelet dysfunction can also lead to hypercoagulable states [49]. Platelet activation occurs through the initiation of angiotensin II type 1 receptor (AT1R) and its release of plasminogen activator inhibitor 1 (PAI-1). Platelets are also triggered by the altered ACE2R function [65]. Another important aspect is that platelets have MRGPCRs that modify thrombosis via NO release, and this also contributes to clot formation. This may be the explanation for the importance of platelet activation in COVID-19 coagulopathy [65].

The interrelation between different factors and pathways involved in the development of arteriopathy and coagulopathy in diabetic patients is presented in Figure 1.

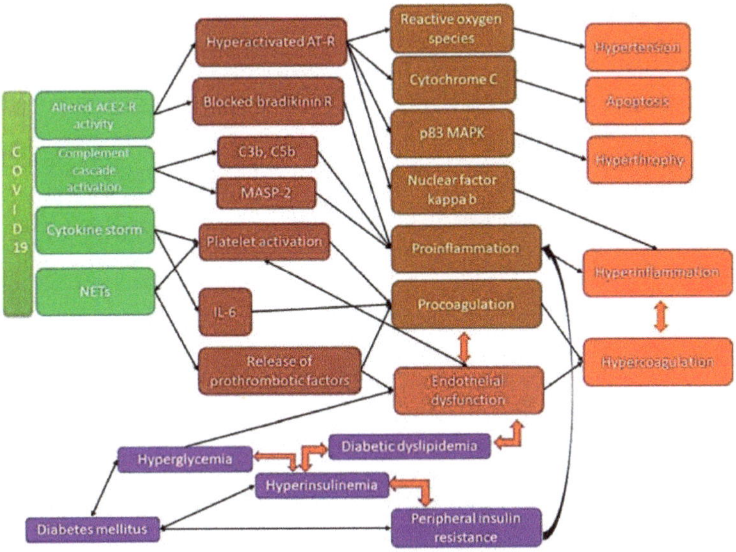

Figure 1. Coagulopathy in DM and COVID-19 infection and the underlying molecular mechanisms.

Hypercoagulability assessment using routine laboratory parameters in COVID-19 and T2DM is listed in Table 1.

Table 1. Laboratory findings of the most assessed parameters in severe COVID-19 and type 2 diabetic patients [59].

Laboratory Parameters	Severe COVID-19 Patient	Type 2 Diabetic Patient
Hemoglobin	Anemia—moderate to severe	Normally unchanged or mild anemia
Platelets	Thrombocytopenia	Normal
Albumin	Hypoalbuminemia	Normal
ALT	Increased	May be increased due to comorbidities (fatty liver disease)
LDH	Increased	May be mildly enhanced due to increased apoptosis
Troponin I	Greater than 28 pg/mL	May be mildly increased due to enhanced apoptosis
D-dimer	Moderately increased	Slightly increased
Prothrombin time	Prolonged	Normal
Activated partial thromboplastin time	Prolonged	Normal
Ferritin	Greater than 300 μg/L	Normal or decreased

In the clinical practice, for rapid assessment of CAC, a highly performant, point-of-care laboratory method was introduced.

Rotational thromboelastometry (ROTEM) is a point-of-care viscoelastic method for whole blood analysis, providing real-time information about clot formation, firmness, and fibrinolysis in severely ill patients and it is useful to identify a hypercoagulable state related to sepsis, COVID-19 [66–68]. Several ROTEM tests can be performed depending on the added substrate along with phospholipids and calcium. The extrinsic coagulation pathway is assessed using rotational thromboelastometry (EXTEM), which is initiated by adding a tissue factor. To assess fibrinolysis, fibrinogen rotational thromboelastometry (FIBTEM) is used, and it differs from EXTEM by using cytochalasin D, which inhibits the platelet cytoskeleton, so the whole clot formation depends on fibrinogen [66].

Point-of-care hemostasis assessment in severe COVID-19 with ROTEM is represented in Table 2 and Figure 2, containing measured parameters, definitions, and levels in severe COVID-19.

Table 2. Results of rotational thromboelastometry (ROTEM) in severe COVID-19 patients.

Parameter, UNIT	Definition	Reference Range	Levels in Severe COVID-19
Clotting time (CT), seconds	The time between the beginning of the coagulation and the increase in the amplitude of the thromboelastogram by at least 2 mm	EXTEM: 38–65 s FIBTEM: 55–87 s	EXTEM: 59 (32–128) mm FIBTEM: 66 (36–178) mm
Clot Formation Time (CFT), seconds	Time from the increase in the amplitude of thromboelastogram from 2 to 20 mm	EXTEM: 42–93 s	EXTEM: 47 (27–157)
Maximum Clot Firmness (MCF), millimeters	Maximum amplitude reached on the thromboelastogram	EXTEM: 53–68 mm FIBTEM: 9–27 mm	EXTEM: 65 (4–74) mm FIBTEM: 28 (9–42) mm
Alpha angle, angle	The slope of the tangent at 2 mm amplitude	EXTEM: 63–83°	EXTEM: 78 (68–83)°
Maximum lysis (ML), percent	The measure of fibrinolysis	EXTEM: 1–12%	EXTEM: 2 (1–13)%

Notes: EXTEM—extrinsically activated test, that is performed by the addition of tissue factor to the sample. FIBTEM—fibrin-based extrinsically activated test, performed with the addition of tissue factor and platelet inhibitor cytochalasin D. CT—clotting time. MCF—maximum clot firmness. CFT—clot formation time.

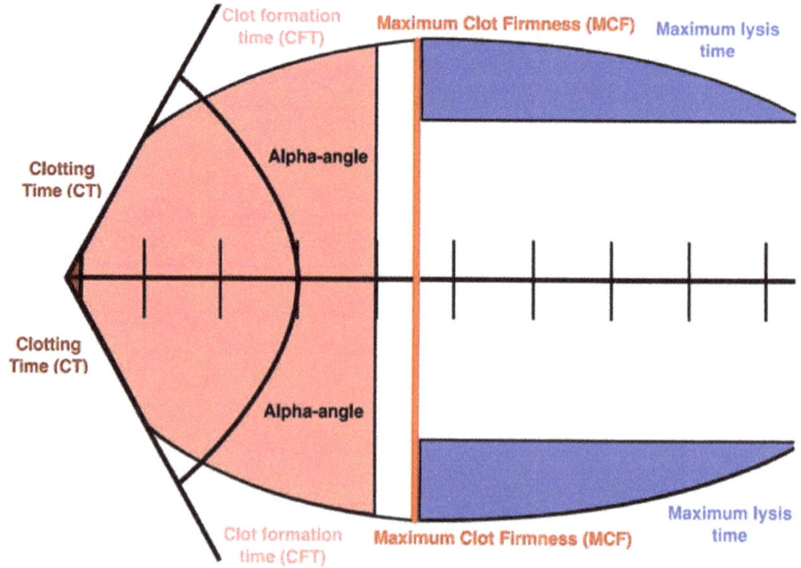

Figure 2. ROTEM parameters in COVID-19 Laboratory parameters and their association with the most frequent pathways in CAC are presented in Table 3.

Table 3. Laboratory findings associated with thrombosis in intensive care unit COVID-19 patients [34,45,59].

Coagulation Biomarkers	Platelet Activation Biomarkers	Inflammation Biomarkers
D-dimer—increased	Thromboxane B2—increased levels associated to thrombosis and higher mortality	Extreme CRP levels—higher in patients with thrombosis compared to those without this complication
Fibrinogen—either increased or decreased	P-selectin- increased levels associated to thrombosis and higher mortality	Procalcitonin—higher in patients with thrombosis compared to those without this complication
Degradation products of fibrin/fibrinogen Increased values	Soluble CD40 ligand—increased levels associated to thrombosis and higher mortality	Erythrocyte sedimentation rate—high levels, higher in patients with thrombosis compared to those without this complication
Von Willebrand Factor Increased values	Mean platelet volume—increased levels associated to thrombosis and higher mortality	Ferritin—higher in patients with thrombosis compared to those without this complication
Prothrombin time, activated partial thromboplastin time—prolonged by 3 s (PT) and by 5 s (APTT)		
Platelet count—thrombocytosis		

The markers of the hypercoagulable state are as follows: shortened CT and higher MCF EXTEM and FIBTEM, shorter than normal EXTEM CFT, and higher alpha-angle [69]. Hypercoagulability could be assessed by ROTEM in 61% of cases [70].

ROTEM would be an appropriate point-of-care method for adequate assessment of coagulopathy, facilitating the work of clinicians to choose the most suitable therapy, applied individually based on the bedside results [66–68,70]. Furthermore, according to Schrick D. et al., ROTEM assays could also reveal platelet reactivity to antiaggregant therapy, and a lower reactivity was found to be associated with higher rates of lethal outcomes in severe COVID-19 cases [71].

2.6. The Importance of Genetic Background

The novel coronavirus breakout and pandemic have intensified the need for genetic investigations related to gene expression for a better understanding of the underlying pathomechanisms of SARS-CoV-2 and its genetic association with different diseases [72,73].

SARS-CoV-2 is a coronavirus of bat origin, causing a disease with various symptoms, from mild fever, cough, and sore throat in some patients or severe pneumonia, ARDS, and even septic shock or MOF in other individuals [74].

The intracellular pathogenicity of viruses makes them dependent on host cells, but it also suggests a virus–host protein–protein interaction (PPI). These PPIs have been the focus of recent analyses. The identification of the most common human proteins known to interact with coronavirus could provide a better understanding of the mechanism of COVID-19 and may suggest therapeutic strategies or drug combinations [75,76].

Using a network-based strategy, which incorporates gene expression profiling, gene ontologies, and PPI analysis, RNA-Seq scientists can identify molecular interactions between virus and host during the development of the infection and establish adequate treatment methods. RNA-Seq is a next-generation sequencing technology to measure gene expression with a high level of accuracy [76].

According to a study conducted by Islam et al. in 2021, cytokine activity and cytokine-mediated signaling pathways were predominant in COVID-19-associated T2DM. Similarly, TNF signaling pathway and cytokine–cytokine receptor interaction were found "enriched" [73].

The most frequently reported pathways were TNF and IL-17 signaling pathways, cytokine–cytokine receptor interactions, and photodynamic therapy-induced NF–κB survival. According to Ouyang et al., the TNF pathway is hyperactivated in severe COVID-19 [77]. On a background of T2DM, there is a direct involvement of TNF-α, through reduction of the insulin metabolism-related GLUT4 expression. Moreover, this phenomenon is also concomitant with insulin receptor inhibition by the serine phosphorylation of insulin receptor substrate-1 (IRS-1) [73]. IL-17, one of the principal triggers of cytokine storm in COVID-19, is released by the activation of the T-helper 17 lymphocyte (Th17) [55,78]. The IL-17 pathway has an insulin resistance-promoting effect, which is worsening the cytokine storm through AT1R excitation, leading to enhanced NO synthesis in diabetes [79,80].

CCL20 was found to have increased levels in the COVID-19-related cytokine storm, obesity, and insulin resistance. In pancreatic β-cells, CCL20 is regulated by NF–κB subunits. FOSL1 TF protein downregulates type I interferon (IFN-1) response, effective in the protection against viral infections [81], thus leading to viral susceptibility.

A study by Islam et al. identified 11 micro-RNAs (miRNAs) with shared pathogenetic potential between COVID-19 and diabetes: *miR-1-3p* and *miR-20a-5p* [73]. The *miR-34a-5p* miRNA decreases the antiapoptotic BCL2 protein, leading to increased glucose-mediated cardiomyocyte apoptosis [82]. Up-regulated *miR-34a-5p* is related to acute myocardial infarction causing heart failure [73]. In COVID-19, some prevalent miRNAs have been found to be associated with asthma (*miR-155-5p, miR-16-5p*) and other lung diseases (*let-7b-5p*). As a response to infection, *miR-146a* expression is induced by NF-κB. This will negatively affect IL-1 and TNF-α receptors so they attenuate inflammation. It has been shown that β-cell miRs are causing islet inflammation, leading to miR-146a-5p expression, which has down-regulated islet inflammation and beta-cell death by impairing NFκB and MAPK signaling [83]. The consequence of downregulated circulating miR-146 is hyper-inflammation in different organs [84]. Donyavi et al. have found that some miRNA can be used as biomarkers for the diagnosis of acute COVID-19 and to distinguish the acute phase from the post-acute form of COVID-19. The identified and suggested miRNAs as biomarkers were: *miR-29a-3p*, *miR-155-5p*, and *miR-146a-3p*. Thus, the connections between transcription factors and miRNAs with the pathogenesis of COVID-19 and diabetes may provide a better understanding of severe COVID-19 in diabetic patients [85,86].

The products of several genes involved in hyperglycemia, cytokine release, hormonal signals, receptor binding, and enzyme activities are interconnected and can influence the pathomechanism of COVID-19 and its complications in diabetic patients [87]. Genetic polymorphisms affecting ACE2 receptors, the cytochrome p450 system, or the cytoprotective heme oxygenase can complicate the treatment of COVID-19 by enhancing a proinflammatory and prooxidant state, increasing the cytokine storm and inducing a prothrombotic state [88].

Iessi et al. suggested that sex-related differences in the immune response may be transmitted via mitochondrial DNA, which could be responsible for the inferior function of male mitochondria and the observed reduced immune response in males [89]. The difference in immune response related to sex may also be explained by the bi-allelic expression [90] of X-linked genes encoding inflammatory mediators or receptors. Viveiros et al. suggested that due to the presence of the ACE2 gene on the X chromosome, which is considered as an X-gene escape, theoretically, women would have a double dose of ACE2, compensating for virus-mediated membrane ACE2 loss. However, ACE2 regulation is under the control of proteolytic cleavage and miRNAs; thus, the expression of ACE2 may not correlate with enzyme activity [90]. Gemmati et al. also hypothesized that women, due to the presence of two X-chromosomes, may have an advantage compared to men, based on their better adaptability to infectious diseases, such as COVID-19 [41].

The role of hyperglycemia in the development of cardiovascular diseases can be partially related to genetic background, although there is limited evidence. More than 150 loci showed association with coronary artery disease in the general population, and some of these loci (such as *9p21*) were clearly demonstrated to be involved in increased cardiovascular risk of diabetic patients, especially in case of poor glycemic control [91].

Certain pathomechanisms of diabetes are closely related to specific genetic and biochemical features, causing inflammation, fibrosis, apoptosis, and the release of ROS enhancing factors. Modified histone proteins, methylation of the genetic material, and modulation of microRNA expression are epigenetic changes which can regulate diabetic vascular complications despite adequate glucose control, or major signaling pathways in T2DM [18,92].

A bidirectional genetic interaction is described in the scientific literature between the human and viral genome during COVID-19. SARS-CoV-2 viral microRNAs can target different genes of the host organism (such as the *ADIPOQ* gene, playing an important role in metabolic syndrome) and human microRNAs were suggested to potentially target viral genes [93].

3. Summary

COVID-19 is characterized by coagulopathy and hemostatic imbalance.

Scientific evidence allows us to formulate the hypothesis that COVID-19-induced coagulopathy in T2DM develops more likely based on pre-existing vascular and metabolic disturbances through the pathomechanisms of the viral infection (intense cytokine release, endothelial dysfunction associated to infection, hyperinflammation, and hypercoagulable state).

Glycemic control will be a priority, not only for CVD protection, but also because ACE2 is present on pancreatic beta-cells as well, and pancreatic inflammation, induced by the cytokine storm, can lead to insulin resistance [94]. Several studies reported higher ACE2 expression in females, and decreasing ACE2 expression in elderly patients, which will be severely altered in the presence of DM. It was also reported that the cytokine storm has a repressing effect on ACE2 leading to severe outcomes [95].

It has been reported that chronic inflammation in T2DM will promote platelet activation leading to hypercoagulability. In T2DM the underlying condition, i.e., excessive level of proinflammatory cytokines and low level of anti-inflammatory cytokines, leading to an immunocompromised state, together with metabolic imbalance may be the explanation for the severe outcome of T2DM patients infected with SARS-CoV-2 [96]. The ROTEM method is a proper diagnostic tool for rapid evaluation of hypercoagulable state in COVID-19-related sepsis, which could be applied on a large scale.

B-cell proliferation is observed in obese patients due to insulin resistance. It occurs as a compensatory response to nondiabetic obesity, when the organism is trying to counteract the insulin resistance by increasing insulin-secreting β-cells [97]. In some cases, the first sign of the onset of DM is in the form of ketoacidosis concomitant with COVID-19, leading to a severe outcome [98]. It has also been reported that those patients who are diabetics at the time of infection with SARS-CoV-2 have a better outcome than those with concomitantly installed DM and COVID-19. Certain studies also reported that patients with DM have a two-fold risk of intensive care unit hospitalization and a two–three-fold risk of hospital mortality than non-diabetic patients [99,100]. Several studies have shown that the infectivity of COVID-19 is not higher in patients with associated diabetes. The prevalence of diabetes in the COVID-19 patient population is not significantly different from the prevalence of diabetes in the general population [101].

Early diagnosis and identification of gene modifications that can influence the course of the disease is a desired aim to prevent further complications and to recognize risk levels for each patient.

The authors concluded that the mechanism of COVID-19, with the virus binding to the ACE2 receptor, might be different in patients in accordance with the individual genetic background or developed susceptibility.

We consider that human genetics plays an important role (inherited predispositions) in COVID-19 management, due to the possibility of identification of gene modifications that contribute to poor prognosis, even more, when pre-existing comorbidities and acquired risk conditions are present.

Comprehensive knowledge of the underlying pathomechanisms of coagulopathy and inflammatory response in diabetes mellitus contributes to a better understanding of the manifestations of angiopathy in this very vulnerable group of patients; thus, they can benefit from a modern, more efficient management.

Author Contributions: Conceptualization, O.-Z.A.-S., S.P.,.K.-I.N., E.N.-N., M.C.T. and Z.S.-S.; methodology, S.P.; E.N.-N., A.-M.F. and Z.S.-S.; formal analysis, M.S.; writing—original draft preparation, O.-Z.A.-S., S.P., K.-I.N., E.N.-N. and Z.S.-S.; editing, E.-G.B., L.D.; visualization, S.P. and Z.S.-S.; critical revision, A.-M.F., L.D., M.S., E.-G.B., M.C.T. and Z.S.-S.; supervision, Z.S.-S. All authors have read and agreed to the published version of the manuscript.

Funding: This research received no external funding.

Institutional Review Board Statement: Not applicable.

Informed Consent Statement: Not applicable.

Data Availability Statement: Not applicable.

Acknowledgments: "George Emil Palade" University of Medicine, Pharmacy, Science, and Technology of Târgu Mureş supported this work by Research Grant nr. 294/6/14.01.2020.

Conflicts of Interest: The authors declare no conflict of interest.

References

1. WHO–Diabetes Mellitus Classification. Available online: https://www.who.int/publications/i/item/classification-of-diabetes-mellitus (accessed on 30 December 2022).
2. WHO–COVID-19. Available online: https://www.who.int/emergencies/diseases/novel-coronavirus-2019 (accessed on 30 December 2022).
3. Arbănași, E.M.; Kaller, R.; Mureșan, V.A.; Voidăzan, S.; Arbănași, E.M.; Russu, E. Impact of COVID-19 Pandemic on Vascular Surgery Unit Activity in Central Romania. *Front. Surg.* **2022**, *9*, 1123. [CrossRef]
4. Xie, L.; Zhang, Z.; Wang, Q.; Chen, Y.; Lu, D.; Wu, W. COVID-19 and Diabetes: A Comprehensive Review of Angiotensin Converting Enzyme 2, Mutual Effects and Pharmacotherapy. *Front. Endocrinol. (Lausanne)* **2021**, *19*, 772865. [CrossRef] [PubMed]
5. Arbănași, E.M.; Halmaciu, I.; Kaller, R.; Mureșan, A.V.; Arbănași, E.M.; Suciu, B.A.; Coșarcă, C.M.; Cojocaru, I.I.; Melinte, R.M.; Russu, E. Systemic Inflammatory Biomarkers and Chest CT Findings as Predictors of Acute Limb Ischemia Risk, Intensive Care Unit Admission, and Mortality in COVID-19 Patients. *Diagnostics* **2022**, *12*, 2379. [CrossRef] [PubMed]
6. Simon, P.; Le Borgne, P.; Lefevbre, F.; Cipolat, L.; Remillon, A.; Dib, C.; Hoffmann, M.; Gardeur, I.; Sabah, J.; Kepka, S.; et al. Platelet-to-Lymphocyte Ratio (PLR) Is Not a Predicting Marker of Severity but of Mortality in COVID-19 Patients Admitted to the Emergency Department: A Retrospective Multicenter Study. *J. Clin. Med.* **2022**, *11*, 4903. [CrossRef]
7. Rose, J.; Suter, F.; Furrer, E.; Sendoel, A.; Stüssi-Helbling, M.; Huber, L.C. Neutrophile-to-Lymphocyte Ratio (NLR) Identifies Patients with Coronavirus Infectious Disease 2019 (COVID-19) at High Risk for Deterioration and Mortality—A Retrospective, Monocentric Cohort Study. *Diagnostics* **2022**, *12*, 1109. [CrossRef]
8. Sarkar, S.; Kannan, S.; Khanna, P.; Singh, A.K. Role of Platelet-to-Lymphocyte Count Ratio (PLR), as a Prognostic Indicator in COVID-19: A Systematic Review and Meta-Analysis. *J. Med. Virol.* **2022**, *94*, 211–221. [CrossRef]
9. Radha, T.P.D.; Arthi, P.S.; Annamalai, S. Diabetes Mellitus and Peripheral Vascular Disease. *Int. J. Contemp. Med. Res.* **2020**, *7*, 10–13. [CrossRef]
10. Klok, F.A.; Kruip, M.J.H.A.; van der Meer, N.J.M.; Arbous, M.S.; Gommers, D.A.M.P.J.; Kant, K.M.; Kaptein, F.H.J.; van Paassen, J.; Stals, M.A.M.; Huisman, M.V.; et al. Incidence of thrombotic complications in critically ill ICU patients with COVID-19. *Thromb. Res.* **2020**, *191*, 145–147. [CrossRef]
11. Jenner, W.J.; Gorog, D.A. Incidence of thrombotic complications in COVID-19. *J. Thromb.* **2021**, *52*, 999–1006. [CrossRef]
12. Atallah, B.; Sadik, Z.G.; Salem, N.; El Nekidy, W.S.; Almahmeed, W.; Park, W.M.; Cherfan, A.; Hamed, F.; Mallat, J. The impact of protocol-based high-intensity pharmacological thromboprophylaxis on thrombotic events in critically ill COVID-19 patients. *Anaesthesia* **2021**, *76*, 327–335. [CrossRef]
13. Zhou, F.; Yu, T.; Du, R.; Fan, G.; Liu, Y.; Liu, Z.; Xiang, J.; Wang, Y.; Song, B.; Gu, X.; et al. Clinical course and risk factors for mortality of adult inpatients with COVID-19 in Wuhan, China: A retrospective cohort study. *Lancet* **2020**, *395*, 1054–1062. [CrossRef] [PubMed]
14. Goshua, G.; Pine, A.B.; Meizlish, M.L.; Chang, C.-H.; Zhang, H.; Bahel, P.; Baluha, A.; Bar, N.; Bona, R.D.; Burns, A.J.; et al. Endotheliopathy in COVID-19-associated coagulopathy: Evidence from a single-centre, cross-sectional study. *Lancet Haematol.* **2020**, *7*, e575–e582. [CrossRef]

15. Moisa, E.; Corneci, D.; Negoita, S.; Filimon, C.R.; Serbu, A.; Negutu, M.I.; Grintescu, I.M. Dynamic Changes of the Neutrophil-to-Lymphocyte Ratio, Systemic Inflammation Index, and Derived Neutrophil-to-Lymphocyte Ratio Independently Predict Invasive Mechanical Ventilation Need and Death in Critically Ill COVID-19 Patients. *Biomedicines* **2021**, *9*, 1656. [CrossRef] [PubMed]
16. Halmaciu, I.; Arbănași, E.M.; Kaller, R.; Mureșan, A.V.; Arbănași, E.M.; Bacalbasa, N.; Suciu, B.A.; Cojocaru, I.I.; Runcan, A.I.; Grosu, F.; et al. Chest CT Severity Score and Systemic Inflammatory Biomarkers as Predictors of the Need for Invasive Mechanical Ventilation and of COVID-19 Patients' Mortality. *Diagnostics* **2022**, *12*, 2089. [CrossRef]
17. Muniyappa, R.; Chen, H.; Montagnani, M.; Sherman, A.; Quon, M.J. Endothelial dysfunction due to selective insulin resistance in vascular endothelium: Insights from mechanistic modeling. *Am. J. Physio. Endocrinol. Metab.* **2020**, *319*, E629–E646. [CrossRef] [PubMed]
18. Munteanu, C.; Rotariu, M.; Turnea, M.A.; Anghelescu, A.; Albadi, I.; Dogaru, G.; Silișteanu, S.C.; Ionescu, E.V.; Firan, F.C.; Ionescu, A.M.; et al. Topical Reappraisal of Molecular Pharmacological Approaches to Endothelial Dysfunction in Diabetes Mellitus Angiopathy. *Curr. Issues Mol. Biol.* **2022**, *44*, 3378–3397. [CrossRef]
19. Love, M.K.; Barrett, E.J.; Malin, S.K.; Reusch, J.E.B.; Regensteiner, J.G.; Liu, Z. Diabetes pathogenesis and management: The endothelium comes of age, *J. Mol. Cell Biol.* **2021**, *13*, 500–512. [CrossRef]
20. Maruhashi, T.; Higashi, Y. Pathophysiological Association between Diabetes Mellitus and Endothelial Dysfunction. *Antioxidants* **2021**, *10*, 1306. [CrossRef]
21. Jung, C.H.; Mok, J.O. Recent updates on vascular complications in patients with type 2 diabetes mellitus. *Endocrinol. Metab.* **2020**, *35*, 260–271. [CrossRef]
22. Galicia-Garcia, U.; Benito-Vicente, A.; Jebari, S.; Larrea-Sebal, A.; Siddiqi, H.; Uribe, K.B.; Ostolaza, H.; Martín, C. Pathophysiology of Type 2 Diabetes Mellitus. *Int. J. Mol. Sci.* **2020**, *21*, 6275. [CrossRef]
23. De Nigris, V.; Prattichizzo, F.; Iijima, H.; Ceriello, A. Dpp-4 inhibitors have different effects on endothelial low-grade inflammation and on the m1-m2 macrophage polarization under hyperglycemic conditions. *Diabetes Metab. Syndr. Obes. Targets Ther.* **2021**, *14*, 1519–1531. [CrossRef] [PubMed]
24. Daryabor, G.; Atashzar, M.R.; Kabelitz, D.; Meri, S.; Kalantar, K. The Effects of Type 2 Diabetes Mellitus on Organ Metabolism and the Immune System. *Front. Immunol.* **2020**, *11*, 1582. [CrossRef]
25. Sen, R.; Sengupta, D.; Mukherjee, A. Mechanical dependency of the SARS-CoV-2 virus and the renin-angiotensin-aldosterone (RAAS) axis: A possible new threat. *Environ. Sci. Pollut. Res. Int.* **2022**, *29*, 62235–62247. [CrossRef] [PubMed]
26. Iacobini, C.; Vitale, M.; Pesce, C.; Pugliese, G.; Menini, S. Diabetic Complications and Oxidative Stress: A 20-Year Voyage Back in Time and Back to the Future. *Antioxidants* **2021**, *10*, 727. [CrossRef]
27. Gusev, E.; Sarapultsev, A.; Hu, D.; Chereshnev, V. Problems of Pathogenesis and Pathogenetic Therapy of COVID-19 from the Perspective of the General Theory of Pathological Systems (General Pathological Processes). *Int. J. Mol. Sci.* **2021**, *22*, 7582. [CrossRef]
28. Hoffmann, M.; Kleine-Weber, H.; Schroeder, S.; Kruger, N.; Herrler, T.; Erichsen, S.; Schiergens, T.S.; Herrler, G.; Wu, N.H.; Nitsche, A.; et al. SARS-CoV-2 Cell Entry Depends on ACE2 and TMPRSS2 and Is Blocked by a Clinically Proven Protease Inhibitor. *Cell* **2020**, *181*, 271–280.e8. [CrossRef]
29. Xu, H.; Zhong, L.; Deng, J.; Peng, J.; Dan, H.; Zeng, X.; Li, T.; Chen, Q. High expression of ACE2 receptor of 2019-nCoV on the epithelial cells of oral mucosa. *Int. J. Oral Sci.* **2020**, *12*, 8. [CrossRef]
30. Pinchera, B.; Scotto, R.; Buonomo, A.; Zappulo, E.; Stagnaro, F.; Gallicchio, A.; Viceconte, G.; Sardanelli, A.; Mercinelli, S.; Villari, R. Diabetes and COVID-19: The potential role of mTOR. *Diabetes Res. Clin. Pract.* **2022**, *186*, 109813. [CrossRef] [PubMed]
31. Calvisi, S.L.; Ramirez, G.A.; Scavini, M.; Da Prat, V.; di Lucca, G.; Laurenzi, A.; Gallina, G.; Cavallo, L.; Borio, G.; Farolfi, F.; et al. Thromboembolism risk among patients with diabetes/stress hyperglycemia and COVID-19. *Metabolism* **2021**, *123*, 154845. [CrossRef]
32. Lumbers, E.R.; Delforce, S.J.; Pringle, K.; Smith, G.R. The Lung, the Heart, the Novel Coronavirus, and the Renin-Angiotensin System; The Need for Clinical Trials. *Front. Med. (Lausanne)* **2020**, *22*, 248. [CrossRef]
33. Scialo, F.; Daniele, A.; Amato, F.; Pastore, L.; Matera, M.G.; Cazzola, M.; Castaldo, G.; Bianco, A. ACE2: The Major Cell Entry Receptor for SARS-CoV-2. *Lung* **2020**, *198*, 867–877. [CrossRef] [PubMed]
34. Ali, M.A.; Spinler, S.A. COVID-19 and thrombosis: From bench to bedside. *Trends Cardiovasc. Med.* **2021**, *31*, 143–160. [CrossRef] [PubMed]
35. Gudowska-Sawczuk, M.; Mroczko, B. The Role of Nuclear Factor Kappa B (NF-κB) in Development and Treatment of COVID-19: Review. *Int. J. Mol. Sci.* **2022**, *23*, 5283. [CrossRef]
36. Iba, T.; Levy, J.H.; Levi, M.; Connors, J.M.; Thachil, J. Coagulopathy of Coronavirus Disease 2019. *Crit. Care Med.* **2020**, *48*, 1358–1364. [CrossRef] [PubMed]
37. Labò, N.; Ohnuki, H.; Tosato, G. Vasculopathy and Coagulopathy Associated with SARS-CoV-2 Infection. *Cells* **2020**, *9*, 1583. [CrossRef]
38. Iba, T.; Warkentin, T.E.; Thachil, J.; Levi, M.; Levy, J.H. Proposal of the Definition for COVID-19-Associated Coagulopathy. *J. Clin. Med.* **2021**, *10*, 191. [CrossRef] [PubMed]
39. Eketunde, A.O.; Mellacheruvu, S.P.; Oreoluwa, P. A review of postmortem findings in patients with COVID-19. *Cureus* **2020**, *12*, e9438. [CrossRef]

40. Smadja, D.M.; Guerin, C.L.; Chocron, R.; Yatim, N.; Boussier, J.; Gendron, N.; Khider, L.; Hadjadj, J.; Goudot, G.; DeBuc, B.; et al. Angiopoietin-2 as a marker of endothelial activation is a good predictor factor for intensive care unit admission of COVID-19 patients. *Angiogenesis* **2020**, *23*, 611–620. [CrossRef]
41. Gemmati, D.; Bramanti, B.; Serino, M.L.; Secchiero, P.; Zauli, G.; Tisato, V. COVID-19 and Individual Genetic Susceptibility/Receptivity: Role of ACE1/ACE2 Genes, Immunity, Inflammation and Coagulation. Might the Double X-chromosome in Females Be Protective against SARS-CoV-2 Compared to the Single X-Chromosome in Males? *Int. J. Mol. Sci.* **2020**, *21*, 3474. [CrossRef]
42. Lazzaroni, M.G.; Piantoni, S.; Masneri, S.; Garrafa, E.; Martini, G.; Tincani, A.; Andreoli, L.; Franceschini, F. Coagulation dysfunction in COVID-19: The interplay between inflammation, viral infection and the coagulation system. *Blood Rev.* **2021**, *46*, 100745. [CrossRef]
43. Savla, S.R.; Prabhavalkar, K.S.; Bhatt, L.K. Cytokine storm associated coagulation complications in COVID-19 patients: Pathogenesis and Management. *Expert Rev. Anti-Infect Ther.* **2021**, *19*, 1397–1413. [CrossRef]
44. Gómez-Mesa, J.E.; Galindo-Coral, S.; Montes, M.C.; Martin, A.J.M. Thrombosis and Coagulopathy in COVID-19. *Curr. Probl. Cardiol.* **2021**, *46*, 100742. [CrossRef]
45. Ragab, D.; Salah Eldin, H.; Taeimah, M.; Khattab, R.; Salem, R. The COVID-19 Cytokine Storm; What We Know So Far. *Front. Immunol.* **2020**, *11*, 1446. [CrossRef] [PubMed]
46. Mascolo, A.; Scavone, C.; Rafaniello, C.; Ferrajolo, C.; Racagni, G.; Berrino, L.; Paolisso, G.; Rossi, F.; Capuano, A. Renin-Angiotensin System and Coronavirus Disease 2019: A Narrative Review. *Front. Cardiovasc. Med.* **2020**, *7*, 143. [CrossRef] [PubMed]
47. Zhang, H.; Penninger, J.M.; Li, Y.; Zhong, N.; Slutsky, A.S. Angiotensin-converting enzyme 2 (ACE2) as a SARS-CoV-2 receptor: Molecular mechanisms and potential therapeutic target. *Intensive Care Med.* **2020**, *46*, 586–590. [CrossRef] [PubMed]
48. Tomerak, S.; Khan, S.; Almasri, M.; Hussein, R.; Abdelati, A.; Aly, A.; Salameh, M.A.; Saed Aldien, A.; Naveed, H.; Elshazly, M.B.; et al. Systemic inflammation in COVID-19 patients may induce various types of venous and arterial thrombosis: A systematic review. *Scand J. Immunol.* **2021**, *94*, e13097. [CrossRef] [PubMed]
49. Kaiafa, G.; Savopoulos, C.; Karlafti, E.; Pantazi, K.; Paramythiotis, D.; Thomaidou, E.; Daios, S.; Ztriva, E.; Gionis, M.; Fyntanidou, V.; et al. Coagulation Profile of COVID-19 Patients. *Life* **2022**, *12*, 1658. [CrossRef]
50. Tomo, S.; Kumar, K.P.; Roy, D.; Sankanagoudar, S.; Purohit, P.; Yadav, D.; Banerjee, M.; Sharma, P.; Misra, S. Complement activation and coagulopathy—An ominous duo in COVID19. *Expert Rev. Hematol.* **2021**, *14*, 155–173. [CrossRef] [PubMed]
51. Conway, E.M.; Pryzdial, E.L.G. Is the COVID-19 thrombotic catastrophe complement-connected? *J. Thromb. Haemost.* **2020**, *18*, 2812–2822. [CrossRef]
52. Pérez-Galarza, J.; Prócel, C.; Cañadas, C.; Aguirre, D.; Pibaque, R.; Bedón, R.; Sempértegui, F.; Drexhage, H.; Baldeón, L. Immune Response to SARS-CoV-2 Infection in Obesity and T2D: Literature Review. *Vaccines* **2021**, *9*, 102. [CrossRef]
53. Hollenberg, M.D.; Epstein, M. The innate immune response, microenvironment proteinases, and the COVID-19 pandemic: Pathophysiologic mechanisms and emerging therapeutic targets. *Kidney Int. Suppl.* **2022**, *12*, 48–62. [CrossRef] [PubMed]
54. Smail, S.W.; Saeed, M.; Alkasalias, T.; Khudhur, Z.O.; Younus, D.A.; Rajab, M.F.; Abdulahad, W.H.; Hussain, H.I.; Niaz, K.; Safdar, M. Inflammation, immunity and potential target therapy of SARS-COV-2: A total scale analysis review. *Food Chem. Toxicol.* **2021**, *150*, 112087. [CrossRef] [PubMed]
55. Megna, M.; Napolitano, M.; Fabbrocini, G. May IL-17 have a role in COVID-19 infection? *Med. Hypotheses* **2020**, *140*, 109749. [CrossRef]
56. Carvelli, J.; Demaria, O.; Vely, F.; Batista, L.; Chouaki Benmansour, N.; Fares, J.; Carpentier, S.; Thibult, M.-L.; Morel, A.; Remark, R.; et al. Association of COVID-19 inflammation with activation of the C5a–C5aR1 axis. *Nature* **2020**, *588*, 146–150. [CrossRef]
57. Ma, L.; Sahu, S.K.; Cano, M.; Kuppuswamy, V.; Bajwa, J.; McPhatter, J.N.; Pine, A.; Meizlish, M.L.; Goshua, G.; Chang, C.-H.; et al. Increased complement activation is a distinctive feature of severe SARS-CoV-2 infection. *Sci. Immunol.* **2021**, *6*, eabh2259. [CrossRef]
58. Zuo, Y.; Zuo, M.; Yalavarthi, S.; Gockman, K.; Madison, J.A.; Shi, H.; Woodard, W.; Lezak, S.P.; Lugogo, N.L.; Knight, J.S.; et al. Neutrophil extracellular traps and thrombosis in COVID-19. *J. Thromb. Thrombolysis* **2021**, *51*, 446–453. [CrossRef] [PubMed]
59. Manolis, A.S.; Manolis, T.A.; Papatheou, D.; Melita, H. COVID-19 Infection: Viral Macro- and Micro-Vascular Coagulopathy and Thromboembolism/Prophylactic and Therapeutic Management. *J. Cardiovasc. Pharmacol. Ther.* **2021**, *26*, 12–24. [CrossRef]
60. Skendros, P.; Mitsios, A.; Chrysanthopoulou, A.; Mastellos, D.C.; Metallidis, S.; Rafailidis, P.; Ntinopoulou, M.; Sertaridou, E.; Tsironidou, V.; Tsigalou, C.; et al. Complement and tissue factor-enriched neutrophil extracellular traps are key drivers in COVID-19 immunothrombosis. *J. Clin. Investig.* **2020**, *130*, 6151–6157. [CrossRef]
61. Shen, S.; Zhang, J.; Fang, Y.; Lu, S.; Wu, J.; Zheng, X.; Deng, F. SARS-CoV-2 interacts with platelets and megakaryocytes via ACE2-independent mechanism. *J. Hematol. Oncol.* **2021**, *14*, 72. [CrossRef]
62. Thierry, A.R.; Roch, B. Neutrophil Extracellular Traps and By-Products Play a Key Role in COVID-19: Pathogenesis, Risk Factors, and Therapy. *J. Clin. Med.* **2020**, *9*, 2942. [CrossRef]
63. Nicolai, L.; Leunig, A.; Brambs, S.; Kaiser, R.; Weinberger, T.; Weigand, M.; Muenchhoff, M.; Hellmuth, J.C.; Ledderose, S.; Schulz, H.; et al. Immunothrombotic Dysregulation in COVID-19 Pneumonia Is Associated With Respiratory Failure and Coagulopathy. *Circulation* **2020**, *142*, 1176–1189. [CrossRef] [PubMed]

64. Wienkamp, A.-K.; Erpenbeck, L.; Rossaint, J. Platelets in the NETworks interweaving inflammation and thrombosis. *Front. Imunol.* **2022**, *13*, 953129. [CrossRef] [PubMed]
65. Ahmed, S.; Zimba, O.; Gasparyan, A.Y. Thrombosis in Coronavirus disease 2019 (COVID-19) through the prism of Virchow's triad. *Clin. Rheumatol.* **2020**, *39*, 2529–2543. [CrossRef]
66. Rubulotta, F.; Soliman-Aboumarie, H.; Filbey, K.; Geldner, G.; Kuck, K.; Ganau, M.; Hemmerling, T.M. Technologies to optimize the care of severe COVID-19 patients for health care providers challenged by limited resources. *Anesth. Analg.* **2020**, *131*, 351–364. [CrossRef]
67. Tejpal Karna, S.; Singh, P.; Ahmad Haq, Z.; Jain, G.; Khurana, A.; Saigal, S.; Prakash Sharma, J.; Waindeskar, V. Role of Thromboelastography and Thromboelastometry in Predicting Risk of Hypercoagulability and Thrombosis in Critically Ill COVID-19 Patients: A Qualitative Systematic Review. *Turk J. Anaesthesiol. Reanim.* **2022**, *50*, 332–339. [CrossRef] [PubMed]
68. Almskog, L.M.; Wikman, A.; Svensson, J.; Wanecek, M.; Bottai, M.; van der Lindeen, J.; Agren, A. Rotational thromboelastometry results are associated with care level in COVID-19. *J. Thromb. Thrombolysis* **2021**, *51*, 437–445. [CrossRef]
69. Bolek, T.; Samoš, M.; Škorňová, I.; Schnierer, M.; Jurica, J.; Bánovčin, P.; Staško, J.; Kubisz, P.; Mokáň, M. ß Rotational thromboelastometry in patients with type 2 diabetes and mild COVID-19 pneumonia: A pilot prospective study. *Medicine* **2022**, *101*, e29738. [CrossRef]
70. Mitrovic, M.; Sabljic, N.; Cvetkovic, Z.; Pantic, N.; Zivkovic Dakic, A.; Bukumiric, Z.; Libek, V.; Savic, N.; Milenkovic, B.; Virijevic, M.; et al. Rotational Thromboelastometry (ROTEM) Profiling of COVID–19 Patients. *Platelets* **2021**, *32*, 690–696. [CrossRef]
71. Schrick, D.; Tőkés-Füzesi, M.; Réger, B.; Molnár, T. Plasma Fibrinogen Independently Predicts Hypofibrinolysis in Severe COVID-19. *Metabolites* **2021**, *11*, 826. [CrossRef]
72. Nashiry, A.; Sumi, S.S.; Islam, S.; Quinn, J.M.W.; Moni, A.M.A. Bioinformatics, and system biology approach to identify the influences of COVID-19 on cardiovascular and hypertensive comorbidities. *Brief Bioinform.* **2021**, *22*, 1387–1401. [CrossRef]
73. Islam, M.B.; Chowdhury, U.N.; Nain, Z.; Uddin, S.; Ahmed, M.B.; Moni, M.A. Identifying molecular insight of synergistic complexities for SARS-CoV-2 infection with pre-existing type 2 diabetes. *Comput. Biol. Med.* **2021**, *136*, 104668. [CrossRef] [PubMed]
74. Huang, C.; Wang, Y.; Li, X.; Ren, L.; Zhao, J.; Hu, Y.; Zhang, L.; Fan, G.; Xu, J.; Gu, X. Clinical features of patients infected with 2019 novel coronavirus in Wuhan, China. *Lancet* **2020**, *395*, 497–506. [CrossRef]
75. Liu, C.; Ma, Y.; Zhao, J.; Nussinov, R.; Zhang, Y.C.; Cheng, F.; Zhang, Z.K. Computational network biology: Data, model, and applications. *Phys. Rep.* **2020**, *846*, 1–66. [CrossRef]
76. Khan, A.A.; Khan, Z. Comparative host–pathogen protein–protein interaction analysis of recent coronavirus outbreaks and important host targets identification. *Brief Bioinform.* **2021**, *22*, 1206–1214. [CrossRef]
77. Ouyang, Y.; Yin, J.; Wang, W.; Shi, H.; Shi, Y.; Xu, B.; Qiao, L.; Feng, Y.; Pang, L.; Wei, F. Down-regulated gene expression spectrum and immune responses changed during the disease progression in COVID-19 patients. *Clin. Infect. Dis.* **2020**, *71*, 2052–2060. [CrossRef] [PubMed]
78. Shibabaw, T. Inflammatory cytokine: IL-17A signaling pathway in patients present with COVID-19 and current treatment strategy. *J. Inflamm. Res.* **2020**, *13*, 673. [CrossRef] [PubMed]
79. Wu, D.; Yang, X.O. TH17 responses in cytokine storm of COVID-19: An emerging target of JAK2 inhibitor fedratinib. *J. Microbiol. Immunol. Infect.* **2020**, *53*, 368–370. [CrossRef]
80. Zhou, Y.; Chi, J.; Lv, W.; Wang, Y. Obesity and diabetes as high-risk factors for severe coronavirus disease 2019 (Covid-19). *Diabetes Metab. Res. Rev.* **2021**, *37*, e3377. [CrossRef]
81. Coperchini, F.; Chiovato, L.; Croce, L.; Magri, F.; Rotondi, M. The cytokine storm in COVID-19: An overview of the involvement of the chemokine/chemokine-receptor system. *Cytokine Growth Factor Rev.* **2020**, *53*, 25–32. [CrossRef]
82. Pan, J.; Zhou, L.; Lin, C.; Xue, W.; Chen, P.; Lin, J. MicroRNA-34a Promotes Ischemia-Induced Cardiomyocytes Apoptosis through Targeting Notch1. *Evid. Based Complement Altern. Med.* **2022**, *2022*, 1388415. [CrossRef]
83. Cerf, M.E. Beta Cell Physiological Dynamics and Dysfunctional Transitions in Response to Islet Inflammation in Obesity and Diabetes. *Metabolites* **2020**, *10*, 452. [CrossRef]
84. Roganović, J. Downregulation of microRNA-146a in diabetes, obesity and hypertension may contribute to severe COVID-19. *Med. Hypotheses* **2021**, *146*, 110448. [CrossRef] [PubMed]
85. Nain, Z.; Rana, H.K.; Liò, P.; Islam, S.M.S.; Summers, M.A.; Moni, M.A. Pathogenetic profiling of COVID-19 and SARS-like viruses. *Brief Bioinform.* **2021**, *22*, 1175–1196. [CrossRef] [PubMed]
86. Donyavi, T.; Bokharaei-Salim, F.; Baghi, H.B.; Khanaliha, K.; Alaei Janat-Makan, M.; Karimi, B.; Sadri Nahand, J.; Mirzaei, H.; Khatami, A.; Garshasbi, S.; et al. Acute and post-acute phase of COVID-19: Analyzing expression patterns of miRNA-29a-3p, 146a-3p, 155-5p, and let-7b-3p in PBMC. *Int. Immunopharmacol.* **2021**, *97*, 107641. [CrossRef]
87. Saik, O.V.; Klimontov, V.V. Gene Networks of Hyperglycemia, Diabetic Complications, and Human Proteins Targeted by SARS-CoV-2: What Is the Molecular Basis for Comorbidity? *Int. J. Mol. Sci.* **2022**, *23*, 7247. [CrossRef] [PubMed]
88. Fakhouri, E.W.; Peterson, S.J.; Kothari, J.; Alex, R.; Shapiro, J.I.; Abraham, N.G. Genetic polymorphisms complicate COVID-19 therapy pivotal role of HO-1 in cytokine storm. *Antioxidants* **2020**, *9*, 636. [CrossRef]
89. Iessi, E.; Cittadini, C.; Anticoli, S.; Fecchi, K.; Matarrese, P.; Ruggieri, A. Sex differences in antiviral immunity in SARS-CoV-2 infection: Mitochondria and mitomiR come into view. *Acta Physiol. (Oxf)* **2021**, *231*, e13571. [CrossRef]

90. Viveiros, A.; Rasmuson, J.; Vu, J.; Mulvagh, S.L.; Yip, C.Y.Y.; Norris, C.M.; Oudit, G.Y. Sex differences in COVID-19: Candidate pathways, genetics of ACE2, and sex hormones. *Am. J. Physiol. Heart Circ. Physiol.* **2021**, *320*, H296–H304. [CrossRef]
91. Cole, J.B.; Florez, J.C. Genetics of diabetes mellitus and diabetes complications. *Nat. Rev. Nephrol.* **2020**, *16*, 377–390. [CrossRef]
92. Lu, J.; Huang, Y.; Zhang, X.; Xu, Y.; Nie, S. Noncoding RNAs involved in DNA methylation and histone methylation, and acetylation in diabetic vascular complications, *Pharmacol. Res.* **2021**, *170*, 105520. [CrossRef]
93. Abedi, F.; Rezaee, R.; Hayes, A.W.; Nasiripour, S.; Karimi, G. MicroRNAs and SARS-CoV-2 life cycle, pathogenesis, and mutations: Biomarkers or therapeutic agents? *Cell Cycle* **2021**, *20*, 143–153. [CrossRef]
94. Ceriello, A.; De Nigris, V.; Prattichizzo, F. Why is hyperglycaemia worsening COVID-19 and its prognosis? *Diabetes Obes. Metab.* **2020**, *20*, 1951–1952. [CrossRef]
95. Perrotta, F.; Corbi, G.; Mazzeo, G.; Boccia, M.; Aronne, L.; D'Agnano, V.; Komici, K.; Mazzarella, G.; Parrella, R.; Bianco, A. COVID-19 and the elderly: Insights into pathogenesis and clinical decision-making. *Aging Clin. Exp. Res.* **2020**, *32*, 1599–1608. [CrossRef]
96. Singh, M.; Barrera Adame, O.; Nickas, M.; Robison, J.; Khatchadourian, C.; Venketaraman, V. Type 2 Diabetes Contributes to Altered Adaptive Immune Responses and Vascular Inflammation in Patients With SARS-CoV-2 Infection. *Front. Immunol.* **2022**, *13*, 833355. [CrossRef]
97. Kusminski, C.M.; Ghaben, A.L.; Morley, T.S.; Samms, R.J.; Adams, A.C.; An, Y.; Johnson, J.A.; Joffin, N.; Onodera, T.; Crewe, C.; et al. A Novel Model of Diabetic Complications: Adipocyte Mitochondrial Dysfunction Triggers Massive β-Cell Hyperplasia. *Diabetes* **2020**, *69*, 313–330. [CrossRef] [PubMed]
98. Unsworth, R.; Wallace, S.; Oliver, N.S.; Yeung, S.; Kshirsagar, A.; Naidu, H.; Kwong, R.M.W.; Kumar, P.; Logan, K.M. New-onset type 1 diabetes in children during COVID-19: Multicenter regional findings in the U.K. *Diabetes Care* **2020**, *43*, e170–e171. [CrossRef] [PubMed]
99. Bode, B.; Garrett, V.; Messler, J.; McFarland, R.; Crowe, J.; Booth, R.; Klonoff, D.C. Glycemic characteristics and clinical outcomes of COVID-19 patients hospitalized in the United States. *J. Diabetes Sci. Technol.* **2020**, *14*, 813–821. [CrossRef] [PubMed]
100. Mantovani, A.; Byrne, C.D.; Zheng, M.H.; Targher, G. Diabetes as a risk factor for greater COVID-19 severity and in-hospital death: A meta-analysis of observational studies. *Nutr. Metab. Cardiovasc. Dis.* **2020**, *30*, 1236–1248. [CrossRef]
101. Fadini, G.P.; Morieri, M.L.; Longato, E.; Avogaro, A. Prevalence and impact of diabetes among people infected with SARS-CoV-2. *J. Endocrinol. Investig.* **2020**, *43*, 867–869. [CrossRef]

International Journal of
Molecular Sciences

MDPI

Review

Monocytic HLA-DR Expression in Immune Responses of Acute Pancreatitis and COVID-19

Shiyu Liu [1,†], Wenjuan Luo [1,†], Peter Szatmary [2], Xiaoying Zhang [1], Jing-Wen Lin [3], Lu Chen [3], Dan Liu [4], Robert Sutton [2], Qing Xia [1], Tao Jin [1,*], Tingting Liu [1,*] and Wei Huang [1]

1 West China Centre of Excellence for Pancreatitis, Institute of Integrated Traditional Chinese and Western Medicine, West China-Liverpool Biomedical Research Centre, West China Hospital, Sichuan University, Chengdu 610041, China
2 Liverpool Pancreatitis Research Group, Institute of Systems, Molecular and Integrative Biology, University of Liverpool, Liverpool L69 3BE, UK
3 State Key Laboratory of Biotherapy, West China Hospital, Sichuan University and Collaborative Innovation Center for Biotherapy, Chengdu 610041, China
4 Department of Respiratory and Critical Care Medicine, Clinical Research Center for Respiratory Disease, West China Hospital, Sichuan University, Chengdu 610041, China
* Correspondence: jintao@wchscu.cn (T.J.); liutingting@wchscu.cn (T.L.)
† These authors contributed equally to this work.

Abstract: Acute pancreatitis is a common gastrointestinal disease with increasing incidence worldwide. COVID-19 is a potentially life-threatening contagious disease spread throughout the world, caused by severe acute respiratory syndrome coronavirus 2. More severe forms of both diseases exhibit commonalities with dysregulated immune responses resulting in amplified inflammation and susceptibility to infection. Human leucocyte antigen (HLA)-DR, expressed on antigen-presenting cells, acts as an indicator of immune function. Research advances have highlighted the predictive values of monocytic HLA-DR (mHLA-DR) expression for disease severity and infectious complications in both acute pancreatitis and COVID-19 patients. While the regulatory mechanism of altered mHLA-DR expression remains unclear, HLA-DR$^{-/low}$ monocytic myeloid-derived suppressor cells are potent drivers of immunosuppression and poor outcomes in these diseases. Future studies with mHLA-DR-guided enrollment or targeted immunotherapy are warranted in more severe cases of patients with acute pancreatitis and COVID-19.

Keywords: acute pancreatitis; COVID-19; HLA-DR; monocytes; immune response; immunosuppression

Citation: Liu, S.; Luo, W.; Szatmary, P.; Zhang, X.; Lin, J.-W.; Chen, L.; Liu, D.; Sutton, R.; Xia, Q.; Jin, T.; et al. Monocytic HLA-DR Expression in Immune Responses of Acute Pancreatitis and COVID-19. *Int. J. Mol. Sci.* **2023**, *24*, 3246. https://doi.org/10.3390/ijms24043246

Academic Editors: Alexandru Schiopu, Emil Arbanasi and Eliza Russu

Received: 22 December 2022
Revised: 1 February 2023
Accepted: 3 February 2023
Published: 7 February 2023

1. Introduction

New insights into the mechanisms of pathology can sometimes arise from similarities between fundamentally different diseases. This effect can be most pronounced during the emergence of a new infectious disease, such as the recent COVID-19 pandemic. One such unlikely pairing is acute pancreatitis (AP) and severe acute respiratory syndrome coronavirus 2 (SARS-CoV-2) infection.

AP is a sterile inflammatory disorder of the pancreas with an increasing global incidence [1] affecting around 2.8 million patients annually [2]. The etiology of AP is diverse and includes gallstones, alcohol excess, hypertriglyceridemia, endoscopic retrograde cholangiopancreatography, certain medicines, and other rarer causes [3]. Most cases of AP patients are mild and uneventful given that supportive care is in time and appropriate. However, some are more severe, which involve local complications (acute pancreatic necrosis or fluid collection; moderately severe acute pancreatitis, MSAP) and/or persistent organ failure (SOFA score of respiratory, circulatory, and renal system equal or more than 2 lasting > 48 h; severe acute pancreatitis, SAP) [4]. Feed-forward auto-amplification of the initial cellular injury in SAP [5,6] results in persistent systemic inflammatory response syndrome (SIRS), multiple organ dysfunction syndrome (MODS), infection, and death. Persistent organ failure [7–10] and infected pancreatic necrosis [11,12], alone or in combination, are key determinants of severity in AP and contribute to an immune anergy, secondary infections, and a mortality of > 30%. Currently, there are no specific therapies effectively targeting the initial cellular injury or determinants that resulting in MODS [13].

COVID-19, on the other hand, is a potentially lethal infectious disease caused by the enveloped, positive-strand RNA, SARS-CoV-2, affecting over 600 million cases globally [14]. The disease spectrum of COVID-19 is also highly variable, ranging from asymptomatic (test-positive) disease to critical illness (respiratory failure, septic shock, and/or MODS) [15,16]. SARS-CoV-2 mainly utilizes the angiotensin-converting enzyme 2 (ACE2) as the human host cell entry receptor [17], which is ubiquitously expressed in the nasal epithelium, lung, heart, intestine, and kidney and rarely expressed on immune cells [18]. ACE2 is also expressed on pancreatic ductal cells, acinar cells, and islet cells, making the pancreas vulnerable to viral infection [19]. Serum pancreatic enzymes are elevated in 25% of patients suffering COVID-19, which is linked to worsened clinical outcomes including mechanical ventilation and mortality even in those without AP [20–22]. Patients with COVID-19 who developed AP during hospitalization also have a more severe clinical course [23], and indeed SARS-CoV-2 may itself precipitate an episode of AP with marked metabolic derangement even in the absence of local complications or organ failure [24]. More importantly, however, patients with severe/critical COVID-19 appear to be increasingly susceptible to secondary infections [25,26] as a result of immune anergy in a similar manner to SAP.

Dysregulated immune responses in SAP and severe/critical COVID-19 have similar patterns of cytokine release and share many pathways of cellular immunity, especially immunosuppression-related monocyte deactivation in the form of downregulated expression of monocytic human leukocyte antigen-DR (HLA-DR) [27,28]. This review summarizes the role of monocytic HLA-DR (mHLA-DR) expression in the development of immunosuppression and organ failure in both SAP and severe/critical COVID-19.

2. Pathogenesis and Immunopathology in AP and COVID-19

2.1. Pathophysiological Mechanisms in AP and COVID-19

Diverse stimuli evoke inflammatory cascades with apparently analogous patterns and clinical manifestations, implying similarities in the pathogenesis and symptomatology of AP and COVID-19 [29]. Cytokines and damage-associated molecular patterns (DAMPs), such as histones, high-mobility group box-1 protein, hyaluronan fragments, mitochondrial DNA, and heat-shock proteins are released from dying or injured cells in the injured pancreas or SARS-CoV-2 infected tissues—particularly lungs. This is associated with and results from a series of molecular events, including premature trypsinogen activation, calcium overload, mitochondria failure, endoplasmic reticulum stress, impaired autophagy, or by SARS-CoV-2 proliferation and release, respectively [6,30–33]. Interaction of DAMPs with pattern-recognition receptors (PRRs), including Toll-like receptors and NLRP3 inflammasome of the adjacent parenchymal cells or immune cells, promotes the production of various pro-inflammatory cytokines and chemokines [31,34–36]. Of note, cell death pathways (e.g., autophagy, NETosis, pyroptosis, apoptosis, necroptosis, and ferroptosis) in surrounding immune cells and stromal cells are activated, fueling the cytokine storm and cultivating a positive cell death-inflammation feedback loop [30,37,38]. In COVID-19, virus particles themselves act as pathogen-associated molecular patterns (PAMPs), which could also be identified by PRRs and activate local inflammation and an innate immune response, evoking the cytokine storm and assembling those induced by DAMPs [29,39]. Activated circulating leukocytes, particularly monocytes, are then recruited to the inflamed pancreas or infected lungs, provoking systemic inflammation and organ failure in AP and COVID-19 alike [29,40–43]. Moreover, monocytes/macrophages could be infected by SARS-CoV-2, triggering massive inflammatory responses in COVID-19 [44].

The involvement of adaptive immunity in AP has been recognized, but its precise role in the sterile inflammatory response seen in AP remains poorly characterized [45].

In contrast, SARS-CoV-2 directly activates specific T cell subsets, initiating an adaptive immune response [46]. Persistent viral stimulation, however, leads to T cell exhaustion, with reduced effector functions and proliferative capacity [47]. This T cell exhaustion phenomenon can also be observed in AP patients [48].

Levels of several circulating pro-inflammatory cytokines are dramatically elevated and closely correlate with the development of SAP or severe/critical COVID-19 [49–52]. Patterns of cytokine alterations in AP and COVID-19 were shown to be remarkably similar in a recent meta-analysis, with tumor necrosis factor-alpha (TNF-α), interleukin (IL)-6, IL-8, and IL-10 concentrations significantly higher in more severe forms than non-severe forms of the two diseases [53]. The crosstalk between excessive inflammatory cytokines, platelet activation, complement activation, and endothelial injury forms a deleterious hyper-inflammatory and hyper-coagulopathy environment which is associated with life-threatening complications (i.e., coagulopathy and vascular immune-thrombosis) of AP and COVID-19 [51,54–58].

Systemic lipotoxicity deserves to be highlighted in this context. In severe/critical COVID-19, lipotoxicity can trigger multiple organ failure and mortality resembling SAP [59]. SARS-CoV-2 can directly infect adipose tissue and promotes the release of several inflammatory cytokines [60]. The pancreas itself is a target of SARS-CoV-2, resulting in the interstitial leakage of pancreatic lipase which induces lipolysis of intrapancreatic adipose tissue and release of excess unsaturated fatty acids (UFAs). These toxic UFAs in turn further directly lead to parenchymal cell injury and provoke the release of pro-inflammatory mediators, driving the cytokine storm and organ failure in SAP and severe/critical COVID-19 [59,61,62]. Lipase inhibitors have been shown to ameliorate lipolysis-induced cytokine storms and mortality [61–64].

In summary, the pathophysiological mechanisms of AP and COVID-19 share many similarities including cell death-inflammation cascade, cytokine storms, enhanced lipolysis, and dysregulated immune responses. These immune responses will be discussed in the next section.

2.2. Altered Immune Responses in AP and COVID-19

Immune anergy, evidenced by the failure of delayed hypersensitivity responses, correlates with the development of sepsis and mortality in trauma and surgical patients [65–67], as well as in SAP [68]. In the first stage of SAP, an excessive pro-inflammatory burst is rapidly followed by an anti-inflammatory reaction that may result in a generalized inflammatory response in sites remote from the initial pancreatic injury site and gives rise to SIRS [69–71]. There is a compensatory response to counteract the overwhelming pro-inflammatory state [72], which may ultimately result in immune suppression [73]. In 1996, Bone termed this immunological phenomenon as "compensatory anti-inflammatory response syndrome" (CARS) [65,66,72].

Unlike SIRS, which is clearly defined by clinical parameters, CARS lacks clinical manifestations and can only be defined molecularly by a combination of immunological alterations. In the landmark paper of Volk's group in 1997, it was described that many septic patients who died from nosocomial infections had associated downregulation of mHLA-DR [74]. Monocytes from these patients had reduced capacity to act in a pro-inflammatory manner by producing TNF-α following stimulation of lipopolysaccharide (LPS) in vitro, termed "immunoparalysis" [74,75]. Where CARS was once thought to follow sequentially from SIRS, current thinking views CARS responses as concomitant to SIRS; balance in both responses restores homeostasis, but an overshoot of the mechanisms of either SIRS or CARS leads to further injury by excessive inflammation or secondary infection and, ultimately, organ failure and death [67,76–83]. Development of CARS results in lymphocyte apoptosis, T lymphocyte anergy, and deactivation of monocytes resulting in reduced mHLA-DR expression. Furthermore, CARS is associated with elevated levels of circulating IL-10, transforming growth factor-beta (TGF-β) and other anti-inflammatory cytokines, which contribute to the risk of secondary infection.

Immune response to SARS-CoV-2 is characterized by the failure of robust type I and type III interferon response and high expression of pro-inflammatory cytokines and chemokines [17]. Like AP, immune alterations, including severe lymphopenia and functional monocyte deactivation, are indicative of immunosuppression in severe/critical COVID-19 patients [84]. Indeed, monocytes exhibit heterogeneous, dynamic, and severity-dependent alterations of transcription and immune phenotype upon acute pathological insults which appear similar in both SAP and severe/critical COVID-19 patients (Figure 1).

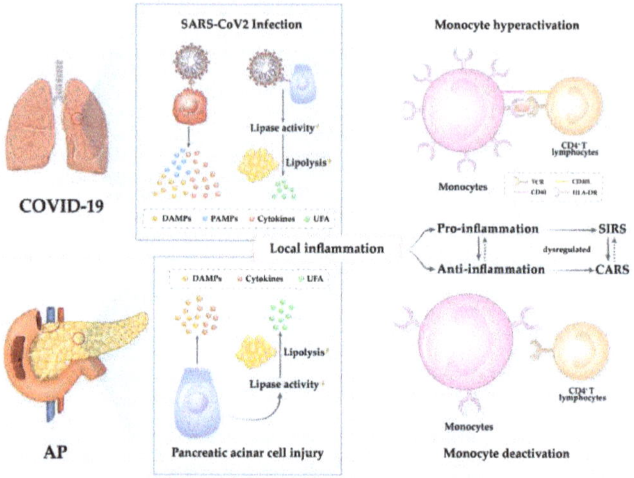

Figure 1. Pathogenesis of inflammation in AP and COVID-19. Acute pathological insults of SARS-CoV-2 infection and pancreatic acinar cell injury elicit local inflammation mediated by cytokines, unsaturated fatty acids (UFAs), damage-associated molecular patterns (DAMPs), and/or pathogen-associated molecular patterns (PAMPs). The pro-inflammatory reaction induces an anti-inflammatory response to restrict inflammation. When the pro-/anti-inflammation is unbalanced and dysregulated, systemic inflammatory response syndrome (SIRS) or compensatory anti-inflammatory response syndrome (CARS) occurs. During SIRS, monocytes are hyperactivated in response to high levels of pro-inflammatory cytokines and chemokines. In contrast, during CARS, monocytes are deactivated, exhibit reduced mHLA-DR expression, and are incapable of presenting antigens to activate $CD4^+$ T lymphocytes.

Inflammatory monocytes are enriched in the lungs of severe/critical COVID-19 patients and are also the most altered pancreatic immune cells during progression and recovery of AP [85,86]. Decreased monocytic expression of HLA-DR has a predictive value for the poor prognosis of patients with sepsis [87,88], and the level of mHLA-DR expression may identify patients who are susceptible to the development of infectious complications after trauma [89], major surgery [90], and burns [91]. Here, we review the utility of mHLA-DR in assessing the state of the immune response in AP and COVID-19 and detail-relevant implications for therapy.

3. Structure and Expression of mHLA-DR

HLA-DR is a type of major histocompatibility complex (MHC) II molecule [92]. It is a heterodimeric glycoprotein composed of the 33–35 kD heavy/α chain and the 27–29 kD light/β chain, assembling into a structure comprising a peptide binding site on top of two immunoglobulin domains [92]. Encoded by adjacent genes, the β chain is polymorphic around the amino acid residues of the peptide-binding site in contrast to the invariant α chain [93].

HLA-DR is mostly expressed on antigen-presenting cells (APCs) such as monocytes, macrophages, dendritic cells, and B cells. The primary function of HLA-DR is to present peptide antigens to the immune system for the purpose of eliciting or suppressing T-(helper)-cell responses, eventually leading to the production of antibodies against the same peptide antigen. HLA-D/DR-controlled antigens play an essential role in the cell-to-cell interactions required to generate an immune response [94,95].

The biosynthesis, trafficking, and recycling of HLA-DR are regulated by multiple factors affecting cell surface expression. Consequently, the tightly regulated level of HLA-DR expression on the surface of monocytes is thought to be an indicator for monocyte function and the state of the immune response, with high levels of mHLA-DR associated with enhanced antigen presenting capacity and immune activation, and low levels associated with immune suppression.

3.1. Measurement of mHLA-DR

Several reviews [67,96,97] have emphasized the importance of flow cytometry as an indicator of immune function in clinical practice. The unit of measurement of HLA-DR via flow cytometer can be the percentage of HLA-DR positive monocytes (%), the mean fluorescence intensity (MFI), the fluorescence unit relative to the monocyte population (RFU), or antibodies per cell (AB/c). Due to the dynamic nature of HLA-DR expression and recycling, it is critical that measurement of expression is standardized. We support the process published by Docke's and Monnaret's groups [98–100], which have been widely tested and published and appear to result in a strong correlation between transcription and cell surface expression of mHLA-DR. It should be highlighted that a percentage of HLA-DR^+ monocytes less than 30% or values of AB/c below 5000 represents immunoparalysis, and values greater than 80% or 15 000 AB/c indicate immunocompetence [99]. The critical features for the sampling and measurement of mHLA-DR from human plasma samples are summarized in Figure 2.

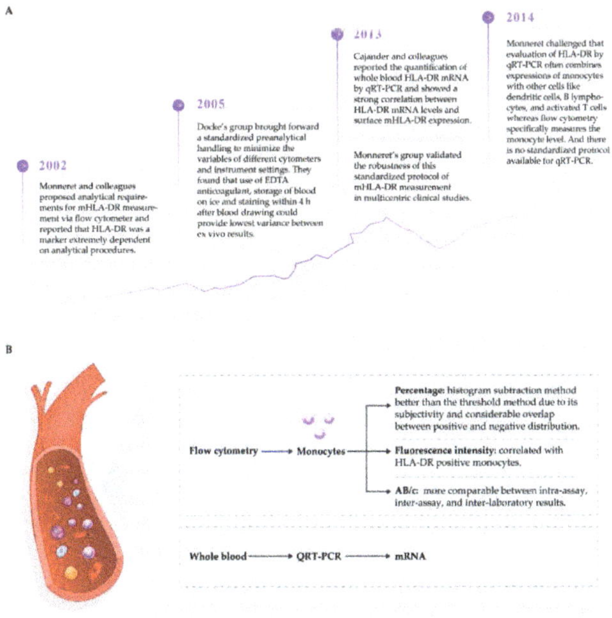

Figure 2. Measurement of mHLA-DR expression. (**A**) Measurement of mHLA-DR expression and requirements for sample handling procedures [97–101]. (**B**) Relationship of units of mHLA-DR expression to different measurement methods.

3.2. Regulation of mHLA-DR Expression

The transcription of mHLA-DR is complex and heterogeneous, mediated by a series of conserved cis-acting regulatory promoter elements and interacting transcription factors [102]. Among these, class II transactivator (CIITA) is the master regulator of HLA-DR transcription [103]. Polymorphisms of CIITA promoter are associated with decreased mHLA-DR expression in patients with septic shock [104]. Besides biosynthesis, the expression of mHLA-DR can be post-translationally regulated by exocytosis, stability, and recycling. The class II-associated Ii peptide (CLIP), generated from cleavage of CD74 (MHC class II invariant chain, Ii) via members of the cathepsin family, is critical for the transport of HLA-DR to the cell surface [105]. In CD74 knockout mice, MHC II molecules are mainly retained in endoplasmic reticulum with reduced levels on the cell surface [106]. Reducing CLIP generation by blocking cysteine protease activity reduced surface MHC II expression, including HLA-DR to 60% on human monocytes in steady state [107]. HLA-DM, the key accessory molecules in the MHC class II loading compartment, catalyzes the dissociation of CLIP in exchange for more stably binding peptides [108]. MHC II molecules on the cell surface are normal in amounts but mainly loaded with CLIP in HLA-DM-deficient mice [109]. HLA-DR loaded with high-affinity peptides are postulated to be more stable than those with CLIP, indicating the role of HLA-DM in regulating mHLA-DR expression [107]. Of note, surface HLA-DR could be internalized, exchanged from lower affinity peptides into other peptides, and rapidly recycled back to the cell surface [110]. In summary, expression of mHLA-DR is finely regulated by multiple steps, including biosynthesis, peptide-loading via cathepsin-induced CLIP and HLA-DM, vesicular transport to the cell surface, and recycling (Figure 3).

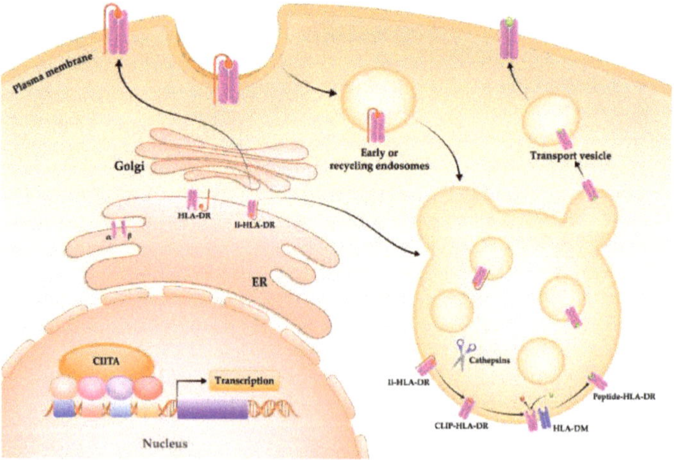

Figure 3. Regulation of mHLA-DR expression. Figure referenced from [105,111]. The transcription of HLA-DR is tightly regulated by a set of cis-acting regulatory promoter elements and transcription factors. Class II transactivator (CIITA) is the master transcriptional regulator. The α- and β-chains of HLA-DR assemble in the endoplasmic reticulum (ER) and then bind with the invariant chain (Ii). The Ii–HLA-DR complexes transport through Golgi complex to the MHC class II compartment (MIIC), directly or via the internalization of the plasma membrane. Ii is degraded into class II-associated Ii peptide (CLIP) via members of cathepsin family. In the aid of chaperone HLA-DM, CLIP is exchanged for antigen peptide. Peptide-HLA-DR complexes are then transported to the plasma membrane for further T cell activation. Interfering with the expression and activity of CIITA, Ii, cathepsins, HLA-DM, as well as the associated vesicle traffic, all result in alteration of the mHLA-DR expression.

Multiple pro- and anti-inflammatory cytokines are reported to dynamically control the expression of mHLA-DR [112]. The main mechanisms of cytokines modulating HLA-DR expression are summarized in Table 1. However, the detailed regulatory mechanisms of various cytokines on mHLA-DR expression remain largely unknown.

Table 1. Cytokine Modulation of HLA-DR Expression.

Cytokines	HLA-DR Expression	Regulatory Mechanisms	References
IL-10	↓	Downregulation of CIITA; Altering vesicular traffic of HLA-DR in exocytosis and recycling	[112,113]
TGF-β	↓	Inhibition of CIITA and downregulation of HLA-DR transcription	[114,115]
IFN-β	↓	Downregulation of CIITA	[116]
IFN-γ	↑	Promotion of HLA-DR and CD74 transcription	[117,118]
GM-CSF	↑	Promoting exocytosis and reducing internalization	[119]
TNF-α, IL-1	↑	Boosting biosynthesis and stability of HLA-DR increasing half-life from about 10 h to over 100 h	[120]
IL-4	↑	Upregulation of CIITA	[113]

Abbreviations: IL, interleukin; CIITA, class II transactivator; TGF-β, transforming growth factor-beta; IFN, interferon; GM-CSF, granulocyte-macrophage colony-stimulating factor; TNF-α, tumor necrosis factor-alpha.

4. The Role of mHLA-DR in AP and COVID-19

Monocytic HLA-DR expression alters dynamically in response to the variation of immune responses in the body during the disease course of AP and COVID-19. Evaluating the dynamic expression of mHLA-DR provides indicative information for diagnosis and prediction of disease severity, infectious complications, and prognosis (Figure 4).

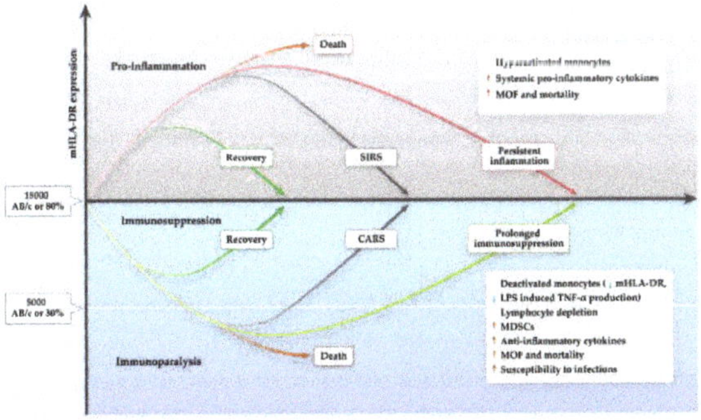

Figure 4. Immune response in AP and COVID-19. Figure referenced from [121,122]. Pro- and anti-inflammatory response are both activated after acute insults of either AP or COVID-19. The initial generalized inflammation is individually heterogeneous. Patients with less intense generalized inflammatory response may survive and restore the immune balance. When inflammation markedly outpaces anti-inflammation, monocytes are hyperactivated, leading to increased systemic release of pro-inflammatory cytokines and resulting in systemic inflammatory response syndrome (SIRS). This cytokine storm and hyperinflammation is associated with multiple organ failure (MOF) and mortality in AP and COVID-19. Conversely, compensatory anti-inflammatory response syndrome (CARS) happens when the anti-inflammatory response is overwhelming. mHLA-DR is an indicator of this, and expression below 15,000 AB/c or 80% characterizes immunosuppression and below 5000 AB/c or 30% characterizes immunoparalysis. In addition to pronouncedly reduced mHLA-DR expression, monocytes are deactivated with TNF-α production upon lipopolysaccharide (LPS) stimulation in CARS. Lymphocytes are depleted, accompanied by a massive release of anti-inflammatory cytokine. This dysregulated and persistent immunosuppression contributes to MOF, death, and infections.

The expression of mHLA-DR on admission was downregulated in AP patients compared to healthy controls; it further decreased on days 1 and 2 with differential degrees depending on severity [123–125]. While mHLA-DR expression recovered rapidly at day 3 and became normal after day 7 in less severe patients, it persisted at low levels for 1–2 weeks in more severe cases [124,126]. Indeed, mHLA-DR expression displays an inverse relationship with severity throughout at least the first three weeks of disease [127], with the lowest expression of mHLA-DR in SAP consistently recorded between 48 and 72 h of disease onset [127,128].

Overall, mHLA-DR expression either increases or decreases slightly in mild COVID-19 patients compared with healthy controls [129,130]. However, a marked and persistent decrease in expression is described in severe/critical COVID-19 patients in most studies [129,131–140]. The immune response to severe COVID-19 can be categorized into three groups according to the kinetics of mHLA-DR expression: (i) hyperactivated monocytes/macrophage phenotype (persistently high mHLA-DR > 30,000 AB/c)—strongly associated with mortality; (ii) prolonged immunodepression (persistently low mHLA-DR < 15,000 AB/c after days 5–7)—strongly correlating with secondary infection; (iii) transient immunodepression (early mHLA-DR < 15,000 AB/c, rising above 15,000 AB/c after 5–7 days)—at risk of secondary infection [141]. Patients with acute respiratory distress syndrome (ARDS) secondary to COVID-19 exhibit either immune dysregulation evidenced by very low mHLA-DR expression (i.e., lower than 5000 AB/c) and depletion of lymphocytes, or macrophage activation syndrome characterized by elevated ferritin, where associated HLA-DR levels might be reduced [142], or comparable to healthy controls [143]. Expression of mHLA-DR may be able to provide some information on disease course and has been observed to normalize upon recovery from critical illness in patients with COVID-19 (from 1–3 days to over 10 days after admission), but continued to fall in a patient who died [136]. Critically ill COVID-19 patients with long hospital stays (>25 days) presented with a more profound reduction in mHLA-DR expression than patients with short hospital stays (<25 days) [140]. Furthermore, convalescent COVID-19 patients exhibit mHLA-DR levels which are higher than those of healthy controls at 6 months, and equal to healthy controls at 9 and 12 months following discharge from the hospital [140,144].

The reduction of HLA-DR expression in COVID-19 patients has been reported in both classical monocytes [144,145], as well as intermediate monocytes and/or non-classical monocytes [132,146,147], although usually in one group or the other, depending on the respective study. Classical monocytes are the first peripheral immune cell type to recover HLA-DR positivity during the recovery of critically ill COVID-19 patients [148].

4.1. Severity Prediction Using mHLA-DR in AP and COVID-19

The predictive values of mHLA-DR for severity and mortality of AP and COVID-19 are summarized in Table 2.

Table 2. Predictive Values of mHLA-DR for severity and mortality in AP and COVID-19.

Disease	Prediction	Sample Size (Incidents/Total)	Measuring Time	Cut-Off Value	AUC	Sensitivity	Specificity	Others
AP [149]	MAP from MSAP/SAP	27/50	Admission	<2274 MFI	0.805	70.4%	82.6%	Combined with classical monocyte proportions (AUC, 0.862)
	SAP from MSAP	9/23		<1094.5 MFI	0.690	85.7%	55.6%	-
AP [150]	SAP	19/58	Admission	<50.8%	0.728	72%	72%	-
			Day 2	<43.35%	0.800	84%	80%	-
			Day 5	<60.8%	0.877	82%	78%	-
AP [151]	Organ failure	29/310	Admission	<78%	0.78	83%	72%	-
				<38 RFU	0.81	69%	84%	-
AP [152]	Mortality	7/25	Day 10	<52.3%	0.944	94.4%	85.7%	-
COVID-19 [136]	Critical COVID-19	9/32	Days 0–3	<81.55%	0.961	100.00%	80.00%	-
COVID-19 [139]	Severe COVID-19	48/97	Admission	<143 MFI	0.9	89.6%	81.6%	Independent predictor of COVID-19 severity (OR = 0.976, 95% CI: 0.955–0.997)
COVID-19 [134]	Mortality	35/124	Days 0–3	<11,312 AB/c	0.64	74%	54%	-
			Days 7–10	<4672 AB/c	0.85	75%	86%	-
COVID-19 [153]	Mortality	1/12	Admission	<270.56 cells/mL	0.875	100.0%	87.5%	-

Abbreviations: AUC, area under the receiver operating characteristic curve; MAP, mild acute pancreatitis; (M)SAP, (moderately) severe acute pancreatitis; MFI, mean fluorescence intensity; RFU, relative fluorescence unit; OR, odds ratio; CI, confidence interval.

MHLA-DR expression is inversely correlated with surrogate biochemical markers of severity (C-reactive protein [CRP], TNF-α, and IL-6) [127,128,154–157], clinical scoring systems (Ranson, Acute Physiology and Chronic Health Evaluation II [APACHE II], and MODS criteria) [128,154,157,158], and actual severity of AP [125,127,128,150,151,156,158–160], and AP patients with low mHLA-DR expression had approximately 2.7 times longer ICU stays than those with normal expression [159]. HLA-DR expressed on classical monocytes was able to distinguish cases of mild from MSAP/SAP and SAP from MSAP on admission [160]. Indeed, mHLA-DR expression on admission, days 2 and 5 all have been shown to have predictive value for SAP [150] and/or the subsequent development of organ failure(s) [151].

The utility of mHLA-DR to predict mortality in AP is more controversial. While several studies have reported differences in mHLA-DR expression between survivors and non-survivors on days 7 [124,128] or 10 after admission [152], others found no difference [127,158,161]. These results might be explained by the differences in the design of the respective clinical studies, or by the heterogeneous and dynamic immune response in the study populations.

Despite one study finding that mHLA-DR expression was irrelevant to severity of COVID-19 [146], most studies demonstrate an inverse relationship [135–137,139]. Low or very low mHLA-DR expression has been described in association with ARDS [162], severe respiratory failure [142], thrombocytopenia, increased antibiotic requirements, and need for extracorporeal membrane oxygenation [134,135,142,153,162]. Similarly to AP, lower levels of mHLA-DR expression correlated with length of hospital stay [140], SOFA score [153], and serum clinical biochemical parameters including D-dimer, lactate dehydrogenase, CRP, procalcitonin, ferritin, IL-6, IL-10, granulocyte colony-stimulating factor, chemokine C-X-C motif ligand 10, chemokine C-C motif ligand 2 (CCL2), and IFN-γ levels [135–137,144,147,153,163]. Although overall mHLA-DR expression does not appear to differ between survivors and non-survivors [141], the lowest levels of mHLA-DR expression can be observed in patients with COVID-19 who died in the ICU [84]. The proportion of mHLA-DR^{+} monocytes was also lower in deceased COVID-19 patients compared with time-matched controls [164]. Expression of mHLA-DR recovers with clinical improvement but continues to fall in patients who do not survive [134,144].

4.2. Prediction of Infectious Complications using mHLA-DR

MHLA-DR regulates the interplay between innate and adaptive immunity and represents an overview of an organism's capacity for antigen presentation, cytokine production, and phagocytosis [165]. HLA-DR downregulation is not only limited to the blood compartment but can also be observed in lymphatic tissue [166]. With standardization of flow cytometry-based measurement of mHLA-DR, a multicenter comparison of obtained results becomes feasible [98]. Therefore, mHLA-DR is now the most frequently utilized biomarker for assessing the development of immunosuppression in critically ill patients, including sepsis, stroke, trauma, and burns [167]. Following the rationale of immunosuppression in severe critical illnesses, mHLA-DR expression levels are predictive of septic complications in AP and COVID-19 using values shown in Table 3.

Table 3. Predictive values of mHLA-DR for septic complications in AP and COVID-19.

Disease	Prediction	Sample Size (Incidents/Total)	Measuring Time	Cut-Off Value	AUC	Sensitivity	Specificity	Others
AP [154]	Sepsis	6/64	Admission	<60%	-	100%	91.3%	Superior to Ranson's score and APACHE II score
			Day 7		-	100%	93.2%	-
			Day 14		-	100%	98.2%	-
AP [128]	Septic complications	11/74	Day 7	<40%	-	73%	94%	-
			Day 10		-	82%	98%	-
			Day 14		-	100%	100%	-
AP [152]	Septic complications	6/25	Day 10	<58%	0.926	76.5%	100%	Comparable to Ranson and APACHE II scores and better than CRP levels (AUC, 0.841, 0.869, and 0.460, respectively)
AP [157]	Secondary infection	11/40	Admission	<35.8%	0.837	81.8%	82.8%	-
COVID-19 [134]	Secondary infection	38/124	Days 0–3	<10,523 AB/c	0.70	76%	60%	-
			Days 7–10	<6804 AB/c	0.62	77%	52%	-

Abbreviations: AUC, area under the receiver operating characteristic curve; APACHE, Acute Physiology and Chronic Health Evaluation; CRP, C-reactive protein.

Failure of the intestinal barrier function is often thought to be responsible for the dysregulated systemic inflammation in AP [126,168]. The proportion of HLA-DR$^+$ monocytes correlated negatively with measures of small intestinal permeability, including the urinary lactulose/mannitol ratio and D(-)-lactate concentrations [126]. AP patients with infectious complications, including sepsis or infected pancreatic necrosis, had lower HLA-DR expression which recovered at a slower rate than those without [127,128,150,152,154,157,169–171]. The relative risk of developing infected pancreatic necrosis in AP patients with low mHLA-DR expression that persisted into the second week of illness was 11.3 (1.6–82.4) [170], and persistently low HLA-DR levels have even been shown to be related to multidrug resistant infection [171]. This ability to identify patients with infectious complications early was as good or superior to routine biochemical markers and clinical scoring systems including CRP and APACHE II [152]. Therefore, a persistently low expression of mHLA-DR might be an effective and reliable indicator of potentially lethal infectious complications in patients with AP that could perhaps be used to identify patients who might benefit from early antimicrobial therapy.

As in AP, persistently low levels of mHLA-DR expression are associated with secondary infection in COVID-19 patients [172]. COVID-19 patients who developed secondary bacterial infections exhibit lower levels of mHLA-DR expression than those without at all time points (days 1, 4, and 7 [173], days 5–7, days 8–10 [141]). MHLA-DR expression (AB/c) on days 0–3 and on days 7–10 have been shown to predict secondary infection in COVID-19 patients in the ICU [134].

4.3. Regulation of mHLA-DR Expression in AP and COVID-19

Both pro- and anti-inflammatory cytokines, including TNF-α, IL-6, IL-8, IL-10, and IL-1RA1, can downregulate—and correlate inversely with—mHLA-DR expression in AP patients [156,160]. IL-6, IL-8, IL-10, and IL-1RA1 inhibit HLA-DR expression on classical monocytes in vitro [160]. TNF-α enhances IL-10 production of monocytes in vitro and downregulates levels of HLA-DR, even in the presence of anti-IL-10 monoclonal antibodies, demonstrating inhibition of mHLA-DR expression via an alternate pathway [156].

The regulatory mechanisms of reduced mHLA-DR expression in severe/critical COVID-19 patients are less well understood, but IL-6 and IL-10 are similarly thought to be possible drivers to reduce mHLA-DR expression in the disease. MHLA-DR expression was strongly reduced by plasma from COVID-19 patients with immune dysregulation but not healthy controls [130,142]; the effect could be partially restored by the addition of the IL-6 blocker Tocilizumab [142]. The highly expressed cytokines in COVID-19 patients included IL-10, IL-6, IL-7, TNF-α, IFN-α, CCL2, and CCL4, but only incubation monocytes with IL-10 downregulated HLA-DR expression [130].

The altered cytokine profiles in sterile or infectious inflammatory diseases including AP and COVID-19 are dynamic and complex, which may affect mHLA-DR expression synergistically or antagonistically. Future studies are needed to investigate the precise role of cytokines in regulating mHLA-DR so as to develop potential therapeutic targets in immune regulation.

4.4. Monocytic Myeloid-Derived Suppressor Cells

A proportion of circulating HLA-DR$^{-/low}$ monocytes seen in both AP and COVID-19 patients have been identified as CD14$^+$CD11b$^+$HLA-DR$^{-/low}$CD15$^-$ monocytic myeloid-derived suppressor cells (M-MDSCs); these cell types may cloud earlier studies on the topic, as they could be misidentified as HLA-DR$^{-/low}$ classical monocytes [174–176]. M-MDSCs are characterized by their potent immunosuppressive effects on other immune cells, especially T cells, through various mechanisms including secretion of arginase-1 (Arg-1), and inducible nitric oxide synthase, production of reactive oxygen and nitrogen species, secretion of cytokines including TGF-β and IL-10, and induction of regulatory T cells [175].

The proportion of M-MDSCs in peripheral blood mononuclear cells correlates with AP severity as reflected by plasma CRP levels, APACHE II score, and length of stay [174].

Increased levels of Arg-1 and ROS can further be observed in AP patients, especially those with a severe clinical course [174]. Similarly, expansion of M-MDSCs was reported together with increased Arg-1 activity in plasma, and these are associated with severity and fatal outcome in COVID-19 patients [175].

Therapeutic approaches aimed at reducing the number, function, and accumulation of M-MDSCs might improve the suppressive state of the immune system and improve complication-free survival in both SAP and severe/critical COVID-19 patients.

5. Conclusions and Future Prospects

MHLA-DR expression serves as a useful biomarker for immune (dys)function in patients with AP and COVID-19. The measurement of patterns and dynamics of mHLA-DR expression in both these diseases can help clinicians to determine the severity and prognosis, and perhaps guide timing and selection of therapy. Monitoring mHLA-DR expression appears to help identify and differentiate patients at higher risk of secondary infections associated with poor outcomes. While immunosuppression in general is thought to represent later stages of both diseases, in actual fact, time course and immune responses can be highly heterogeneous and variable [127,177]. MHLA-DR modulation occurs over several days [178], necessitating multiple, consecutive mHLA-DR measurements following a standardized assessment procedure of flow cytometry in patients from point of admission. MHLA-DR measurement should be prioritized for patients with clinically severe presentations with rapidly worsening organ dysfunctions or who are in need of invasive treatments or are at high risk of infectious complications with poor prognosis [179–181].

Examples of potential mHLA-DR-directed interventions that could find utility in AP and COVID-19 include several immunostimulatory agents, including IFN-γ [155,182–184], recombinant IL-7 [185], and granulocyte-macrophage colony-stimulating factor [155]. Thymosin alpha 1 (Tα1), a peptide hormone used to stimulate the T-cell mediated immune response, has been tested in patients with predicted for necrotizing pancreatitis (presumably immunocompromised), but results are so far disappointing [186]; thus far, there has been no demonstrable reduction in the incidence of infected pancreatic necrosis, new-onset organ failure, or any other complications. Defining immunosuppression, for example, by using the measurement of mHLA-DR expression to guide participant selection and/or tailor the treatment dose, may be required to demonstrate effective immune-stimulatory therapy.

The complex and highly variable immune alterations seen in severe acute inflammation and infection warrant stratified immunotherapy. MHLA-DR expression provides supportive information in determining the timing and strategies of individual immune treatments, including anti-inflammatory, immune-stimulatory or immune-modulatory agents at different disease stages, something that has been demonstrated in both acute pancreatitis and COVID-19. The emergence of a new global pandemic disease has provided valuable insights into the mechanisms of a long-established illness, with considerable potential to draw insights into one disease from the other. There is a need for a simple, cheap, and effective universal immune assessment tool, combining mHLA-DR with established clinical markers of disease severity and possibly other circulating immune cell profiles to aid assessment of the disease course of illnesses with a systemic inflammatory component in order to predict outcomes and to guide treatment decisions.

Author Contributions: Conceptualization, S.L., W.H.; investigation, S.L., W.L.; writing original draft preparation, S.L.; writing-review and editing, S.L., W.L., P.S., X.Z., W.H.; visualization, S.L., W.L., R.S., W.H.; supervision, P.S., X.Z., J.-W.L., L.C., D.L., R.S.; project administration, Q.X., T.J., T.L., W.H. All authors have read and agreed to the published version of the manuscript.

Funding: This research was funded by the Program of Science and Technology Department of Sichuan Province (No. 2022YFS0419 to T.L.); Sichuan Science and Technology Plan Projects—Key Research and Development Program (23ZDYF1772, awarded to T.J.; awarded to W.H.); National Natural Science Foundation of China (No. 82274321 to Q.X.; No. 81973632 to W.H.); National Institute for Health Research Senior Investigator Award, an EME Award (15/20/01), an MRC Award (MR/T002220/1) and the TransBioLine Consortium (all to R.S.).

Institutional Review Board Statement: The study did not require ethical approval.

Informed Consent Statement: Not applicable.

Data Availability Statement: Not applicable.

Acknowledgments: Not applicable.

Conflicts of Interest: The authors declare no conflict of interest.

References

1. Iannuzzi, J.P.; King, J.A.; Leong, J.H.; Quan, J.; Windsor, J.W.; Tanyingoh, D.; Coward, S.; Forbes, N.; Heitman, S.J.; Shaheen, A.A.; et al. Global incidence of acute pancreatitis is increasing over time: A systematic review and meta-analysis. *Gastroenterology* **2022**, *162*, 122–134. [CrossRef]
2. Li, C.L.; Jiang, M.; Pan, C.Q.; Li, J.; Xu, L.G. The global, regional, and national burden of acute pancreatitis in 204 countries and territories, 1990–2019. *BMC Gastroenterol.* **2021**, *21*, 332. [CrossRef] [PubMed]
3. Szatmary, P.; Grammatikopoulos, T.; Cai, W.; Huang, W.; Mukherjee, R.; Halloran, C.; Beyer, G.; Sutton, R. Acute pancreatitis: Diagnosis and treatment. *Drugs* **2022**, *82*, 1251–1276. [CrossRef] [PubMed]
4. Banks, P.A.; Bollen, T.L.; Dervenis, C.; Gooszen, H.G.; Johnson, C.D.; Sarr, M.G.; Tsiotos, G.G.; Vege, S.S.; Acute Pancreatitis Classification Working Group. Classification of acute pancreatitis–2012: Revision of the Atlanta classification and definitions by international consensus. *Gut* **2013**, *62*, 102–111. [CrossRef] [PubMed]
5. Linkermann, A.; Stockwell, B.R.; Krautwald, S.; Anders, H.J. Regulated cell death and inflammation: An auto-amplification loop causes organ failure. *Nat. Rev. Immunol.* **2014**, *14*, 759–767. [CrossRef] [PubMed]
6. Barreto, S.G.; Habtezion, A.; Gukovskaya, A.; Lugea, A.; Jeon, C.; Yadav, D.; Hegyi, P.; Venglovecz, V.; Sutton, R.; Pandol, S.J. Critical thresholds: Key to unlocking the door to the prevention and specific treatments for acute pancreatitis. *Gut* **2021**, *70*, 194–203. [CrossRef] [PubMed]
7. Guo, Q.; Li, A.; Xia, Q.; Liu, X.; Tian, B.; Mai, G.; Huang, Z.; Chen, G.; Tang, W.; Jin, X.; et al. The role of organ failure and infection in necrotizing pancreatitis: A prospective study. *Ann. Surg.* **2014**, *259*, 1201–1207. [CrossRef] [PubMed]
8. Sternby, H.; Bolado, F.; Canaval-Zuleta, H.J.; Marra-López, C.; Hernando-Alonso, A.I.; Del-Val-Antoñana, A.; García-Rayado, G.; Rivera-Irigoin, R.; Grau-García, F.J.; Oms, L.; et al. Determinants of severity in acute pancreatitis: A nation-wide multicenter prospective cohort study. *Ann. Surg.* **2019**, *270*, 348–355. [CrossRef] [PubMed]
9. Schepers, N.J.; Bakker, O.J.; Besselink, M.G.; Ahmed Ali, U.; Bollen, T.L.; Gooszen, H.G.; van Santvoort, H.C.; Bruno, M.J. Impact of characteristics of organ failure and infected necrosis on mortality in necrotising pancreatitis. *Gut* **2019**, *68*, 1044–1051. [CrossRef]
10. Shi, N.; Liu, T.; de la Iglesia-Garcia, D.; Deng, L.; Jin, T.; Lan, L.; Zhu, P.; Hu, W.; Zhou, Z.; Singh, V.; et al. Duration of organ failure impacts mortality in acute pancreatitis. *Gut* **2020**, *69*, 604–605. [CrossRef]
11. Petrov, M.S.; Shanbhag, S.; Chakraborty, M.; Phillips, A.R.; Windsor, J.A. Organ failure and infection of pancreatic necrosis as determinants of mortality in patients with acute pancreatitis. *Gastroenterology* **2010**, *139*, 813–820. [CrossRef]
12. Werge, M.; Novovic, S.; Schmidt, P.N.; Gluud, L.L. Infection increases mortality in necrotizing pancreatitis: A systematic review and meta-analysis. *Pancreatology* **2016**, *16*, 698–707. [CrossRef]
13. Moggia, E.; Koti, R.; Belgaumkar, A.P.; Fazio, F.; Pereira, S.P.; Davidson, B.R.; Gurusamy, K.S. Pharmacological interventions for acute pancreatitis. *Cochrane Database Syst. Rev.* **2017**, *4*, Cd011384. [CrossRef] [PubMed]
14. WHO Coronavirus (COVID-19) Dashboard. Available online: https://covid19.who.int/ (accessed on 20 September 2022).
15. *Coronavirus Disease 2019 (COVID-19) Treatment Guidelines*; National Institutes of Health (US): Bethesda, MD, USA, 2021.
16. Zuo, Y.; Yalavarthi, S.; Shi, H.; Gockman, K.; Zuo, M.; Madison, J.A.; Blair, C.; Weber, A.; Barnes, B.J.; Egeblad, M.; et al. Neutrophil extracellular traps in COVID-19. *JCI Insight* **2020**, *5*, e138999. [CrossRef]
17. Carvalho, T.; Krammer, F.; Iwasaki, A. The first 12 months of COVID-19: A timeline of immunological insights. *Nat. Rev. Immunol.* **2021**, *21*, 245–256. [CrossRef] [PubMed]
18. Chung, J.Y.; Thone, M.N.; Kwon, Y.J. COVID-19 vaccines: The status and perspectives in delivery points of view. *Adv. Drug Deliv. Rev.* **2021**, *170*, 1–25. [CrossRef] [PubMed]
19. Liu, F.; Long, X.; Zhang, B.; Zhang, W.; Chen, X.; Zhang, Z. ACE2 expression in pancreas may cause pancreatic damage after SARS-CoV-2 infection. *Clin. Gastroenterol. Hepatol. Off. Clin. Pract. J. Am. Gastroenterol. Assoc.* **2020**, *18*, 2128–2130.e2. [CrossRef] [PubMed]
20. Yang, F.; Xu, Y.; Dong, Y.; Huang, Y.; Fu, Y.; Li, T.; Sun, C.; Pandanaboyana, S.; Windsor, J.A.; Fu, D. Prevalence and prognosis of increased pancreatic enzymes in patients with COVID-19: A systematic review and meta-analysis. *Pancreatology* **2022**, *22*, 539–546. [CrossRef]
21. Goyal, H.; Sachdeva, S.; Perisetti, A.; Mann, R.; Inamdar, S.; Tharian, B. Hyperlipasemia and potential pancreatic injury patterns in COVID-19: A marker of severity or innocent bystander? *Gastroenterology* **2021**, *160*, 946–948.e2. [CrossRef]
22. Kiyak, M.; Düzenli, T. Lipase elevation on admission predicts worse clinical outcomes in patients with COVID-19. *Pancreatology* **2022**, *22*, 665–670. [CrossRef] [PubMed]
23. Kumar, V.; Barkoudah, E.; Souza, D.A.T.; Jin, D.X.; McNabb-Baltar, J. Clinical course and outcome among patients with acute pancreatitis and COVID-19. *Eur. J. Gastroenterol. Hepatol.* **2021**, *33*, 695–700. [CrossRef]

24. Szatmary, P.; Arora, A.; Thomas Raraty, M.G.; Joseph Dunne, D.F.; Baron, R.D.; Halloran, C.M. Emerging phenotype of severe acute respiratory syndrome-coronavirus 2-associated pancreatitis. *Gastroenterology* **2020**, *159*, 1551–1554. [CrossRef] [PubMed]
25. De Bruyn, A.; Verellen, S.; Bruckers, L.; Geebelen, L.; Callebaut, I.; De Pauw, I.; Stessel, B.; Dubois, J. Secondary infection in COVID-19 critically ill patients: A retrospective single-center evaluation. *BMC Infect. Dis.* **2022**, *22*, 207. [CrossRef] [PubMed]
26. Ripa, M.; Galli, L.; Poli, A.; Oltolini, C.; Spagnuolo, V.; Mastrangelo, A.; Muccini, C.; Monti, G.; De Luca, G.; Landoni, G.; et al. Secondary infections in patients hospitalized with COVID-19: Incidence and predictive factors. *Clin. Microbiol. Infect.* **2021**, *27*, 451–457. [CrossRef] [PubMed]
27. Gallo, C.G.; Fiorino, S.; Posabella, G.; Antonacci, D.; Tropeano, A.; Pausini, E.; Pausini, C.; Guarniero, T.; Hong, W.; Giampieri, E.; et al. COVID-19, what could sepsis, severe acute pancreatitis, gender differences, and aging teach us? *Cytokine* **2021**, *148*, 155628. [CrossRef] [PubMed]
28. Huang, B.Z.; Sidell, M.A.; Wu, B.U.; Setiawan, V.W.; Chen, Z.; Xiang, A.H. Pre-existing pancreatitis and elevated risks of COVID-19 severity and mortality. *Gastroenterology* **2022**, *162*, 1758–1760.e3. [CrossRef]
29. Karki, R.; Kanneganti, T.D. The 'cytokine storm': Molecular mechanisms and therapeutic prospects. *Trends Immunol.* **2021**, *42*, 681–705. [CrossRef]
30. Guéant, J.L.; Guéant-Rodriguez, R.M.; Fromonot, J.; Oussalah, A.; Louis, H.; Chery, C.; Gette, M.; Gleye, S.; Callet, J.; Raso, J.; et al. Elastase and exacerbation of neutrophil innate immunity are involved in multi-visceral manifestations of COVID-19. *Allergy* **2021**, *76*, 1846–1858. [CrossRef]
31. de Vries, F.; Huckriede, J.; Wichapong, K.; Reutelingsperger, C.; Nicolaes, G.A.F. The role of extracellular histones in COVID-19. *J. Intern. Med.* **2022**, *293*, 275–292. [CrossRef]
32. Lee, P.J.; Papachristou, G.L. New insights into acute pancreatitis. *Nat. Rev. Gastroenterol. Hepatol.* **2019**, *16*, 479–496. [CrossRef]
33. Szatmary, P.; Huang, W.; Criddle, D.; Tepikin, A.; Sutton, R. Biology, role and therapeutic potential of circulating histones in acute inflammatory disorders. *J. Cell Mol. Med.* **2018**, *22*, 4617–4629. [CrossRef] [PubMed]
34. Vora, S.M.; Lieberman, J.; Wu, H. Inflammasome activation at the crux of severe COVID-19. *Nat. Rev. Immunol.* **2021**, *21*, 694–703. [CrossRef] [PubMed]
35. Naqvi, I.; Giroux, N.; Olson, L.; Morrison, S.A.; Llanga, T.; Akinade, T.O.; Zhu, Y.; Zhong, Y.; Bose, S.; Arvai, S.; et al. DAMPs/PAMPs induce monocytic TLR activation and tolerance in COVID-19 patients; nucleic acid binding scavengers can counteract such TLR agonists. *Biomaterials* **2022**, *283*, 121393. [CrossRef] [PubMed]
36. Zheng, L.; Xue, J.; Jaffee, E.M.; Habtezion, A. Role of immune cells and immune-based therapies in pancreatitis and pancreatic ductal adenocarcinoma. *Gastroenterology* **2013**, *144*, 1230–1240. [CrossRef]
37. Karki, R.; Sharma, B.R.; Tuladhar, S.; Williams, E.P.; Zalduondo, L.; Samir, P.; Zheng, M.; Sundaram, B.; Banoth, B.; Malireddi, R.K.S.; et al. Synergism of TNF-α and IFN-γ triggers inflammatory cell death, tissue damage, and mortality in SARS-CoV-2 infection and cytokine shock syndromes. *Cell* **2021**, *184*, 149–168.e17. [CrossRef] [PubMed]
38. Li, X.; Zhang, Z.; Wang, Z.; Gutiérrez-Castrellón, P.; Shi, H. Cell deaths: Involvement in the pathogenesis and intervention therapy of COVID-19. *Signal Transduct. Target. Ther.* **2022**, *7*, 186. [CrossRef]
39. Yamada, T.; Takaoka, A. Innate immune recognition against SARS-CoV-2. *Inflamm. Regen.* **2023**, *43*, 7. [CrossRef] [PubMed]
40. Habtezion, A.; Gukovskaya, A.S.; Pandol, S.J. Acute pancreatitis: A multifaceted set of organelle and cellular interactions. *Gastroenterology* **2019**, *156*, 1941–1950. [CrossRef]
41. Garg, P.K.; Singh, V.P. Organ failure due to systemic injury in acute pancreatitis. *Gastroenterology* **2019**, *156*, 2008–2023. [CrossRef]
42. Xue, J.; Sharma, V.; Habtezion, A. Immune cells and immune-based therapy in pancreatitis. *Immunol. Res.* **2014**, *58*, 378–386. [CrossRef]
43. Liu, S.; Szatmary, P.; Lin, J.W.; Wang, Q.; Sutton, R.; Chen, L.; Liu, T.; Huang, W.; Xia, Q. Circulating monocytes in acute pancreatitis. *Front. Immunol.* **2022**, *13*, 1062849. [CrossRef]
44. Felsenstein, S.; Herbert, J.A.; McNamara, P.S.; Hedrich, C.M. COVID-19: Immunology and treatment options. *Clin. Immunol.* **2020**, *215*, 108448. [CrossRef] [PubMed]
45. Fonteh, P.; Smith, M.; Brand, M. Adaptive immune cell dysregulation and role in acute pancreatitis disease progression and treatment. *Arch. Immunol. Et Ther. Exp.* **2018**, *66*, 199–209. [CrossRef] [PubMed]
46. Li, G.; Fan, Y.; Lai, Y.; Han, T.; Li, Z.; Zhou, P.; Pan, P.; Wang, W.; Hu, D.; Liu, X.; et al. Coronavirus infections and immune responses. *J. Med. Virol.* **2020**, *92*, 424–432. [CrossRef] [PubMed]
47. Anka, A.U.; Tahir, M.I.; Abubakar, S.D.; Alsabbagh, M.; Zian, Z.; Hamedifar, H.; Sabzevari, A.; Azizi, G. Coronavirus disease 2019 (COVID-19): An overview of the immunopathology, serological diagnosis and management. *Scand. J. Immunol.* **2021**, *93*, e12998. [CrossRef]
48. Pietruczuk, M.; Dabrowska, M.I.; Wereszczynska-Siemiatkowska, U.; Dabrowski, A. Alteration of peripheral blood lymphocyte subsets in acute pancreatitis. *World J. Gastroenterol.* **2006**, *12*, 5344–5351. [CrossRef] [PubMed]
49. Norman, J. The role of cytokines in the pathogenesis of acute pancreatitis. *Am. J. Surg.* **1998**, *175*, 76–83. [CrossRef]
50. Makhija, R.; Kingsnorth, A.N. Cytokine storm in acute pancreatitis. *J. Hepato-Biliary-Pancreat. Surg.* **2002**, *9*, 401–410. [CrossRef]
51. To, K.K.; Sridhar, S.; Chiu, K.H.; Hung, D.L.; Li, X.; Hung, I.F.; Tam, A.R.; Chung, T.W.; Chan, J.F.; Zhang, A.J.; et al. Lessons learned 1 year after SARS-CoV-2 emergence leading to COVID-19 pandemic. *Emerg. Microbes Infect.* **2021**, *10*, 507–535. [CrossRef]
52. Lucas, C.; Wong, P.; Klein, J.; Castro, T.B.R.; Silva, J.; Sundaram, M.; Ellingson, M.K.; Mao, T.; Oh, J.E.; Israelow, B.; et al. Longitudinal analyses reveal immunological misfiring in severe COVID-19. *Nature* **2020**, *584*, 463–469. [CrossRef]

53. Hegyi, P.; Szakács, Z.; Sahin-Tóth, M. Lipotoxicity and cytokine storm in severe acute pancreatitis and COVID-19. *Gastroenterology* **2020**, *159*, 824–827. [CrossRef] [PubMed]
54. Pena, A.L.B.; Oliveira, R.A.; Severo, R.G.; Simões, E.S.A.C. COVID-19 related coagulopathy: What is Known Up to Now. *Curr. Med. Chem.* **2021**, *28*, 4207–4225. [CrossRef] [PubMed]
55. Subramaniam, S.; Kothari, H.; Bosmann, M. Tissue factor in COVID-19-associated coagulopathy. *Thromb. Res.* **2022**, *220*, 35–47. [CrossRef]
56. Bettac, L.; Denk, S.; Seufferlein, T.; Huber-Lang, M. Complement in pancreatic disease-perpetrator or savior? *Front. Immunol.* **2017**, *8*, 15. [CrossRef] [PubMed]
57. Dumnicka, P.; Maduzia, D.; Ceranowicz, P.; Olszanecki, R.; Drożdż, R.; Kuśnierz-Cabala, B. The interplay between inflammation, coagulation and endothelial injury in the early phase of acute pancreatitis: Clinical implications. *Int. J. Mol. Sci.* **2017**, *18*, 354. [CrossRef]
58. Kakafika, A.; Papadopoulos, V.; Mimidis, K.; Mikhailidis, D.P. Coagulation, platelets, and acute pancreatitis. *Pancreas* **2007**, *34*, 15–20. [CrossRef] [PubMed]
59. El-Kurdi, B.; Khatua, B.; Rood, C.; Snozek, C.; Cartin-Ceba, R.; Singh, V.P. Mortality from coronavirus disease 2019 increases with unsaturated fat and may be reduced by early calcium and albumin supplementation. *Gastroenterology* **2020**, *159*, 1015–1018.e4. [CrossRef] [PubMed]
60. Saccon, T.D.; Mousovich-Neto, F.; Ludwig, R.G.; Carregari, V.C.; Dos Anjos Souza, A.B.; Dos Passos, A.S.C.; Martini, M.C.; Barbosa, P.P.; de Souza, G.F.; Muraro, S.P.; et al. SARS-CoV-2 infects adipose tissue in a fat depot- and viral lineage-dependent manner. *Nat. Commun.* **2022**, *13*, 5722. [CrossRef]
61. Patel, K.; Trivedi, R.N.; Durgampudi, C.; Noel, P.; Cline, R.A.; DeLany, J.P.; Navina, S.; Singh, V.P. Lipolysis of visceral adipocyte triglyceride by pancreatic lipases converts mild acute pancreatitis to severe pancreatitis independent of necrosis and inflammation. *Am. J. Pathol.* **2015**, *185*, 808–819. [CrossRef] [PubMed]
62. de Oliveira, C.; Khatua, B.; Noel, P.; Kostenko, S.; Bag, A.; Balakrishnan, B.; Patel, K.S.; Guerra, A.A.; Martinez, M.N.; Trivedi, S.; et al. Pancreatic triglyceride lipase mediates lipotoxic systemic inflammation. *J. Clin. Investig.* **2020**, *130*, 1931–1947. [CrossRef]
63. Navina, S.; Acharya, C.; DeLany, J.P.; Orlichenko, L.S.; Baty, C.J.; Shiva, S.S.; Durgampudi, C.; Karlsson, J.M.; Lee, K.; Bae, K.T.; et al. Lipotoxicity causes multisystem organ failure and exacerbates acute pancreatitis in obesity. *Sci. Transl. Med.* **2011**, *3*, 107ra110. [CrossRef] [PubMed]
64. Baek, Y.B.; Kwon, H.J.; Sharif, M.; Lim, J.; Lee, I.C.; Ryu, Y.B.; Lee, J.I.; Kim, J.S.; Lee, Y.S.; Kim, D.H.; et al. Therapeutic strategy targeting host lipolysis limits infection by SARS-CoV-2 and influenza A virus. *Signal Transduct. Target. Ther.* **2022**, *7*, 367. [CrossRef] [PubMed]
65. Meakins, J.L.; Pietsch, J.B.; Bubenick, O.; Kelly, R.; Rode, H.; Gordon, J.; MacLean, L.D. Delayed hypersensitivity: Indicator of acquired failure of host defenses in sepsis and trauma. *Ann. Surg.* **1977**, *186*, 241–250. [CrossRef]
66. MacLean, L.D.; Meakins, J.L.; Taguchi, K.; Duignan, J.P.; Dhillon, K.S.; Gordon, J. Host resistance in sepsis and trauma. *Ann. Surg.* **1975**, *182*, 207–217. [CrossRef]
67. Monneret, G.; Gossez, M.; Aghaeepour, N.; Gaudilliere, B.; Venet, F. How clinical flow cytometry rebooted sepsis immunology. *Cytom. Part A J. Int. Soc. Anal. Cytol.* **2019**, *95*, 431–441. [CrossRef] [PubMed]
68. Garcia-Sabrido, J.L.; Valdecantos, E.; Bastida, E.; Tellado, J.M. The anergic state as a predictor of pancreatic sepsis. *Zent. Fur Chir.* **1989**, *114*, 114–120.
69. Mayerle, J.; Dummer, A.; Sendler, M.; Malla, S.R.; van den Brandt, C.; Teller, S.; Aghdassi, A.; Nitsche, C.; Lerch, M.M. Differential roles of inflammatory cells in pancreatitis. *J. Gastroenterol. Hepatol.* **2012**, *27* (Suppl. 2), 47–51. [CrossRef]
70. Jain, S.; Midha, S.; Mahapatra, S.J.; Gupta, S.; Sharma, M.K.; Nayak, B.; Jacob, T.G.; Shalimar; Garg, P.K. Interleukin-6 significantly improves predictive value of systemic inflammatory response syndrome for predicting severe acute pancreatitis. *Pancreatology* **2018**, *18*, 500–506. [CrossRef] [PubMed]
71. Bhatia, M. Acute pancreatitis as a model of SIRS. *Front. Biosci. (Landmark Ed.)* **2009**, *14*, 2042–2050. [CrossRef]
72. Bone, R.C. Sir Isaac Newton, sepsis, SIRS, and CARS. *Crit. Care Med.* **1996**, *24*, 1125–1128. [CrossRef]
73. Zhulai, G.A.; Oleinik, E.K.; Ostrovskii, K.A.; Oleinik, V.M.; Kravchenko, P.N.; Churov, A.V. Alterations of lymphocyte subsets and indicators of immune suppression in patients with acute pancreatitis. *Eksp. Klin. Gastroenterol.* **2014**, *9*, 21–25.
74. Döcke, W.D.; Randow, F.; Syrbe, U.; Krausch, D.; Asadullah, K.; Reinke, P.; Volk, H.D.; Kox, W. Monocyte deactivation in septic patients: Restoration by IFN-gamma treatment. *Nat. Med.* **1997**, *3*, 678–681. [CrossRef]
75. Volk, H.D.; Reinke, P.; Krausch, D.; Zuckermann, H.; Asadullah, K.; Müller, J.M.; Döcke, W.D.; Kox, W.J. Monocyte deactivation–rationale for a new therapeutic strategy in sepsis. *Intensive Care Med.* **1996**, *22* (Suppl. 4), S474–S481. [CrossRef] [PubMed]
76. Venet, F.; Lepape, A.; Monneret, G. Clinical review: Flow cytometry perspectives in the ICU-from diagnosis of infection to monitoring of injury-induced immune dysfunctions. *Crit. Care* **2011**, *15*, 231–239. [CrossRef] [PubMed]
77. Hotchkiss, R.S.; Monneret, G.; Payen, D. Immunosuppression in sepsis: A novel understanding of the disorder and a new therapeutic approach. *Lancet Infect. Dis.* **2013**, *13*, 260–268. [CrossRef] [PubMed]
78. Leentjens, J.; Kox, M.; van der Hoeven, J.G.; Netea, M.G.; Pickkers, P. Immunotherapy for the adjunctive treatment of sepsis: From immunosuppression to immunostimulation. Time for a paradigm change? *Am. J. Respir. Crit. Care Med.* **2013**, *187*, 1287–1293. [CrossRef] [PubMed]

79. Giamarellos-Bourboulis, E.J. What is the pathophysiology of the septic host upon admission? *Int. J. Antimicrob. Agents* **2010**, *36* (Suppl. 2), S2–S5. [CrossRef] [PubMed]
80. Minkov, G.A.; Halacheva, K.S.; Yovtchev, Y.P.; Gulubova, M.V. Pathophysiological mechanisms of acute pancreatitis define inflammatory markers of clinical prognosis. *Pancreas* **2015**, *44*, 713–717. [CrossRef]
81. Zhuang, Y.G.; Peng, H.; Chen, Y.Z.; Zhou, S.Q.; Chen, Y.Q. Dynamic monitoring of monocyte HLA-DR expression for the diagnosis, prognosis, and prediction of sepsis. *Front. Biosci.-Landmrk* **2017**, *22*, 1344–1354.
82. Li, J.; Yang, W.-J.; Huang, L.-M.; Tang, C.-W. Immunomodulatory therapies for acute pancreatitis. *World J. Gastroenterol.* **2014**, *20*, 16935–16947. [CrossRef] [PubMed]
83. Misra, A.K.; Levy, M.M.; Ward, N.S. Biomarkers of Immunosuppression. *Crit. Care Clin.* **2020**, *36*, 167–176. [CrossRef]
84. Benlyamani, I.; Venet, F.; Coudereau, R.; Gossez, M.; Monneret, G. Monocyte HLA-DR measurement by flow cytometry in COVID-19 patients: An interim review. *Cytom. Part A J. Int. Soc. Anal. Cytol.* **2020**, *97*, 1217–1221. [CrossRef] [PubMed]
85. Manohar, M.; Jones, E.K.; Rubin, S.J.S.; Subrahmanyam, P.B.; Swaminathan, G.; Mikhail, D.; Bai, L.; Singh, G.; Wei, Y.; Sharma, V.; et al. Novel circulating and tissue monocytes as well as macrophages in pancreatitis and recovery. *Gastroenterology* **2021**, *161*, 2014–2029.e14. [CrossRef] [PubMed]
86. Napoli, C.; Benincasa, G.; Criscuolo, C.; Faenza, M.; Liberato, C.; Rusciano, M. Immune reactivity during COVID-19: Implications for treatment. *Immunol. Lett.* **2021**, *231*, 28–34. [CrossRef] [PubMed]
87. Volk, H.D.; Thieme, M.; Heym, S.; Döcke, W.D.; Ruppe, U.; Tausch, W.; Manger, D.; Zuckermann, S.; Golosubow, A.; Nieter, B.; et al. Alterations in function and phenotype of monocytes from patients with septic disease–predictive value and new therapeutic strategies. *Behring. Inst. Mitt.* **1991**, *88*, 208–215.
88. Lin, R.Y.; Astiz, M.E.; Saxon, J.C.; Rackow, E.C. Altered leukocyte immunophenotypes in septic shock. Studies of HLA-DR, CD11b, CD14, and IL-2R expression. *Chest* **1993**, *104*, 847–853. [CrossRef] [PubMed]
89. Ditschkowski, M.; Kreuzfelder, E.; Rebmann, V.; Ferencik, S.; Majetschak, M.; Schmid, E.N.; Obertacke, U.; Hirche, H.; Schade, U.F.; Grosse-Wilde, H. HLA-DR expression and soluble HLA-DR levels in septic patients after trauma. *Ann. Surg.* **1999**, *229*, 246–254. [CrossRef]
90. Wakefield, C.H.; Carey, P.D.; Foulds, S.; Monson, J.R.; Guillou, P.J. Changes in major histocompatibility complex class II expression in monocytes and T cells of patients developing infection after surgery. *Br. J. Surg.* **1993**, *80*, 205–209. [CrossRef] [PubMed]
91. Sachse, C.; Prigge, M.; Cramer, G.; Pallua, N.; Henkel, E. Association between reduced human leukocyte antigen (HLA)-DR expression on blood monocytes and increased plasma level of interleukin-10 in patients with severe burns. *Clin. Chem. Lab. Med.* **1999**, *37*, 193–198. [CrossRef] [PubMed]
92. Kaufman, J.F.; Auffray, C.; Korman, A.J.; Shackelford, D.A.; Strominger, J. The class II molecules of the human and murine major histocompatibility complex. *Cell* **1984**, *36*, 1–13. [CrossRef]
93. Unanue, E.R.; Turk, V.; Neefjes, J. Variations in MHC Class II antigen processing and presentation in health and disease. *Annu. Rev. Immunol.* **2016**, *34*, 265–297. [CrossRef]
94. Crux, N.B.; Elahi, S. Human leukocyte antigen (HLA) and immune regulation: How do classical and non-classical HLA alleles modulate immune response to human immunodeficiency virus and hepatitis C virus infections? *Front. Immunol.* **2017**, *8*, 832. [CrossRef]
95. Mosaad, Y.M. Clinical role of human leukocyte antigen in health and disease. *Scand. J. Immunol.* **2015**, *82*, 283–306. [CrossRef]
96. Monneret, G.; Venet, F. Sepsis-induced immune alterations monitoring by flow cytometry as a promising tool for individualized therapy. *Cytom. B Clin. Cytom.* **2016**, *90*, 376–386. [CrossRef]
97. Monneret, G.; Venet, F. Monocyte HLA-DR in sepsis: Shall we stop following the flow? *Crit. Care* **2014**, *18*, 102. [CrossRef]
98. Monneret, G.; Elmenkouri, N.; Bohe, J.; Debard, A.L.; Gutowski, M.C.; Bienvenu, J.; Lepape, A. Analytical requirements for measuring monocytic human lymphocyte antigen DR by flow cytometry: Application to the monitoring of patients with septic shock. *Clin. Chem.* **2002**, *48*, 1589–1592. [CrossRef] [PubMed]
99. Docke, W.D.; Hoflich, C.; Davis, K.A.; Rottgers, K.; Meisel, C.; Kiefer, P.; Weber, S.U.; Hedwig-Geissing, M.; Kreuzfelder, E.; Tschentscher, P.; et al. Monitoring temporary immunodepression by flow cytometric measurement of monocytic HLA-DR expression: A multicenter standardized study. *Clin. Chem.* **2005**, *51*, 2341–2347. [CrossRef] [PubMed]
100. Demaret, J.; Walencik, A.; Jacob, M.C.; Timsit, J.F.; Venet, F.; Lepape, A.; Monneret, G. Inter-laboratory assessment of flow cytometric monocyte HLA-DR expression in clinical samples. *Cytom. B Clin. Cytom.* **2013**, *84*, 59–62. [CrossRef] [PubMed]
101. Cajander, S.; Backman, A.; Tina, E.; Stralin, K.; Soderquist, B.; Kallman, J. Preliminary results in quantitation of HLA-DRA by real-time PCR: A promising approach to identify immunosuppression in sepsis. *Crit. Care* **2013**, *17*, R223. [CrossRef] [PubMed]
102. van den Elsen, P.J. Expression regulation of major histocompatibility complex class I and class II encoding genes. *Front. Immunol.* **2011**, *2*, 48. [CrossRef]
103. Steimle, V.; Otten, L.A.; Zufferey, M.; Mach, B. Complementation cloning of an MHC class II transactivator mutated in hereditary MHC class II deficiency (or bare lymphocyte syndrome). *Cell* **1993**, *75*, 135–146. [CrossRef] [PubMed]
104. Miatello, J.; Lukaszewicz, A.C.; Carter, M.J.; Faivre, V.; Hua, S.; Martinet, K.Z.; Bourgeois, C.; Quintana-Murci, L.; Payen, D.; Boniotto, M.; et al. CIITA promoter polymorphism impairs monocytes HLA-DR expression in patients with septic shock. *iScience* **2022**, *25*, 105291. [CrossRef] [PubMed]
105. Pishesha, N.; Harmand, T.J.; Ploegh, H.L. A guide to antigen processing and presentation. *Nat. Rev. Immunol.* **2022**, *22*, 751–764. [CrossRef] [PubMed]

106. Viville, S.; Neefjes, J.; Lotteau, V.; Dierich, A.; Lemeur, M.; Ploegh, H.; Benoist, C.; Mathis, D. Mice lacking the MHC class II-associated invariant chain. *Cell* **1993**, *72*, 635–648. [CrossRef] [PubMed]
107. Wolk, K.; Kunz, S.; Crompton, N.E.; Volk, H.D.; Sabat, R. Multiple mechanisms of reduced major histocompatibility complex class II expression in endotoxin tolerance. *J. Biol. Chem.* **2003**, *278*, 18030–18036. [CrossRef] [PubMed]
108. Alfonso, C.; Karlsson, L. Nonclassical MHC class II molecules. *Annu. Rev. Immunol.* **2000**, *18*, 113–142. [CrossRef] [PubMed]
109. Fung-Leung, W.P.; Surh, C.D.; Liljedahl, M.; Pang, J.; Leturcq, D.; Peterson, P.A.; Webb, S.R.; Karlsson, L. Antigen presentation and T cell development in H2-M-deficient mice. *Science* **1996**, *271*, 1278–1281. [CrossRef]
110. Pinet, V.; Vergelli, M.; Martin, R.; Bakke, O.; Long, E.O. Antigen presentation mediated by recycling of surface HLA-DR molecules. *Nature* **1995**, *375*, 603–606. [CrossRef]
111. Neefjes, J.; Jongsma, M.L.M.; Paul, P.; Bakke, O. Towards a systems understanding of MHC class I and MHC class II antigen presentation. *Nat. Rev. Immunol.* **2011**, *11*, 823–836. [CrossRef]
112. Koppelman, B.; Neefjes, J.J.; de Vries, J.E.; de Waal Malefyt, R. Interleukin-10 down-regulates MHC class II alphabeta peptide complexes at the plasma membrane of monocytes by affecting arrival and recycling. *Immunity* **1997**, *7*, 861–871. [CrossRef]
113. Ting, J.P.; Trowsdale, J. Genetic control of MHC class II expression. *Cell* **2002**, *109* (Suppl. 1), S21–S33. [CrossRef]
114. Czarniecki, C.W.; Chiu, H.H.; Wong, G.H.; McCabe, S.M.; Palladino, M.A. Transforming growth factor-beta 1 modulates the expression of class II histocompatibility antigens on human cells. *J. Immunol.* **1988**, *140*, 4217–4223. [CrossRef]
115. Piskurich, J.F.; Wang, Y.; Linhoff, M.W.; White, L.C.; Ting, J.P. Identification of distinct regions of 5′ flanking DNA that mediate constitutive, IFN-gamma, STAT1, and TGF-beta-regulated expression of the class II transactivator gene. *J. Immunol.* **1998**, *160*, 233–240. [CrossRef]
116. Lu, H.T.; Riley, J.L.; Babcock, G.T.; Huston, M.; Stark, G.R.; Boss, J.M.; Ransohoff, R.M. Interferon (IFN) beta acts downstream of IFN-gamma-induced class II transactivator messenger RNA accumulation to block major histocompatibility complex class II gene expression and requires the 48-kD DNA-binding protein, ISGF3-gamma. *J. Exp. Med.* **1995**, *182*, 1517–1525. [CrossRef] [PubMed]
117. Hershman, M.J.; Appel, S.H.; Wellhausen, S.R.; Sonnenfeld, G.; Polk, H.C., Jr. Interferon-gamma treatment increases HLA-DR expression on monocytes in severely injured patients. *Clin Exp Immunol* **1989**, *77*, 67–70. [PubMed]
118. Blanar, M.A.; Boettger, E.C.; Flavell, R.A. Transcriptional activation of HLA-DR alpha by interferon gamma requires a trans-acting protein. *Proc. Natl. Acad. Sci. USA* **1988**, *85*, 4672–4676. [CrossRef] [PubMed]
119. Pierre, P.; Turley, S.J.; Gatti, E.; Hull, M.; Meltzer, J.; Mirza, A.; Inaba, K.; Steinman, R.M.; Mellman, I. Developmental regulation of MHC class II transport in mouse dendritic cells. *Nature* **1997**, *388*, 787–792. [CrossRef] [PubMed]
120. Cella, M.; Engering, A.; Pinet, V.; Pieters, J.; Lanzavecchia, A. Inflammatory stimuli induce accumulation of MHC class II complexes on dendritic cells. *Nature* **1997**, *388*, 782–787. [CrossRef] [PubMed]
121. Hotchkiss, R.S.; Monneret, G.; Payen, D. Sepsis-induced immunosuppression: From cellular dysfunctions to immunotherapy. *Nat. Rev. Immunol.* **2013**, *13*, 862–874. [CrossRef] [PubMed]
122. Cao, C.; Yu, M.; Chai, Y. Pathological alteration and therapeutic implications of sepsis-induced immune cell apoptosis. *Cell Death Dis.* **2019**, *10*, 782. [CrossRef] [PubMed]
123. Kylanpaa-Back, M.L.; Takala, A.; Kemppainen, E.; Puolakkainen, P.; Kautiainen, H.; Jansson, S.E.; Haapiainen, R.; Repo, H. Cellular markers of systemic inflammation and immune suppression in patients with organ failure due to severe acute pancreatitis. *Scand. J. Gastroenterol.* **2001**, *36*, 1100–1107.
124. Richter, A.; Nebe, T.; Wendl, K.; Schuster, K.; Klaebisch, G.; Quintel, M.; Lorenz, D.; Post, S.; Trede, M. HLA-DR expression in acute pancreatitis. *Eur. J. Surg.* **1999**, *165*, 947–951. [CrossRef] [PubMed]
125. Turunen, A.; Kuuliala, A.; Penttilä, A.; Kaukonen, K.M.; Mustonen, H.; Pettilä, V.; Puolakkainen, P.; Kylänpää, L.; Kuuliala, K. Time course of signaling profiles of blood leukocytes in acute pancreatitis and sepsis. *Scand. J. Clin. Lab. Investig.* **2020**, *80*, 114–123. [CrossRef] [PubMed]
126. Li, J.P.; Yang, J.; Huang, J.R.; Jiang, D.L.; Zhang, F.; Liu, M.F.; Qiang, Y.; Gu, Y.L. Immunosuppression and the infection caused by gut mucosal barrier dysfunction in patients with early severe acute pancreatitis. *Front. Biosci. (Landmark Ed.)* **2013**, *18*, 892–900. [PubMed]
127. Mentula, P.; Kylanpaa, M.L.; Kemppainen, E.; Jansson, S.E.; Sarna, S.; Puolakkainen, P.; Haapiainen, R.; Repo, H. Plasma anti-inflammatory cytokines and monocyte human leucocyte antigen-DR expression in patients with acute pancreatitis. *Scand. J. Gastroenterol.* **2004**, *39*, 178–187. [CrossRef] [PubMed]
128. Yu, W.K.; Li, W.Q.; Li, N.; Li, J.S. Mononuclear histocompatibility leukocyte antigen-DR expression in the early phase of acute pancreatitis. *Pancreatology* **2004**, *4*, 233–243. [CrossRef]
129. Walter, L.O.; Cardoso, C.C.; Santos-Pirath, Í.M.; Costa, H.Z.; Gartner, R.; Werle, I.; Mohr, E.T.B.; da Rosa, J.S.; Felisberto, M.; Kretzer, I.F.; et al. The relationship between peripheral immune response and disease severity in SARS-CoV-2-infected subjects: A cross-sectional study. *Immunology* **2022**, *165*, 481–496. [CrossRef] [PubMed]
130. Yang, Q.; Wen, Y.; Qi, F.; Gao, X.; Chen, W.; Xu, G.; Wei, C.; Wang, H.; Tang, X.; Lin, J.; et al. Suppressive monocytes impair MAIT cells response via IL-10 in patients with severe COVID-19. *J. Immunol.* **2021**, *207*, 1848–1856. [CrossRef] [PubMed]
131. Gatti, A.; Radrizzani, D.; Viganò, P.; Mazzone, A.; Brando, B. Decrease of non-classical and intermediate monocyte subsets in severe acute SARS-CoV-2 infection. *Cytom. Part A J. Int. Soc. Anal. Cytol.* **2020**, *97*, 887–890. [CrossRef]

132. Mudd, P.A.; Crawford, J.C.; Turner, J.S.; Souquette, A.; Reynolds, D.; Bender, D.; Bosanquet, J.P.; Anand, N.J.; Striker, D.A.; Martin, R.S.; et al. Distinct inflammatory profiles distinguish COVID-19 from influenza with limited contributions from cytokine storm. *Sci. Adv.* **2020**, *6*, eabe3024. [CrossRef]
133. Xu, G.; Qi, F.; Li, H.; Yang, Q.; Wang, H.; Wang, X.; Liu, X.; Zhao, J.; Liao, X.; Liu, Y.; et al. The differential immune responses to COVID-19 in peripheral and lung revealed by single-cell RNA sequencing. *Cell Discov.* **2020**, *6*, 73. [CrossRef]
134. Bonnet, B.; Cosme, J.; Dupuis, C.; Coupez, E.; Adda, M.; Calvet, L.; Fabre, L.; Saint-Sardos, P.; Bereiziat, M.; Vidal, M.; et al. Severe COVID-19 is characterized by the co-occurrence of moderate cytokine inflammation and severe monocyte dysregulation. *EBioMedicine* **2021**, *73*, 103622. [CrossRef] [PubMed]
135. Christensen, E.E.; Jørgensen, M.J.; Nore, K.G.; Dahl, T.B.; Yang, K.; Ranheim, T.; Huse, C.; Lind, A.; Nur, S.; Stiksrud, B.; et al. Critical COVID-19 is associated with distinct leukocyte phenotypes and transcriptome patterns. *J. Intern. Med.* **2021**, *290*, 677–692. [CrossRef] [PubMed]
136. Qin, S.; Jiang, Y.; Wei, X.; Liu, X.; Guan, J.; Chen, Y.; Lu, H.; Qian, J.; Wang, Z.; Lin, X. Dynamic changes in monocytes subsets in COVID-19 patients. *Hum. Immunol.* **2021**, *82*, 170–176. [CrossRef] [PubMed]
137. Zenarruzabeitia, O.; Astarloa-Pando, G.; Terrén, I.; Orrantia, A.; Pérez-Garay, R.; Seijas-Betolaza, I.; Nieto-Arana, J.; Imaz-Ayo, N.; Pérez-Fernández, S.; Arana-Arri, E.; et al. T cell activation, highly armed cytotoxic cells and a shift in monocytes CD300 receptors expression is characteristic of patients with severe COVID-19. *Front. Immunol.* **2021**, *12*, 655934. [CrossRef] [PubMed]
138. Cizmecioglu, A.; Emsen, A.; Sumer, S.; Ergun, D.; Akay Cizmecioglu, H.; Turk Dagi, H.; Artac, H. Reduced monocyte subsets, their HLA-DR expressions, and relations to acute phase reactants in severe COVID-19 cases. *Viral Immunol.* **2022**, *35*, 273–282. [CrossRef] [PubMed]
139. Hammad, R.; Kotb, H.G.; Eldesoky, G.A.; Mosaad, A.M.; El-Nasser, A.M.; Abd El Hakam, F.E.; Eldesoky, N.A.; Mashaal, A.; Farhoud, H. Utility of monocyte expression of HLA-DR versus T lymphocyte frequency in the assessment of COVID-19 outcome. *Int. J. Gen. Med.* **2022**, *15*, 5073–5087. [CrossRef] [PubMed]
140. Venet, F.; Gossez, M.; Bidar, F.; Bodinier, M.; Coudereau, R.; Lukaszewicz, A.C.; Tardiveau, C.; Brengel-Pesce, K.; Cheynet, V.; Cazalis, M.A.; et al. T cell response against SARS-CoV-2 persists after one year in patients surviving severe COVID-19. *EBioMedicine* **2022**, *78*, 103967. [CrossRef]
141. Marais, C.; Claude, C.; Semaan, N.; Charbel, R.; Barreault, S.; Travert, B.; Piloquet, J.E.; Demailly, Z.; Morin, L.; Merchaoui, Z.; et al. Myeloid phenotypes in severe COVID-19 predict secondary infection and mortality: A pilot study. *Ann. Intensive Care* **2021**, *11*, 111. [CrossRef]
142. Giamarellos-Bourboulis, E.J.; Netea, M.G.; Rovina, N.; Akinosoglou, K.; Antoniadou, A.; Antonakos, N.; Damoraki, G.; Gkavogianni, T.; Adami, M.E.; Katsaounou, P.; et al. Complex immune dysregulation in COVID-19 patients with severe respiratory failure. *Cell Host Microbe* **2020**, *27*, 992–1000.e3. [CrossRef]
143. Moser, D.; Biere, K.; Han, B.; Hoerl, M.; Schelling, G.; Choukér, A.; Woehrle, T. COVID-19 impairs immune response to candida albicans. *Front. Immunol.* **2021**, *12*, 640644. [CrossRef]
144. Utrero-Rico, A.; González-Cuadrado, C.; Chivite-Lacaba, M.; Cabrera-Marante, O.; Laguna-Goya, R.; Almendro-Vazquez, P.; Díaz-Pedroche, C.; Ruiz-Ruigómez, M.; Lalueza, A.; Folgueira, M.D.; et al. Alterations in circulating monocytes predict COVID-19 severity and include chromatin modifications still detectable six months after recovery. *Biomedicines* **2021**, *9*, 1253. [CrossRef] [PubMed]
145. Mairpady Shambat, S.; Gómez-Mejia, A.; Schweizer, T.A.; Huemer, M.; Chang, C.C.; Acevedo, C.; Bergada-Pijuan, J.; Vulin, C.; Hofmaenner, D.A.; Scheier, T.C.; et al. Hyperinflammatory environment drives dysfunctional myeloid cell effector response to bacterial challenge in COVID-19. *PLoS Pathog.* **2022**, *18*, e1010176. [CrossRef] [PubMed]
146. Boumaza, A.; Gay, L.; Mezouar, S.; Bestion, E.; Diallo, A.B.; Michel, M.; Desnues, B.; Raoult, D.; La Scola, B.; Halfon, P.; et al. Monocytes and macrophages, targets of severe acute respiratory syndrome coronavirus 2: The clue for coronavirus disease 2019 immunoparalysis. *J. Infect. Dis.* **2021**, *224*, 395–406. [CrossRef]
147. Laing, A.G.; Lorenc, A.; Del Molino Del Barrio, I.; Das, A.; Fish, M.; Monin, L.; Muñoz-Ruiz, M.; McKenzie, D.R.; Hayday, T.S.; Francos-Quijorna, I.; et al. A dynamic COVID-19 immune signature includes associations with poor prognosis. *Nat. Med.* **2020**, *26*, 1623–1635. [CrossRef] [PubMed]
148. Penttilä, P.A.; Van Gassen, S.; Panovska, D.; Vanderbeke, L.; Van Herck, Y.; Quintelier, K.; Emmaneel, A.; Filtjens, J.; Malengier-Devlies, B.; Ahmadzadeh, K.; et al. High dimensional profiling identifies specific immune types along the recovery trajectories of critically ill COVID19 patients. *Cell Mol. Life Sci.* **2021**, *78*, 3987–4002. [CrossRef]
149. Zhang, R.; Shi, J.; Zhang, R.; Ni, J.; Habtezion, A.; Wang, X.; Hu, G.; Xue, J. Expanded CD14(hi)CD16(-) Immunosuppressive monocytes predict disease severity in patients with acute pancreatitis. *J. Immunol.* **2019**, *202*, 2578–2584. [CrossRef]
150. Minkov, G.; Dimitrov, E.; Yovtchev, Y.; Enchev, E.; Lokova, R.; Halacheva, K. Prognostic value of peripheral blood CD14+HLA-DR+ monocytes in patients with acute pancreatitis. *J. Immunoass. Immunochem.* **2021**, *42*, 478–492. [CrossRef] [PubMed]
151. Mentula, P.; Kylanpaa-Back, M.L.; Kemppainen, E.; Takala, A.; Jansson, S.E.; Kautiainen, H.; Puolakkainen, P.; Haapiainen, R.; Repo, H. Decreased HLA (human leucocyte antigen)-DR expression on peripheral blood monocytes predicts the development of organ failure in patients with acute pancreatitis. *Clin. Sci.* **2003**, *105*, 409–417. [CrossRef]
152. Ho, Y.P.; Sheen, I.S.; Chiu, C.T.; Wu, C.S.; Lin, C.Y. A strong association between down-regulation of HLA-DR expression and the late mortality in patients with severe acute pancreatitis. *Am. J. Gastroenterol.* **2006**, *101*, 1117–1124. [CrossRef]

153. Yang, M.; Liu, Z.; Kang, K.; Yu, K.; Wang, C. Letter to the Editor: CD14(+)HLA-DR(+) Cells in patients may be a biomarker reflecting the progression of COVID-19. *Viral Immunol.* **2021**, *34*, 579–581. [CrossRef] [PubMed]
154. Satoh, A.; Miura, T.; Satoh, K.; Masamune, A.; Yamagiwa, T.; Sakai, Y.; Shibuya, K.; Takeda, K.; Kaku, M.; Shimosegawa, T. Human leukocyte antigen-DR expression on peripheral monocytes as a predictive marker of sepsis during acute pancreatitis. *Pancreas* **2002**, *25*, 245–250. [CrossRef]
155. Kylanpaa, M.L.; Mentula, P.; Kemppainen, E.; Puolakkainen, P.; Aittomaki, S.; Silvennoinen, O.; Haapiainen, R.; Repo, H. Monocyte anergy is present in patients with severe acute pancreatitis and is significantly alleviated by granulocyte-macrophage colony-stimulating factor and interferon-gamma in vitro. *Pancreas* **2005**, *31*, 23–27. [CrossRef] [PubMed]
156. Ho, Y.P.; Chiu, C.T.; Sheen, I.S.; Tseng, S.C.; Lai, P.C.; Ho, S.Y.; Chen, W.T.; Lin, T.N.; Lin, C.Y. Tumor necrosis factor-alpha and interleukin-10 contribute to immunoparalysis in patients with acute pancreatitis. *Hum. Immunol.* **2011**, *72*, 18–23. [CrossRef] [PubMed]
157. Lin, Z.Q.; Guo, J.; Xia, Q.; Yang, X.N.; Huang, W.; Huang, Z.W.; Xue, P. Human leukocyte antigen-DR expression on peripheral monocytes may be an early marker for secondary infection in severe acute pancreatitis. *Hepatogastroenterology* **2013**, *60*, 1896–1902. [PubMed]
158. Gotzinger, P.; Sautner, T.; Spittler, A.; Barlan, M.; Wamser, P.; Roth, E.; Jakesz, R.; Fugger, R. Severe acute pancreatitis causes alterations in HLA-DR and CD14 expression on peripheral blood monocytes independently of surgical treatment. *Eur. J. Surg.* **2000**, *166*, 628–632. [PubMed]
159. Wolk, K.; Hoflich, C.; Zuckermann-Becker, H.; Docke, W.D.; Volk, H.D.; Sabat, R. Reduced monocyte CD86 expression in postinflammatory immunodeficiency. *Crit. Care Med.* **2007**, *35*, 458–467. [CrossRef] [PubMed]
160. Zhang, Y.; Wang, C.; Yu, M.; Zhao, X.; Du, J.; Li, Y.; Jing, H.; Dong, Z.; Kou, J.; Bi, Y.; et al. Neutrophil extracellular traps induced by activated platelets contribute to procoagulant activity in patients with colorectal cancer. *Thromb. Res.* **2019**, *180*, 87–97. [CrossRef] [PubMed]
161. Ferat-Osorio, E.; Wong-Baeza, I.; Esquivel-Callejas, N.; Figueroa-Figueroa, S.; Duarte-Rojo, A.; Guzman-Valdivia-Gomez, G.; Rodea-Rosas, H.; Torres-Gonzalez, R.; Sanchez-Fernandez, P.; Arriaga-Pizano, L.; et al. Triggering receptor expressed on myeloid cells-1 expression on monocytes is associated with inflammation but not with infection in acute pancreatitis. *Crit. Care* **2009**, *13*, R69. [CrossRef] [PubMed]
162. Hue, S.; Beldi-Ferchiou, A.; Bendib, I.; Surenaud, M.; Fourati, S.; Frapard, T.; Rivoal, S.; Razazi, K.; Carteaux, G.; Delfau-Larue, M.H.; et al. Uncontrolled innate and impaired adaptive immune responses in patients with COVID-19 acute respiratory distress syndrome. *Am. J. Respir. Crit. Care Med.* **2020**, *202*, 1509–1519. [CrossRef] [PubMed]
163. Peruzzi, B.; Bencini, S.; Capone, M.; Mazzoni, A.; Maggi, L.; Salvati, L.; Vanni, A.; Orazzini, C.; Nozzoli, C.; Morettini, A.; et al. Quantitative and qualitative alterations of circulating myeloid cells and plasmacytoid DC in SARS-CoV-2 infection. *Immunology* **2020**, *161*, 345–353. [CrossRef] [PubMed]
164. Wang, F.; Hou, H.; Yao, Y.; Wu, S.; Huang, M.; Ran, X.; Zhou, H.; Liu, Z.; Sun, Z. Systemically comparing host immunity between survived and deceased COVID-19 patients. *Cell Mol. Immunol.* **2020**, *17*, 875–877. [CrossRef] [PubMed]
165. Pfortmueller, C.A.; Meisel, C.; Fux, M.; Schefold, J.C. Assessment of immune organ dysfunction in critical illness: Utility of innate immune response markers. *Intensive Care Med. Exp.* **2017**, *5*, 49. [CrossRef] [PubMed]
166. Boomer, J.S.; To, K.; Chang, K.C.; Takasu, O.; Osborne, D.F.; Walton, A.H.; Bricker, T.L.; Jarman, S.D., 2nd; Kreisel, D.; Krupnick, A.S.; et al. Immunosuppression in patients who die of sepsis and multiple organ failure. *JAMA* **2011**, *306*, 2594–2605. [CrossRef] [PubMed]
167. Monneret, G.; Lepape, A.; Venet, F. A dynamic view of mHLA-DR expression in management of severe septic patients. *Crit. Care* **2011**, *15*, 198. [CrossRef]
168. Wu, L.M.; Sankaran, S.J.; Plank, L.D.; Windsor, J.A.; Petrov, M.S. Meta-analysis of gut barrier dysfunction in patients with acute pancreatitis. *Br. J. Surg.* **2014**, *101*, 1644–1656. [CrossRef]
169. Qin, Y.; Pinhu, L.; You, Y.; Sooranna, S.; Huang, Z.; Zhou, X.; Yin, Y.; Song, S. The role of Fas expression on the occurrence of immunosuppression in severe acute pancreatitis. *Dig. Dis. Sci.* **2013**, *58*, 3300–3307. [CrossRef] [PubMed]
170. Sharma, D.; Jakkampudi, A.; Reddy, R.; Reddy, P.B.; Patil, A.; Murthy, H.V.V.; Rao, G.V.; Reddy, D.N.; Talukdar, R. Association of systemic inflammatory and anti-inflammatory responses with adverse outcomes in acute pancreatitis: Preliminary results of an ongoing study. *Dig. Dis. Sci.* **2017**, *62*, 3468–3478. [CrossRef]
171. Yu, Z.X.; Chen, X.C.; Zhang, B.Y.; Liu, N.; Gu, Q. Association between HLA-DR expression and multidrug-resistant infection in patients with severe acute pancreatitis. *Curr. Med. Sci.* **2018**, *38*, 449–454. [CrossRef] [PubMed]
172. Giamarellos-Bourboulis, E.J. Complex immune deregulation in severe COVID-19: More than a mechanism of pathogenesis. *EBioMedicine* **2021**, *73*, 103673. [CrossRef]
173. Loftus, T.J.; Ungaro, R.; Dirain, M.; Efron, P.A.; Mazer, M.B.; Remy, K.E.; Hotchkiss, R.S.; Zhong, L.; Bacher, R.; Starostik, P.; et al. Overlapping but disparate inflammatory and immunosuppressive responses to SARS-CoV-2 and bacterial sepsis: An immunological time course analysis. *Front. Immunol.* **2021**, *12*, 792448. [CrossRef]
174. Ding, L.; Wan, M.; Wang, D.; Cao, H.; Wang, H.; Gao, P. Myeloid-derived suppressor cells in patients with acute pancreatitis with increased inhibitory function. *Front. Immunol.* **2022**, *13*, 840620. [CrossRef] [PubMed]
175. Grassi, G.; Notari, S.; Gili, S.; Bordoni, V.; Casetti, R.; Cimini, E.; Tartaglia, E.; Mariotti, D.; Agrati, C.; Sacchi, A. Myeloid-derived suppressor cells in COVID-19: The paradox of good. *Front. Immunol.* **2022**, *13*, 842949. [CrossRef]

176. Falck-Jones, S.; Österberg, B.; Smed-Sörensen, A. Respiratory and systemic monocytes, dendritic cells and myeloid-derived suppressor cells in COVID-19: Implications for disease severity. *J. Intern. Med.* **2022**, *293*, 130–143. [CrossRef]
177. Kylänpää, M.L.; Repo, H.; Puolakkainen, P.A. Inflammation and immunosuppression in severe acute pancreatitis. *World J. Gastroenterol.* **2010**, *16*, 2867–2872. [CrossRef] [PubMed]
178. Monneret, G.; Venet, F.; Meisel, C.; Schefold, J.C. Assessment of monocytic HLA-DR expression in ICU patients: Analytical issues for multicentric flow cytometry studies. *Crit. Care* **2010**, *14*, 432. [CrossRef] [PubMed]
179. De Waele, J.; Vogelaers, D.; Decruyenaere, J.; De Vos, M.; Colardyn, F. Infectious complications of acute pancreatitis. *Acta Clin. Belg.* **2004**, *59*, 90–96. [CrossRef] [PubMed]
180. Leppäniemi, A.; Tolonen, M.; Tarasconi, A.; Segovia-Lohse, H.; Gamberini, E.; Kirkpatrick, A.W.; Ball, C.G.; Parry, N.; Sartelli, M.; Wolbrink, D.; et al. 2019 WSES guidelines for the management of severe acute pancreatitis. *World J. Emerg. Surg.* **2019**, *14*, 27. [CrossRef]
181. Estella, Á.; Vidal-Cortés, P.; Rodríguez, A.; Andaluz Ojeda, D.; Martín-Loeches, I.; Díaz, E.; Suberviola, B.; Gracia Arnillas, M.P.; Catalán González, M.; Álvarez-Lerma, F.; et al. Management of infectious complications associated with coronavirus infection in severe patients admitted to ICU. *Med. Intensiv.* **2021**, *45*, 485–500. [CrossRef] [PubMed]
182. Dickel, S.; Grimm, C.; Amschler, K.; Schnitzler, S.U.; Schanz, J.; Moerer, O.; Payen, D.; Tampe, B.; Winkler, M.S. Case report: Interferon-γ restores monocytic human leukocyte antigen receptor (mHLA-DR) in severe COVID-19 with acquired immunosuppression syndrome. *Front. Immunol.* **2021**, *12*, 645124. [CrossRef]
183. van Laarhoven, A.; Kurver, L.; Overheul, G.J.; Kooistra, E.J.; Abdo, W.F.; van Crevel, R.; Duivenvoorden, R.; Kox, M.; Ten Oever, J.; Schouten, J.; et al. Interferon gamma immunotherapy in five critically ill COVID-19 patients with impaired cellular immunity: A case series. *Med (N. Y.)* **2021**, *2*, 1163–1170.e2. [CrossRef] [PubMed]
184. Nguyen, L.S.; Ait Hamou, Z.; Gastli, N.; Chapuis, N.; Pène, F. Potential role for interferon gamma in the treatment of recurrent ventilator-acquired pneumonia in patients with COVID-19: A hypothesis. *Intensive Care Med.* **2021**, *47*, 619–621. [CrossRef] [PubMed]
185. Laterre, P.F.; François, B.; Collienne, C.; Hantson, P.; Jeannet, R.; Remy, K.E.; Hotchkiss, R.S. Association of interleukin 7 immunotherapy with lymphocyte counts among patients with severe coronavirus disease 2019 (COVID-19). *JAMA Netw. Open* **2020**, *3*, e2016485. [CrossRef] [PubMed]
186. Ke, L.; Zhou, J.; Mao, W.; Chen, T.; Zhu, Y.; Pan, X.; Mei, H.; Singh, V.; Buxbaum, J.; Doig, G.; et al. Immune enhancement in patients with predicted severe acute necrotising pancreatitis: A multicentre double-blind randomised controlled trial. *Intensive Care Med.* **2022**, *48*, 899–909. [CrossRef] [PubMed]

MDPI
St. Alban-Anlage 66
4052 Basel
Switzerland
www.mdpi.com

International Journal of Molecular Sciences Editorial Office
E-mail: ijms@mdpi.com
www.mdpi.com/journal/ijms

www.ingramcontent.com/pod-product-compliance
Lightning Source LLC
LaVergne TN
LVHW070449100526
838202LV00014B/1688
9783725809646